UNDERSTANDING HOSPITAL BILLING AND CODING

Second Edition

UNDERSTANDING HOSPITAL BILLING AND CODING

Debra P. Ferenc
BS, CPC, CPC-I, CPC-H, CMSCS, PCS, FCS

Senior Consultant/Educator MRCE
Medical Insurance, Billing, and Coding Program
Director–Everest University
Founder, Past President and Education Officer–Gulf to Bay Local Chapter of the AAPC

SECOND EDITION

ELSEVIER
SAUNDERS

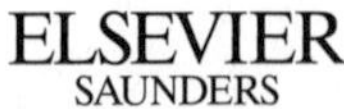

3251 Riverport Lane
St. Louis, Missouri 63043

UNDERSTANDING HOSPITAL BILLING AND CODING ISBN: 978-1-4377-2251-2

Notice

Knowledge and best practice in this field are constantly changing. As new research and experience broaden our understanding, changes in research methods, professional practices, or medical treatment may become necessary.

Practitioners and researchers must always rely on their own experience and knowledge in evaluating and using any information, methods, compounds, or experiments described herein. In using such information or methods they should be mindful of their own safety and the safety of others, including parties for whom they have a professional responsibility.

With respect to any drug or pharmaceutical products identified, readers are advised to check the most current information provided (i) on procedures featured or (ii) by the manufacturer of each product to be administered, to verify the recommended dose or formula, the method and duration of administration, and contraindications. It is the responsibility of practitioners, relying on their own experience and knowledge of their patients, to make diagnoses, to determine dosages and the best treatment for each individual patient, and to take all appropriate safety precautions.

To the fullest extent of the law, neither the Publisher nor the authors, contributors, or editors, assume any liability for any injury and/or damage to persons or property as a matter of products liability, negligence or otherwise, or from any use or operation of any methods, products, instructions, or ideas contained in the material herein.

Library of Congress Cataloging-in-Publication Data

Ferenc, Debra P.
Understanding hospital billing and coding / Debra P. Ferenc.—2nd ed.
p. ; cm.
Includes bibliographical references and index.
ISBN 978-1-4377-2251-2 (pbk. : alk. paper)
1. Hospitals—Accounting. 2. Health insurance claims—Code numbers. I. Title.
[DNLM: 1. Hospital Charges—classification. 2. Financial Management, Hospital. 3. Forms and Records Control—methods. 4. Insurance, Health, Reimbursement. 5. Patient Credit and Collection—methods. WX 157.1 F349u 2011]
RA971.3.F47 2011
657'.8322—dc22

2010020457

Acquisitions Editor: Susan Cole
Developmental Editor: Elizabeth Fergus
Publishing Services Manager: Gayle May
Project Manager: Stephen Bancroft
Design Direction: Teresa McBryan

Printed in the United States of America

Last digit is the print number: 9 8 7 6 5 4 3 2 1

To my husband, David, *who is a kind, loving, supportive, and caring man, for providing support, encouragement, and love during the time it took me to write this text, and to Agnes Ferenc, our mother, a special thank you for your support and for bringing David into this world.*

To my family and dearest friends
Thank you for all the support and encouragement you have given me through the years and understanding my absence while writing this text.

Knowledge is power
Without it one lives in a world where no logic can be found.
With it one can find logic and move through the maze of life with confidence.
It is the sharing of knowledge that contributes to positive life transitions.

To all my mentors and instructors
Thank you taking an interest in my learning and contributing greatly to my success through sharing knowledge with passion and compassion.

To all students *who are committed to achieving success through hard work, learning, and integrity*
Continue to strive to be the best you can be and continue learning throughout life

To all instructors
When the day is long and the task is endless remember the positive contributions you make to the life of your students.
Strength, encouragement, confidence, and knowledge to be all they can be—this is your contribution.

Preface

ABOUT THE AUTHOR

One of my first jobs out of high school was in the medical field. As a child I did not dream about working in the health insurance billing and coding industry, it just happened that way. I started out as an administrative assistant to the chairman of a department in a teaching hospital. After several years I was promoted to department administrator. During the 1980s, when hospitals began to develop hospital-based private practices, I assumed the role of setting up the billing system for my department and this led to my career in the field. I have served the health care industry for over 30 years in progressive leadership positions. With a primary background in private and hospital-based practice administration I gained extensive experience in practice management, insurance billing and coding, claims processing, reimbursement strategies, documentation requirements, auditing and consulting. The challenges presented by the health insurance billing and coding industry required constant evolution and the quest for knowledge. I obtained the Certified Professional Coder (CPC), Certified Professional Coder—Hospital (CPC-H), Certified Multi-Specialty Coding Specialist (CMSCS) status as well as Certified Professional Coder—Instructor. The most difficult challenge for practice managers is hiring individuals with health insurance billing and coding knowledge and experience. To accomplish this, I became involved with a local vocational school that offered medical insurance billing and coding courses. The school required students to complete an externship. I was thrilled to provide externship opportunities for these students in my primary care and urgent care clinics. Through externship placements I was able to hire individuals with a solid foundation in medical insurance billing and coding.

In 1996, I founded Medical Recovery & Consulting Experts, Inc. (MRCE). MRCE's primary focus was to act as a patient advocate and audit hospital bills for individuals and third-party payers. Soon after MRCE was founded I began teaching medical insurance billing and coding at the local vocational school. I continued to focus on patient advocacy, auditing, and consulting and expanded MRCE's mission to include education of health care professionals seeking certifications. Over the years I have expanded my teaching role to health insurance billing and coding programs as well as certification workshops and review classes to assist individuals in achieving their Certified Professional Coding status through the American Academy of Professional Coding (AAPC).

Many individuals looking to change paths in their health care careers or to enter the health care industry enrolled in programs to learn health insurance billing and coding. Schools that offered a certificate or a degree program in health insurance billing and coding often concentrated on physician and outpatient billing and coding. This concentration makes sense considering the number of jobs available in the physician and outpatient arena are greater than those available in the hospital sector. Despite these statistics, changes in reimbursement methods and increasing focus on fraud and abuse have contributed to the rising demand for individuals with formal training or certification in hospital billing and coding.

In a quest to provide such training for potential or current hospital personnel, a hospital billing course was added to the curriculum. As I continued to enhance this course, I went on a futile search for a text that addressed hospital billing and coding. I found books that contained hospital billing or hospital coding, but none that contained both. For this reason, I began to develop my own material to teach hospital billing and coding.

Welcome to the second edition of Understanding Hospital Billing and Coding. This text is designed to provide individuals seeking employment in the hospital billing and coding industry with a solid foundation and understanding of billing and coding in a hospital setting.

The driving force behind the development of this book was the need for instructional material required to teach all aspects of hospital billing and coding. This text is the first to provide a basic understanding of various aspects of hospital billing and coding including the history of hospitals, the hospital regulatory environment, structure and function of hospital departments, patient accounts and data flow, the billing process, accounts receivable management, coding, claim forms, payers, reimbursement, and HIPAA. This text was developed on the premise that students have an understanding of health insurance billing and coding concepts relative to physician and outpatient billing and coding. The text is designed to transition the student's knowledge from the physician or outpatient environment to the hospital environment. Features of this text include a direct approach to learning, repetition of skills as concepts presented in one chapter are utilized in future chapters, test your knowledge exercises that are provided after the presentation of concepts to reinforce the concepts, chapter review exercises added at the end of each chapter to further reinforce chapter concepts, and actual hospital cases designed to provide students with an opportunity to apply concepts. Other instructional resources include an instructor's curriculum, and a computer program designed to provide application of registration, charge entry, coding, claim form preparation, and review of APC and MS-DRG assignments.

ORGANIZATION OF THIS TEXTBOOK

The text is organized in six sections designed to present concepts in an order that is similar to the hospital billing process. Appendices are provided at the end of the text that include vital information required to understand and apply concepts presented in the text.

Section One is designed to present concepts relating to the hospital environment including hospital introduction, the hospital regulatory environment, and hospital organizational structure and function.

Section Two advances the concepts introduced in the first section to provide an understanding of patient accounts and data flow in the hospital, the hospital billing process, and accounts receivable management.

Section Three presents concepts on coding patient conditions (diagnosis coding) and coding procedures, services, and items (procedure coding). This section also includes a chapter on coding guidelines and applications to provide an opportunity for students to apply knowledge presented in the section.

Section Four utilizes all the information in the first three sections to provide an explanation of claim form preparation and submission.

Section Five provides information regarding third-party payers, government payers, and Prospective Payment Systems.

Section Six is an overview of the Privacy, Security, and Administrative Simplifications provisions outlined under the Health Insurance Portability and Accountability (HIPAA).

EVOLVE COURSE MANAGEMENT SYSTEM

The Evolve site is a free, interactive learning resource site that works in coordination with the textbook material. It provides Internet-based course management tools for the instructor, and content related resources for the student. Some of the functions include the following:

- Post the class syllabus, outline, and lecture notes
- Set up "virtual office hours" and e-mail communication
- Share important dates and information through the online class calendar
- Encourage student participation through chat rooms and discussion boards

The learning resources for the student include:

- Self-assessment quizzes to evaluate the student's mastery through multiple choice, true-false, fill-in-the-blank, and matching questions. Instant scoring and feedback are available at the click of a button.
- Weblinks: Web sites that have been carefully gathered to supplement the content of the text, and that are updated regularly.
- Technical updates to keep up with changes in government regulations, codes, and other industry changes.
- Student software with exercises to accompany the information in the textbook.

INSTRUCTOR'S RESOURCE MANUAL

The Instructor's Resource Manual is available in printed form and on the Evolve site. This resource allows the instructor the flexibility to quickly adapt the textbook for his or her individual classroom needs and to gauge students' understanding. The Instructor's Resource Manual features the following:

- Guidelines for establishing a medical insurance course
- Answer keys to the Test Your Knowledge boxes and discussion-leading critical thinking questions.
- Lesson suggestions for each chapter
- Suggested classroom activities

The Evolve site includes all of the information in the printed Instructor's Resource Manual, plus the following:

- An image collection of forms and summaries of important chapter concepts from the textbook for use as overheads or as PowerPoint slides. A PowerPoint presentation will capture attention and create lively lectures to assist in learning and retention.
- A test bank with more than 1200 questions to assist the instructor in test construction. It gives a variety of testing formats, such as multiple choice, true or false, short answer, matching, fill-in-the-blank, and coding. The tests can be customized, revised, and printed.

FERENC STUDENT SOFTWARE

The student software available on the Evolve site contains 10 software cases that allow students to work from different source documents to produce a completed UB-04 claim form. These source documents, the Coding Worksheet and the Patient Face Sheet (found in the 10 cases in Appendix A), must be completed prior to working on the software cases. Working from the completed documents the student experiences how the various source information flows into a completed UB-04 claim form. This software serves to simulate the patient registration and charge entry function to show how patient billing information from multiple sources is entered correctly on the UB-04. Students use the software to complete a UB-04 form, edit as required, and submit the printed form to their instructor.

Acknowledgments

This text was developed in collaboration with many professionals in the health insurance billing and coding industry and at Elsevier. The text was reviewed by instructors and hospital billing and coding professionals. Excellent feedback was provided and incorporated into this text.

Thank you to all my peers who assisted with this project for taking pride in this text and taking the time to share your knowledge to ensure that this text will provide individuals with the solid foundations required to embark on or advance in their careers in hospital billing and coding.

I also want to express my thanks to everyone at Elsevier for all your hard work, direction, support, and encouragement throughout the development of this text.

A special thank you to my team members who were involved in the development of this text in research, content, editorial, technical, and coding specialist capacities.

Russell Dowling, LPN, CPC, CPC-H, CCS, CMC, CMSCS	Content expert and coding specialist
Karen Fair, CRNA	Clinical content assistant
William Jahn	Historical research specialist
Donna Long, CPC, CPC-H, CBCS	Content expert and coding specialist
Mandi Nagy, AS, CPC, CPC-H	Editorial, content, technical expert, and coding specialist
Tamara Waluk, CPC, CBCS	Research, editorial, and coding specialist
Andrea Waldman, BA, CPC, CPC-H, CMC, CMIS	Editorial, content, and coding specialist

Editorial Review Board

Contents

SECTION ONE

Hospital Overview

Hospital Introduction

Hospital Regulatory Environment

Hospital Organizational Structure and Function

Chapter 1

Hospital Introduction

The purpose of this chapter is to provide an understanding of how hospitals evolved into the complex health care systems we know today. Over the centuries, hospitals evolved from ancient healing centers to facilities designed to care for the sick. The evolution of hospitals was greatly influenced by religious, environmental, and economic factors. Advances in medicine also contributed to the growth and development of hospitals. This chapter explores some of the most significant factors that influenced the evolution of hospitals from ancient times to today. An overview of how advances in medicine contributed to the evolution of hospitals leads us to a discussion of the purpose and types of hospitals as well as the services provided in a hospital. A review of the history and evolution of hospitals will provide a basis for understanding the status of hospitals today and the challenges they face.

Chapter Objectives

- Define terms, phrases, abbreviations, and acronyms related to history and evolution of hospitals.
- Demonstrate an understanding of how hospitals evolved from ancient times to today.
- Provide an overview of the influence of advances made in medicine on hospital evolution.
- Briefly discuss three areas of economic influence on hospital development.
- Describe how changes in reimbursement systems affected hospital development.
- Discuss the difference between a primary care network and an integrated delivery system.
- Explain the purpose of a hospital.
- Differentiate among diagnostic, therapeutic, palliative, and preventive services.
- Describe three levels of care provided at hospitals.
- Provide an explanation of the difference between a for-profit and a not-for-profit hospital.
- Demonstrate an understanding of different types of hospitals.

Outline

Key Terms

Accounts receivable
Acute care facility
Ambulatory surgery
American College of Surgeons (ACS)
American Hospital Association (AHA)
American Medical Association (AMA)
Blue Cross
Coding
Community hospital
Demographic information
Diagnostic service
Emergency Department
Evaluation and management (E/M)
Fee-for-service
General hospital
Group health insurance
Hill-Burton Act
Hospital
Hospital Standardization Program
Indigent
Inpatient
Insurance information
Integrated delivery system
Managed care plan
Medicaid
Medicare
Medicare Severity Diagnosis Related Groups (MS-DRG)
Non-patient
Observation
Outpatient
Palliative service
Payers
Peer review
Per diem
Percentage of accrued charges
Prepaid health plan
Preventive service
Primary care network
Primary care physician (PCP)
Private hospital
Prospective Payment System (PPS)
Quality Improvement Organization (QIO)
Social Security Act
Specialty hospital
Teaching hospital
Tertiary care hospital
The Joint Commission (TJC)
Therapeutic service
Third-party payer
Trauma center
Utilization management (UM)
Utilization review (UR)

Acronyms and Abbreviations

ACS—American College of Surgeons
AHA—American Hospital Association
AMA—American Medical Association
E/M—evaluation and management
MS-DRG—Medicare Severity Diagnosis Related Groups
PPS—Prospective Payment System
QIO—Quality Improvement Organization
TJC—The Joint Commission
UM—utilization management
UR—utilization review

HOSPITAL INTRODUCTION

The term *hospital* comes from a Latin word *hospitalis*. *Hospitalis* means "a house or institution for guests." This definition describes the hospital when it served as housing for traveling guests such as the pilgrims who traveled to distant lands. Today's definition of **hospital** is "an institution where the sick or injured receive medical or surgical care." A hospital is a facility where patients with health care problems go to seek diagnosis and treatment of condition(s). A hospital may be housed in one building or in many buildings on a campus. Some hospitals are affiliated with medical universities that train medical personnel. Hospitals today have five major characteristics:

1. A network of highly specialized personnel organized into departments designed to carry out clinical, administrative, and operational tasks required to provide effective and efficient patient care services.
2. A medical staff representing many specialties, organized to provide health care services from an interdisciplinary approach.
3. Provision of diagnostic, therapeutic, palliative, and preventive services.
4. Inpatient beds for patients who require care for periods greater than 24 hours.
5. Nursing services provided 24 hours a day.

The major purpose of a hospital is to diagnose and treat illness. Hospitals are providers of medical care, and they provide diagnostic and therapeutic medical care to patients with various types of illness. Patient illness can range from a simple fracture to a condition that requires the patient to have an organ transplant. Administrative, financial, operational, and clinical departments within

BOX 1-1 ■ KEY POINTS

Characteristics of Today's Hospital

Network of highly specialized personnel organized into departments
A medical staff representing many specialties
Diagnostic, therapeutic, palliative, and preventive services
Inpatient care for periods greater than 24 hours
24-hour nursing services

the hospital are coordinated to ensure that patient care is efficient and effective. The names of the departments may vary from hospital to hospital, but the functions are generally the same.

Hospitals maintain financial stability through the billing process. Medical care provided to a patient must be processed for billing to the patient or other payers. **Payers** are insurance companies or government programs that pay health benefits for patient care services. The complex process of billing health care payers and patients begins when patient demographic and insurance information is obtained. Patient **demographic information** includes the patient's name, address, date of birth, sex, and Social Security number. **Insurance information** consists of the plan identification number, plan name and number, and group name and number.

Services and items provided must be recorded in the patient's medical record. The medical record is used to record pertinent information regarding the patient's condition and treatment. It improves communication among providers and it serves as supporting documentation for charges billed. Patient conditions, services, and items are coded in preparation for submission of the charges to payers. **Coding** is the process of translating written descriptions of services, items, and patient conditions into numeric or alphanumeric codes. A claim form containing information about the services provided and the patient's condition is used to submit charges to payers. Each payer conducts a review of the claim to determine payment or denial of the claim. Patient statements outlining charges, payments, and the outstanding balance are prepared and mailed as appropriate.

The final stage of the billing process involves the collection of outstanding account balances. **Accounts receivable** is the term that describes monies owed to the hospital from patients, insurance companies, and government programs.

Hospital departmental functions and the billing process will be discussed at length later in the text. To gain an understanding of the structure and function of today's hospital, it is necessary to explore historical factors that influenced the development and growth of hospitals. The evolution of hospitals was greatly influenced by advances in medicine that came in response to cultural and environmental factors affecting health care. The following review of hospital history, from antiquity to the 20th century, will highlight some of the major factors that contributed to the growth and development of hospitals.

EVOLUTION OF HOSPITALS

The evolution of hospitals began in ancient times when some of the first institutions utilized for the sick were temples built in Egypt, Greece, and Rome. These institutions evolved to serve as a place for worshipers of gods, treat injured soldiers, isolate those with contagious disease, offer rest for weary travelers, and finally to address health care needs of individuals. The worldwide growth and development of hospitals was influenced by religious, environmental, and economic factors. Throughout history, the spread of infectious disease and the need to care for injured soldiers contributed to the pursuit of new cures and treatments. These pursuits led to medical advances that greatly influenced the growth and development of hospitals.

Ancient Medicine and Healing Centers

The practice of medicine dates back to ancient times. There is evidence of primitive procedures such as boring a hole into the skull, (trephining), and the use of medicinal herbs and fungi dating back to 10,000 B.C. or earlier (Figure 1-1). These procedures and natural

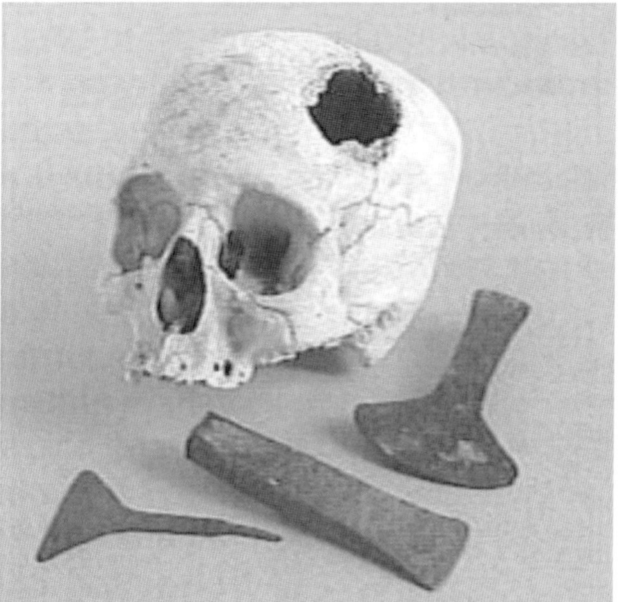

Figure 1-1 Trephining is a procedure performed in ancient times that involves boring a hole into the skull. It is believed this procedure was performed to release evil spirits. *(From World Book:* World book encyclopedia, *vol 2, Chicago, 2000, World Book.)*

remedies appeared to be effective, and research has shown that the treatment of disease and wounds was very "modern" in approach. Despite the "modern" approach, medicine and healing was heavily influenced by religious beliefs and mythical magic.

Ancient temples built in Egypt, Greece, and Rome were said to be the first institutions built for those with an illness. The temples were dedicated to the worship of healer gods. Healer gods, such as Aesculapius, were thought to be responsible for the cure of illness. Priests provided comfort to the sick while waiting for guidance from the gods. Temples were often referred to as healing centers.

Research indicates that the first hospital-like institutions were built between the 5th and 2nd centuries B.C. in places such as India, Ireland, and Rome. Some of these hospitals were built specifically to provide care for the sick. The first hospital in India was established in Sri Lanka by the 5th century B.C. Buddhism was introduced in India by the 3rd century B.C., and the Buddhist King Asoka was said to have established 18 Brahmanic hospitals. These hospitals were established to meet the health care needs of the population in the region. Some scholars believe that during this time Indian hospitals began to resemble modern-day hospitals. Physicians and nurses provided care, following principals of sanitation and performing various surgical procedures such as skin grafting. The first hospital in Ireland was established in the 4th century B.C. The hospital was called Broin Bearg, which also means "house of sorrows." Princess Macha founded this hospital for use by the Red Branch Knights. It also served as the royal residence in Ulster through the 4th century A.D. Roman military hospitals were established by the 2nd century B.C. These hospitals were used to provide medical care to the sick and injured soldiers. However, medical care during this period was dominated by religious beliefs, and healing was intertwined with spiritual and ritualistic ceremonies. It was only with the rise of the Greek civilization that the principles of medicine shifted to a holistic and realistic approach.

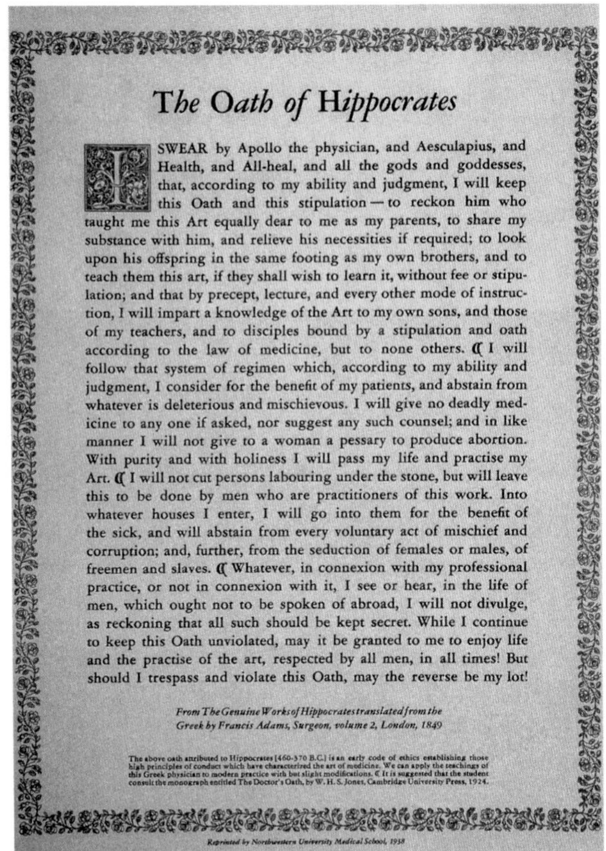

The Oath of Hippocrates

I SWEAR by Apollo the physician, and Aesculapius, and Health, and All-heal, and all the gods and goddesses, that, according to my ability and judgment, I will keep this Oath and this stipulation — to reckon him who taught me this Art equally dear to me as my parents, to share my substance with him, and relieve his necessities if required; to look upon his offspring in the same footing as my own brothers, and to teach them this art, if they shall wish to learn it, without fee or stipulation; and that by precept, lecture, and every other mode of instruction, I will impart a knowledge of the Art to my own sons, and those of my teachers, and to disciples bound by a stipulation and oath according to the law of medicine, but to none others. ℭ I will follow that system of regimen which, according to my ability and judgment, I consider for the benefit of my patients, and abstain from whatever is deleterious and mischievous. I will give no deadly medicine to any one if asked, nor suggest any such counsel; and in like manner I will not give to a woman a pessary to produce abortion. With purity and with holiness I will pass my life and practise my Art. ℭ I will not cut persons labouring under the stone, but will leave this to be done by men who are practitioners of this work. Into whatever houses I enter, I will go into them for the benefit of the sick, and will abstain from every voluntary act of mischief and corruption; and, further, from the seduction of females or males, of freemen and slaves. ℭ Whatever, in connexion with my professional practice, or not in connexion with it, I see or hear, in the life of men, which ought not to be spoken of abroad, I will not divulge, as reckoning that all such should be kept secret. While I continue to keep this Oath unviolated, may it be granted to me to enjoy life and the practise of the art, respected by all men, in all times! But should I trespass and violate this Oath, may the reverse be my lot!

From The Genuine Works of Hippocrates translated from the Greek by Francis Adams, Surgeon, volume 2, London, 1849

The above oath attributed to Hippocrates [460-370 B.C.] is an early code of ethics establishing those high principles of conduct which have characterized the art of medicine. We can apply the teachings of this Greek physician to modern practice with but slight modifications. ℭ It is suggested that the student consult the monograph entitled The Doctor's Oath, by W. H. S. Jones, Cambridge University Press, 1924.

Reprinted by Northwestern University Medical School, 1938

Figure 1-2 The Hippocratic Oath. *(From Young AP:* Kinn's administrative medical assistant, *ed 5, St Louis, 2003, Saunders.)*

Classic Greece and Rome

Contributions of the high cultures of classic Greece and Rome are considered to be the foundations of modern medicine as we know it today.

Classic Greece

In the historical view, credit for the birth of medicine is given to Hippocrates, an ancient Greek physician (460 to 379 B.C.). He is credited with changing theories of medicine from those based on supernatural beliefs to those with a scientific foundation. Hippocrates did not believe illness was caused by evil spirits. He believed that illness came in response to poor environment, diet, and hygiene. Hippocrates's approach to medicine involved observation through physical examination and conservative treatment. If diet and exercise did not succeed, then medicines formulated from minerals and plants were used. Surgery was performed only if treatments with diet and medicine were not successful.

Hippocrates also laid the foundations for the development of the Hippocratic Oath. The Hippocratic Oath (Figure 1-2) outlines standards for medical and ethical behavior that physicians follow today. Hippocrates traveled throughout Greece practicing his medicine. He founded a medical school in Greece and began teaching his ideas. Hippocrates is known as the "Father of Medicine" because his philosophies and methods formed the foundations of medicine and treatment we recognize today.

Classic Rome

Classic Rome is a culmination of Greek and Roman civilizations. Rome developed superior armies that eventually conquered Greece by 133 B.C. Many elements of Greek civilization were adopted and modified by Rome. Hippocratic foundations of medicine were advanced by a physician from Asia named Claudius Galen. Galen assumed the role of primary physician in

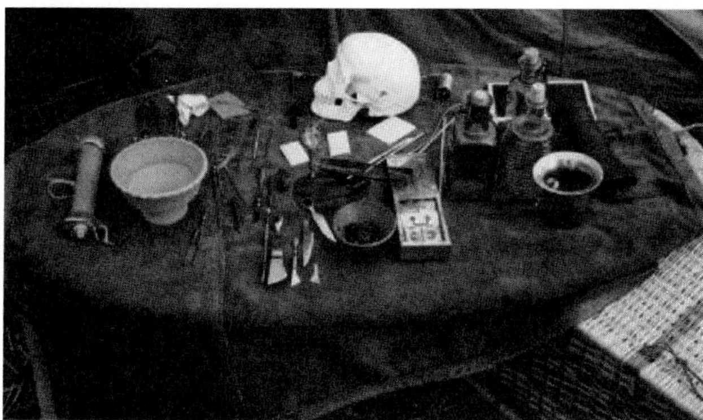

Figure 1-3 Instruments found in a Roman legion's field kit included suture kits, scalpels, wound spreaders, and splints. *(Courtesy I. Roemercohorte Opladen.)*

Rome, and his teachings carried into the modern age of medicine. Rome's contribution to the advancement of medical care was enormous. Roman hospitals were primarily found in military settlements, commonly referred to as field hospitals. Medical care provided in field hospitals showed evidence of the first systemized approach to medical care emphasizing diet, sanitation, and hygiene. Advances in medical treatments and instruments were made using knowledge gained from treating injured soldiers through many wars. Instruments found in a Roman legion's field kit included suture kits, scalpels, wound spreaders, and splints (Figure 1-3). The drugs known to clean and promote healing were similar to those used today. The Roman model of medical care was maintained for hundreds of years until the fall of Rome.

BOX 1-2 ■ KEY POINTS

Ancient Medicine and Healing Centers in Classic Greece and Rome

Evidence of primitive medicine back to 10,000 B.C.
Medicine based on religious beliefs and mythical magic
Temples built for worship of healer gods
First hospital-like institutions established
Military hospitals established
Hippocrates (460 to 379 B.C.)
Roman physician Galen advances Hippocratic theories
Roman military hospitals advance medical knowledge

Middle Ages

The Middle Ages was a period marked by the chaos of war and the global spread of disease. The growth of hospitals was stimulated as the Roman Empire was converted to Christianity. By decree of Emperor Constantine in 335 A.D., Pagan hospitals were abolished, and Christian hospitals were affiliated with monasteries. War and the global spread of disease also contributed to the establishment of many hospitals. Lazar houses (hospitals) were built to isolate lepers from the public. Military hospitals continued to be established to treat injured soldiers. This was also a period that witnessed a shift of scientific and medical knowledge from Europe to the Arab countries.

Early Middle Ages (475 to 1000 A.D.)

The fall of the Roman Empire had a profound effect on all aspects of life, including medicine, throughout the Middle Ages. Barbarians overran the Roman Empire; however, disease was also thought to have contributed to the fall of the empire. As established health and hygiene standards vanished, disease continued to spread. The centers of medicine and learning decayed and were eventually lost in Europe. However, the growth of hospitals in Europe continued into the early Middle Ages as a result of the Christian commitment to caring for the sick and poor and the need to treat soldiers of war.

One of the oldest institution-like facilities, the Hôtel Dieu, was founded in 542 A.D. in Lyon, France. The focus of care at the Hôtel Dieu was not to cure illness but rather to heal the patient's soul. The Hôtel Dieu is still in existence today.

For many centuries after the fall of the Roman Empire, the Arab world was the center of scientific and medical knowledge. Texts from Greece and Rome were translated into Arabic and studied by Islamic scholars. They developed and refined Hippocratic theories, and Islamic physicians began to use the regulation of diet and exercise and the prescription of medicinal herbs to treat their patients. Arabic pharmacists became skilled in the formulation of medicines from plants and minerals. It is said that many efficient hospitals were developed in Arab countries during the Middle Ages. The first hospitals were established in Persia and Baghdad in the 8th century A.D. Hospitals were not just for the wealthy. They treated rich and poor alike. Islamic hospitals of this time would not look out of place today. They had medical and surgical wards as well as operating theatres and pharmacies for the dispensing of medicine. By 931 A.D., large hospitals were involved in the training and licensing of doctors and pharmacists. Growth and development of medicine and hospitals continued in the Arab world throughout history.

High Middle Ages (1000 to 1350 A.D.)

Two major factors influencing growth and development during this period were the Crusades and the global spread of disease. This period of the Middle Ages marked the high point of medieval civilization. Population growth, the flourishing of towns and farms, the emergence of merchant classes, and the development of governmental bureaucracies were part of the cultural and economic revival during this period. The church underwent reform that strengthened the place of the

Pope in church and society. This led to a clash between the Pope and the Holy Roman Emperor, resulting in the Crusades, which had a major influence on the growth and development of hospitals during this period. The Crusades began when Christian armies traveled to Jerusalem and entered into battle to seize the Holy Land from the Muslims. Thousands of knights followed the call of the Church to join the Crusades, which took place from the 11th to the 13th centuries. During this time many military hospitals were built to care for the injured soldiers of the Crusades. The hospital established by the Knights Hospitallers of the Order of St. John in Jerusalem in 1099 is said to be one of the first specialized hospitals developed.

A more significant factor in the growth in the number of hospitals during this period was the epidemic spreading of contagious diseases. The living conditions in Europe were very unhealthy. There was no sewage system, the streets were covered with refuse, drinking water was not clean, people did not bathe, and animals roamed the streets. It is said that the lack of sanitation and poor hygiene caused infectious diseases such as the black plague, or "Black Death." By 1348, the black plague had killed a large percentage of the total European population.

Hospitals became well known as places where people with contagious diseases were isolated and cured because of good care. Many hospitals became involved in teaching physicians. It was during this period that the title "doctor" was adopted through legislative implementation of curriculum and state licensing requirements for physicians. The practice of medicine was now an official profession. Over time schools and universities were organized for the purpose of training individuals in the field of medicine. The church controlled the hospitals, but citizens managed them. Hospital expansion continued as a result of the growing population and the continued spread of diseases such as the plague, which were at epidemic proportions.

BOX 1-3 ■ KEY POINTS

Hospitals in the Early to High Middle Ages (475 to 1350 A.D.)

Early Middle Ages

Global spread of disease
Lazar houses and other hospitals (Hôtel Dieu)
Fall of Rome—medicine, education, and sanitation lost
Hospital growth influenced by Christianity
Center of scientific medicine shifts to the Arab world

High Middle Ages

Population growth and governmental bureaucracies
Crusades
Knights Hospitallers Order of St. John
Global spread of diseases such as the "Black Death"

Renaissance (1350 to 1650 A.D.)

The Renaissance period was marked by the establishment of commercial enterprise and a rekindling of the scientific spirit. As commercial enterprise flourished, a shift from villages and feudal estates to cities occurred. The growing economy and increasing population of the cities led to the need for more hospitals. The establishment and endowment of hospitals was accomplished through contributions from municipalities, guilds, and public individuals.

The last 200 years of this period were marked by widespread abuse and disorder. Hospital revenues were lost, confiscated, or distributed by the magistrates and used for purposes other than caring for the sick. This continued misappropriation of funds from endowments and charities came to light, which led to a major upheaval. Monasteries were dissolved, which left the church with little or no support for charity work and caring for the sick. The responsibility for management of institutions that were founded to care for the sick and injured began to shift to secular authorities.

Enlightenment (1650 to 1890 A.D.)

Throughout the Enlightenment period, the patterns established in the Middle Ages continued as towns and cities throughout Europe built hospitals for the purpose of caring for victims of contagious diseases and also to care for the poor. Toward the end of the Renaissance period, hospitals began to be operated by nonreligious organizations rather than religious orders. The voluntary hospital movement started with the establishment of a voluntary hospital in England in 1718. These hospitals were funded through voluntary contributions and managed by representatives appointed by the contributors. Many other voluntary hospitals were established from 1719 to 1729. By the close of the century, hospital direction had been assumed by private interests with land and funds. By the 18th century, hospitals had been constructed in the new lands colonized in the Americas.

BOX 1-4 ■ KEY POINTS

Hospitals in the Renaissance to the Enlightenment (1350 to 1890 A.D.)

Commercial enterprise established
Rekindling of scientific spirit
Hospitals established with endowments funds
Shift of hospital ownership and management to secular authorities
Hospitals built by towns and cities
First three voluntary hospitals established in the United States

TEST YOUR *Knowledge* BOX 1-1

HOSPITAL INTRODUCTION; EVOLUTION OF HOSPITALS

1. Define today's hospital.
2. List the five characteristics of a hospital.
3. What is the major purpose of a hospital?
4. Name four categories of hospital departments.
5. Describe the purpose of billing in hospitals.
6. What patient information is considered demographic?
7. How does documentation in the medical record affect the billing process?
8. Explain the relationship between billing and coding.
9. Discuss the stages of the billing process from when patient demographic and insurance information is obtained to the collection of outstanding accounts.
10. Define accounts receivable.
11. When did the evolution of hospitals begin?
12. Describe early institutions utilized for the sick.
13. Provide an example of primitive medicine during ancient times.
14. List where the first hospital-like institutions were built between the 5th and 2nd centuries B.C.
15. Briefly describe the influence of classic Greece on medicine.
16. Discuss Hippocrates's approach to medicine.
17. How did Roman hospitals influence future hospital growth?
18. List two major factors that influenced the expansion of hospitals during the High Middle Ages.
19. Provide an overview of the two factors influencing hospitals during the Renaissance period.
20. What changes in hospital operations took place during the Enlightenment period?

HISTORY OF HOSPITALS IN THE UNITED STATES

With the discovery and conquest of new lands came many of the same health care problems experienced in foreign lands. With the early settlers in America came contagious diseases. The population in early American colonies grew rapidly, and disease continued to spread. Soldiers with wartime injuries required medical care. The need to treat injured soldiers, care for the sick and poor, and isolate those with contagious disease led to the establishment of American hospitals. Early institutions were primarily military hospitals, almshouses for the poor, and places to isolate those with contagious disease. Hospitals were later established specifically to care for the sick. American hospitals later took the form of modern-day hospitals. These hospitals became teaching and research environments that contributed greatly to advances made in medicine and ultimately the growth and development of hospitals.

Public Health Status

The health status of the early American population was like that of the countries from which its settlers came. Contagious diseases were brought in. The population in early American colonies grew from around 2,000 in the year 1620 to more than 1 million by 1760 (Figure 1-4). Settlers lived in primitive housing situated near waterways. There were no sanitation systems, and eventually the water became contaminated by human waste. The rapid growth of the population made it impossible to provide healthy food and living conditions. The population was stricken with diseases such as malaria, smallpox, yellow fever, cholera, and typhoid. Table 1-1 illustrates the outbreaks of various diseases from the period 1620 to 1760. A limited number of educated physicians had traveled to America; however, there were no known cures for these diseases. It was difficult to obtain care because the population was spread over large areas, and physicians would travel to patients' homes to treat them. The health status of early American populations did not improve greatly until the 19th century.

Medical Practice

The practice of medicine in early colonial America was based largely on religious superstitions and rituals, and it was heavily reliant on home cures and folk remedies. It was believed that an imbalance of the body's humors (blood, phlegm, yellow bile or choler, and black bile or gall) was responsible for illness. Medical care was provided by a few trained physicians and others who were self-taught or learned through apprenticeships. Despite the training of some physicians, there were no known cures for many of the diseases seen in those days. Medical treatment focused on treating the symptom. Treatments used to bring the humors into balance included bleeding, purging, and trephining. Herbs and other natural remedies were also used. Access to medical treatment expanded in the late 1700s as more hospitals became established.

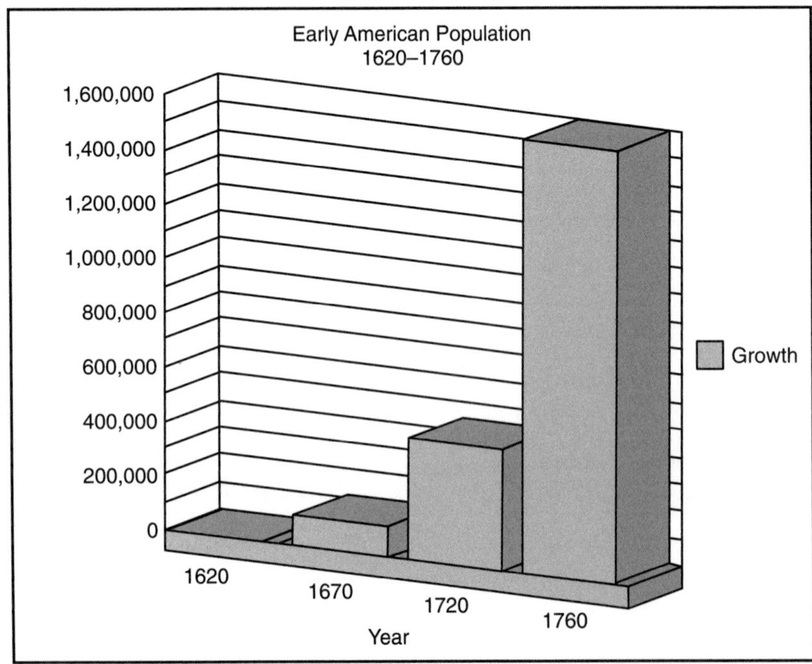

Figure 1-4 The early American population grew from 2,300 to 1,593,625 between 1620 and 1760. *(Data from Middleton R:* Colonial america: a history, 1565–1776, *ed 3, Malden, Mass., 2002, Blackwell.)*

TABLE 1-1 Outbreak of Diseases, 1620 to 1760

Year	Disease	Location
1607–1612	Typhus, dysentery	Jamestown, VA
1617–1624	Typhus, dysentery	James River Valley, VA
1638	Smallpox	Massachusetts (few deaths)
1647	Influenza/smallpox	Massachusetts, Connecticut (90 deaths)
1648–1649	Whooping cough	Massachusetts
1657	Measles	Boston (few deaths)
1658	Typhoid fever	New Amsterdam, New England
1659	Diphtheria, whooping cough	Massachusetts
1660–1661	Influenza	New England (few deaths)
1665	Influenza	New England (few deaths)
1666	Smallpox	New England (about 40 deaths)
1677–1678	Smallpox	Boston (more than 200 died)
1678–1679	Influenza	New England (few deaths)
1687–1688	Measles	Massachusetts
1688	Influenza	Virginia
1689	Diphtheria	New London, CT (many deaths)
1689–1690	Smallpox	New England and New York (at least 320 deaths)
1693	Yellow fever	Boston
1693	Measles	Virginia
1696	Smallpox	Jamestown, VA
1697–1698	Smallpox	South Carolina (more than 200 deaths)
1699	Yellow fever	Charles Town, SC (179 deaths) and Philadelphia (220 deaths)
1697–1698	Influenza	New England (heavy mortality)
1699	Influenza	New England (heavy mortality)
1702	Smallpox	New York City
1702	Yellow fever	New York City (570 deaths)
1702–1703	Smallpox and scarlet fever	Boston (about 300 deaths)
1707	Yellow fever	Charles Town, SC
1710	Influenza	Connecticut (250 deaths)
1711–1712	Smallpox	Charles Town, SC
1713–1714	Measles	New England (at least 150 deaths)
1715–1718	Measles	Mid-Atlantic colonies
	Smallpox	New York, New Jersey
1717	Measles	Virginia
1721	Smallpox	Boston (844 deaths)
1724	Diphtheria or scarlet fever	Charles Town, SC
1727	Typhoid fever	Norwich (40 deaths) and Woodbury, CT
1728	Yellow fever	Charles Town, SC
1728	Influenza	South Carolina
1729	Measles	Boston (15 deaths)
1730–1732	Smallpox	New York City
1731–1732	Smallpox	Boston (about 500 deaths), New York (549 deaths in New York City, about 300 in rural areas), Pennsylvania, New Jersey
1732–1734	Influenza	New England, mid-Atlantic colonies
1732	Yellow fever	Charles Town, SC
1732	Dysentery	Salem, MA
1732	Smallpox	Wallingford, CT (14 deaths)
1732	Yellow fever	New York City (70 deaths)
1734	Typhoid fever	New Haven, CT
1734	Dysentery	Boston and New London, CT
1735–1741	Diphtheria	New England, New York, New Jersey (as many as 20,000 deaths)
1735–1736	Scarlet fever	Boston (100 deaths)
1736	Scarlet fever	Newport, RI

Continued

TABLE 1-1 Outbreak of Diseases, 1620 to 1760—*cont'd*

Year	Disease	Location
1736–1737	Smallpox	Philadelphia
1737	Typhoid fever	Worcester County, MA
1737	Smallpox	Charles Town, SC (311 deaths)
1737–1738	Smallpox	Martha's Vineyard, MA (12 deaths)
1738	Whooping cough	South Carolina
1738–1739	Smallpox	New York City (1,550 cases)
1739	Yellow fever	Charles Town, SC
1739	Smallpox	Newport, RI (17 deaths)
1739	Measles	Massachusetts and Connecticut
1741	Yellow fever	Philadelphia (200 deaths)
1741	Typhoid fever	Suttun, MA (19 deaths) and New London, CT
1742	Dysentery	New London, CT and New York City (217 deaths)
1743	Yellow fever	Massachusetts
1744–1745	Diphtheria	New Hampshire and New York
1745	Dysentery	Shrewsbury, MA (several deaths)
1745	Typhoid fever	Stamford, CT (70 deaths)
1745	Yellow fever	New York City
1745	Yellow fever	Charles Town, SC
1746	Typhoid fever	Albany, NY
1746	Diphtheria	Pennsylvania, Delaware, and New Jersey
1746	Typhoid fever	Albany, NY
1747	Smallpox	Harwich, MA (9 deaths), New York, New Jersey, Delaware, and Maryland
1747	Typhoid fever	New York City
1747	Yellow fever	Charles Town, SC
1747–1748	Diphtheria	Massachusetts
	Measles	Massachusetts, Connecticut, and New York
1748	Smallpox	Pennsylvania and South Carolina
1748	Yellow fever	Williamsburg,VA, and Charles Town, SC
1748–1749	Influenza or pneumonia	Atlantic seaboard
1749	Typhus and dysentery	Connecticut (at least 150 deaths)
1749–1750	Influenza or pneumonia	Mid-Atlantic and southern colonies
1750–1751	Diphtheria or scarlet fever	South Carolina
1750–1755	Diphtheria or scarlet fever	New England and New York
1751	Smallpox	Boston (569 deaths)
1752	Smallpox	New York and New Jersey
1753	Smallpox	New London, CT (4 deaths)
1755	Mumps	Brookfield, MA (several deaths)
1755–1756	Smallpox	New York
1756	Smallpox	Philadelphia
1756	Dysentery	New England
1756–1757	Smallpox	Annapolis, MD
1759	Smallpox	Widespread in colonies
1759	Whooping cough	New Jersey, South Carolina
1760	Smallpox	Charles Town, SC (730 deaths)
1760–1761	Smallpox	New England
1761	Influenza	Atlantic seaboard
1762–1763	Yellow fever	Philadelphia
	Diphtheria	Massachusetts and Connecticut
1763	Typhus	Nantucket, MA (222 Indians died)
1763	Smallpox	South Carolina
1763	Diphtheria	Philadelphia

From Middleton R: Colonial america: a history, 1565–1776, *ed 3, Malden, Mass., 2002, Blackwell.*

BOX 1-5 ■ KEY POINTS

History of Hospitals in the United States

Contagious diseases were carried to the United States
American colonies grew rapidly
Early institutions were military hospitals and almshouses
Medicine was heavily reliant on home cures and folk remedies
Later hospitals mirrored modern-day practices
Medicine shifted to a scientific basis

EARLY DEVELOPMENT OF UNITED STATES HOSPITALS

It is said that the first hospital established in the United States was a military hospital on Manhattan Island, New York (Figure 1-5). The Dutch founded this hospital in 1663 to care for wounded soldiers. It was referred to as the "hospital for soldiers." In addition to military hospitals, there were almshouses to care for the poor and places used to isolate those with contagious disease. In 1713, William Penn established one of the first almshouses, in Philadelphia. The growing population and spread of disease resulted in a growing awareness of the need for hospitals to care for the sick.

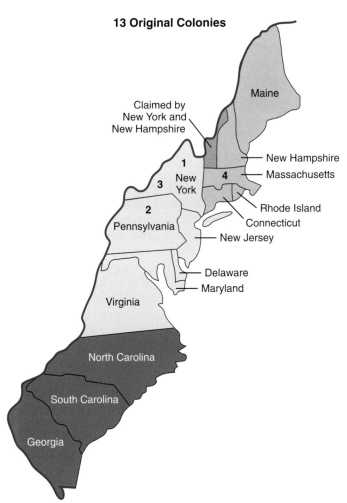

Figure 1-5 The first hospitals established in Colonial America. *1*, Military Hospital, Manhattan, 1663. *2*, Pennsylvania Hospital, 1751. *3*, New York Hospital, 1775. *4*, Massachusetts General, 1804. *(Modified from World Book:* World book encyclopedia, *Vol 4, Chicago, 2000, World Book.)*

Voluntary hospitals were the first institutions established in the United States specifically to care for the sick. These hospitals were funded with monies collected from voluntary contributions. Physicians served without pay, and patients were required to pay for services. Those who could not pay donated time to perform various duties such as cleaning and assisting others. Three of the first voluntary hospitals were Pennsylvania Hospital in 1751, New York Hospital in 1775, and Massachusetts General Hospital in 1804. The nation's first incorporated hospital was the Pennsylvania Hospital founded by Benjamin Franklin and Dr. Thomas Bond to care for the "sick-poor and insane of Philadelphia." It was funded by voluntary contributions from the public and by matching government funds. The hospital was governed by 12 board members who established policies such as those for admissions and selection of physicians. The contributors met annually to elect members to serve on the board. The Pennsylvania Hospital, the New York Hospital, and the Massachusetts General Hospital served as models for modern-day hospitals and teaching institutions.

The establishment of hospitals continued throughout the United States. However, the cause of disease was unknown, so the death rate of hospital patients was very high. Sanitation conditions in hospitals were not as they are today, which resulted in the spread of infection within the hospital. With this came the stigma that admission to a hospital was a last resort. Hospitals were not thought to be a safe place where someone could get well. It was not until scientific advances were made that hospital conditions were improved.

Scientific Advances

The 17th century is known as the era of scientific revolution. The focus of medicine shifted to research and scientific exploration of the cause of disease. Many of the discoveries made at that time regarding the structure and function of the human body as well as disease processes are essential parts of the practice of modern medicine. Discoveries in technology led to the invention of new diagnostic tools used in the identification and treatment of disease. Diagnostic, technological, and therapeutic advances made in medicine through the 20th century contributed to the growth of hospitals.

Diagnostic Advances in Medicine

Progress made in diagnosing patient conditions came as the result of research in the areas of anatomy, body

TABLE 1-2 Diagnostic Advances in Medicine

Anatomy	A greater understanding of anatomy and physiology was gained through autopsies: • The ability to perform autopsies enhanced the study of structure and function of the body. • Autopsies were also instrumental in the identification and classification of disease. Drawings of anatomy were created based on visualizations during autopsies.
Body systems	A greater understanding of various body systems such as the circulatory, respiratory, digestive, and nervous systems was gained: • Blood circulates through the body via a complex system of vessels. • Oxygen is added to blood through the lungs. • Dietary habits were realized to be related to specific conditions. Study of the nervous system focused on the brain, and theories about the relationship between the brain and mechanical functions of the body were explored.
Contagious diseases	Knowledge of how infections were spread increased as theories of contagious diseases were developed: • Specific organisms were identified. • Germs had a connection to various diseases. • Bacteria were identified and determined to be the cause of specific diseases (bacteriology). Specific cures were needed for specific diseases.
Prevention of disease	The reality that sanitation and hygiene were directly related to disease brought about changes in attitudes toward public health.

TABLE 1-3 Technological Advances in Medicine

Microscopic innovation	Provided a way to examine anatomical tissue and other living organisms
The creation of gunpowder	Resulted in the need to identify ways to treat gunshot wounds and was instrumental in the development of advanced surgical procedures
Development of techniques for measurement of blood pressure and temperature	Enhanced the ability to monitor a patient's status by measuring the patient's vital signs, including pulse and respiratory rate
Advanced exploration in the science chemistry	Discovered various laboratory tests to diagnose specific conditions
Introduction of anesthetic agents	Allowed the performance of more complex surgical procedures through the alleviation of pain
Discovery of X-ray technology	Provided ways to diagnose various internal conditions such as foreign body presence and fractures
Invention of the printing press	Increased ability to document and distribute medical information

systems, contagious disease, and prevention of disease. Table 1-2 highlights some of the major advances in diagnosing patient conditions. The study of anatomy through autopsies provided greater opportunities to learn about the body internally. Exploration of the human anatomy provided graphic descriptions of body parts that were used to develop principles of the structure and functions of body systems. These principles were applied and used to identify organisms that contribute to dysfunction in those systems. Ultimately, the study of anatomy contributed to the ability to identify, classify, treat, and prevent disease. These advances were made possible with new technologies.

Technological Advances in Medicine

Technological advances made medical advances possible. These included new equipment used to study disease and also to distribute medical knowledge. Table 1-3 highlights some of these advances. The invention of the microscope allowed for the examination of anatomical tissue and other living organisms. New surgical procedures were developed to treat soldiers inflicted with gunshot wounds, which came after the creation of gunpowder. Equipment developed to measure and monitor blood pressure and body temperature enhanced the ability to monitor the patient's vital signs, which were seen as an indicator of health status. The exploration of chemistry led to the discovery of various laboratory tests used to diagnose specific conditions. More complex surgical procedures were performed after the introduction of anesthetic agents. Diagnostic and therapeutic procedures were improved with the advent of X-ray technology. The sharing of new medical knowledge was greatly improved with the invention of the printing press.

Therapeutic Advances in Medicine

Much progress was made in the treatment of conditions as a result of the medical and technological advances. Table 1-4 outlines some of the most significant therapeutic advances. Advanced studies of plants led to the identification and categorization of many new medications such as antibiotics, insulin, and those used for birth control. Vaccinations for diseases such as small-

TABLE 1-4	Therapeutic Advances in Medicine
Medications	Through the study of plants, various drugs were developed and categorized: • Antibiotics (penicillin) • Insulin • Birth control
Vaccinations	The development of vaccinations prevented thousands of deaths from: • Smallpox • Diphtheria • Typhoid fever • Measles • Chickenpox
Surgery	The treatment option of surgery enhanced the ability to cure more complex conditions: • Surgical removal of cancerous tissue and organs • Open heart surgery, leading to the ability to bypass clogged arteries • Transplantations of organs to replace diseased, nonfunctional organs

pox, diphtheria, typhoid, measles, and chickenpox prevented thousands of deaths. Surgery became a more viable option with anesthetics, and more complex conditions were treated through the performance of new surgical techniques. Advanced surgical procedures included removal of cancerous tissue, open heart surgery, and organ transplants.

Medical Standards and Accreditation

The development of hospitals in the United States was greatly influenced by scientific progress. Early European and U.S. hospitals were developed without knowledge of bacteria and how disease spread. Sanitary measures did not exist. The spread of disease continued, and postsurgical infections were common. It was later realized that disease and infection could be prevented through the use of disinfectants and antiseptics. These discoveries led to a changing view toward sanitation and hygiene. A great contributor to the development of standards of hygiene and sanitation was Florence Nightingale, a nurse who trained at a hospital in Europe. After completion of her training she worked throughout Europe in military hospitals that were dirty and unsanitary. She improved standards of hygiene and sanitation in military hospitals during the 19th century. She later developed standards for nursing that included sanitary measures, which had not existed up to that point. Hospital units, clothing, linen, and surgical instruments were cleaned regularly. The reality that more sterile environments prevented infections led to a general acceptance of hospitals as a place to receive medical care.

As medicine became more scientific, the need for trained physicians and nurses was highlighted. U.S. hospitals, such as the Pennsylvania Hospital, offered apprentice opportunities for physicians. Hospitals contributed significantly to medical education by providing access to a large number of patients available for observation. Many medical schools were opened, most of which were proprietary. By the 19th century, there were more than 400 medical schools in the United States. A group of U.S. physicians formed the **American Medical Association (AMA)** in 1847, with a mission to improve the standards of medical education. It is said that the AMA's efforts in raising medical standards led to the creation of the first state licensing boards.

Medical care during early American history improved; however, the quest to raise standards continued. As the role of hospitals changed, it was realized that standards for care provided in the hospital must also be developed. An organization called the Association of Hospital Superintendents was formed in 1898 to provide a forum for hospital superintendents to discuss areas of concerns and to share ideas. Membership in this organization was later expanded to include other hospital personnel, and the name was changed to the **American Hospital Association (AHA)** in 1906. The mission of the organization was to promote public welfare by providing better health care in hospitals. The AHA conducted inspections of hospitals and, over time, established standards for the provision of care in hospital facilities.

Standards for medical education came to the forefront again in 1910 when Abraham Flexner conducted a study on the quality of medical education. The Flexner Report identified problems in medical education and outlined a model of standards for medical education. The AMA initiated an accreditation process that ranked schools according to their performance based on a model for medical education established by the Flexner Report. This model is still used in many schools today.

During the 1900s the expansion of hospitals continued throughout the United States, and thus the need for standardization in hospitals was highlighted. The **American College of Surgeons (ACS)** was established in 1913 for the purpose of developing hospital standards by collecting patient care data. These standards were tested in 692 hospitals. The ACS reported that only 89 hospitals met the standards. The ACS was at the forefront of developing and maintaining standards for hospital medical care, which were referred to as the **Hospital Standardization Program**. Hospitals that met the standards of care outlined by the ACS were recognized.

The Hospitalization Standardization Program established by the ACS was adopted by the newly formed **Joint Commission on Accreditation of Health-Care Organizations (JCAHO)** in 1952, which was founded

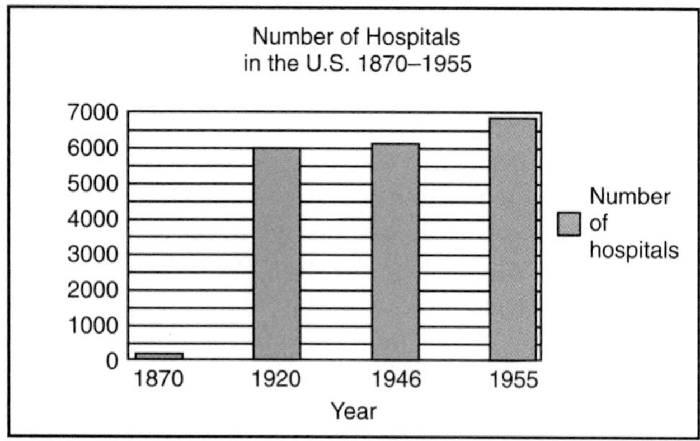

Figure 1-6 Number of hospitals in the United States, 1870 to 1955. *(Data from Abdelhak M, Grostick S, Hanken MA, Jacobs E (editors):* Health information: management of a strategic resource, *ed 2, St Louis, 2001, Saunders.)*

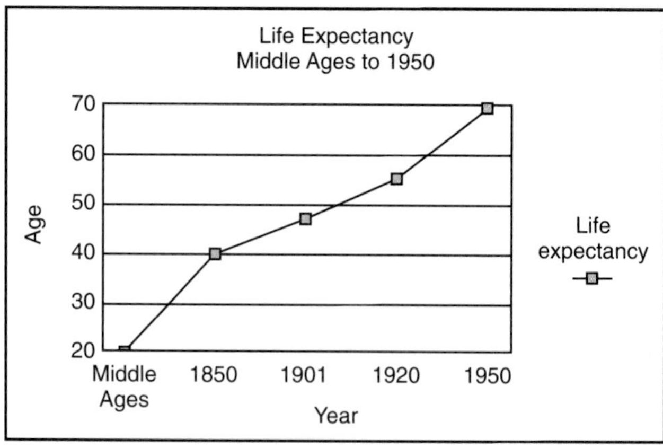

Figure 1-7 Life expectancy from the Middle Ages to 1950. *(Data from Abdelhak M, Grostick S, Hanken MA, Jacobs E (editors):* Health information: management of a strategic resource, *ed 2, St Louis, 2001, Saunders, and Mitchell J, Haroun L:* Introduction to health care, *ed 1, Albany, N.Y., 2001, Delmar.)*

for the purpose of developing guidelines for hospitals and other health care organizations. The JCAHO announced their name change to **The Joint Commission (TJC)** in 2007. TJC evaluates and accredits health care organizations based on established standards of quality for operations and medical services. Accreditation will be discussed further in Chapter 2 of this text.

Economic Influences on Hospital Development

Advanced medical treatments and standards of care contributed to an increase in the number of patients seen in hospitals, which created a demand for more personnel and equipment, which in turn caused the cost of care provided in the hospital to rise. As the cost of hospital care increased, individuals and hospitals began to experience financial difficulties. Figure 1-6 shows the increase in the number of hospitals from 1870 to 1955.

Rising Health Care Costs

The rising cost of hospital care created a financial burden for people who could not afford it. Individuals and hospitals continued to experience financial difficulty, especially after the Great Depression. In an effort to deal the with financial difficulty experienced by individuals and hospitals, a third-party payer, **Blue Cross**, introduced one of the first prepaid health plans in 1929 to provide coverage for hospital care. A **thirdparty payer** is an organization or entity other than the patient or provider that pays for health care services. A **prepaid health plan** provides health benefits for specified medical services in exchange for prepayment of monthly or annual premiums. Prepaid insurance spreads the financial burden of hospital care among a large group of members, thus reducing the individual cost. The Blue Cross prepaid health plan provided coverage for 21 days of hospitalization. A group of school teachers at Baylor University Hospitals purchased the plan from Blue Cross at a monthly payment of 50 cents. The prepaid insurance helped people protect themselves against the cost of hospitalization, and it helped to improve the financial position of hospitals, as they could now receive payment for the care provided. During World War II employers began to offer full-time employees group health insurance as an incentive for employment. Wages could not be increased because of the wage freeze; therefore, pretax dollars were used to purchase the insurance. **Group health insurance** provides coverage for medical services to members of a group, such as an employer group or association.

Hospital Overcrowding

By the 1930s and 1940s, as a result of advanced medical care, medications, and technologies, the life expectancy of an individual had increased dramatically (as illustrated in Figure 1-7) from less than 20 years during the Middle Ages to 70 in the 1950s. As the population aged, people began to require more hospital care.

Hospitals became overcrowded as the number of patients increased due to the growing elderly population, military involvement, and medical advances. Legislative action was taken, and the Hospital Construction and Survey Act, otherwise known as the **Hill-Burton Act**, was passed in 1946. The Act made funding available, based on state need, through government grants to modernize existing hospitals and build new hospitals. Hospitals receiving the government funds were required to provide care to individuals who were unable to pay, at reduced rates or for free. The Hill-Burton Act provided funding for the growth and development of hospitals for many years.

Many other factors through this period and into the 1960s contributed to the rising cost of health care. One significant factor was the growing elderly population. The field of medicine began to see more chronic disease, and the need for hospitalization continued to rise. Hospitals expanded services and began to provide laboratory tests, X-rays, and other therapies in outpatient clinics. Another factor included government-sponsored programs created to address the growing concern about the number of uninsured and underinsured individuals among the elderly population.

Government Health Care Programs

While hospitals continued to expand services, the growing concern over rising health care costs and limited access to care for the poor and elderly required government action. In 1965, through an amendment of the **Social Security Act** of 1935, health insurance for the aged was implemented. The program, called **Medicare**, provides coverage for health expenses to individuals over age 65 and other eligible groups, such as the disabled. Another program, **Medicaid**, was implemented to provide coverage for health expenses to medically indigent people. Both of these programs will be discussed in greater detail in Chapter 12. Through the implementation of these programs, the federal government became one of the largest payers of health care services.

BOX 1-6 ■ KEY POINTS

Early Development of United States Hospitals

First hospitals
- Military hospital on Manhattan Island, New York, in 1663
- Almshouse established by William Penn in 1713
- Voluntary hospitals in Pennsylvania, New York, and Massachusetts

Medical and technological advances contribute to the growth and development of hospitals

Medical standards and accreditation

Economic factors influence hospital growth
- Rising health care costs
- Hospital overcrowding
- Government health care programs

TEST YOUR *Knowledge* BOX 1-2

HISTORY OF HOSPITALS IN THE UNITED STATES; EARLY DEVELOPMENT OF UNITED STATES HOSPITALS

1. What led to the establishment of the first hospital in the United States?
2. Explain how medical and technological advances contributed to the growth and development of hospitals.
3. Who was Florence Nightingale and what did she do?
4. The American Medical Association (AMA) was formed for what purpose?
5. Explain why the American Hospital Association (AHA) was formed.
6. The Joint Commission guidelines outline standards for what areas?
7. How did Blue Cross have a positive impact on hospitals in the 1920s?
8. Discuss how the Hill-Burton Act contributed to the growth and development of hospitals.
9. List four factors that contributed to hospital overcrowding.
10. What factors influenced the rise in health care cost during the 1900s?

MODERN-DAY HOSPITAL DEVELOPMENT

Toward the close of the 20th century, our health care delivery system had evolved into a maze of services, providers, and settings. Health care services advanced through new technologies and treatments. Providers diversified into specific areas of medicine, referred to as specialties. Patient care services are delivered in a variety of different environments such as offices, hospitals, ambulatory care centers, and long-term care and mental health facilities. Insurance benefits varied from plan to plan. The cost of providing care under this health system was rising at an alarming rate (Figure 1-8). The number of uninsured or underinsured individuals was also rising at an alarming rate. The federal government became a major player in controlling the cost of health care services and ensuring the provision of quality health care services for patients under the Medicare and Medicaid programs. Politicians, interest groups, and consumers applied pressure on the legislature and demanded that the system be reformed to provide quality health care while controlling costs. It was during this period that a shift toward managed care plans occurred.

Managed Care

Managed care plans were thought to be one solution to improving access to care and containing health care costs. They were designed to provide comprehensive health care services effectively and cost efficiently. **Managed care plans** are prepaid health insurance plans that incorporate the provision of coordinated health care services and cost containment measures to monitor and manage health care services provided to members of the plan. Hospitals, physicians, and other providers enter into an agreement with a managed care organization to provide health care services to its members at predetermined fixed rates. Coordination of health care service is accomplished through the use of a **primary care physician (PCP)** who monitors and manages the services provided. Cost containment is accomplished through the implementation of utilization management procedures.

Primary Care Physician (PCP)

A managed care patient selects a PCP, who is considered the "gatekeeper" for the patient. The PCP is responsible for monitoring and managing all health ser-

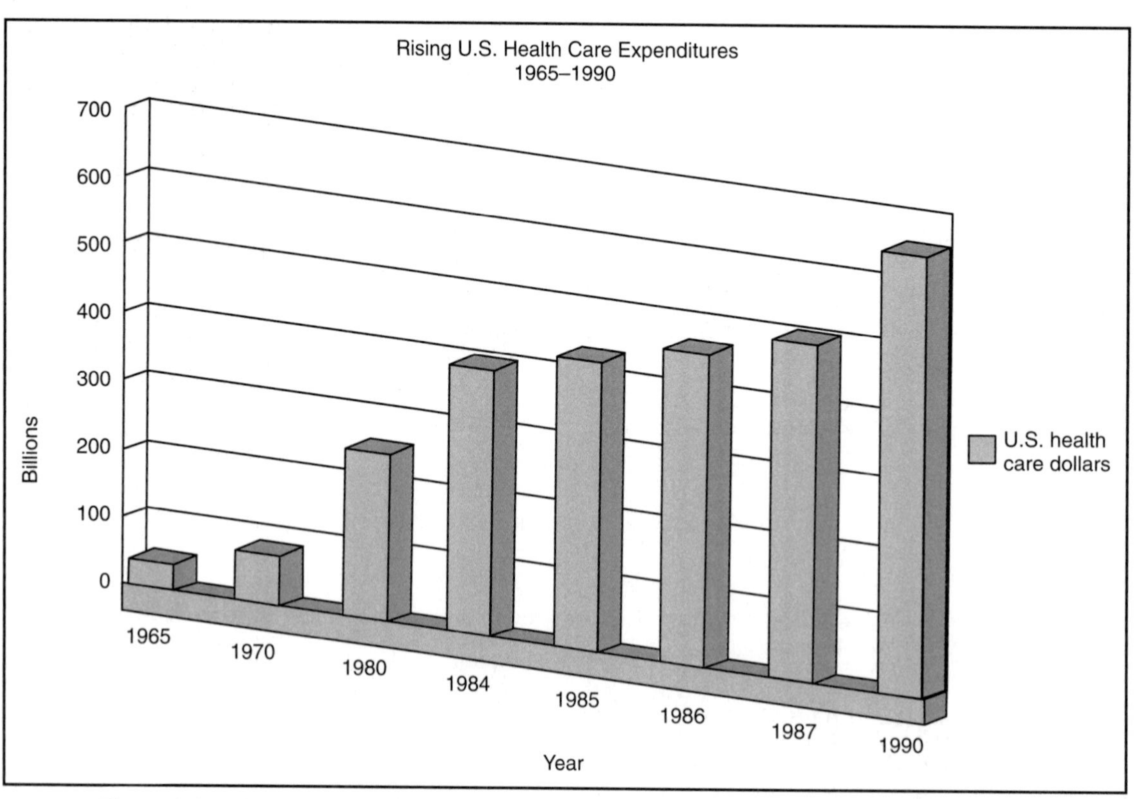

Figure 1-8 Rising U.S. health care expenditures from 1965 to 1990. *(From Marshall RW:* The U.S. health system: origins and functions, *Albany, N.Y., 2001, Delmar.)*

vices required by the patient. Managed care plans also contain measures to monitor utilization of services. These measures affect how federal government programs reimburse hospitals for patient care.

Utilization Management (UM)

Utilization management (UM) is the term used to describe the procedures implemented to manage the utilization of health care services. The purpose of UM is to ensure that services provided to patients are appropriate in response to their medical condition. Medicare requires hospitals to conduct **utilization reviews (URs)** of hospital cases involving Medicare patients. The UR process involves a **peer review**, which is a review conducted by a physician. All records pertinent to the patient stay are reviewed within a specified period after the patient is discharged. The patient record is reviewed to determine whether the care provided during the hospital stay was appropriate based on the patient diagnosis. Later, **quality improvement organizations (QIOs)** were created to conduct Utilization Reviews. These organizations were charged with the determination of appropriateness of care, and they had the authority to deny payment for hospital services provided to Medicare patients that were considered inappropriate based on criteria developed. Managed care will be discussed further in Chapters 11 and 12.

Reimbursement Systems

In another effort to control health care costs, Medicare reimbursement for hospital inpatient services changed from the traditional **fee-for-service** or **percentage of accrued charges**, where payment was made based on charges submitted. Reimbursement changed to the **per diem** method, where payment was based on a daily rate for the inpatient stay. Reimbursement is not provided for services that are not considered appropriate or medically necessary. Many of the services that were typically provided in a hospital setting were no longer considered appropriate, and therefore reimbursement was not provided. The government implemented a new reimbursement method under the **Prospective Payment System (PPS)** in 1983 called Diagnosis Related Groups (DRGs). Under the DRG system of reimbursement, hospitals are paid a fixed amount for the inpatient hospital stay regardless of the amount of charges accrued. The DRG system was replaced with **Medicare Severity Diagnosis Related Groups (MS-DRG)** effective October 1, 2007. The MS-DRG payment is driven by the patient's condition (diagnosis) and the medical severity of that condition. Implementation of UM provisions and changes in reimbursement methods for hospital services drastically reduced hospital revenue. At the same time, hospitals began to lose a market share of patients to physician offices, clinics, urgent care centers, ambulatory care centers, imaging centers, and laboratories outside the traditional hospital; thus inpatient admissions decreased.

Complex Hospital Systems

Over the years, hospitals have experienced tremendous changes. Years ago, institutions were a place where those with diseases were isolated. Over time, hospitals evolved into a place where people could go for treatment of illness. Hospitals concentrated on providing services within the hospital focusing primarily on emergency and inpatient care. Government programs, third-party payers, and patients made payment for services. The cost of health care continued to escalate. Statistics on the national health expenditures indicate an increase from $41.9 billion in 1965 to $647.3 billion in 1990 (see Figure 1-8).

The changes that occurred in health care throughout the 20th century required hospitals to restructure to regain market share, increase admissions, and operate in a cost-effective manner. To accomplish this, many hospitals began to develop primary care networks and integrated delivery systems. The purpose of these systems was to provide total care to patients in inpatient and outpatient settings.

Primary Care Network

A **primary care network** is a network of physicians focused on providing primary care services to patients. Primary care refers to the initial point of contact with a patient for a particular illness. The PCP assesses the patient's condition and determines a plan of treatment. The PCP is responsible for overseeing care provided to the patient by other providers. Primary care networks can be owned by a hospital, a group of physicians, or an insurance company.

Integrated Delivery Systems

An **integrated delivery system** is an organization consisting of a network of providers that are organized within a health system to offer patients a full range of managed health care services. Integrated delivery systems can be owned by an organization such as a hospital, insurance company, or physician group.

Figure 1-9 illustrates a sample hospital-based integrated health care delivery system. Hospital-based physician practices, imaging centers, and ambulatory surgery centers emerged. Expansion of hospital-based services into organized systems such as the one illustrated provides the hospital an opportunity to increase patient market share and to share risks and costs while providing total care to patients.

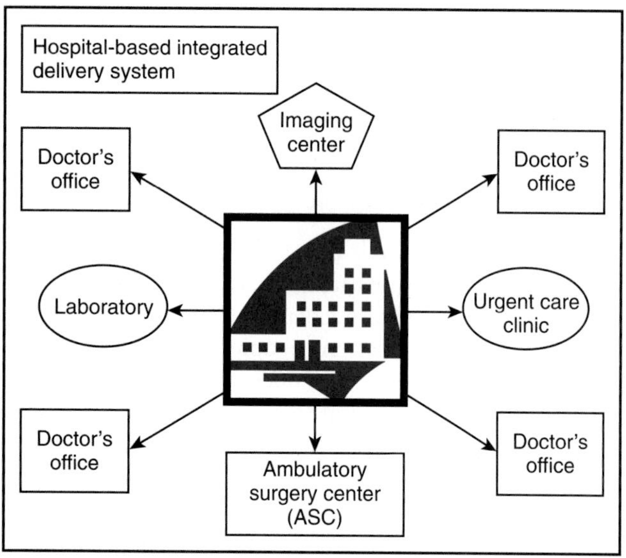

Figure 1-9 Integrated delivery system.

BOX 1-7 ■ KEY POINTS

Modern-Day Hospital Development

Government a major player in controlling cost of health care
Pressure to reform health care system
Shift to managed care plans
Changing reimbursement systems
Development of complex hospital systems
- Primary care network
- Integrated delivery systems

Before we begin our discussion of hospital billing and coding, we will explore the purpose of a hospital in today's health care environment.

PURPOSE OF A HOSPITAL

The purpose of a hospital is to diagnose and treat patient illness, injury, and/or disease. A hospital provides diagnostic, therapeutic, palliative, or preventive services.

TEST YOUR *Knowledge* BOX 1-3

MODERN-DAY HOSPITAL DEVELOPMENT

1. Explain changes in the health care system that contributed to the evolution of hospitals toward the close of the 20th century.
2. Define managed care.
3. How did managed care impact hospitals?
4. What is utilization management?
5. Discuss the utilization review process.
6. Outline changes in reimbursement that affected hospitals.
7. What is a primary care network?
8. Define the integrated delivery system.
9. Explain the difference between an integrated delivery system and a primary care network.
10. List steps taken by hospitals to regain market share.

Hospital Services

Diagnostic Services

Diagnostic services are performed to diagnose a patient's condition. A patient arrives at the hospital with a sign, symptom, illness, injury, or disease. Medical personnel at the hospital obtain a history. The provider reviews the history and performs an examination. Laboratory studies, X-ray studies, or even a surgical procedure such as an arthroscopy or laparoscopy may be required to diagnose the patient's condition. These procedures are referred to as diagnostic services because they are performed to determine the patient's condition.

After the examination and diagnostic studies are complete, the provider evaluates the results to assess the patient's condition and determine a diagnosis. The provider develops a plan of care to treat the patient's condition or alleviate acute symptoms. The process of taking a history, performing an examination, and making a decision about the patient's condition and care is referred to as an **evaluation and management (E/M)** service.

Therapeutic Services

Therapeutic services are performed to treat the patient's condition. The hospital treatment of a patient's condition may involve a range of therapeutic measures such as medication management, therapy, or surgical procedures. These services are considered therapeutic because they are performed to treat the patient's condition.

Palliative Services

Palliative services are performed to minimize the acute symptoms of chronic terminal illnesses such as cancer. These services can include pain management, social services, and other procedures such as surgery.

Preventive Services

Preventive services are provided to promote wellness and prevent illness. They include services performed to detect and treat conditions early and to minimize the effect of disease or disability.

Hospital Service Levels

Diagnostic, therapeutic, palliative, and preventive services can be performed at different levels within the hospital—outpatient, inpatient, and non-patient.

Outpatient

Outpatient is the term used when patient care services are provided and the patient is released within 24 hours. These services do not require the patient to stay in the hospital overnight. Hospitals provide a wide range of services on an outpatient basis such as observation, Emergency Department, and ambulatory surgery.

Observation

An attending physician may see the need to monitor a patient closely for 24 hours or more based on the severity of the patient's illness. The patient may be admitted for observation in these cases. Observation care is considered an outpatient service. Generally the decision to discharge or admit a patient is made within 24 hours; however, some payers may allow observation services for up to 72 hours, when medically necessary.

Emergency Department

Emergency Department services are provided to patients who present with conditions that they believe require immediate attention. The Emergency Department physician assesses the patient's condition and performs services required to stabilize the patient and to treat the acute condition. Emergency Department services are considered outpatient services.

Ambulatory Surgery

Ambulatory surgery is a surgery that is performed on the same day the patient is released. It is an outpatient service.

Inpatient

Inpatient is the term used when patient care services are provided to a patient who is admitted to the hospital for more than 24 hours. The admitting physician orders an inpatient admission. The patient is assigned a bed in a room and receives 24-hour nursing care.

Non-Patient

Non-patient services are performed when a patient's specimen is received by the hospital for processing. Specimens can be blood, fluids, feces, and tissue. The patient is not present when the specimen is processed.

HOSPITAL CLASSIFICATIONS

Hospital Organizations

Hospitals can be classified by how the corporation is formed: for-profit or not-for-profit organization. These designations are defined under state and federal laws and they indicate how the corporation is taxed (Figure 1-10).

Not-for-Profit

As defined under law, a not-for-profit organization is not formed for the sole purpose of making money. It is formed for the purpose of providing some service that is designed to benefit the community. The not-for-profit organization is considered tax exempt. Not-for-profit organizations can make money; however, the profits are put back into the organization. Not-for-profit hospitals are required by law to see indigent patients.

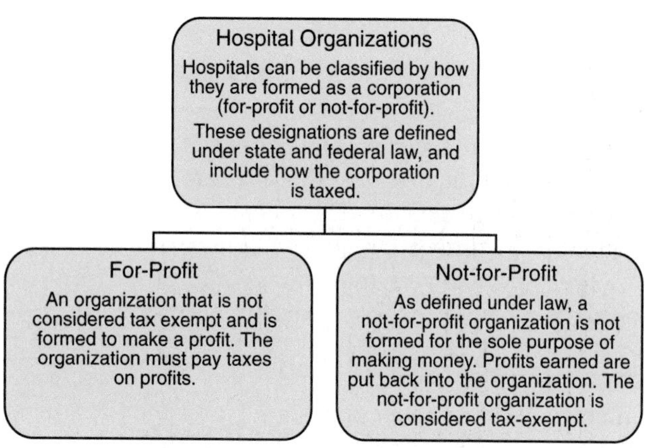

Figure 1-10 Hospital classifications.

They are not allowed to turn patients away based on the status of coverage or their ability to pay. An **indigent** person is one who has no means of paying for medical services or treatments and is not eligible for benefits under Medicaid or other public assistance programs. Local hospital authorities or religious organizations generally operate not-for-profit organizations.

For-Profit

A for-profit organization is not considered tax exempt and is formed to make a profit. Profits are distributed to shareholders. There are no provisions in the law requiring for-profit organizations to see indigent patients, except in cases that are life threatening. There are provisions in the law that require hospitals receiving federal funds to treat anyone who presents in the emergency room, regardless of their ability to pay.

Hospital Types

Hospitals can be further classified by the type of facility. Common classifications used to describe the various types of hospital facilities are acute care facility, community hospital, general hospital, private hospital, specialty hospital, teaching hospital, trauma center, and tertiary care hospital (Figure 1-11). These hospitals may be private or publicly held.

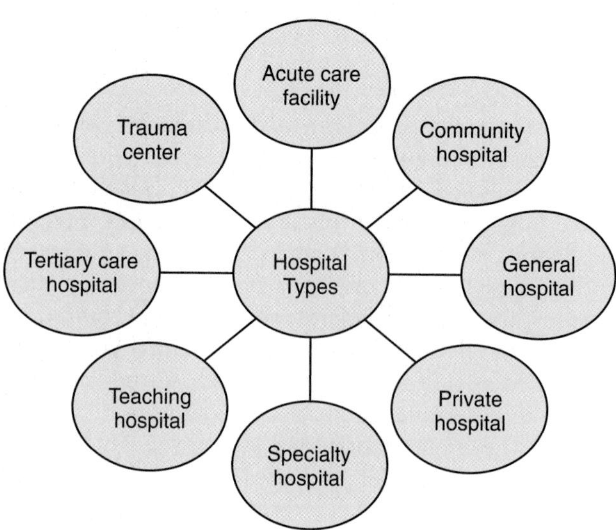

Figure 1-11 Hospital types.

Acute Care Facility

Acute care facilities see patients who have a sudden onset of a condition, illness, or disease. The patient is diagnosed and treated. The patient's stay at the hospital is short term, generally less than 30 days.

Community Hospital

A **community hospital** provides patient services to individuals in a specific community. Unlike other hospitals that only accept certain patient groups, community hospitals are open to anyone. Community hospitals may be non-profit or for-profit. If the community hospital is non-profit, it is required under state and federal guidelines to accept indigent (needy) patients.

General Hospital

A **general hospital** is designed to provide medical, surgical, and emergency services required to treat a wide range of illnesses and injuries.

Private Hospital

A **private hospital**, such as Shriner's Hospital, is privately owned by an individual(s) or by a corporation. Private hospitals are generally for-profit organizations.

Specialty Hospital

A **specialty hospital** provides medical care for specific illnesses, such as a cancer center, children's hospital, or psychiatric center.

Teaching Hospital

A **teaching hospital** provides patient care services and clinical experiences for students from a medical school and graduates of medical schools. The hospital and medical school typically enter into an agreement outlining the arrangement. Graduates of medical school work in a hospital for a period of time to complete what is referred to as a residency program. The number of years of residency varies depending on the medical specialty that is being pursued by the resident. The hospital may also agree to provide clinical experience to other health professionals, such as nurses.

Tertiary Care Hospital

A **tertiary care hospital** works with patients who have complex conditions. Very often these patients are transferred from other hospitals. Highly specialized board-certified physicians with expertise in their specialty area conduct extensive diagnostic testing to determine the patient's condition and develop a treatment plan.

Trauma Center

Patients who have been severely injured due to a major trauma or who are critically ill may be admitted to a **trauma center**. The trauma facility has specialized equipment and staff to handle trauma cases on a 24-hour basis. Trauma patients are generally brought in by life-flight or medivac helicopter and received through the emergency room.

BOX 1-8 ■ KEY POINTS

Purpose and Classification of Hospitals

Hospital Services

- Diagnostic
- Therapeutic
- Palliative
- Preventative

Hospital Service Levels

- Outpatient
- Inpatient
- Non-patient

Hospital Classifications

- Not-for-profit
- For profit

Hospital Types

- Acute care facility
- Community hospital
- General hospital
- Private hospital
- Specialty hospital
- Teaching hospital
- Tertiary care hospital
- Trauma center

CHAPTER SUMMARY

A review of the evolution of hospitals from ancient times to the 20th century highlights the significant factors that influenced the development and growth of hospitals. The spread of infectious disease and the need to care for the sick, the poor, and injured soldiers increased the need for hospitals. Hippocrates laid the foundations of modern medicine. The Middle Ages was marked by war and the spread of contagious disease. These issues were carried by early settlers to the United States. Population growth and the spread of contagious disease continued in the United States through the Renaissance period. The first hospitals were established in the United States by the 1700s. The focus of medicine shifted to research and scientific exploration of the cause of disease. This led to discoveries in medicine and technology that contributed greatly to the growth of hospitals. The continued growth of the population and medical advances contributed to the rising cost of health care, hospital overcrowding, and eventually to the creation of government health care programs.

By the close of the 20th century, the cost of health care was rising at an alarming rate. The demand for health care reform led to a shift to managed care plans and changes in reimbursement systems for government-sponsored health care. The number of hospitals declined drastically as a result of reduced reimbursements and utilization review measures that carefully scrutinized services provided. Hospitals underwent major transformations during this period to regain market share, increase admissions, and operate in a cost-effective manner. Hospitals began to develop primary care networks and integrated delivery systems to provide quality health care services in a cost-efficient manner. The hospital regulatory environment is evidence of the efforts to improve access to health care and control costs. Now that we have an understanding of the history, evolution, and purpose of a hospital, we can begin discussion of the hospital regulatory environment in the next chapter.

TEST YOUR *Knowledge* BOX 1-4

PURPOSE OF A HOSPITAL; HOSPITAL CLASSIFICATIONS

1. Explain the purpose of a hospital today.
2. Name four categories of service that can be provided in a hospital.
3. What is the difference between diagnostic services and therapeutic services?
4. Palliative services are performed to minimize what?
5. Define preventive services.
6. What is an evaluation and management (E/M) service?
7. Name three levels of care provided in a hospital.
8. Distinguish between inpatient and outpatient services.
9. Describe a situation in which palliative services may be required.
10. Explain observation services.
11. Provide an explanation of non-patient care.
12. Explain the difference between for-profit and not-for-profit organizations.

MATCH THE DEFINITIONS IN QUESTIONS 13 TO 20 WITH THE TERMS AT RIGHT

13. ___ Severely injured or critically ill patients are admitted to this type of hospital for care.
14. ___ Hospital that works with patients who have highly complex conditions.
15. ___ Facility owned by an individual or organization
16. ___ Handles patients who have conditions with sudden onset.
17. ___ Hospital that provides clinical experiences to medical students in addition to providing medical care to patients.
18. ___ Patients in a specific area are treated by this hospital.
19. ___ Organization formed to provide services that benefit a specific community; generally considered tax exempt.
20. ___ Organization formed for the purpose of providing services and making a profit that would be taxed.

A. Community hospital
B. Private hospital
C. For-profit
D. Trauma center
E. Acute care facility
F. Tertiary care hospitals
G. Teaching hospital
H. Not-for-profit

CHAPTER REVIEW 1-1

True/False

1. Departments in hospitals are categorized as: Medical, Operations, and Billing. T F
2. Accounts receivable means money owed to a hospital by patients and insurance companies and government programs. T F
3. Hospitals provide 24-hour nursing service. T F
4. A facility that provides diagnostic, therapeutic, palliative, and preventive services to patients is called a hospital. T F
5. Documentation provides a description of services and diagnosis and it is not utilized for billing purposes. T F

Fill in the Blank

6. What legislative action was passed in 1946 that contributed to the expansion of hospitals?

   ____________________.

7. The organization that was founded for the purpose of setting standards for medical practice and physician ethics is called ____________________.
8. The process where a physician reviews services to determine whether they are appropriate and medically necessary in response to the patient's condition is ____________________.
9. Service performed to evaluate a patient's condition, determine the patient's diagnosis, and develop a treatment plan is ____________________.
10. The difference between an inpatient visit and outpatient visit is ____________________.

Match the Following Definitions With the Terms at Right

11. ___ A facility that is designed to treat problems that have sudden onset.
12. ___ Specific characteristic information about a patient: name, address, date of birth, sex, and Social Security number.
13. ___ A person who has no means of paying for medical services or treatments and is not eligible for benefits under Medicaid or other public assistance programs.
14. ___ A payment method used by various payers that reimburses providers for a daily rate for services.
15. ___ Health plan that covers specific medical services in exchange for an annual or monthly payment that is predetermined.

A. Indigent
B. Prepaid health plan
C. Acute care facility
D. Per diem
E. Demographic Information

Research Project

Utilize information in this chapter and conduct research as required to develop a timeline for the evolution of hospitals in:

1. Europe during the Middle Ages and Renaissance.
2. The United States from the 17th century to today.

GLOSSARY

Accounts receivable The term that describes monies owed to the hospital from patients, insurance companies, and government programs.

Acute care facility A facility designed to treat patients who have sudden onset of a condition, illness, or disease.

Ambulatory surgery A surgery that is performed on the same day the patient is released.

American College of Surgeons (ACS) Organization formed in 1913 for the purpose of developing hospital standards by collecting patient care data.

American Hospital Association (AHA) Organization formed in 1906 to promote public welfare by improving health care provided in hospitals.

American Medical Association (AMA) Organization formed in 1847, with a mission to improve standards of medical education.

Blue Cross Organization that introduced one of the first prepaid health plans in 1929 to provide coverage for hospital care.

Coding The process of translating written descriptions of diagnoses, services, and items into numeric or alphanumeric codes.

Community hospital A hospital that provides care to members of a specific community.

Demographic information Specific characteristic information about a patient including: name, address, date of birth, sex, and Social Security number.

Diagnostic service A service performed to diagnose a patient's condition.

Emergency Department Services are provided to patients who present with conditions that they believe require immediate attention.

Evaluation and management (E/M) A service performed to evaluate and manage a patient's condition, which includes a history, exam, and medical decision making by the provider.

Fee-for-service A payment method used by various payers that reimburses providers based on charges submitted.

General hospital Designed to provide medical, surgical, and emergency services required to treat a wide range of illness and injury.

Group health insurance Health insurance to provide coverage for medical services to members of a group. Group health insurance is often sold to employer groups or associations.

Hill-Burton Act Legislation implemented in 1946 that made funding available to modernize existing hospitals and build new ones.

Hospital A facility where patients with health care problems can go to seek diagnosis and treatment of their condition(s).

Hospital Standardization Program Program designed by the American College of Surgeons (ACS) in 1913 to establish standards for hospital medical care.

Indigent A person who has no means of paying for medical services or treatments and who is not eligible for benefits under Medicaid or other public assistance program.

Inpatient Patient care services are provided to a patient who is admitted to the hospital for more than 24 hours.

Insurance information Information regarding the insurance plan or government program that the patient is insured under including: plan name and number, identification number, group name.

Integrated delivery system An organization consisting of a network of providers that are affiliated within the system to offer patients a full range of managed health care services.

Joint Commission on Accreditation of Healthcare Organizations (JCAHO) A national commission formed in 1952 to develop guidelines for hospitals and other health care organizations. JCAHO changed its name to The Joint Commission (TJC) in 2007. TJC evaluates and accredits health care organizations based on established standards of quality for operations and medical services.

Managed care plans Prepaid health insurance plans that incorporate the provision of coordinated health care services and cost containment measures to monitor and manage health care services provided to members of the plan.

Medicaid Federal program administered at the state level established under title XIX of the SSA to provide health care benefits for medically indigent people.

Medicare A government program that provides coverage for health expenses to individuals over age 65 and other eligible groups such as the disabled.

Medicare Severity Diagnosis Related Groups (MS-DRG) A reimbursement method implemented under PPS that pays hospitals a fixed amount for a hospital stay based on the patient's diagnosis and the severity of that condition. MS-DRG replaced DRG in 2007.

Non-patient A laboratory or pathology service is performed on specimens received at the hospital. The patient is not present when the service is performed.

Observation A patient is admitted to a facility for the purpose of being observed and is generally released within 24 hours.

Outpatient Patient care services are provided and the patient is released within 24 hours.

Palliative service A service provided to chronically ill patients to help alleviate symptoms of their illness.

Payer Insurance company or government program that pays health benefits for patient care services.

Peer review A review of a medical case conducted by a physician to determine or assess the medical services.

Per diem A payment method used by various payers that reimburses providers for a daily rate for services.

Percentage of accrued charges A reimbursement method that calculates payment based on a percentage of total charges submitted.

Prepaid health plan Health plan that provides health benefits for specified medical services in exchange for prepayment of an annual or monthly premium.

Preventive service A service provided to promote wellness and prevent illness.

Primary care network A network of physicians focused on providing primary care services to patients. Primary care refers to the initial point of contact with a patient for a particular illness.

Primary care physician (PCP) The physician, selected by the plan member, who is considered "the gatekeeper." The PCP is responsible for monitoring and managing all care for the patient.

Private hospital A hospital that is privately owned by an individual, individuals, or a corporation.

Prospective Payment System (PPS) Reimbursement systems services provided to Medicare beneficiaries by which payment is based on a predetermined, fixed amount.

Quality Improvement Organization (QIO) An organization that conducts medical reviews to determine whether the quality of care, medical necessity, and appropriateness of service criteria were met.

Specialty hospital Provides medical care for specific illnesses.

Teaching hospital Hospital that provides clinical experiences to medical students in addition to providing medical care to patients.

Tertiary care hospital A hospital that provides highly specialized care to patients who have complex conditions.

Therapeutic service A service performed to treat the patient's condition.

Third-party payer An organization or entity other than the patient or provider that pays for health care services.

Trauma center A facility that is designed to receive and treat patients who have been severely injured due to a major trauma or who are critically ill.

Utilization management (UM) The term used to describe the procedures implemented to manage the utilization of health care services.

Utilization review (UR) The process of reviewing a medical case to determine whether the care provided was appropriate.

Chapter 2

Hospital Regulatory Environment

The purpose of this chapter is to provide an overview of the hospital regulatory environment. Hospitals are regulated in accordance with various federal and state statutes. Federal regulations are designed to address specific health care issues including patient care activities and the cost of health care. In addition to federal regulations, states have implemented regulations regarding licensure of health care facilities, such as hospitals. State licensing regulations outline specific operating conditions required for hospitals to be licensed. Compliance with all federal and state regulations is of critical importance. These regulations also have an impact on hospital personnel and the hospital's credentialing requirements. This chapter will provide a review of some of the most significant federal and state regulations that have an impact on the structure and function of hospitals today, and will close with a discussion of nonclinical personnel and credentials.

Outline

Chapter Objectives

- Define terms, phrases, abbreviations, and acronyms related to the hospital regulatory environment, federal and state regulations, accreditation, and nonclinical credentials.
- Describe factors that led to the government's expanded role in regulating health care.
- Demonstrate an understanding of federal and state legislation implemented to address health care issues and the impact of the legislation on the hospital's regulatory environment.
- Discuss how the creation of Medicare and Medicaid enhanced the government's role in health care regulation.
- Provide a brief overview of federal and state regulatory agencies involved in health care regulation.
- Demonstrate an understanding of state licensing requirements and how they have an impact on the hospital's structure and function.
- State the purpose of accreditation and explain why it is important.
- Provide an overview of the history of accreditation.
- Demonstrate an understanding of accreditation organizations and the survey process.
- Explain the relationship between federal and state regulations and accreditation.
- Discuss various credentials required for hospital billing and coding personnel.

Key Terms

Accreditation
Admitting privileges
Agency for Health Care Administration (AHCA)
American Academy of Professional Coders (AAPC)
American Health Information Management Association (AHIMA)
American Osteopathic Association (AOA)
Centers for Medicare and Medicaid Services (CMS)
Civil Monetary Penalties Law (CMPL)
Consolidated Omnibus Budget Reconciliation Act (COBRA)
Conditions of Participation (COP)
Continuing education units (CEUs)
Credentialing
Department of Health (DOH)
Department of Health and Human Services (DHHS)
Department of Health, Education, and Welfare (HEW)
Emergency Medical Treatment and Labor Act (EMTALA)
Federal False Claims Act
Federal Register
Health Information Management (HIM)
Health Insurance Portability and Accountability Act (HIPAA)
Medicaid
Medicare
Occupational Safety and Health Administration (OSHA)
Office of Inspector General (OIG)
Patient Self-Determination Act (PSDA)
Peer Review Organization (PRO)
Professional Standards Review Organization (PSRO)
Prospective Payment System (PPS)
Quality Improvement Organization (QIO)
Tax Equity and Fiscal Responsibility Act (TEFRA)
The Joint Commission (TJC)

Acronyms and Abbreviations

AAHAM—American Association of Healthcare Administrative Management
AAPC—American Academy of Professional Coders
AHCA—Agency for Health Care Administration
AHIMA—American Health Information Management Association
AOA—American Osteopathic Association
CCA—Certified Coding Associate
CCS—Certified Coding Specialist
CCS-P—Certified Coding Specialist-Physician
CEUs—continuing education units
CMPL—Civil Monetary Penalties Law
CMS—Centers for Medicare and Medicaid Services
COBRA—Consolidated Omnibus Budget Reconciliation Act
COP—Conditions of Participation
CPC—Certified Professional Coder
CPC-A—Certified Professional Coder-Apprentice
CPC-H—Certified Professional Coder-Hospital
DHHS—Department of Health and Human Services
DOH—Department of Health
EMTALA—Emergency Medical Treatment and Labor Act
HEW—Department of Health, Education, and Welfare
HIM—Health Information Management
HIPAA—Health Insurance Portability and Accountability Act
OSHA—Occupational Safety and Health Administration
OIG—Office of Inspector General
PCP—Primary care physician
PFS—Patient Financial Services
PPS—Prospective Payment System
PRO—Peer Review Organization
PSDA—Patient Self-Determination Act
PSRO—Professional Standards Review Organization
PPS—Prospective Payment System
QIO—Quality Improvement Organization
RHIT—Registered Health Information Technician
TJC—The Joint Commission
UM—utilization management
UR—utilization review

HOSPITAL REGULATORY ENVIRONMENT INTRODUCTION

Throughout history, the health care industry has experienced tremendous change. Many changes were in response to specific needs related to health and human welfare and the control of health care costs. As discussed in Chapter 1, cultures have faced issues relating to disease and the need to improve health care since before the significant advances in health care that occurred during the Middle Ages. Medicine evolved scientifically, and discoveries of new treatments and technology led to the development of standards for medical practice, education, and health care professionals. The development of standards resulted in increased regulatory activities by various governmental entities.

The government's role as regulator expanded as health care issues arose. The federal government moved to the forefront as one of the largest payers for health care services with the creation of the Medicare and Medicaid programs, signed into law in 1965. As the largest payer, the government inherited the responsibility of ensuring that quality patient care is provided, improving public health, and controlling rising health care costs. A review of some of the legislation dealing with these issues will provide an understanding of how the regulatory environment came to be what it is today.

BOX 2-1 ■ KEY POINTS

Hospital Regulatory Environment

Government Regulation

- Federal
- State
- Local

Nongovernmental Regulations

- Accreditation organizations

FEDERAL LEGISLATION

The federal government's influence on the health care industry stems from its role in funding health care, ownership of facilities, and responsibility for implementing legislation. Throughout history, laws have been passed with a view toward governing and controlling specific areas of health care. Health care legislation is created in response to issues that face the public.

BOX 2-2 ■ KEY POINTS

Federal Regulatory Capacity

Funding health care programs
Ownership of facilities
Implementation of federal legislation

Figure 2-1 shows the U.S. government's legislative branches and departments. The federal legislature (Congress) enacts laws commonly referred to as statutes. The executive branch (president) is responsible for the enforcement of the laws. The president delegates the responsibility and authority to administer and enforce the laws to various departments such as the Departments of Defense, Labor, Veterans Affairs, and Health and Human Services. These departments enforce the laws through regulatory activity and legal processes through the judicial Branch (Supreme Court, Court of Appeals, and District Courts) when required.

The primary focus of health care legislation passed from 1946 to 1996 was to improve access to and quality of health care as well as to address other issues relating to the health, education, and welfare of the public. Figure 2-2 provides an overview of selected health care legislation passed over the years, highlighting some of the major laws designed to address health care issues such as the following:

- Access to and quality of health care
- Health, education, and welfare of the public
- Control of the rising cost of health care

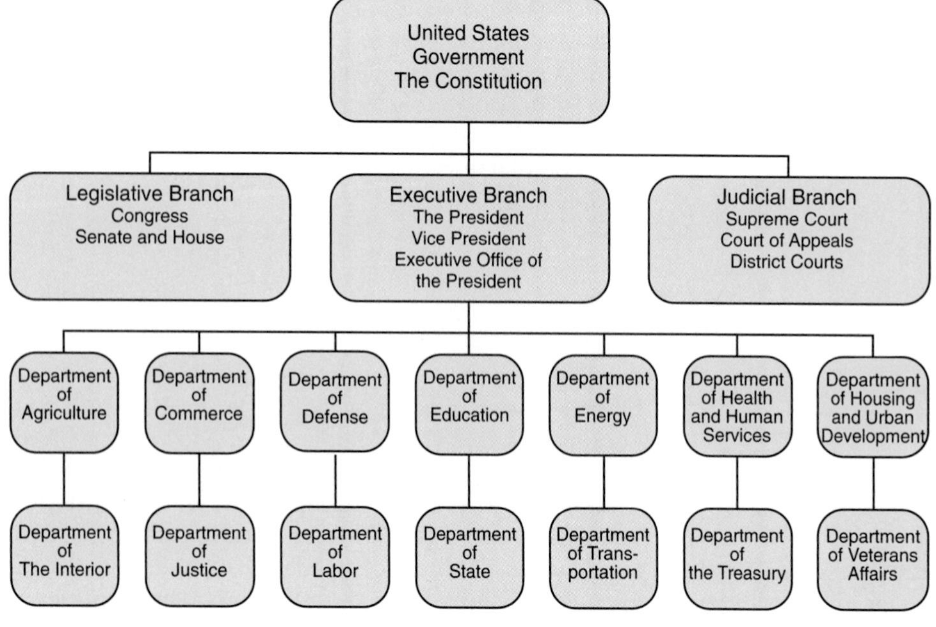

Figure 2-1 U.S. government branches and departments. *(From Oran D: Oran's dictionary of the law, ed 3, Clifton Park, N.Y., 1999, Delmar.)*

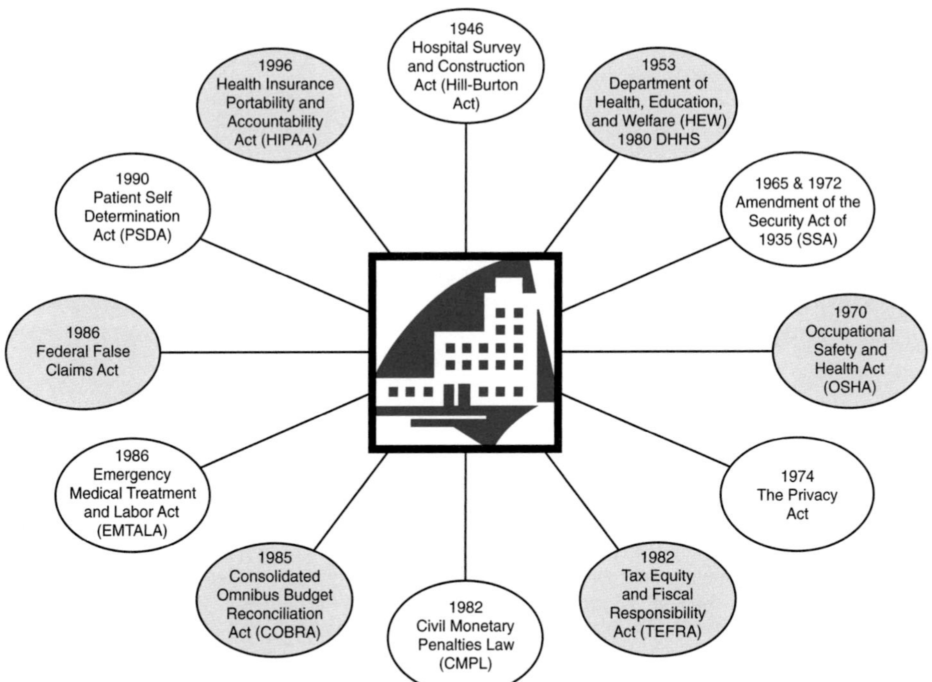

Figure 2-2 Selected federal health care legislation (1946 to 1996).

Access to and Quality of Health Care

1946, Hospital Survey and Construction Act (Hill-Burton Act)

The Hill-Burton Act was passed to provide funding for the construction and modernization of hospitals. The act authorized the provision of federal grants to states for the purpose of assessing health care needs and building additional facilities when needed. States conducted surveys of their hospitals and public health centers to assess construction needs and developed plans for building additional facilities. Existing facilities were modernized and new ones built with Hill-Burton funding. Federal hospital construction funds were allocated on the basis of population and per capita income. The states with lower income received more per capita than the wealthier states. Hospitals that received Hill-Burton funding were required to provide health care services to individuals in the community who could not afford health care. Individuals who qualified for services under this act could not be covered by any insurance or government program and had to meet specific income requirements.

BOX 2-3 ■ KEY POINTS

Federal Legislation 1946 to 1996: Focus Areas

Access to and quality of health care
Health, education, and welfare
Control of rising health care costs

For many years the Hill-Burton Act contributed greatly to the expansion of hospitals. A survey conducted in 1984 estimated that more than 9,200 medical facilities had been constructed or renovated with funds provided by or through this legislation. Many of these hospitals still exist today and are required to continue fulfilling their "community service obligation." They must comply with basic requirements outlined in the Community Service Assurance section under Title VI of the Public Health Service Act. These basic requirements can be viewed on the Web site of the Department of Health and Human Service (DHHS) at http://www.os.dhhs.gov (Figure 2-3).

1965, Amendment to the Social Security Act (SSA) of 1935

Two government programs were created through this amendment. **Medicare**, under Title XVIII of the SSA, provides health care benefits for individuals over age 65, the disabled, and other qualified individuals. President Lyndon Johnson signed Medicare into law in 1965 and at the same time enrolled former President Harry Truman, who received the first Medicare card (Figure 2-4). **Medicaid**, under Title XIX of the SSA, is a federal program administered at the state level that provides health care benefits for indigent people (Figure 2-5). As the federal government became a major payer of health care services with the creation of these programs, the government's role as regulator expanded. Regulations were outlined and guidelines implemented to ensure that Medicare and Medicaid beneficiaries received appropriate care as needed.

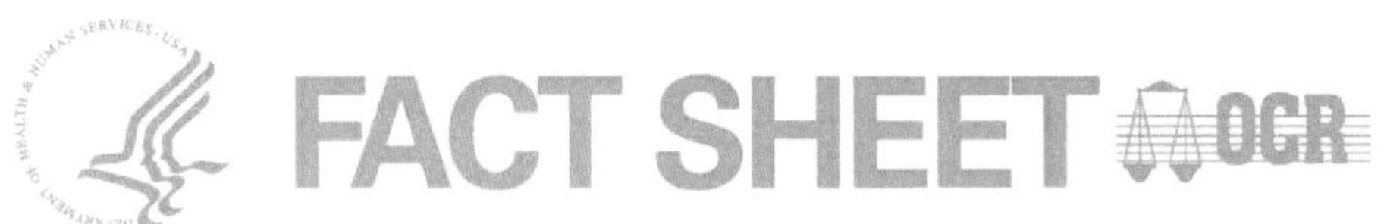

U.S. Department of Health and Human Services • Office for Civil Rights • Washington, D.C. 20201 • (202) 619-0403

YOUR RIGHTS UNDER THE COMMUNITY SERVICE ASSURANCE PROVISION OF THE HILL-BURTON ACT

What Is Hill-Burton?

The Hill-Burton Act authorizes assistance to public and other nonprofit medical facilities such as acute care general hospitals, special hospitals, nursing homes, public health centers, and rehabilitation facilities. **The Community Service Assurance under Title VI of the Public Health Service Act requires recipients of Hill-Burton funds to make services provided by the facility available to persons residing in the facility's service area without discrimination on the basis of race, color, national origin, creed, or any other ground unrelated to the individual's need for the service or the availability of the needed service in the facility. These requirements also apply to persons employed in the service area of the facility if it was funded under Title XVI of the Public Health Service Act.** Please note that the community service obligation is different from the uncompensated care provision. The community service obligation does not require the facility to make non-emergency services available to persons unable to pay for them. It does, however, require the facility to make emergency services available without regard to the person's ability to pay.

There are several basic requirements that every Hill-Burton hospital or other facility must comply with to fulfill the community service obligation:

- ✔ A person residing in the Hill-Burton facility's service area has the right to medical treatment at the facility without regard to race, color, national origin or creed.
- ✔ Hill-Burton facilities must participate in the Medicare and Medicaid programs unless they are ineligible to participate.
- ✔ Hill-Burton facilities must make arrangements for reimbursement for services with principal State and local third-party payors that provide reimbursement that is not less than the actual cost of the services
- ✔ A Hill-Burton facility must post notices informing the public of its community service obligations in English and Spanish. If 10 percent or more of the households in the service area usually speak a language other than English or Spanish, the facility must translate the notice into that language and post it as well
- ✗ A Hill-Burton facility may not deny emergency services to any person residing in the facility's service area on the grounds that the person is unable to pay for those services
- ✗ A Hill-Burton facility may not adopt patient admissions policies that have the effect of excluding persons on grounds of race, color, national origin, creed or any other ground unrelated to the patient's need for the service or the availability of the needed service.

The entire U.S. Department of Health and Human Services Hill-Burton regulation can be found at 42 CFR Part 124.

For information on how to file a complaint of discrimination, or to obtain information of a civil rights nature, please contact us. Office for Civil Rights (OCR) employees will make every effort to provide prompt service.

Hotlines: 1-800-368-1019(Voice) **1-800-537-7697 (TDD**
E-Mail: ocrmail@hhs.gov **Website:** http://www.hhs.gov/ocr

Figure 2-3 DHHS Hill-Burton basic requirements for hospital compliance. *(Modified from U. S. Department of Health and Human Services:* Your Rights Under the Community Assurance Provision of the Hill-Burton Act, *http://www.hhs.gov/ocr/civilrights/resources/factsheets/hillburton.pdf.)*

TITLE XVIII—HEALTH INSURANCE FOR THE AGED AND DISABLED

TABLE OF CONTENTS OF TITLE

Sec. 1801. Prohibition against any Federal interference
Sec. 1802. Free choice by patient guaranteed
Sec. 1803. Option to individuals to obtain other health insurance protection
Sec. 1804. Notice of medicare benefits: medicare and medigap information
Sec. 1805. Medicare payment advisory commission
Sec. 1806. Explanation of medicare benefits

Part A—Hospital Insurance Benefits for the Aged and Disabled

Sec. 1811. Description of program
Sec. 1812. Scope of benefits
Sec. 1813. Deductibles and coinsurance
Sec. 1814. Conditions of and limitations on payment for services
Sec. 1815. Payment to providers of services
Sec. 1818. Hospital insurance benefits for uninsured elderly individuals not otherwise eligible
Sec. 1818A Hospital insurance benefits for disabled individuals who have exhausted other entitlement

Part B—Supplementary Medical Insurance Benefits for the Aged and Disabled

488-40-6969-A
APPLICATION FOR ENROLLMENT in the Supplementary Medical Insurance Program Under the Social Security Act
PLEASE READ THE ENCLOSED LEAFLET
Harry S Truman
Independence, Missouri
Do not write in the space above

TO GET MEDICAL INSURANCE → CHECK [X] YES
The Federal Government will pay half the cost of this insurance. Your share of the cost ($3) will be deducted from your monthly social security benefits.
IF YOU DO NOT WANT THIS MEDICAL INSURANCE → CHECK [ ] NO
SIGN HERE
Signature by mark (X) must be witnessed below.
SIGNATURE OF WITNESS
ADDRESS OF WITNESS

Figure 2-4 1965 Amendment of the SSA of 1935: Title XVIII, creation of the Medicare program. *(Modified from Social Security Administration: Health Insurance for the Aged and Disabled, www.ssa.gov.)*

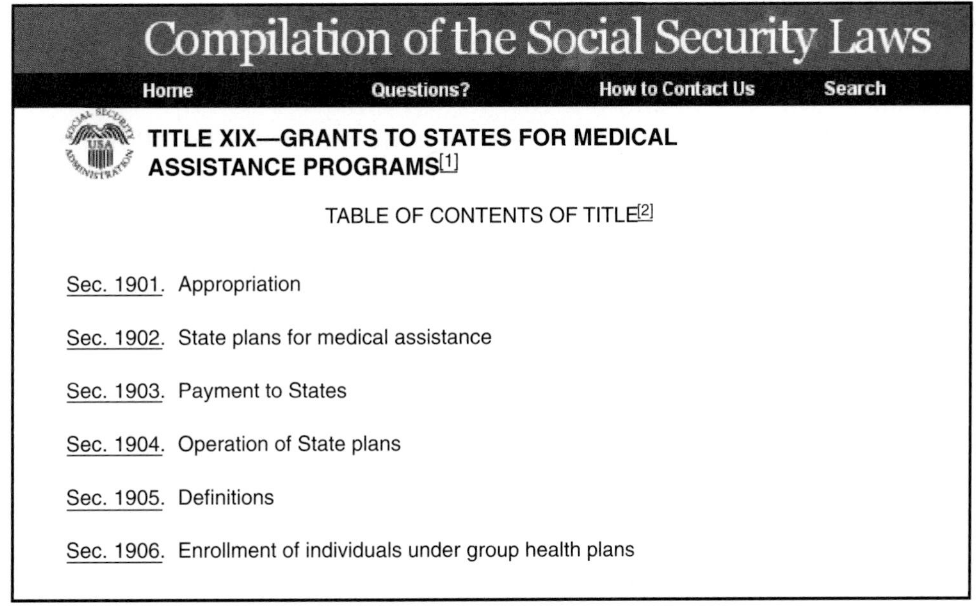

Compilation of the Social Security Laws

Home | Questions? | How to Contact Us | Search

TITLE XIX—GRANTS TO STATES FOR MEDICAL ASSISTANCE PROGRAMS[1]

TABLE OF CONTENTS OF TITLE[2]

Sec. 1901. Appropriation
Sec. 1902. State plans for medical assistance
Sec. 1903. Payment to States
Sec. 1904. Operation of State plans
Sec. 1905. Definitions
Sec. 1906. Enrollment of individuals under group health plans

Figure 2-5 1965 Amendment of the SSA of 1935: Title XIX, creation of the Medicaid program. *(Modified from Social Security Administration: Health Insurance for the Aged and Disabled, www.ssa.gov.)*

1972, Amendment to the Social Security Act (SSA) of 1935

Under Title XI of the SSA, **Professional Standards Review Organizations (PSROs)** were created for the purpose of reviewing and evaluating "hospital inpatient resource utilization, quality of care, and medical necessity" (Figure 2-6). PSROs are organizations that contract with Medicare to conduct reviews to determine the appropriateness and medical necessity of services provided. PSROs have full authority to deny reimbursement for health care services provided to Medicare patients when the services are deemed inappropriate. The PSROs were later replaced by peer review organizations (PROs) under the Tax Equity and Fiscal Responsibility Act. The name PRO was changed to Quality Improvement Organization (QIO) in 2001 in accordance with a quality initiative launched by the DHHS.

1985, Consolidated Omnibus Budget Reconciliation Act (COBRA)

COBRA was passed to prevent inappropriate transfer or discharge of patients from one facility to another, commonly referred to as "dumping." This legislation is known as the antidumping statute, as it established criteria for the transfer and discharge of Medicare and Medicaid patients. This legislation also contained provisions allowing employees to maintain health insurance coverage after termination of employment, and it pro-

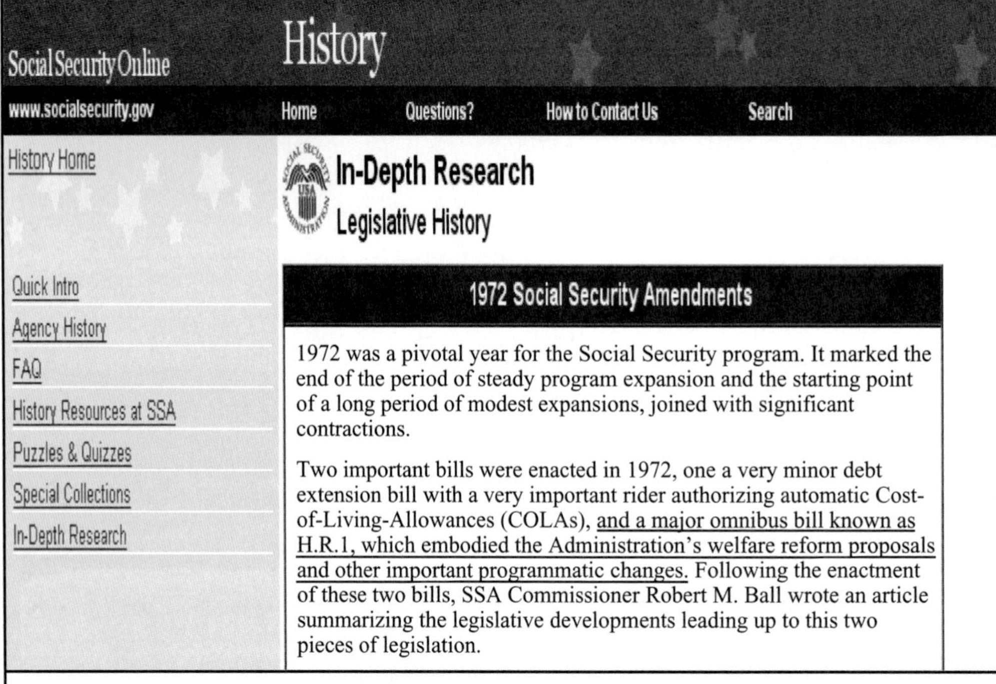

This legislation resulted in many programmatic changes. The following excerpts from the SSA Web page describe two significant changes:

Establishment of a peer review system through the use of organizations representing a substantial number of practicing physicians in local areas to be called Professional Standards Review Organizations (PSROs) (these organizations would assume responsibility for comprehensive and ongoing review of services provided under Medicare and Medicaid).

Establishment of an Office of Inspector General for Health Administration within the Department of Health, Education, and Welfare having the responsibility to review and audit Medicare and other health programs on a continuing and comprehensive basis and the authority to suspend any regulation, practice, or procedure employed in the administration of such programs if he determines that the suspension will promote efficiency and economy of administration or that the regulation, practice, or procedure involved is contrary to or does not carry out the objectives and purposes of applicable provisions of law.

Figure 2-6 1972 SSA amendments (establishment of PSROs and the OIG). *(Modified from Social Security Administration: 1972 Social Security Amendments, http://www.ssa.gov.)*

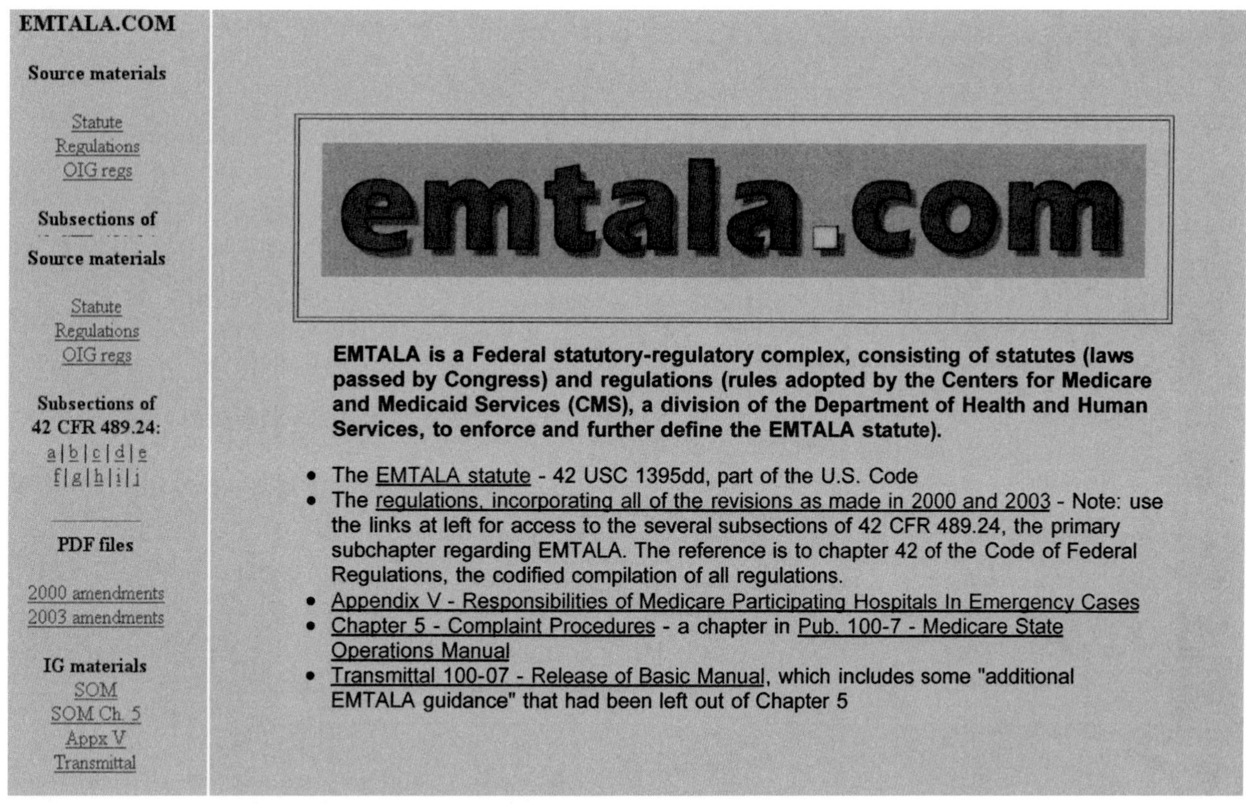

Figure 2-7 EMTALA 1986 legislation Web page. *(Modified from www.emtala.com.)*

vided Medicare with the authority to deny payments to providers for substandard care.

1986, Emergency Medical Treatment and Labor Act (EMTALA)

EMTALA was passed by Congress to ensure public access to emergency services regardless of ability to pay. Section 1867 of the SSA imposes specific obligations on Medicare-participating hospitals that offer emergency services. Medicare-participating hospitals are required to provide a medical screening examination when requested for an emergency medical condition. Hospitals are then required to provide stabilizing treatment for patients with emergency medical conditions. A patient may be transferred if the hospital is unable to stabilize the patient with its resources or if the patient requests a transfer. Information regarding EMTALA can be found on the Centers for Medicare and Medicaid Services (CMS) Web site and at http://www.emtala.com (Figure 2-7).

1996, Health Insurance Portability and Accountability Act (HIPAA)

HIPAA was implemented in phases from 1996 to 2009 to address several issues including continuity of health insurance, prevention and detection of fraud and abuse, limited coverage, access to long-term care, simplification of the administration of health insurance standards for the claims process, and protection of the privacy of health information (Figure 2-8). HIPAA has had a major impact on the health care industry. This legislation extends provisions regarding the privacy of patient information to the electronic transfer of private health information. HIPAA will be discussed in detail in Chapter 14.

BOX 2-4 ■ KEY POINTS

Federal Legislation 1946 to 1996 (Access to and Quality of Health Care)

- 1946, Hospital Survey and Construction Act (Hill-Burton Act)
- 1965 and 1972, Amendments to the SSA of 1935
- 1985, Consolidated Omnibus Budget Reconciliation Act (COBRA)
- 1986, Emergency Medical Treatment and Labor Act (EMTALA)
- 1996, Health Insurance Portability and Accountability Act (HIPAA)

Health, Education, and Welfare

1953, Department of Health, Education, and Welfare (HEW)

HEW was formed for the purpose of addressing issues related to the health, education, and welfare of the

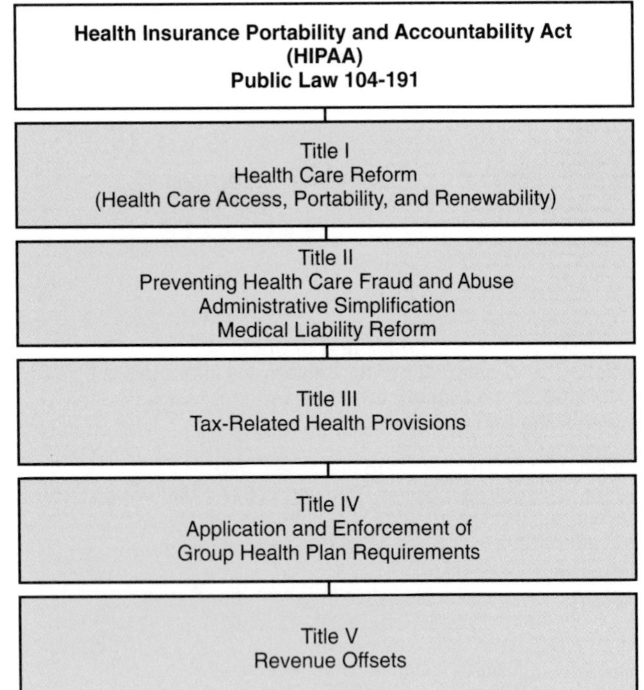

Figure 2-8 HIPAA legislation PL 104-191.

History of the Department of Health, Education, and Welfare 1953

The Department of Health, Education, and Welfare was created when Reorganization Plan No. 1 of 1953 became effective.

President Eisenhower signed HEW legislation into law on April 11, 1953.

HEW thus became the first new Cabinet-level department since the Department of Labor was created in 1913. The Reorganization Plan abolished the Federal Security Agency and transferred all of its functions to the Secretary of Health, Education, and Welfare and all components of the Agency to the Department. The first Secretary of HEW was Oveta Culp Hobby, a native of Texas, who had served as Commander of the Women's Army Corps in World War II and was editor and publisher of the *Houston Post*. Sworn in on April 11, 1953, as Secretary, she had been FSA Administrator since January 21, 1953.

Figure 2-9 Creation of the Department of Health, Education, and Welfare. *(Modified from U. S. Department of Health and Human Services: History of the Department of Health, Education, and Welfare 1953, www.hhs.gov/about/hhshist.html.)*

people of the United States (Figure 2-9). HEW was reorganized into the DHHS in 1980. The DHHS will be discussed later in this chapter.

1970, Occupational Safety and Health Administration (OSHA)

OSHA was created under the Occupational Safety and Health Act for the purpose of developing standards and conducting site visits to determine compliance with safety standards. The legislation was passed to protect employees from working in environments that are not healthy and are considered unsafe. This law requires employers to comply with health and safety standards by creating a work environment that prevents injury and health hazards.

1974, Privacy Act

The Privacy Act was designed to address the rights of individuals to privacy. It contains provisions for individuals to have access to and control over information collected by the federal government. The provisions acknowledge the rights of individuals to determine what information is collected for the purpose of review and correction and to provide authorization for disclosure of such information.

1990, Patient Self-Determination Act (PSDA)

PSDA was implemented to ensure that individuals are informed of their rights regarding health care decisions. The act requires facilities to provide patients with information regarding a living will, durable power of attorney, and advance directives. Health care facilities are also required to maintain such documents in the patient's record when provided.

BOX 2-5 ■ KEY POINTS

Federal Legislation 1946 to 1996 (Health, Education, and Welfare)

1953, Department of Health, Education, and Welfare (HEW)
1970, Occupational Safety and Health Act (OSHA)
1974, Privacy Act
1990, Patient Self-Determination Act (PSDA)

Control of the Rising Cost of Health Care

1982, Tax Equity and Fiscal Responsibility Act (TEFRA)

Many changes that occurred in the Medicare program were implemented under **TEFRA** in 1982. TEFRA mandated a total restructuring of reimbursement methods used for Medicare services. One of the most significant changes was the implementation of the **Prospective Payment System (PPS)** in 1983. PPS is a reimbursement system for inpatient services provided to Medicare beneficiaries that provides a predetermined payment based on the patient's diagnosis and procedures performed. TEFRA mandated a change in payment methods for hospital inpatient services over a 4-year period. Under TEFRA, the reimbursement system changed from the historical cost-based payment type to one that provides a predetermined reimbursement. This system of reimbursement was known as Diagnosis Related Groups (DRG), which were later replaced with Medicare Severity Diagnosis Related Groups (MS-DRG). Reimbursement systems will be discussed in detail in later chapters.

TEFRA provisions also required that PSROs be replaced by PROs. The Health Care Financing Administration (HCFA), now known as the CMS, established a national network of PROs. The name of PROs was later changed to Quality Improvement Organization (QIO).

BOX 2-6 ▪ KEY POINTS

Tax Equity and Fiscal Responsibility Act of 1982 (TEFRA)

Implementation of Prospective Payment Systems (PPS)—Diagnosis Related Groups (DRG)

Required replacement of Professional Services Organizations (PSRO) with Peer Review Organizations (PRO)

1983, Civil Monetary Penalties Law (CMPL)

CMPL of 1983 was passed for the purpose of prosecuting cases of Medicare and Medicaid fraud (Figure 2-10). This law contains provisions regarding the sanctions that can be imposed on individuals or organizations convicted of fraudulent activities as defined by law. Sanctions that may be imposed under CMPL are as follows:

1. A penalty of up to $2,000 for each item or service wrongfully listed on a claim submitted to Medicare or Medicaid
2. An assessment of up to twice the total amount improperly claimed
3. Suspension from government programs for a period defined by DHHS

1986, Federal False Claims Act

The **Federal False Claims Act** was passed to prevent overuse of services and to uncover fraudulent activities in the Medicare and Medicaid programs. The act also contains provisions to offer financial incentives to informants who report providers suspected of defrauding the federal government.

BOX 2-7 ▪ KEY POINTS

Federal Legislation 1946 to 1996 (Control of Rising Health Care Costs)

1982, Tax Equity and Fiscal Responsibility Act (TEFRA)
1983, Civil Monetary Penalties Law (CMPL)
1986, Federal False Claims Act

Social Security Online — Compilation of the Social Security Laws

www.socialsecurity.gov | Home | Questions? | How to Contact Us | Search

CIVIL MONETARY PENALTIES

SEC. 1128A *[42 U.S.C. 1320a-7a]* (a) Any person (including an organization, agency, or other entity, but excluding a beneficiary, as defined in subsection (i)(5)) that—

(1) knowingly presents or causes to be presented to an officer, employee, or agent of the United States, or of any department or agency thereof, or of any State agency (as defined in subsection (i)(1)), a claim (as defined in subsection (i)(2)) that the Secretary determines—

(A) is for a medical or other item or service that the person knows or should know was not provided as claimed, including any person who engages in a pattern or practice of presenting or causing to be presented a claim for an item or service that is based on a code that the person knows or should know will result in a greater payment to the person than the code the person knows or should know is applicable to the item or service actually provided,

(B) is for a medical or other item or service and the person knows or should know the claim is false or fraudulent,

(C) is presented for a physician's service (or an item or service incident to a physician's service) by a person who knows or should know that the individual who furnished (or supervised the furnishing of) the service—

(i) was not licensed as a physician,

(ii) was licensed as a physician, but such license had been obtained through a misrepresentation of material fact (including cheating on an examination required for licensing), or

(iii) represented to the patient at the time the service was furnished that the physician was certified in a medical specialty by a medical specialty board when the individual was not so certified.

Figure 2-10 Civil Monetary Penalties Law (CMPL). Sec. 1128A. *[42 U.S.C. 1320a-7a]* (a). Grants the Secretary of Health and Human Services authority to impose civil monetary penalties (CMPs) for violations specified. *(Modified from Social Security Administration: Civil Monetary Penalties, http://www.socialsecurity.gov/OP_Home/ssact/title11/1128A.htm)*

BOX 2-8 ■ KEY POINTS

Civil Monetary Penalties Law (CMPL), 1983

Sanctions that may be imposed under CMPL are as follows:

- A penalty of up to $2,000 for each item or service wrongfully listed on a claim submitted to Medicare or Medicaid
- An assessment of up to twice the total amount improperly claimed
- Suspension from government programs for a period of time defined by the DHHS

FEDERAL REGULATORY AGENCIES

Regulatory departments and agencies write rules and regulations that explain the details regarding implementation of and compliance with all legislative provisions. Rules and regulations of the agencies are published in the ***Federal Register*** (Figure 2-11), which is the official publication for federal regulations and legal notices. Regulatory activity to enforce health care legislation is performed by various departments within the federal government (Figure 2-12). The Department of Labor, Department of Veterans Affairs, Department of

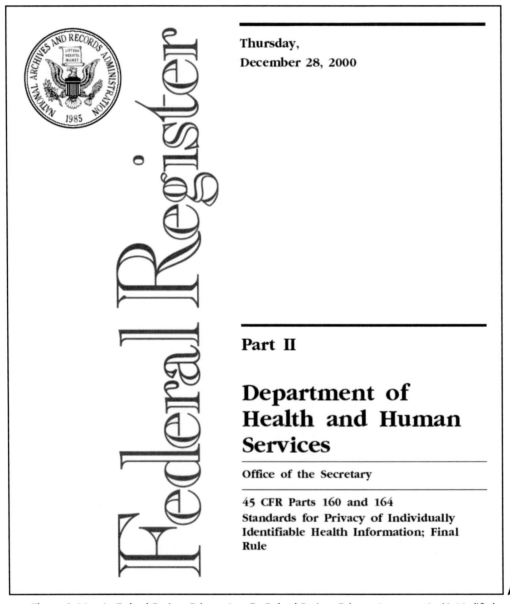
Federal Register

Thursday,
December 28, 2000

Part II

Department of Health and Human Services

Office of the Secretary

45 CFR Parts 160 and 164
Standards for Privacy of Individually Identifiable Health Information; Final Rule

A

Figure 2-11 A, *Federal Register* Privacy Act. B, *Federal Register* Privacy Act, page 1. *(A Modified from Social Security Administration*: Federal Register, *www.gpoaccess.gov/fr.)*

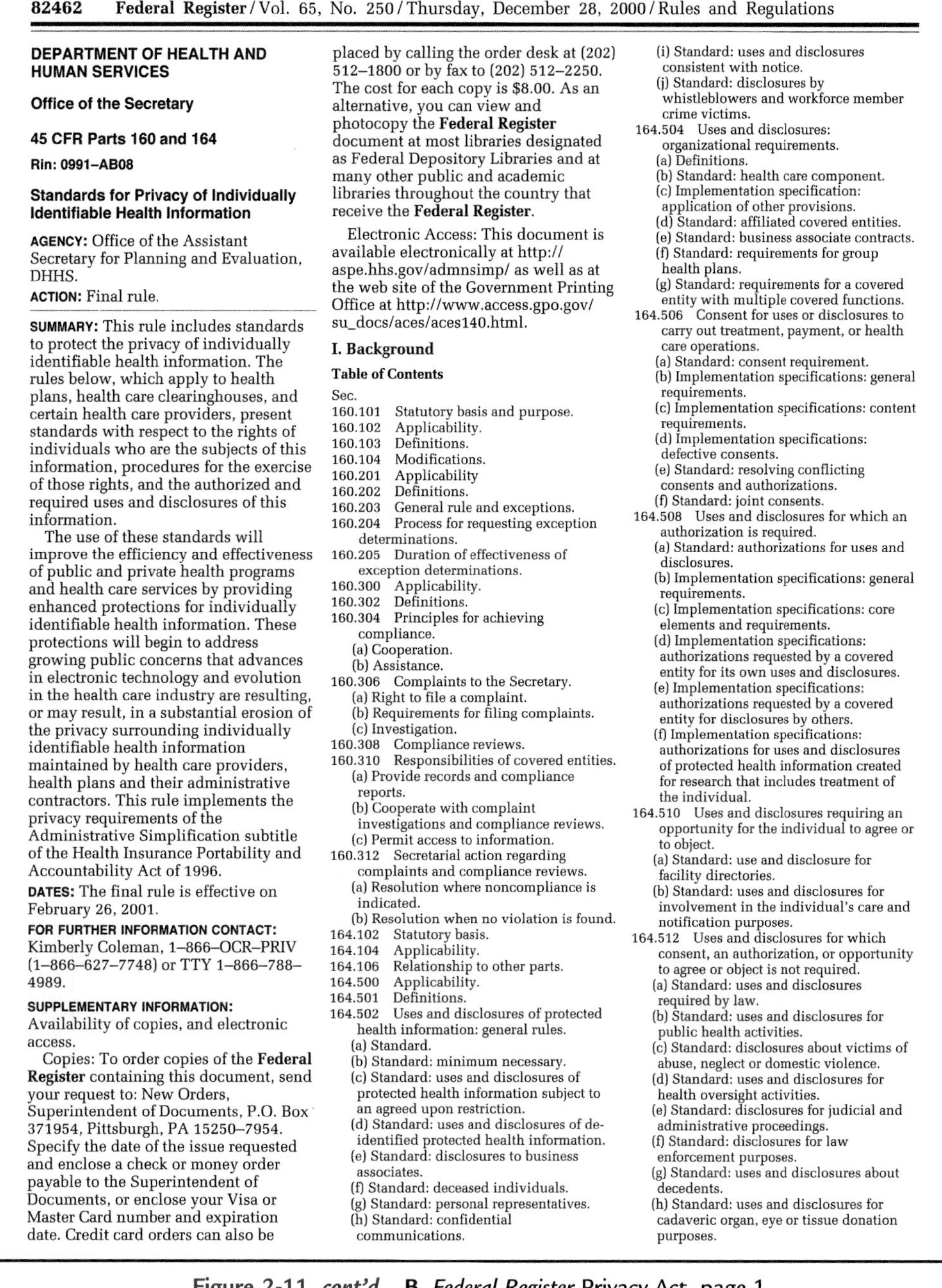

82462 **Federal Register**/Vol. 65, No. 250/Thursday, December 28, 2000/Rules and Regulations

DEPARTMENT OF HEALTH AND HUMAN SERVICES

Office of the Secretary

45 CFR Parts 160 and 164

Rin: 0991–AB08

Standards for Privacy of Individually Identifiable Health Information

AGENCY: Office of the Assistant Secretary for Planning and Evaluation, DHHS.

ACTION: Final rule.

SUMMARY: This rule includes standards to protect the privacy of individually identifiable health information. The rules below, which apply to health plans, health care clearinghouses, and certain health care providers, present standards with respect to the rights of individuals who are the subjects of this information, procedures for the exercise of those rights, and the authorized and required uses and disclosures of this information.

The use of these standards will improve the efficiency and effectiveness of public and private health programs and health care services by providing enhanced protections for individually identifiable health information. These protections will begin to address growing public concerns that advances in electronic technology and evolution in the health care industry are resulting, or may result, in a substantial erosion of the privacy surrounding individually identifiable health information maintained by health care providers, health plans and their administrative contractors. This rule implements the privacy requirements of the Administrative Simplification subtitle of the Health Insurance Portability and Accountability Act of 1996.

DATES: The final rule is effective on February 26, 2001.

FOR FURTHER INFORMATION CONTACT: Kimberly Coleman, 1–866–OCR–PRIV (1–866–627–7748) or TTY 1–866–788–4989.

SUPPLEMENTARY INFORMATION: Availability of copies, and electronic access.

Copies: To order copies of the **Federal Register** containing this document, send your request to: New Orders, Superintendent of Documents, P.O. Box 371954, Pittsburgh, PA 15250–7954. Specify the date of the issue requested and enclose a check or money order payable to the Superintendent of Documents, or enclose your Visa or Master Card number and expiration date. Credit card orders can also be placed by calling the order desk at (202) 512–1800 or by fax to (202) 512–2250. The cost for each copy is $8.00. As an alternative, you can view and photocopy the **Federal Register** document at most libraries designated as Federal Depository Libraries and at many other public and academic libraries throughout the country that receive the **Federal Register**.

Electronic Access: This document is available electronically at http://aspe.hhs.gov/admnsimp/ as well as at the web site of the Government Printing Office at http://www.access.gpo.gov/su_docs/aces/aces140.html.

I. Background

Table of Contents

B

Figure 2-11, ***cont'd*** **B,** ***Federal Register*** **Privacy Act, page 1.**

Defense, and Department of Health and Human Services are some of the agencies most commonly involved in health care regulatory activities. Table 2-1 outlines some of the agencies under these departments and the health-related regulatory functions they perform.

Department of Labor

OSHA is an agency within the Department of Labor that is responsible for the regulation of health and safety in the workplace. Hospitals are required to follow established standards to ensure that employees have a healthy and safe work environment. OSHA develops standards and conducts site visits to determine the hospital's compliance with health and safety regulations.

Department of Veterans Affairs

The Department of Veterans Affairs maintains a network of facilities and services for armed service veterans and in some cases their dependents. Primary facilities designed to provide medical care to veterans are known as Veterans Administration (VA) hospitals. The Department of Veterans Affairs also negotiates with other providers and health insurance programs to provide medical services to veterans.

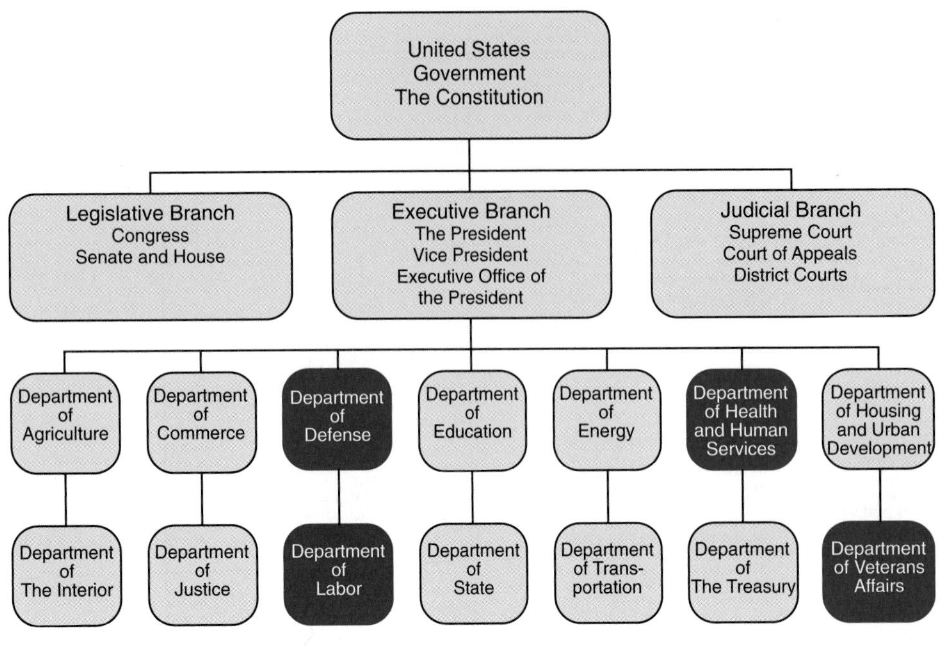

Figure 2-12 U.S. government departments most commonly involved in health care regulation (*dark red*).

TABLE 2-1 Health-Related Functions of Government Agencies

Department	Agency	Function
Department of Labor	Occupational Safety and Health Administration (OSHA)	Regulates workplace health and safety
Department of Veterans Affairs	Veterans Affairs Facilities	Maintains a network of facilities and services for armed services veterans and sometimes their dependents
Department of Defense	Health Affairs	Maintains a network of health care providers and facilities for service personnel and their dependents
	TRICARE management activity	Coordinates and administers the TRICARE Program
DHHS	Centers for Medicare and Medicaid Services (CMS)	Oversees Medicare, Medicaid, and other government programs
	Office of Inspector General (OIG)	Conducts and audits investigations to identify fraudulent activities within government programs
	Centers for Disease Control and Prevention (CDC)	Provides a system of health surveillance to monitor and prevent outbreak of diseases
	Health Resources and Services Administration (HRSA)	Helps provide health resources for medically underserved populations

Modified from Davis N, LaCour M: Introduction to health information technology, *ed 1, St Louis, 2002, Saunders.*

Department of Defense (DOD)

The Health Affairs agency of the DOD maintains a network of health care providers and facilities for personnel and their dependents. Tasks and responsibilities required for the administration of various programs are referred to as field activities. The DOD creates agencies to conduct field activities as well as various tasks and responsibilities required for the operation of the DOD. One agency created by the DOD is called TRICARE Management Activity (TMA), created to oversee the TRICARE program.

TRICARE Management Activity (TMA)

TMA is organized under the DOD's Health Affairs agency to coordinate and administer the TRICARE program. The organizational structure of the DOD field activity agencies, including TMA, is outlined in Figure 2-13. TMA is responsible for the management of all financial matters of the department's medical and dental programs and the execution of policies issued by the Assistant Secretary of Defense for the administration of those programs. TRICARE will be discussed in detail in Chapter 12.

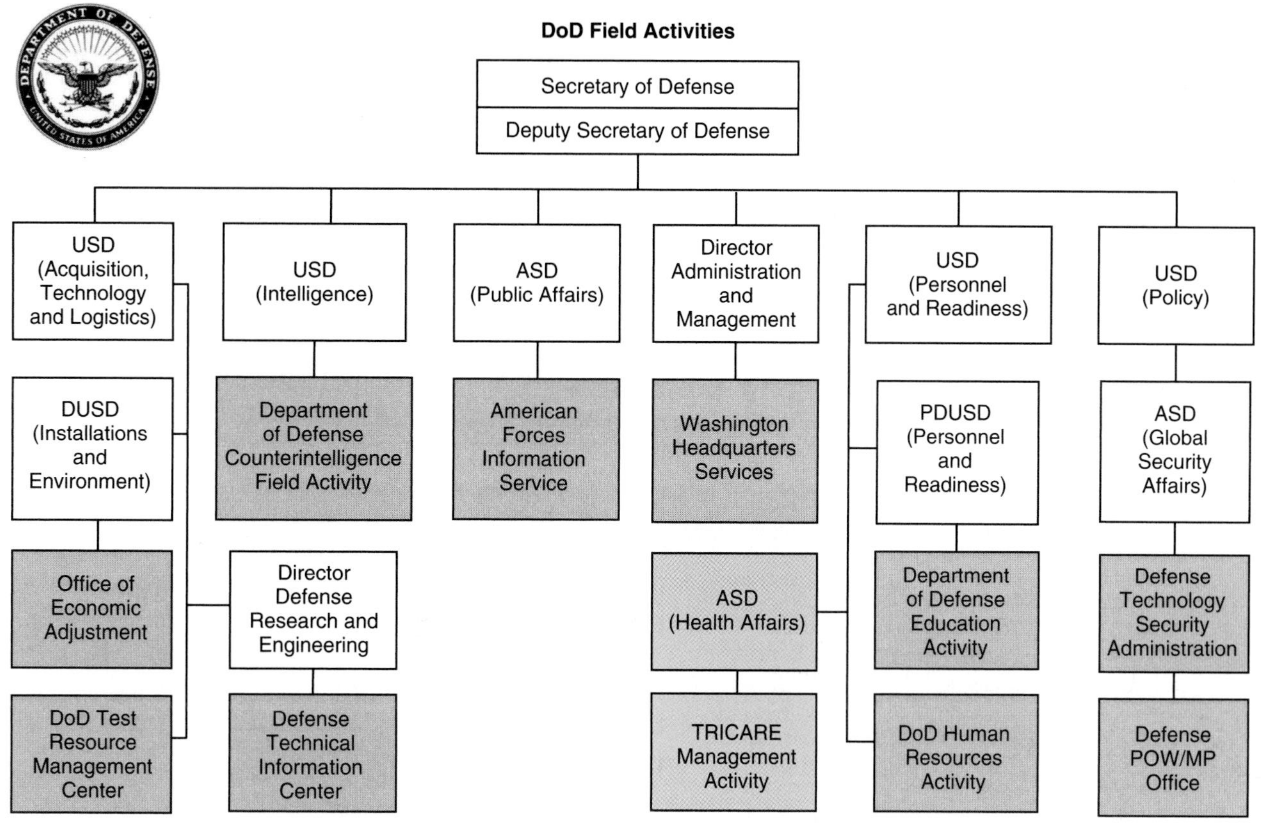

Figure 2-13 Department of Defense organizational chart. TRICARE management administers the TRICARE program. *(Modified from U. S. Department of Defense: Guide Book, http://odam.defense.gov/omp/pubs/GuideBook/pdf/FldAct.pdf.)*

Department of Health and Human Services (DHHS)

The DHHS is a federal department responsible for health issues, including controlling the rising cost of health care, the health and welfare of various populations, occupational safety, and income security plans. DHHS is a product of the reorganization of the HEW department that occurred in 1980. Many health care programs are regulated by DHHS, which is a branch of the federal government. Several agencies under DHHS are involved in health care regulatory activities, such as the CMS, Office of Inspector General (OIG), Centers for Disease Control and Prevention (CDC), and Health Resources and Services Administration (HRSA). The CMS and OIG are two agencies under DHHS that have significant regulatory influence on health care (Figure 2-14).

Centers for Medicare and Medicaid Services (CMS)

The **CMS** oversees the federal responsibilities for the Medicare and Medicaid programs. CMS was formerly known as the Health Care Financing Administration (HCFA). A facility cannot receive reimbursement from the federal government unless it is certified under Medicare's **Conditions of Participation (COP)**. COP contains CMS rules and regulations that govern the Medicare program. Providers of service are required to follow regulations outlined in COP implemented under the Code of Federal Regulations, Title 42 (Figure 2-15). The Code of Federal Regulations indicates that "hospitals participating in Medicare must meet certain specified requirements and the Secretary may impose additional requirements if they are found necessary in the interest of the health and safety of the individuals who are involved with health care delivery in hospitals." COP outlines standards to be followed in areas such as patients' rights, quality assurance, medical staff, nursing services, medical record services, radiology services, utilization review, physical environment, discharge planning, and emergency services. The provisions in COP are vast guidelines that are specific to billing and coding and will be referenced as we progress through this chapter and the rest of the text.

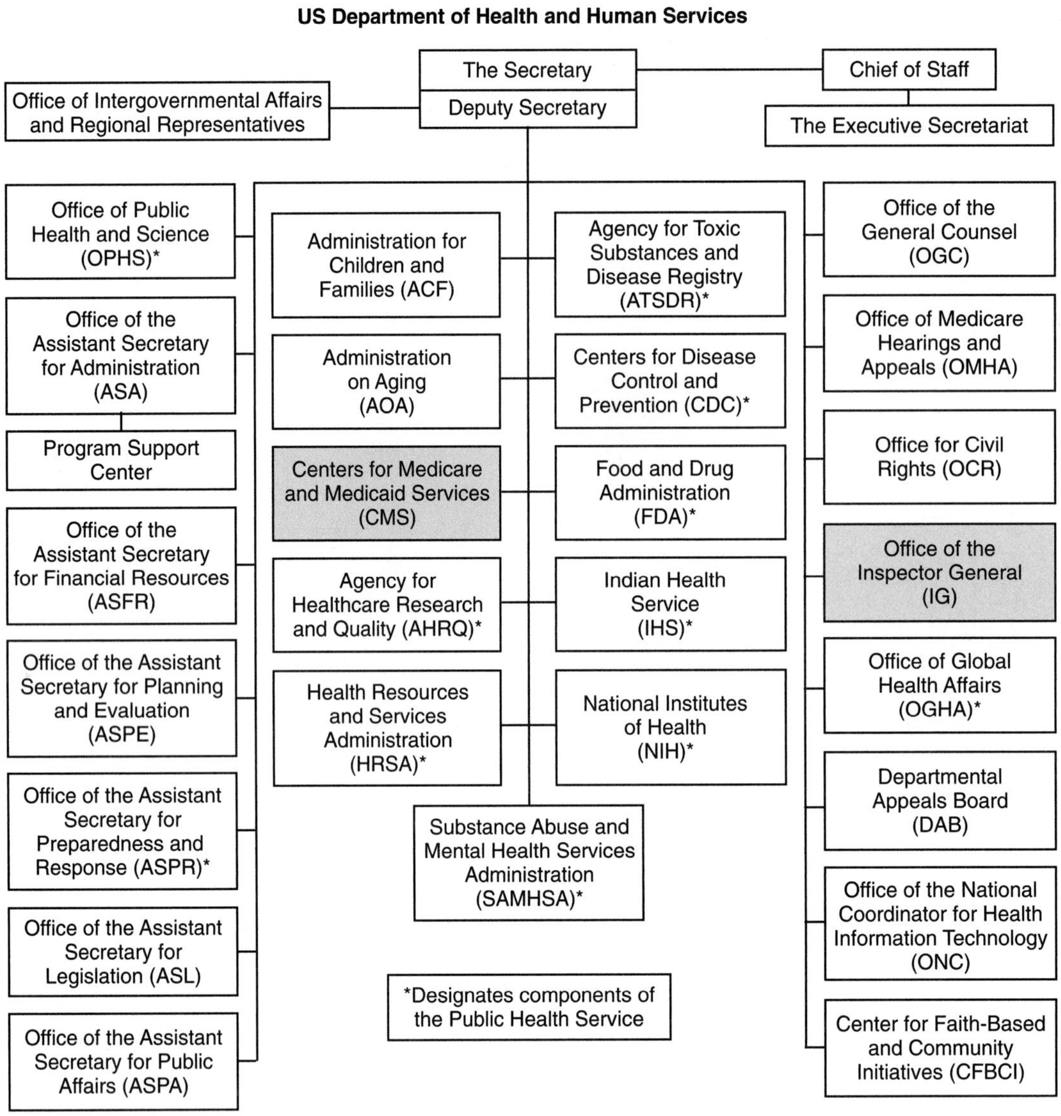

US Department of Health and Human Services

The Secretary
Deputy Secretary
Chief of Staff
The Executive Secretariat
Office of Intergovernmental Affairs and Regional Representatives

Office of Public Health and Science (OPHS)*
Office of the Assistant Secretary for Administration (ASA)
Program Support Center
Office of the Assistant Secretary for Financial Resources (ASFR)
Office of the Assistant Secretary for Planning and Evaluation (ASPE)
Office of the Assistant Secretary for Preparedness and Response (ASPR)*
Office of the Assistant Secretary for Legislation (ASL)
Office of the Assistant Secretary for Public Affairs (ASPA)

Administration for Children and Families (ACF)
Administration on Aging (AOA)
Centers for Medicare and Medicaid Services (CMS)
Agency for Healthcare Research and Quality (AHRQ)*
Health Resources and Services Administration (HRSA)*

Agency for Toxic Substances and Disease Registry (ATSDR)*
Centers for Disease Control and Prevention (CDC)*
Food and Drug Administration (FDA)*
Indian Health Service (IHS)*
National Institutes of Health (NIH)*

Substance Abuse and Mental Health Services Administration (SAMHSA)*

*Designates components of the Public Health Service

Office of the General Counsel (OGC)
Office of Medicare Hearings and Appeals (OMHA)
Office for Civil Rights (OCR)
Office of the Inspector General (IG)
Office of Global Health Affairs (OGHA)*
Departmental Appeals Board (DAB)
Office of the National Coordinator for Health Information Technology (ONC)
Center for Faith-Based and Community Initiatives (CFBCI)

Figure 2-14 DHHS organizational chart highlighting CMS and OIG. *(Modified from U. S. Department of Health and Human Services: Department of Health and Human Services Organizational Chart, http://www.hhs.gov/ABOUT/ORGCHART/#TEXT)*

Office of Inspector General (OIG)

The **OIG** is a federal agency under the DHHS that is responsible for protecting the integrity of DHHS programs, such as Medicare and Medicaid. The primary focus of the OIG is to prevent fraud and abuse in the Medicare and Medicaid programs. Fraud and abuse prevention activities include conducting audits and investigating potential improprieties in the programs. The OIG develops and publishes a work plan annually. The work plan highlights focus areas for the current year. For example, evaluation and management services may be on the OIG's target list for this year. The OIG's work plan for the current year can be viewed on the OIG's Web page at http://oig.hhs.gov/publications/workplan.asp.

BOX 2-9 ■ KEY POINTS

Federal Regulatory Agencies

Department of Labor

- Occupational Safety and Health Administration (OSHA)

Department of Veterans Affairs

- Veterans Administration (VA)

Department of Defense

- TRICARE Management Activity (TMA)

Department of Health and Human Services (DHHS)

- Centers for Medicare and Medicaid Services (CMS)
- Office of Inspector General (OIG)

STATE REGULATIONS

Government involvement in the regulatory process is carried down from the federal level to the state level. State rules and regulations, which vary among states, are often more stringent than federal laws. City rules and regulations may be more stringent than state requirements. Regulations can vary within a state based on the location of the facility—"urban" or "rural." States are involved in all phases of health care legislation as a result of the following responsibilities of state government:

- Each state has hospitals that are owned and operated by the state.
- States are involved in the funding for teaching hospitals and medical education.
- States are responsible for public health departments.
- Certification and licensing of health care facilities is performed at the state level.

BOX 2-10 KEY POINTS

State Regulatory Capacity

State-owned facilities
Funding of teaching hospitals and education
Oversight of Department of Health
Certification and licensing of health care facilities

Code of Federal Regulations, Title 42-Public Health, Part 482

Chapter IV–Health Care Financing Administration, Department of Health and Human Services (Center for Medicare and Medicaid Services)

Part 482–Conditions of Participation for Hospitals

482.1	Basis and scope.
482.2	Provision of emergency services by nonparticipating hospitals.
482.11	Condition of participation: Compliance with Federal, State and local laws.
482.12	Condition of participation: Governing body.
482.13	Condition of participation: Patients' rights.
482.21	Condition of participation: Quality assurance.
482.22	Condition of participation: Medical staff.
482.23	Condition of participation: Nursing services.
482.24	Condition of participation: Medical record services.
482.25	Condition of participation: Pharmaceutical services.
482.26	Condition of participation: Radiologic services.
482.27	Condition of participation: Laboratory services.
482.28	Condition of participation: Food and dietetic services.
482.30	Condition of participation: Utilization review.
482.41	Condition of participation: Physical environment.
482.42	Condition of participation: Infection control.
482.43	Condition of participation: Discharge planning.
482.45	Condition of participation: Organ, tissue, and eye procurement.
482.51	Condition of participation: Surgical services.
482.52	Condition of participation: Anesthesia services.
482.53	Condition of participation: Nuclear medicine services.
482.54	Condition of participation: Outpatient services.
482.55	Condition of participation: Emergency services.
482.56	Condition of participation: Rehabilitation services.
482.57	Condition of participation: Respiratory care services.
482.60	Special provisions applying to psychiatric hospitals.
482.61	Condition of participation: Special medical record requirements for psychiatric hospitals.
482.62	Condition of participation: Special staff requirements for psychiatric hospitals.
482.66	Special requirements for hospital providers of long-term care services ("swing-beds").

Figure 2-15 *Code of Federal Regulations,* Title 42-Public Health Part 482 (conditions of Medicare participation for hospitals). *(Modified from U.S. Government Printing Office: Code of Federal Regulations, www.access.gpo.gov.)*

State Regulatory Agencies

All states have regulatory agencies that are responsible for the oversight and investigation of hospitals and other health care providers. Regulatory agencies for the health care industry vary from state to state; however, they share a common mission, which is to ensure that efficient quality health care services are accessible to members of their state. The Department of Health and the Agency for Health Care Administration are examples of Florida state agencies that are involved in regulating hospitals in Florida (Figure 2-16).

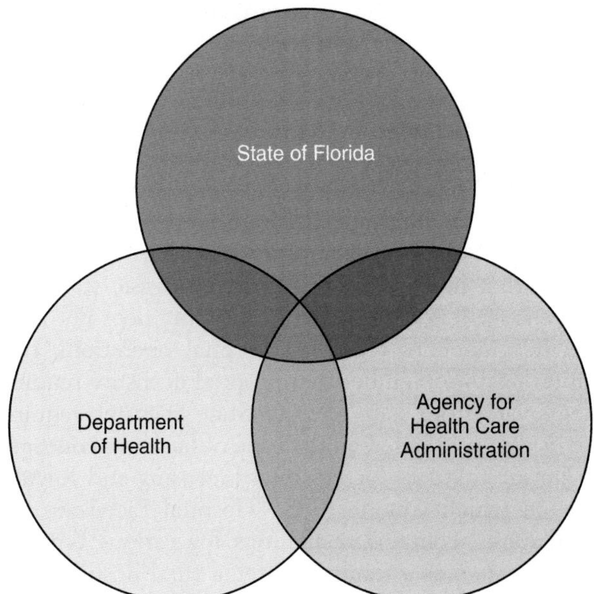

Figure 2-16 State of Florida health care regulatory agencies.

Department of Health (DOH)

Each state has a **DOH** that is involved in health care initiatives within the state. The mission of the DOH includes promoting public health and health safety of all state residents through disease prevention and ensuring that quality medical care is provided. Health departments provide health care services to individuals within the state who are poor or do not have access to health care services. The organization of state health departments varies from state to state but is a joint venture between the state and the local communities. The health care provided is usually directed toward maternal and child care as well as communicable and chronic diseases. The maternal and child health care services usually provide obstetric care, family planning, well-baby checkups, vaccinations, and other services.

Agency for Health Care Administration (AHCA)

Another regulatory agency in Florida is **ACHA**. The AHCA may also regulate hospitals in other states. The ACHA was created in 1992 under the Health Care Reform Act of 1992. The purpose of this agency is to ensure that efficient, quality health care services are accessible to all Floridians. The ACHA's mission extends to improving the state's efficiency in addressing health care issues and to controlling health care costs. The AHCA investigates complaints about hospitals and other health care facilities in the state of Florida. It has the authority to review medical records and interrogate any involved entities in order to aid in the determination of the validity of the charges. Information on the AHCA can be viewed on the home page at http://www.fdhc.state.fl.us/index.shtml.

State governments are generally involved in regulating health care in various areas from employment to provision of health care services. State governments are also involved in many other aspects of health care regulation, from zoning regulations, record retention, and human resources to licensing of facilities.

BOX 2-11 ■ KEY POINTS

State Regulatory Agencies: Florida
Department of Health (DOH)
Agency for Health Care Administration (AHCA)

Florida Statutes, Title XXIX, Public Health

Part I	Hospitals and other licensed facilities (ss. 395.001-395.3041)
Part II	Trauma (ss. 395.40-395.51)
Part III	Rural hospitals (ss. 395.602-395-6061)
Part IV	Public medical assistance trust fund (ss. 395.701-395.7016)
Part V	Family practice teaching hospitals (ss. 395.805-395.807)

Figure 2-17 Florida statutes, Chapter 395, Hospital Licensing and Regulations. *(Modified from The Florida Legislature: The 2004 Florida Statutes, www.leg.state.fl.us.)*

STATE HOSPITAL LICENSING REQUIREMENTS

Health care facilities must be licensed to operate within each state. State licensing requirements are designed to ensure that health care facilities meet basic standards. A license will not be granted if a facility does not meet specific guidelines regarding hospital operations. It is important to remember that hospital licensure requirements vary from state to state. State licensing requirements also vary based on the type of facility, as outlined in Florida Statutes for Hospital Licensing and Regulation, in which Chapter 395, "Hospital Licensing and Regulation," contains regulations for various types of facilities such as a trauma center, a rural hospital, or a family practice teaching hospital (Figure 2-17).

Hospital standards for licensure are outlined under state statutes, and the authority to enforce the statutes is delegated to the appropriate agency within the state. Some states delegate authority to regulate hospitals to the DOH or other agencies like the state of Florida's AHCA. AHCA has the authority to grant a license to hospitals in the state of Florida that meet basic requirements as outlined in Chapter 59A-3 of the Florida Administrative Code titled "Hospital Licensing and Regulation" (Figure 2-18).

BOX 2-12 ■ KEY POINTS

Florida State Hospital Licensing and Regulation
Florida statutes Title XXIX Chapter 395
Florida Administrative Code Chapter 59A-3
Regulatory agency: Agency for Health Care Administration (AHCA)

Minimum Hospital Licensing Requirements, Subsection 2

Subsection 2 states that, in addition to the other requirements outlined in Chapter 59A-3, "all hospitals shall have at least the following:

a. Inpatient beds.
b. A governing authority legally responsible for the conduct of the hospital.
c. A chief executive officer and other similarly titled officials, to whom the governing authority delegates the full-time authority for the operation of the hospital in accordance with the established policy of the governing authority.
d. An organized medical staff, to which the governing authority delegates responsibility for maintaining proper standards for medical and other health care.
e. A current and complete medical record for each patient admitted to the hospital.
f. A policy requiring that all patients are admitted on the authority of and under the care of a member of the organized medical staff.
g. Facilities and professional staff available to provide food to patients to meet their nutritional needs.

TEST YOUR *Knowledge* BOX 2-1

HOSPITAL REGULATORY ENVIRONMENT INTRODUCTION; FEDERAL LEGISLATION AND FEDERAL REGULATORY AGENCIES

1. Provide a brief explanation of how the evolution of medicine contributed to the increase in governmental regulatory activity.

2. Discuss how the creation of Medicare and Medicaid expanded the government's role in regulating health care.

3. List three focus areas of governmental responsibility related to health care.

4. The government's influence on health care expanded with the creation of what programs?

5. Provide a brief overview of the federal legislature's role in the implementation and enforcement of health care legislation.

6. Outline five legislative actions designed to address the access and quality of health care. Provide the year the legislation was implemented.

7. Provide a brief explanation of issues addressed by HIPAA legislation.

8. Outline four legislative actions designed to address the health, education, and welfare of the public. Provide the year the legislation was implemented.

9. Outline three legislative actions designed to address the rising cost of health care. Provide the year the legislation was implemented.

10. Discuss briefly four federal regulatory agencies involved in the regulation of health care in hospitals.

11. List the department that is responsible for facilities and services provided to armed service veterans.

12. List the agency under the Department of Defense that is responsible for oversight of the TRICARE Program.

13. Discuss the role of CMS in health care regulation.

14. List two agencies under the DHHS that are involved in the regulation of health care.

15. Name the federal agency that investigates fraud and abuse issues.

Chapter 59A-3, Florida Administrative Code

Subsection 2–Minimum Requirements
a. Inpatient beds
b. A governing authority legally responsible for the conduct of the hospital
c. A chief executive officer and other similarly titled official to whom the governing authority delegates the full-time authority for the operation of the hospital in accordance with the established policy of the governing authority
d. An organized medical staff to which the governing authority delegates responsibility for maintaining proper standards for medical and other health care
e. A current and complete medical record for each patient admitted to the hospital
f. A policy requiring that all patients be admitted on the authority of and under the care of a member of the organized medical staff
g. Facilities and professional staff available to provide food to patients to meet their nutritional needs
h. A procedure for providing care in emergency cases
i. A method and policy for infection control
j. An ongoing organized program to enhance the quality of patient care and review the appropriateness of utilization of services

Subsection 3–Additional Requirements
a. One licensed registered nurse on duty at all times on each floor or similarly titled part of the hospital for rendering patient care services
b. A pharmacy supervised by a licensed pharmacist either in the facility or by contract sufficient to meet patient needs
c. Diagnostic imaging services either in the facility or by contract sufficient to meet patient needs
d. Clinical laboratory services either in the facility or by contract sufficient to meet patient needs
e. Operating room services
f. Anesthesia service

Figure 2-18 Hospital Licensing and Regulation, Florida Administrative Code Chapter 59A-3. (*Modified from Agency for Health Care Administration: Hospitals & Outpatient Services Unit, www.fdhc.state.fl.us.*)

h. A procedure for providing care in emergency cases.
i. A method and policy for infection control.
j. An ongoing organized program to enhance the quality of patient care and review the appropriateness of utilization of services."

BOX 2-13 ■ KEY POINTS

Minimum State Hospital Licensing Requirements in Florida

Requirement	*Statute 395 Section Chapter 59 A-3*
Licensed physician	Subsection 2 "d"
Nursing services	Subsection 3 "a"
Patient medical record	Subsection 2 "e"
Admitting process	Subsections 2 and 3
Discharge process	Subsections 2 and 3
Financial policies and procedures	Section 59A-3.218

Additional Hospital Licensing Requirements, Subsection 3

Subsection 3 of Chapter 59A-3 of the Florida hospital licensing requirements states that, in addition to the requirements of Subsection 2 and other requirements, "general hospitals shall have at least the following additional requirements:

a. One licensed registered nurse on duty at all times on each floor or similarly titled part of the hospital for rendering patient care services.
b. A pharmacy supervised by a licensed pharmacist, either in the facility or by contract, sufficient to meet patient needs.
c. Diagnostic imaging services, either in the facility or by contract, sufficient to meet patient needs.
d. Clinical laboratory services, either in the facility or by contract, sufficient to meet patient needs.
e. Operating room services.
f. Anesthesia service."

The licensing requirements outlined above apply to general hospitals seeking a license to operate in the state of Florida; they are not inclusive, but they do provide an overview of the requirements listed in Chapter 59A-3, "Hospital Licensing and Regulations." Florida's hospital licensing requirements can be found on AHCA's Web page at http://www.fdhc.state.fl.us (Figure 2-19). It is important to remember that licensing requirements vary by state and by type of facility.

Hospitals are required to meet requirements regarding staffing, operations, and other policies and procedures to obtain state licensure. Compliance with these requirements also contributes to a smooth and efficient patient care process. The patient care process is complex. Standards and procedures must be in place to provide effective and efficient patient care services and maintain financial stability (Figure 2-20). Many requirements outlined in Statute 395, Chapter 59A-3 include provisions regarding licensed physicians, nursing services, patient medical records, admitting process, discharge process, and a billing process. The following section explores some of these staffing requirements and procedures and the primary departments involved in each area. Hospital departments and functions will be discussed in detail in Chapter 3.

Licensed Physician

In accordance with Subsection 2 of Chapter 59A-3 "d," hospitals must have an organized medical staff, and patients are to be admitted under the care of a member of the organized medical staff. Services provided in a hospital setting are performed under the supervision of a licensed physician to ensure that quality patient care is provided. The admitting physician manages patient care during a hospital stay. A patient cannot be admit-

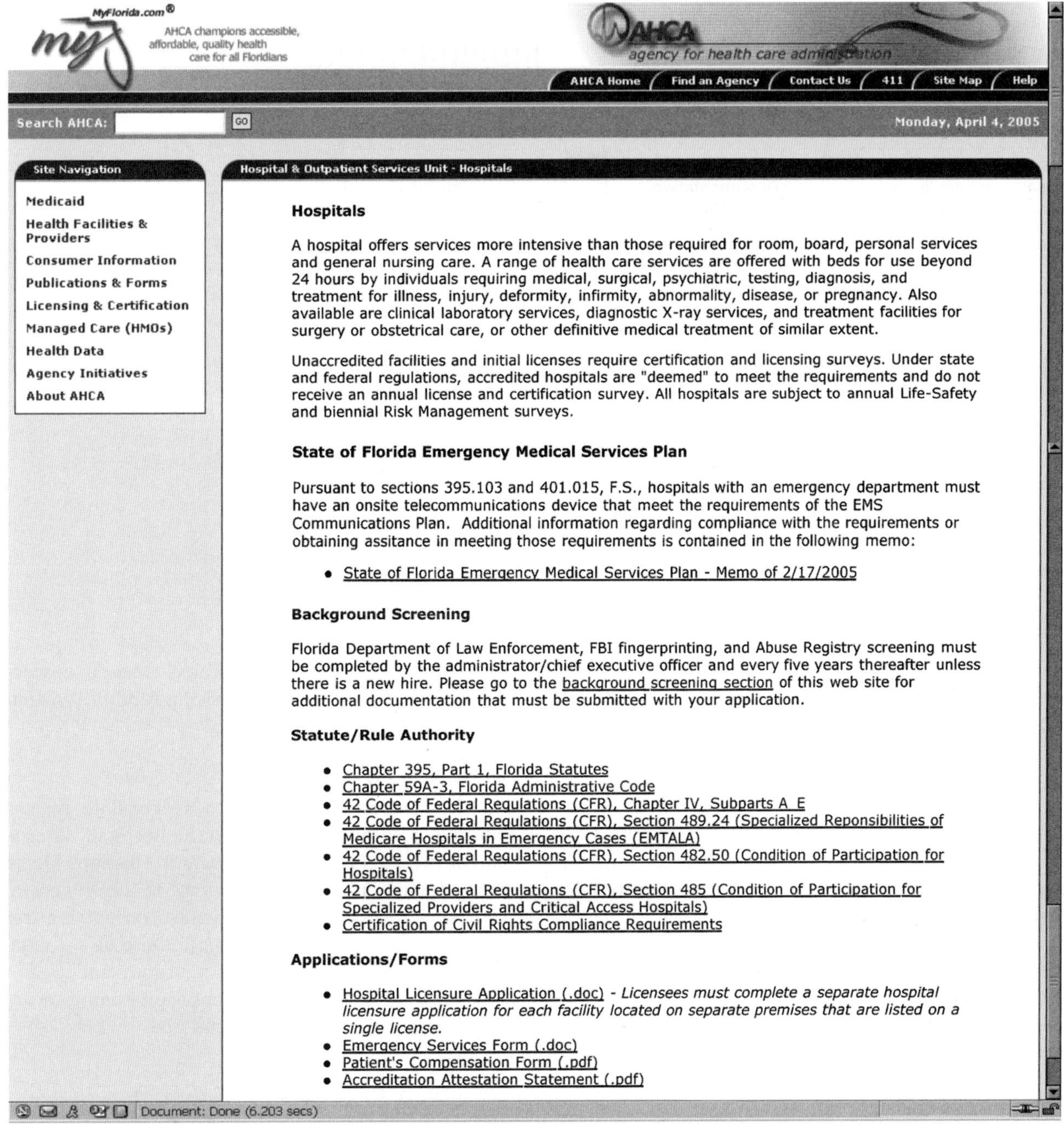

Hospitals

A hospital offers services more intensive than those required for room, board, personal services and general nursing care. A range of health care services are offered with beds for use beyond 24 hours by individuals requiring medical, surgical, psychiatric, testing, diagnosis, and treatment for illness, injury, deformity, infirmity, abnormality, disease, or pregnancy. Also available are clinical laboratory services, diagnostic X-ray services, and treatment facilities for surgery or obstetrical care, or other definitive medical treatment of similar extent.

Unaccredited facilities and initial licenses require certification and licensing surveys. Under state and federal regulations, accredited hospitals are "deemed" to meet the requirements and do not receive an annual license and certification survey. All hospitals are subject to annual Life-Safety and biennial Risk Management surveys.

State of Florida Emergency Medical Services Plan

Pursuant to sections 395.103 and 401.015, F.S., hospitals with an emergency department must have an onsite telecommunications device that meet the requirements of the EMS Communications Plan. Additional information regarding compliance with the requirements or obtaining assitance in meeting those requirements is contained in the following memo:

- State of Florida Emergency Medical Services Plan - Memo of 2/17/2005

Background Screening

Florida Department of Law Enforcement, FBI fingerprinting, and Abuse Registry screening must be completed by the administrator/chief executive officer and every five years thereafter unless there is a new hire. Please go to the background screening section of this web site for additional documentation that must be submitted with your application.

Statute/Rule Authority

- Chapter 395, Part 1, Florida Statutes
- Chapter 59A-3, Florida Administrative Code
- 42 Code of Federal Regulations (CFR), Chapter IV, Subparts A E
- 42 Code of Federal Regulations (CFR), Section 489.24 (Specialized Reponsibilities of Medicare Hospitals in Emergency Cases (EMTALA)
- 42 Code of Federal Regulations (CFR), Section 482.50 (Condition of Participation for Hospitals)
- 42 Code of Federal Regulations (CFR), Section 485 (Condition of Participation for Specialized Providers and Critical Access Hospitals)
- Certification of Civil Rights Compliance Requirements

Applications/Forms

- Hospital Licensure Application (.doc) - *Licensees must complete a separate hospital licensure application for each facility located on separate premises that are listed on a single license.*
- Emergency Services Form (.doc)
- Patient's Compensation Form (.pdf)
- Accreditation Attestation Statement (.pdf)

Figure 2-19 The Agency for Health Care Administration's Hospital Licensing Statutes, Chapter 59A-3. *(Modified from Agency for Health Care Administration: Hospital Licensing and Regulation, www.fdhc.state.fl.us.)*

ted without an order from the admitting physician. The physician's order outlines the plan of care for the patient during the admission, including required medications, diagnostic and therapeutic services to be performed, and other patient care needs such as diet. Physician orders can be written or verbal.

Medical Staff Department

The medical staff department is responsible for overseeing patient care services. These departments are commonly referred to as clinical departments, as they are involved in the clinical aspects of patient care services. The department consists of licensed physicians and other health care professionals representing a variety of medical specialties. All providers in a hospital setting must be credentialed. **Credentialing** is the process followed by hospitals and other organizations for evaluation of physicians to determine whether they should be granted admitting privileges. **Admitting privileges** are granted to health care professionals to define what

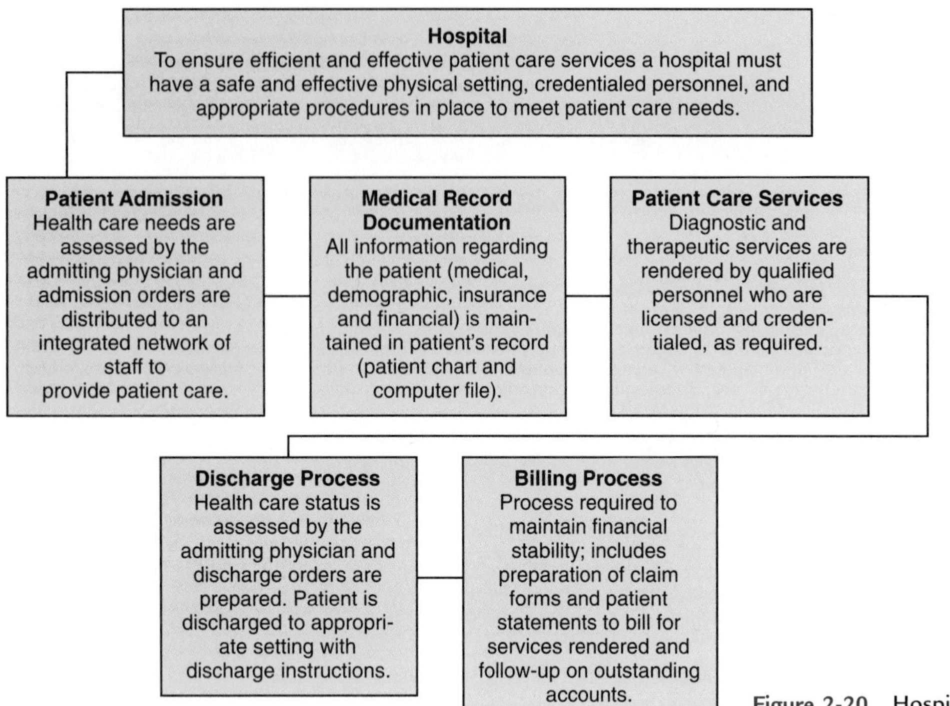

Hospital
To ensure efficient and effective patient care services a hospital must have a safe and effective physical setting, credentialed personnel, and appropriate procedures in place to meet patient care needs.
Patient Admission
Health care needs are assessed by the admitting physician and admission orders are distributed to an integrated network of staff to provide patient care.
Medical Record Documentation
All information regarding the patient (medical, demographic, insurance and financial) is maintained in patient's record (patient chart and computer file).
Patient Care Services
Diagnostic and therapeutic services are rendered by qualified personnel who are licensed and credentialed, as required.
Discharge Process
Health care status is assessed by the admitting physician and discharge orders are prepared. Patient is discharged to appropriate setting with discharge instructions.
Billing Process
Process required to maintain financial stability; includes preparation of claim forms and patient statements to bill for services rendered and follow-up on outstanding accounts.

Figure 2-20 Hospital patient care process.

categories of patients can be seen by the professional along with the type of services and procedures that can be performed within the hospital.

Nursing Services

In accordance with Subsection 3 of Chapter 59A-3 "a," hospitals must have one licensed registered nurse on duty at all times on each floor. Hospital patients require nursing care, particularly patients who are admitted on an inpatient basis and require 24-hour nursing care. Licensing requirements state that "each hospital shall employ a registered nurse on a full time basis who shall have the authority and responsibility for managing nursing services."

Nursing Department

The nursing department is responsible for supervision and coordination of all nursing services provided in the hospital. The nursing department consists of registered nurses, licensed practical nurses, and other advanced nursing professionals such as nurse practitioners. Nursing services are provided in accordance with the physician's order and standards of medical care.

Admitting Process

Admittance to the hospital requires a procedure ensuring that standards (Subsections 2 and 3 of Chapter 59A-3) regarding the management of patient care services and medical care are met. The required information must be obtained to assess the patient's medical needs and also to process patient charges. The process begins when the admitting physician submits written or verbal orders for the admission.

Admissions Department

The Admissions Department is responsible for tasks required to admit the patient to the hospital. When the patient presents for admission, the Admissions Department obtains medical, demographic, insurance, and financial information. The patient's consent for treatment and the release of information are also obtained during the admission process. A room and bed are assigned to the patient on the appropriate unit or floor, and patient care services are rendered.

Patient Medical Record

In accordance with Subsection 2 of Chapter 59A-3 "e," hospitals are required to have a current and complete medical record for each patient admitted to the hospital. All information regarding patient care must be recorded in the patient's medical record to ensure continuity of care and to adhere to documentation requirements. Hospital personnel in various departments are involved in recording information regarding the patient's condition at each encounter, including progress, medications given, tests performed, and supplies provided (Figure 2-21).

Health Information Management (HIM)

The **HIM** Department is responsible for the organization, maintenance, production, storage, retention, dis-

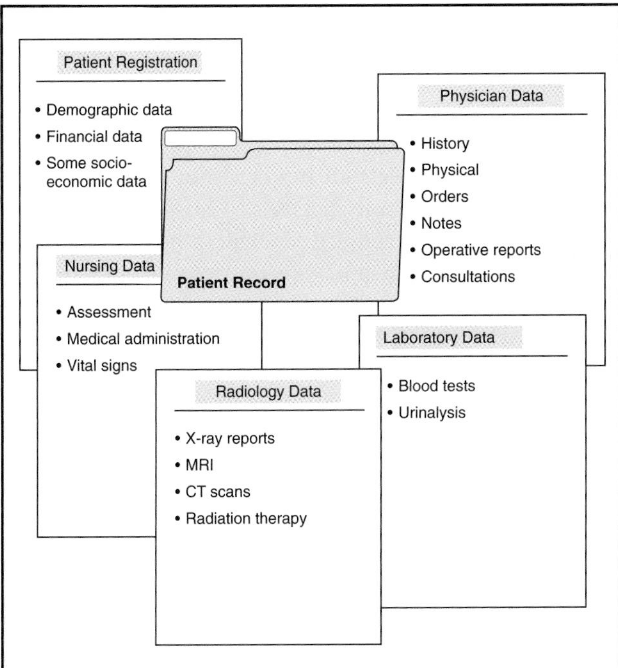

Figure 2-21 Patient medical record. *(From Davis N, LaCour M: Introduction to health information technology, ed 1, St Louis, 2002, Saunders.)*

semination, and security of patient information. Patient information can be categorized as follows:

- **Medical information** includes all information related to the patient's medical condition, including history, current medical status, and treatment. All information related to care provided during the hospital stay must be recorded in the patient's medical record, including diagnostic and therapeutic procedures and the patient's response to treatment.
- **Demographic information** is statistical information about the patient such as name, address, date of birth, sex, and Social Security number.
- **Insurance and financial information** includes all information regarding the patient's insurance, including plan name, number, group name and number, identification number, and the policyholder or other individual who has obtained the insurance coverage, such as a spouse or parent. Additional financial information such as income, expenses, and assets may be required if the patient is unable to pay for services rendered. This information may be used to assist the patient in finding other sources of funding for care.

BOX 2-14 ■ KEY POINTS

Medical Record: Categorized Patient Information

Medical information
Demographic information
Insurance and financial information

Discharge Process

In accordance with Section 59A-3.218, hospitals are required to have policies and procedures on discharge planning. Subsection 2 of Chapter 59A-3 "j," requires hospitals to have an ongoing, organized program to enhance the quality of patient care and to review the appropriateness of utilization of service. This standard applies to all patient care services rendered during admission. Additionally, a process must be followed to ensure that the patient is discharged at an appropriate time and to an appropriate setting.

Utilization Management (UM)

The **UM** Department is responsible for managing the utilization of health care resources. Patient care services are reviewed at admission and during the hospital stay to determine the appropriateness of services provided. The UM Department is also involved in the discharge planning process to ensure that the patient is discharged at an appropriate time and to an appropriate environment. For example, a patient who has a brain injury and cannot perform daily activities of living should not be discharged to home, unless someone is available to assist the patient with daily activities. The department may also be involved in planning and coordinating medical and financial resources required for the patient's discharge.

Billing Process

In accordance with Section 59A-3.218, hospitals are required to have financial policies and procedures. These policies and procedures include provisions regarding billing for patient care services. Hospitals employ highly qualified staff to provide patient care services, and they operate equipment that is very expensive. The cost of care provided to a patient per day must be recovered in an appropriate time period in order for the hospital to maintain financial stability. The billing process is required to obtain reimbursement for services rendered. The process requires the collection of necessary information to submit charges to third-party payers and patients. The billing process begins when the patient is admitted. The Admissions Department collects the information required for billing purposes. The preparation of patient statements and insurance claims is performed by the Patient Financial Services Department (PFS).

Patient Financial Services (PFS) Department

The PFS Department is responsible for preparing patient statements and insurance claim forms for submission of charges to patients and other payers. This department is often referred to as the Billing Department or Patient

BOX 2-15 ■ KEY POINTS

Hospital Billing Process

The billing process is critical to maintaining the financial stability of the hospital.

The billing process is required to obtain and process information for submission of charges for reimbursement from patients and third-party payers.

Accounts Department. The billing process includes preparation and submission of patient statements and claim forms, recording patient care transactions such as payments and adjustments, and follow-up on outstanding patient account balances.

Hospitals must comply with all licensing requirements and maintain compliance with provisions discussed above to be licensed to operate within the state. A hospital license is granted after an application is submitted and appropriate surveys are conducted to ensure that the hospital meets all standards. In Florida, AHCA is the agency that grants licenses to hospitals that meet standards. All states require renewal of hospital licenses. Some require annual renewal, but many states require renewal every 2 years. An application for renewal must be submitted, and the process to determine the facility's compliance with standards must be accomplished as well. Many states include provisions in the statutes that say "under state and federal regulations, accredited hospitals are 'deemed' to meet the requirements and do not require an annual license and certification survey."

TEST YOUR *Knowledge* BOX 2-2

STATE REGULATIONS; STATE LICENSING REQUIREMENTS

1. Describe state governmental responsibilities that contribute to the government's involvement in regulating health care.
2. Name a common mission of many state health care regulatory agencies.
3. Name two state agencies involved in regulating hospitals in Florida.
4. Provide a brief explanation of the state's involvement in regulating health care facilities.
5. Explain the purpose of state licensing of hospitals.
6. Explain how state licensing requirements vary.
7. Briefly discuss minimum state licensing requirements related to hospital medical staff and list the hospital department that is involved in ensuring that the requirements are met.
8. Briefly discuss minimum state licensing requirements related to the patient's medical record and list the hospital department that is involved in ensuring that the requirements are met.
9. Briefly discuss minimum state licensing requirements related to patient admissions and list the hospital department that is involved in ensuring that the requirements are met.
10. Briefly discuss additional state hospital licensing requirements that relate to the billing process.

Accreditation is the process by which an organization or agency performs an external review and grants recognition to a program of study or institution that meets certain predetermined standards. Hospitals are not required to obtain accreditation; however, accreditation plays a significant role in the development and enforcement of hospital standards. Therefore, it is necessary to understand the history, purpose, and process of accreditation.

BOX 2-16 ■ KEY POINTS

State Licensing Requirements

State licensing requirements are designed to ensure that health care facilities meet basic standards.
All states require hospitals to obtain a license.
License requirements vary by state and by type of facility.
Licensing/regulatory agency varies by state.

HISTORY AND PURPOSE OF ACCREDITATION

Accreditation efforts began in 1848, when the American Hospital Association (AHA) was founded to improve services provided in a hospital. Accreditation efforts were advanced through efforts of the American College of Surgeons (ACS) from 1913 to 1917. The ACS originally developed the Hospital Standardization Program. Under the program, hospitals were evaluated for the purpose of measuring hospital performance against standards outlined in the program. From 1917 to 1919, the ACS evaluated hospitals and accumulated information to identify various elements required for the provision of quality patient care in hospitals. The elements identified were adopted as Minimum Standards for "proper care and treatment of hospital patients." The Joint Commission on Accreditation of Hospitals (JCAH) was established in 1952. JCAH adopted the Hospital Standardization Program from the ACS and assumed the new name of Joint Commission on Accreditation of Healthcare Organizations (JCAHO) in 1987 (Figure 2-22). JCAHO changed its name to The Joint Commission (TJC) in 2007.

The purpose of accreditation of health care facilities is to identify facilities that do not meet standards of care guidelines and to provide endorsement to facilities that do meet certain specified standards. Accreditation is not mandated under federal and state laws. However, many hospitals voluntarily seek accreditation to assist them in determining compliance with state and federal guidelines. Table 2-2 outlines many benefits to obtaining accreditation, including improved patient care, facilitation of Medicare and Medicaid certification, and meeting the requirements of other third-party payers. Federal and state regulators seek accreditation of organizations, as it demonstrates that the organization has met specific

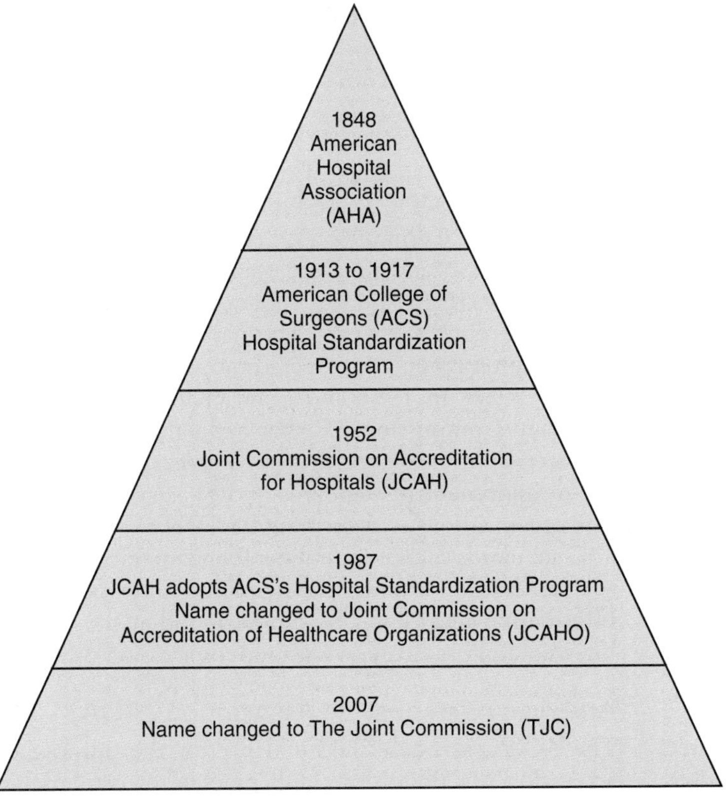

Figure 2-22 History of accreditation, 1848 to 2007.

TABLE 2-2 **Benefits of Accreditation**

Improves care	Joint Commission standards focus on state-of-the-art performance improvement strategies that help health care organizations continuously improve the safety and quality of care provided to individuals.
Strengthens community confidence	Accreditation highlights an organization's commitment to providing safe, quality care to the community it serves. Achieving accreditation makes a strong statement to the community about an organization's efforts to provide the highest quality services.
Provides professional advice and enhances staff education	The survey process is designed to be educational, not punitive. Joint Commission surveyors are experienced health care professionals trained to provide expert advice and education during the survey.
Offers ongoing support	Through its not-for-profit affiliate, Joint Commission Resources, each year the Joint Commission offers hundreds of educational seminars and publications about performance improvement and other standards-related topics. In addition, staff from each accreditation program and from the Standards Interpretation Group can provide immediate assistance and suggestions on survey process and standards compliance.
Enhances staff recruitment	The Accreditation Council for Graduate Medical Education recommends that postgraduate medical residents be placed in accredited hospitals. Joint Commission accreditation can also help attract qualified personnel who prefer to serve in an accredited organization.
Facilitates Medicare and Medicaid certification	Accreditation can help lessen the burdens imposed by duplicative federal and state regulatory agency surveys. Some accredited health care organizations may qualify for Medicare and Medicaid certification without undergoing a separate government quality inspection.
Meets insurer and other third-party requirements	Increasingly, accreditation is becoming a prerequisite to eligibility for insurance reimbursement, to participation in managed care plans, and to bidding on contracts.
Attracts professional referrals	Case managers and other health care professionals frequently use accreditation as a benchmark of quality when placing individuals in health care organizations.
Improves liability insurance coverage	By enhancing risk management efforts, accreditation may improve access to and reduce the cost of liability insurance coverage.
Provides a competitive advantage	Exposure of accreditation status may provide a marketing advantage in a competitive health care marketplace.
Meets lender conditions	Joint Commission accreditation is often helpful to health care organizations in meeting lender conditions for securing financing.

Data from www.jointcommission.org.

standards. Accreditation can be achieved through several organizations by meeting the standards developed by the organizations.

Accrediting Organizations

There are several organizations involved in accreditation, such as TJC, American Osteopathic Association, Accreditation Association for Ambulatory Health Care, Commission on Accreditation of Rehabilitation Facilities, National Committee for Quality Assurance, Community Health Accreditation Program, and the Utilization Review Accreditation Commission.

The following section will focus on two major organizations that provide accreditation to hospitals: TJC and the American Osteopathic Association.

The Joint Commission

The Joint Commission is a national commission formed to evaluate and accredit health care organizations based on established standards of quality for operations and medical services. TJC was established in 1952 under the name of Joint Commission on Accreditation of Hospitals to develop and measure standards by conducting accreditation visits and has enhanced the accreditation process through the years. The name was changed to Joint Commission on Accreditation of Healthcare Organizations in 1987 and again changed in 2007 to The Joint Commission. TJC has had a major impact on the accreditation of health care organizations through the development of standards and by surveying health care organizations to determine the level of compliance. TJC standards incorporate federal and state regulations such as the Conditions of Participation under Medicare. Information regarding TJC can be found at the following web address http://www.jointcommission.org

American Osteopathic Association (AOA)

The **AOA** was established in 1997 for the purpose of advancing the philosophy and practice of osteopathic medicine. Osteopathic medicine is based on the theory that the human body is a vital organism in which structural and functional states are of equal importance and that the body is able to rectify toxic conditions when it has favorable environmental circumstances and satisfactory nourishment. Physicians who have a degree in osteopathy use the designation D.O. The Healthcare Facilities Accreditation Program (HFAP) was established under the AOA to evaluate osteopathic hospitals for the purpose of ensuring quality of patient care. Information regarding the AOA can be viewed on the AOA Web page at www.osteopathic.org or www. do-online.org.

BOX 2-17 ■ KEY POINTS

Accreditation Organizations

The Joint Commission (TJC)
American Osteopathic Association (AOA)
Accreditation Association for Ambulatory Health Care
Commission on Accreditation of Rehabilitation Facilities (CARF)
National Committee on Quality Assurance (NCQA)
Community Health Accreditation Program
Utilization Review Accreditation Commission

TABLE 2-3 The Accreditation Process

Opening conference	Introduces the survey team and reviews agenda
Document review	Committee reviews documents and reports and provides orientation to hospital functions
Interviews with hospital leaders	Chief executive officer, medical staff, nursing staff, and department directors
Visit to patient care settings	Survey team identifies patient care settings to be included in their visit, such as: inpatient units, ambulatory areas, pathology, laboratory, radiology, emergency, rehabilitation, and operating areas
Focus interviews	Survey team interviews selected staff members
Feedback session	Survey team shares observations with the medical staff
Leadership exit conference	Last day of survey; survey team provides a preliminary report, which includes recommended accreditation decision

Data from www.jointcommission.org.

ACCREDITATION PROCESS

The accreditation process involves evaluation of health care organizations to ensure that standards are met for the provision of quality patient care services. Accreditation standards are designed to meet government regulations and to be customer focused. The evaluation focuses on all areas of hospital operations and patient care delivery including physical environment, patient care activities, admission and discharge procedures, and utilization management.

The accreditation process begins with the submission of specified documents detailing hospital operations including policies and procedures. A survey team visits the hospital to evaluate all aspects of operations further, including patient care delivery. At the end of the visit the survey team provides an overview of its findings. The accreditation process is outlined in Table 2-3.

Accreditation visits focus on all areas of hospital operations, from the physical setting to the provision of care and discharge planning (Figure 2-23). The accreditation team reviews all policies and procedures, medical record documentation, health information management systems, and patient care, to name just a few areas. Reviews are conducted to determine standards on assessment of and addressing patient care needs, providing patients with information required to make health care decisions, medical necessity for treatment, appropriate medication administration, appropriateness of admission and discharge, environmental safety for employees and patients, accommodations for physical impairments and infection control, quality improvement, and information management. The survey usually lasts a week. An exit interview is conducted at the end of the survey, and the accreditation team will review the survey findings with the hospital's administration. Accreditation

Accreditation Focus Areas

I. Hospital operations and physical environment
- Safety
- Human Resources

II. Patient Care Activities
- Health Information Management
- Patient medical record
- Patient care assessment
- Patient education
- Quality improvement

III. Admission and discharge procedures

IV. Utilization management

Note: This list is not all inclusive.

Figure 2-23 The accreditation process involves evaluation of all areas of hospital operations and patient care activities.

organizations may grant one of several accreditations or denials of accreditation, as outlined below:

Accreditation	*Denial*
Full accreditation granted	Accreditation denied
Provisional accreditation	Preliminary denial of accreditation
Conditional accreditation	Accreditation watch
Preliminary accreditation	

If deficiencies are identified, the accreditation organization grants a 60-day period for hospitals to prepare and submit a report on how the deficiencies will be corrected.

BOX 2-18 ■ KEY POINTS

Accreditation Decisions

Accreditation Granted

- Full accreditation
- Provisional accreditation
- Conditional accreditation
- Preliminary accreditation

Accreditation Denied

- Preliminary denial of accreditation
- Denial of accreditation
- Accreditation watch

A review of state and federal regulations and accreditation standards illustrates the specific requirements hospitals must comply with in many areas, including operations, the provision of patient care, and health information. Health care professionals who provide patient care services are required to have specified credentials and licensing through State Boards and other organizations. For example, hospital physicians and nursing personnel are required to have specified levels of education and the appropriate certifications and licenses. Nonclinical personnel, who are involved in billing, coding, and health information management, are also required to have specified levels of education and the appropriate certifications. The next section will focus on some of the billing and coding certifications and major organizations that provide these certifications.

NONCLINICAL CREDENTIALS

Many of the federal and state regulations implemented are related to the patient medical record, the coding of medical records, and the billing process. Nonclinical roles within hospitals have evolved from the clerk who performed scheduling and filing functions to roles involving technical aspects of the medical record, coding, and billing. Career opportunities for nonclinical personnel in hospitals have increased significantly. Figure 2-24 provides an overview of some billing and coding positions available in hospitals today. Billing and coding functions are directly related to reimbursement and compliance. Hospitals have employment requirements outlining levels of education and required certifications for billing and coding positions such as patient account technician, collection representative, or coder. Although not all hospitals require these certifications, the likelihood of securing employment in the field is enhanced for certified professionals. Hospital billing and coding professionals are advancing their knowledge and achieving certifications. The purpose of certification is to demonstrate competence in specific areas. Some of the most common billing and coding credentials that hospitals require are Registered Health Information Technician, Certified Coder, Patient Account Technician, and Healthcare Collection Specialist. Three nationally accepted credentialing organizations are the American Academy of Professional Coders (AAPC), the American Health Information Management Association (AHIMA), and the American Association of Health Care Administrative Management (AAHAM) (Table 2-4).

Community General Hospital Open Positions

Health Information Technician
Responsibilities include but are not limited to: data collection, analysis and retention of data, abstracting and coding from medical records.

Certified Coding Specialist/Certified Professional Coder
Responsibilities include but are not limited to: abstracting from medical records and translating written description of services, items, and diagnoses into codes.

Reimbursement Specialist
Responsibilities include monitoring and follow-up on outstanding accounts, contact with insurance companies/government payers regarding claims issues.

Figure 2-24 Sample of hospital employment opportunities.

American Academy of Professional Coders (AAPC)

The **AAPC** is a national organization founded for the purpose of elevating medical coding standards by providing ongoing education, networking opportunities, certification, and recognition of health insurance billing and coding professionals. AAPC has a membership base of over 85,000 members. Certifications offered by the AAPC include Certified Professional Coder (CPC), Certified Professional Coder-Hospital (CPC-H), and Certified Professional Coder-Apprentice (CPC-A). Information regarding the AAPC's certification examinations can be found on their Web page at http://www.aapc.com.

Certified Professional Coder (CPC)

Individuals who are involved in coding physician and outpatient services pursue the CPC certification. The

TEST YOUR *Knowledge* BOX 2-3

HISTORY AND PURPOSE OF ACCREDITATION; ACCREDITATION PROCESS

1. Provide an outline of the history of accreditation.
2. Explain the purpose of accreditation.
3. Why is accreditation important to hospitals?
4. Describe how accreditation is related to federal and state regulations.
5. List two organizations involved in the accreditation of hospitals.
6. State why The Joint Commission was formed.
7. Provide an overview of the accreditation process.
8. Identify four areas of focus for an accreditation evaluation.
9. Describe how accreditation affects hospital personnel credentialing requirements.
10. Explain how deficiencies identified during an accreditation survey are handled.

examination measures competencies in medical concepts, CPT, ICD-9-CM, and HCPCS coding for physician and outpatient services.

Qualifications to sit for the examination are a high school diploma or GED equivalent, 2 years of CPT, ICD-9-CM, and HCPCS coding experience, or 1 year of experience and the completion of an approved coding educational program.

Certified Professional Coder-Hospital (CPC-H)

Professionals involved in hospital outpatient coding pursue the CPC-H certification. The CPC-H measures competencies in medical concepts and CPT, ICD-9-CM, and HCPCS coding for hospital outpatient services.

Qualifications to sit for the examination are a high school diploma or GED equivalent, 2 years of CPT, ICD-9-CM, and HCPCS coding experience, or 1 year of experience and the completion of an approved coding educational program.

Certified Professional Coder-Apprentice (CPC-A)

Individuals who do not meet the 2-year experience requirement can obtain the CPC-A. The CPC-A examination measures competencies in medical concepts and CPT, ICD-9-CM, and HCPCS coding for physician and outpatient services.

Qualifications to sit for the examination are a high school diploma or GED equivalent. A CPC-A designation may be changed to CPC after 2 years of work experience have been achieved or 1 year of experience and the completion of an approved coding educational program.

TABLE 2-4 Organizations and Credentials Offered

Organization	Credentials
American Academy of Professional Coders (AAPC)	Certified Professional Coder (CPC) Certified Professional Coder-Hospital (CPC-H) Certified Professional Coder-Apprentice (CPC-A)
American Health Information Management Association (AHIMA)	Registered Health Information Technician (RHIT) Certified Coding Associate (CCA) Certified Coding Specialist (CCS) Certified Coding Specialist-Physician(CCS-P)
American Association of Healthcare Administration Management (AAHAM)	Certified Patient Account Technician (CPAT) Certified Clinic Account Technician (CCAT) Certified Patient Accounts Manager (CPAM)

American Health Information Management Association (AHIMA)

AHIMA is a national organization founded for the purpose of setting national standards in health information management, certification, and the provision of support to health information management professionals. AHIMA has a membership base of over 50,000 health information management professionals. It offers a variety of coding and health information certifications. The most common AHIMA certifications required for coding professionals are Registered Health Information Technician (RHIT), Certified Coding Associate (CCA), Certified Coding Specialist (CCS), and Certified Coding Specialist-Physician (CCS-P). Information regarding AHIMA certifications can be found on their Web page at http://www.ahima.org.

Registered Health Information Technician (RHIT)

An RHIT is responsible for coding services and conditions provided by hospitals and verifying the completeness, accuracy, and proper entry of medical information into the computer system. They may also use computer applications to assemble and analyze patient data for the purpose of improving patient care or controlling costs. RHIT professionals often specialize in coding diagnoses and procedures from patient records for reimbursement and research. RHIT professionals may serve as cancer registrars who compile and maintain data on cancer patients. With experience, the RHIT credential holds solid potential for advancement to management positions, especially if it is combined with a bachelor's degree.

The RHIT examination measures various competencies including those in the areas of health care data, information technology, organization, and supervision and coding. Qualifications to sit for the examination are a 2-year degree from an accredited program for health information technology or a certificate of completion of AHIMA's independent study program.

Certified Coding Associate (CCA)

CCA professionals are entry-level coders who perform basic coding tasks. The CCA examination measures basic CPT, ICD-9-CM, and HCPCS coding, other health care data, and information technology competencies. To take the CCA examination, candidates must have earned a U.S. high school diploma or the equivalent. Although it is not required, it is strongly recommended that candidates have at least 6 months of experience in a health care organization applying ICD-9-CM and CPT coding conventions and guidelines or have completed either an AHIMA-approved coding certificate program or another formal coding training program. The CCA examination is not linked to any formal education or training in coding.

Certified Coding Specialist (CCS)

Hospital coding professionals are responsible for various aspects of coding patient services and diagnoses including the review of patient medical records for the purpose of assigning the appropriate diagnosis and procedure codes. The CCS examination measures competencies in CPT, ICD-9-CM, and HCPCS coding of inpatient and ambulatory services. Eligibility to sit for the examination includes a high school diploma or equivalent, and the recommended amount of experience in inpatient and ambulatory medical record coding is 3 or more years.

Certified Coding Specialist-Physician (CCS-P)

Physicians and outpatient-based professionals are responsible for coding various physician and outpatient services. The CCS-P examination measures competencies in CPT, ICD-9-CM, and HCPCS coding for physician and outpatient services. Eligibility to sit for the examination includes a high school diploma or equivalent, and the recommended amount of experience in coding physician and outpatient services is 3 or more years.

American Association of Healthcare Administrative Management (AAHAM)

AAHAM was founded in 1968 as the American Guild of Patient Account Management. Initially formed to serve the interests of hospital patient account managers, AAHAM has evolved into a national membership association that represents a broad-based constituency of health care professionals. AAHAM offers several billing-related certifications such as the Certified Patient Account Technician (CPAT), the Certified Clinic Account Technician (CCAT), and the Certified Patient Accounts Manager (CPAM). Information regarding AAHAM and the certifications offered can be viewed on their Web site at http://www.aaham.org.

Certified Patient Account Technician

The CPAT is one of two technical certifications offered by AAHAM. This certification measures the proficiency of clerical staff involved in the processing of patient accounts on the hospital side of patient accounting. The examination covers the following topics: patient access services and communications, third-party billing regulations, credit and collection laws, and third-party follow-up. The recommendation of experience for this examination is 1 year of inpatient accounting.

Certified Clinic Account Technician

The CCAT is the second technical certification offered by AAHAM. This certification measures the proficiency of clerical staff involved in the processing of patient accounts on the physician/clinical side of patient accounting. The examination covers the following topics: patient access services and communications, third-party billing regulations, credit and collection laws, and third-party follow-up. The recommended experience for this examination is 1 year in patient accounting.

Certified Patient Accounts Manager

The CPAM certification is for individuals who work in the hospital administrative management side of patient accounts with a minimum of 4 years of health care experience, or 2 years of health care experience and a 2-year college or university associate degree. The CPAM is an extensive written examination covering all aspects of patient account management.

The health insurance billing and coding industry experiences daily changes in guidelines and procedures that require professionals in the field to maintain a current knowledge base. Credentialing organizations recognize the significance of maintaining a current knowledge base, and they offer various educational programs for professionals. Credentialing organizations also require individuals to obtain a specific number of **continuing education units (CEUs)** per year in order to maintain certification. CEUs are earned by individuals when they attend an educational function. Organizations generally grant 1 CEU for each hour attended. Continuing education functions provide an opportunity for professionals to gain new knowledge and maintain credentials.

BOX 2-19 ■ KEY POINTS

Nonclinical Credentials

American Academy of Professional Coders (AAPC)

- CPC
- CPC-H
- CPC-A

American Health Information Management Association (AHIMA)

- RHIT
- CCA
- CCS
- CCS-P

American Association of Health Administrative Management (AAHAM)

- CPAT
- CCAT
- CPAM

CHAPTER SUMMARY

Hospitals are greatly influenced by federal and state regulations. Regulations regarding a hospital's physical setting, patient care, health information, billing and coding, reimbursement, and human resource management have contributed to the development of a hospital structure from the departments to staffing. Regulations drive hospital procedures. An awareness of the regulations affecting health care in hospitals is necessary to ensure compliance with such regulations. Accrediting organizations assist with this through evaluation of hospitals based on established standards. A detailed discussion of hospital departments, functions, and procedures will follow in the next chapter.

TEST YOUR *Knowledge* BOX 2-4

NONCLINICAL CREDENTIALS

1. Provide an explanation of why credentials benefit nonclinical personnel.
2. List six acronyms for coding credentials available through the AHIMA and AAPC.
3. Describe the purpose of certification.
4. Name two national organizations that provide credentials for coding professionals.
5. State three various career opportunities for billing and coding professionals in a hospital.
6. Explain the difference between the CCS and the CCS-P.
7. Explain the difference between the CPC and the CPC-H.
8. Provide a description of the responsibilities of an RHIT.
9. Briefly describe the functions of a CCS or CPC.
10. Provide an explanation of the purpose of CEUs.

CHAPTER REVIEW 2-1

True/False

1. The Health Insurance Portability and Accountability Act was implemented for the sole purpose of simplifying the administration of health insurance standards. T F
2. Rules and regulations regarding health care legislation are published in the *Federal Register*. T F
3. Health care regulatory agencies have a primary focus on quality of care. T F
4. Hospital coding personnel can possess the RHIT, CCS, CCA, or CCS-P certification. T F
5. The purpose of accreditation is to develop standards. T F

Fill in the Blank

6. Hospitals must obtain a ____________________ from the state in order to operate within a particular state.
7. Three organizations offering certification examinations for billing and coding professionals are ____________________, ____________________ and ____________________.
8. The CPC xamination measures competencies in coding for ____________________ and ____________________ services.
9. Facilities voluntarily seek ____________________ to demonstrate their compliance with state and federal regulations.
10. Accrediting organizations provide hospitals with a specific time period in which to submit a plan of corrective action for deficiencies. What is the time period? ____________________

Match the Following Definitions With the Terms at Right

11. ___ An agency created for the purpose of overseeing Medicare and Medicaid programs.
12. ___ Office under the DHHS that is responsible for conducting audits and investigating potential improprieties in programs regulated by the DHHS.
13. ___ Conditions established for providers to participate in the Medicare program.
14. ___ Federal program established under Title XVIII of the SSA to provide health care benefits for individuals over age 65.
15. ___ The official publication in which federal regulations and legal notices are published.

A. Medicare
B. *Federal Register*
C. CMS
D. OIG
E. Conditions of Participation

Research Project

Research the legislation for the Social Security Act of 1965, Tax Equity and Fiscal Responsibility Act of 1982, and the Federal False Claims Act of 1986 and answer the following questions.

1. What impact does each of these acts have on provision of hospital services?
2. How do these acts affect the role of billing and coding professionals?
3. Why do these acts make it critical for hospitals to employ certified billing and coding professionals?
4. What are the consequences of non-compliance with guidelines and regulations under these legislative actions?
5. What are specific ways in which billing and coding professionals maintain current knowledge to ensure they are following guidelines?

GLOSSARY

Accreditation The process by which an organization or agency performs an external review and grants recognition to a program of study or institution that meets certain predetermined standards.

Admitting privileges Granted to health care professionals to define what categories of patients can be seen by the professional along with the type of services and procedures that can be performed within the hospital.

Agency for Health Care Administration (AHCA) A regulatory agency in Florida created in 1992 under the Health Care Reform Act of 1992 for the purpose of ensuring that efficient quality health care services are accessible to all Floridians.

American Academy of Professional Coders (AAPC) National organization founded for the purpose of elevating medical coding standards by providing ongoing education, networking opportunities, certification, and recognition of health insurance billing and coding professionals.

American Health Information Management Association (AHIMA) National organization founded for the purpose of setting national standards in health information management and certification and providing support to health information management professionals.

American Osteopathic Association (AOA) An organization established in 1997 for the purpose of advancing the philosophy and practice of osteopathic medicine.

Centers for Medicare and Medicaid Services (CMS) Agency under the Department of Health and Human Services that oversees the federal responsibilities for the Medicare and Medicaid programs. CMS was formerly known as the Health Care Financing Administration (HCFA).

Civil Monetary Penalties Law (CMPL) A law passed in 1983 for the purpose of prosecuting cases of Medicare and Medicaid fraud.

Conditions for Participation (COP) Conditions established for providers to participate in the Medicare program. Medicare's COP contains CMS rules and regulations that govern the Medicare program. Providers of service are required to follow regulations outlined in the COP implemented under the Code of Federal Regulations, Title 42.

Consolidated Omnibus Budget Reconciliation Act (COBRA) Legislation passed to prevent inappropriate transfer or discharge of patients from one facility to another, commonly referred to as "dumping."

Continuing education units (CEUs) Credits earned by individuals when they attend an educational function. Organizations generally grant 1 CEU for each hour attended.

Credentialing The process followed by hospitals and other organizations for evaluating physicians to determine whether they should be granted admitting privileges.

Department of Health (DOH) Agency within each state that is involved in the state's health care initiatives, including promoting public health and health safety of all state residents through disease prevention and ensuring that quality medical care is provided.

Department of Health and Human Services (DHHS) Federal department responsible for health issues, including controlling the rising cost of health care, the health and welfare of various populations, occupational safety, and income security plans.

Emergency Medical Treatment and Labor Act (EMTALA) Legislation passed by Congress to ensure public access to emergency services regardless of ability to pay.

Federal False Claims Act Legislation passed to prevent overuse of services and uncover fraudulent activities in the Medicare and Medicaid programs.

Federal Register The official publication in which federal regulations and legal notices are published.

Health, Education, and Welfare (HEW) A governmental agency formed for the purpose of addressing issues related to health, education, and welfare of the people of the United States.

Health Information Management (HIM) A hospital department responsible for the organization, maintenance, production, storage, retention, dissemination, and security of patient information.

Health Insurance Portability and Accountability Act (HIPAA) Legislation implemented in phases from 1996 to 2009 to address several issues: continuity of health insurance, prevention and detection of fraud and abuse, limited coverage, access to long-term care, simplification of the administration of health insurance standards for the claims process, and protection of the privacy of health information.

Joint Commission on the Accreditation of Health Care Organizations (JCAHO) A National Commission formed in 1952 to develop guidelines for hospitals and other health care organizations. JCAHO changed its name to The Joint Commission (TJC) in 2007. TJC evaluates and accredits health care organizations based on establish standards of quality for operations and medical services.

Medicaid Federal program administered at the state level established under Title XIX of the SSA to provide health care benefits for medically indigent people.

Medicare Government program created under Title XVIII of the Social Security Act that provides health care benefits for medical services provided to individuals over age 65, the disabled, and other qualified individuals.

Occupational Safety and Health Administration (OSHA) Agency under the Department of Labor created under the OSHA Act for the purpose of developing standards and conducting site visits to determine compliance with safety standards.

Office of Inspector General (OIG) A federal agency under the DHHS that is responsible for protecting the integrity of DHHS programs, such as Medicare and Medicaid.

Patient Self-Determination Act (PDSA) Legislation passed in 1990 for the purpose of ensuring that individuals are informed of their rights regarding health care decisions. The act requires facilities to provide patients with information regarding a living will, durable power of attorney, and advanced directives.

Prospective Payment System (PPS) A reimbursement system implemented in 1983 as mandated under TEFRA for inpatient services provided to Medicare beneficiaries that provides a predetermined payment based on the patient's diagnosis and procedures performed.

Quality Improvement Organization (QIO) Organizations that contract with Medicare to conduct reviews to determine the appropriateness and medical necessity of services provided. IROs have full authority to deny reimbursement for health care services provided to Medicare patients if the services are deemed inappropriate IRO replaced Peer Review Organizations (PROs). Peer Review Organizations replaced the Professional Standard Review Organizations (PSRO).

Registered Health Information Technician (RHIT) Responsible for coding services and conditions provided by hospitals and verifying the completeness, accuracy, and proper entry of medical information into computer systems.

Tax Equity and Fiscal Responsibility Act (TEFRA) Legislation passed in 1982 that mandated a total restructuring of reimbursement methods used for Medicare services. One of the most significant changes was the implementation of the Prospective Payment System of reimbursement in 1983.

Chapter 3

Hospital Organizational Structure and Function

The purpose of this chapter is to provide an overview of the internal workings of a hospital. A review of the organizational structure and departmental functions will provide a basis for understanding how departments and personnel work together to accomplish organizational goals. A description of departmental roles and responsibilities will provide a greater understanding of how the internal network of a hospital functions to provide patient care services. We will then explore various services provided by the hospital and discuss the departments involved in providing those services.

Outline

Chapter Objectives

- Define terms, phrases, abbreviations, and acronyms related to hospital functions and departments.
- Discuss hospital organizational structures and how they are designed to contribute to the accomplishment of a hospital's goals and mission.
- Explain why organizational structures may vary.
- List and describe four categories of functions in a hospital.
- Describe functions performed by various departments.
- Discuss the importance of the Compliance Department in a hospital.
- Provide an explanation of how financial departments contribute to maintaining the financial stability of a hospital.
- Discuss the relationship among the Health Information Management (HIM) Department, medical record documentation, and submission of charges.
- Explain the purpose of medical record documentation and what significant information is maintained in the medical record.
- Identify and discuss three service levels where patient care services are rendered in a hospital.

Key Terms

Accounts receivable
Acute
Admission process
Ancillary services
Census
Clinical
Emergency Department (ED)
Health Information Management (HIM)
Health Information Systems
History and Physical (H&P)
Inpatient
Medical record documentation
Outpatient
Professional component
Technical component
Utilization Management (UM)

Acronyms and Abbreviations

ASC—ambulatory surgery center
CRNA—Certified Registered Nurse Anesthetist
ED—Emergency Department
EHR—Electronic Health Record
ER—Emergency Room
E/M—Evaluation and Management
HIM—Health Information Management
H&P—History and Physical
PA—Physician Assistant
PFS—Patient Financial Services
QA—Quality Assurance
UR—Utilization Review
UM—Utilization Management

INTRODUCTION

The purpose of this chapter is to provide an overview of a hospital's organizational structure and how a hospital functions. The complex network of personnel in a hospital is designed to contribute to the accomplishment of hospital goals. The mission of a hospital is to provide effective and efficient patient care. The survival of a hospital is directly related to carrying out the hospital mission and to maintaining a sound financial base. It is essential for personnel to understand how they contribute to the organization's mission. Billing and coding professionals play a significant role in maintaining a sound financial base through accurate coding and billing. Additionally, billing and coding personnel play an important role in ensuring that the hospital is in compliance with billing, coding, and documentation guidelines.

HOSPITAL ORGANIZATIONAL STRUCTURES

Hospital organizational structures have changed over time in response to new medical treatments, technologies, and government regulations. Various departments and specialized personnel work together to accomplish patient care tasks. Hospitals are required to operate in compliance with federal guidelines. Many departments in the hospital were created to ensure compliance with regulatory guidelines. For example, departments such as quality assurance and utilization management were developed as a direct result of the implementation of federal regulations relative to ensuring quality of patient care and assessing resources utilized in hospitals.

Organizational structures, department names, and functions vary from hospital to hospital. The hospital's organizational chart illustrates the complex network of a hospital. Figure 3-1 illustrates a sample organizational chart. It is important to remember that such charts vary according to each hospital's organizational structure.

Variations in organizational charts may be a result of the type of services offered. For example, some hospitals may not have a Satellite Development Department because they do not have satellite clinics. Clinical services provided vary based on the type of hospital. For example, a tertiary care center may have more specific clinical departments as a result of the highly specialized services provided. Variations may also be a result of the reporting structure of various departments. For example, the Health Information Management Department may report to the Finance Director, or the Compliance Department may report to the Operations Director. Despite the variations in hospital design, many of the departments and functions outlined below are consistent from hospital to hospital.

Hospital services are provided through the coordinated efforts of various hospital departments. Coding and billing personnel code medical records and process charges for hospital services. An understanding of hospital departments and services provided by each department will ensure that coding and billing functions for hospital services are performed accurately. The following is a review of the categories of hospital functions. Reference to the sample organizational chart in Figure 3-1 should be made during this review.

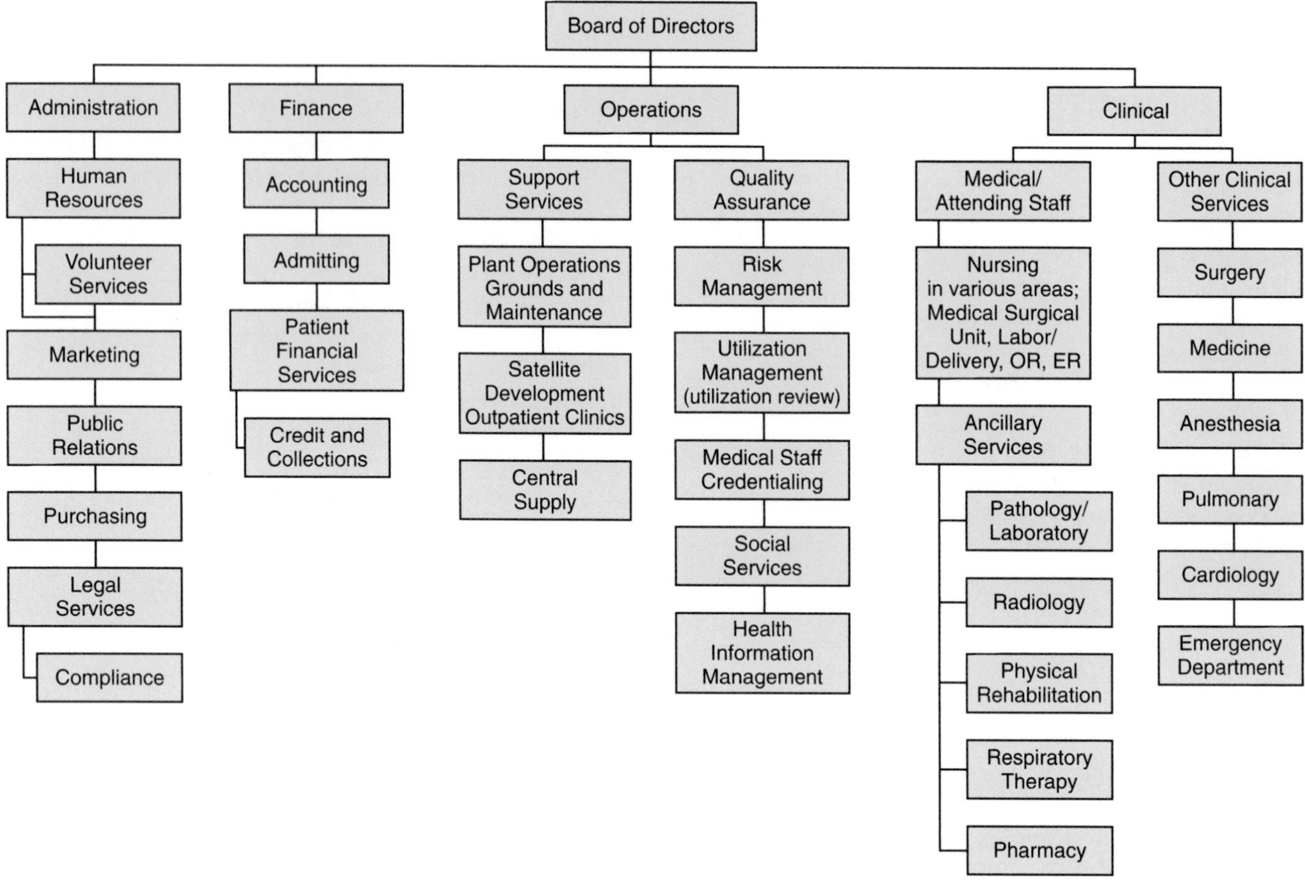

Figure 3-1 Sample hospital organizational chart.

HOSPITAL FUNCTIONS CATEGORIZED

An efficient organizational design is critical to accomplishing organizational goals. Performance of functions to reach organizational goals requires overall management. Management involves coordinating, supervising, and monitoring functions. Effective management design typically groups functions into like categories. This is referred to as departmentalization. Personnel, equipment, and space are selected based on specific needs for each functional category.

As discussed earlier in this chapter, hospital mission statements outline their major purpose, which is to provide effective and efficient patient care services (Figure 3-2). To fulfill this mission, hospitals must maintain a sound financial base. Tasks required to accomplish the hospital's mission and maintain a sound financial base are distributed in a methodical manner among various departments.

Hospital functions are generally categorized according to a grouping of specific tasks. These tasks can generally be categorized into four major areas of functions: Administrative, Financial, Operational, and Clinical (Figure 3-3).

BOX 3-1 ▪ KEY POINTS

Efficient Organizational Design

Departmentalization (groups functions into like categories):

- Administrative
- Financial
- Operational
- Clinical

Community General Hospital

Mission Statement

To provide the highest quality care to the members of our community and distant communities effectively and efficiently with compassion, integrity, and kindness through maintaining excellence in health care professions

Figure 3-2 Hospital functional statement.

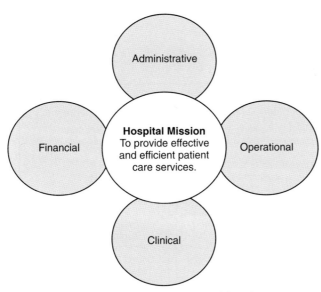

Figure 3-3 Categories of hospital functions.

Administrative

Administrative functions involve various tasks related to the direction and management of services to support the provision of patient care. Administrative functions are relative to the various areas of business including human resources, marketing, public relations, purchasing, and legal services.

Financial

Financial functions involve the overall management of the hospital's finances. Financial management involves functions such as planning, organizing, and controlling the hospital's finances including income and expenses of the organization. Functions relating to financial management include accounting, admitting, patient financial services, and credit and collections.

Operational

Operational functions entail tasks related to the operation and physical environment of the hospital. Some of the functions in operations include support services, plant operations, satellite development, quality assurance, risk management, utilization management, medical staff credentialing, social services, and health information management.

Clinical

Clinical functions consist of various patient care tasks performed by personnel in specialized departments. Clinical personnel in each department are trained and qualified to perform specific patient care services such as nursing, radiology, pathology/laboratory, physical rehabilitation, and social services. Specialized personnel such as nurses, radiology or pathology/laboratory technicians, physical therapists, and social workers perform clinical functions. Clinical departments include medical staff, nursing, surgery, medicine, anesthesia, pulmonary, cardiology, emergency, and ancillary service departments such as radiology and pathology/laboratory.

The internal hospital system consists of various departments and personnel within those departments, working together to achieve patient care objectives. Departments are designed based on specialized tasks that are required. Each department performs specific functions relative to administration, finance, operations, and clinical care. Staff and equipment needs are determined based on the area of specialization. Roles and responsibilities related to daily management, operation, finance, and provision of clinical services are departmentalized according to each of the four categories.

BOX 3-2 ■ KEY POINTS

Categories of Hospital Functions

Hospital Administrative Functions

Direction and management of services to support the provision of patient care including human resource management, marketing, public relations, purchasing, and legal issues.

Hospital Financial Functions

Overall management (planning, organization, and control) of hospital finances, including accounting, admitting, patient financial services, and credit and collections.

Hospital Operational Functions

Tasks related to the operation and physical environment of the hospital including support services, plant operations, satellite development, quality assurance, utilization management, medical staff credentialing, and social services.

Hospital Clinical Functions

Patient care tasks performed by clinical personnel in specialized departments including Nursing, Radiology, Pathology/Laboratory, Physical Rehabilitation, and Social Services.

DEPARTMENTAL FUNCTIONS

Hospital departments are developed to perform specialized administrative, financial, operational, and clinical tasks. To gain an understanding of how the hospital functions, it is necessary to look at how tasks are distributed into functional areas. A review of some of the most common departmental functions for each of the four categories is outlined in this section (Figure 3-4). Although this is not a complete review of all functions, it will provide a basic understanding of the

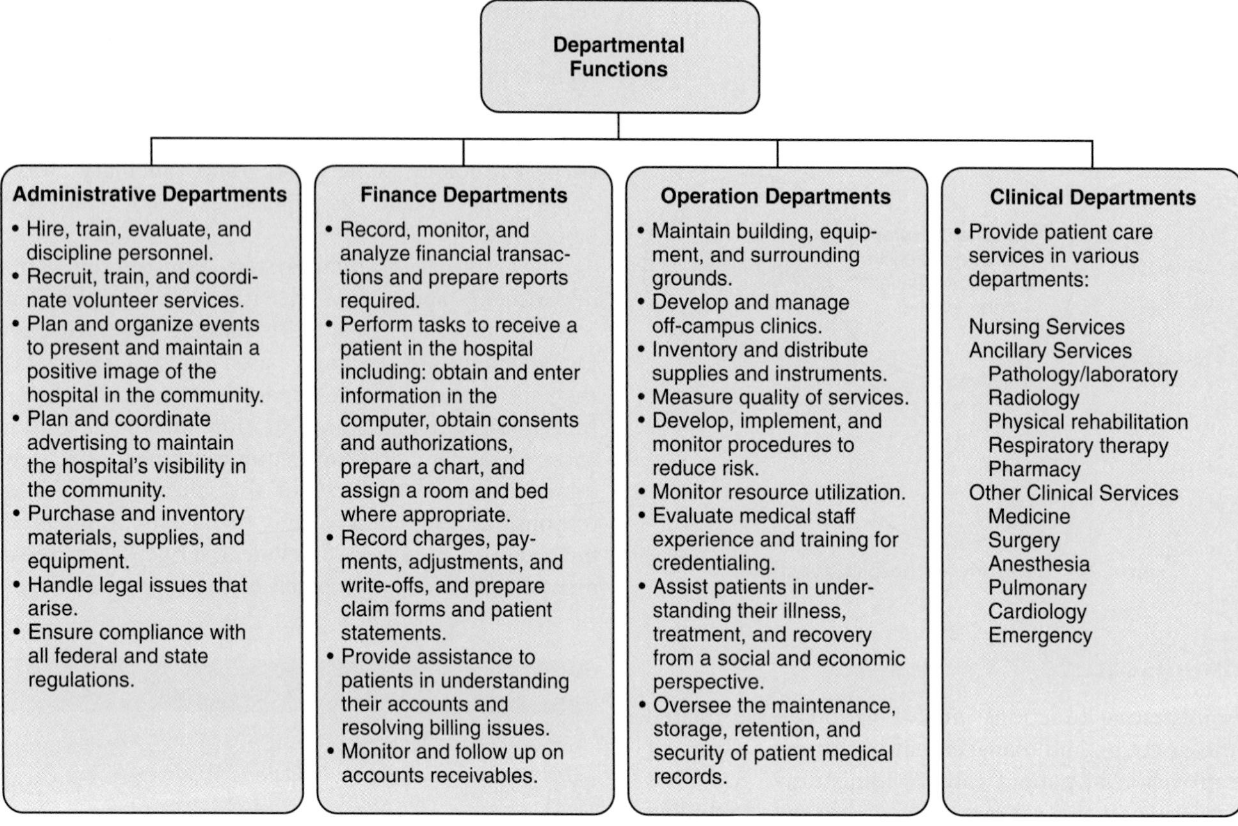

Departmental Functions
Administrative Departments
• Hire, train, evaluate, and discipline personnel.
• Recruit, train, and coordinate volunteer services.
• Plan and organize events to present and maintain a positive image of the hospital in the community.
• Plan and coordinate advertising to maintain the hospital's visibility in the community.
• Purchase and inventory materials, supplies, and equipment.
• Handle legal issues that arise.
• Ensure compliance with all federal and state regulations.
Finance Departments
• Record, monitor, and analyze financial transactions and prepare reports required.
• Perform tasks to receive a patient in the hospital including: obtain and enter information in the computer, obtain consents and authorizations, prepare a chart, and assign a room and bed where appropriate.
• Record charges, payments, adjustments, and write-offs, and prepare claim forms and patient statements.
• Provide assistance to patients in understanding their accounts and resolving billing issues.
• Monitor and follow up on accounts receivables.
Operation Departments
• Maintain building, equipment, and surrounding grounds.
• Develop and manage off-campus clinics.
• Inventory and distribute supplies and instruments.
• Measure quality of services.
• Develop, implement, and monitor procedures to reduce risk.
• Monitor resource utilization.
• Evaluate medical staff experience and training for credentialing.
• Assist patients in understanding their illness, treatment, and recovery from a social and economic perspective.
• Oversee the maintenance, storage, retention, and security of patient medical records.
Clinical Departments
• Provide patient care services in various departments:
Nursing Services
Ancillary Services
Pathology/laboratory
Radiology
Physical rehabilitation
Respiratory therapy
Pharmacy
Other Clinical Services
Medicine
Surgery
Anesthesia
Pulmonary
Cardiology
Emergency

Figure 3-4 Administrative, Financial, Operational, and Clinical departmental functions.

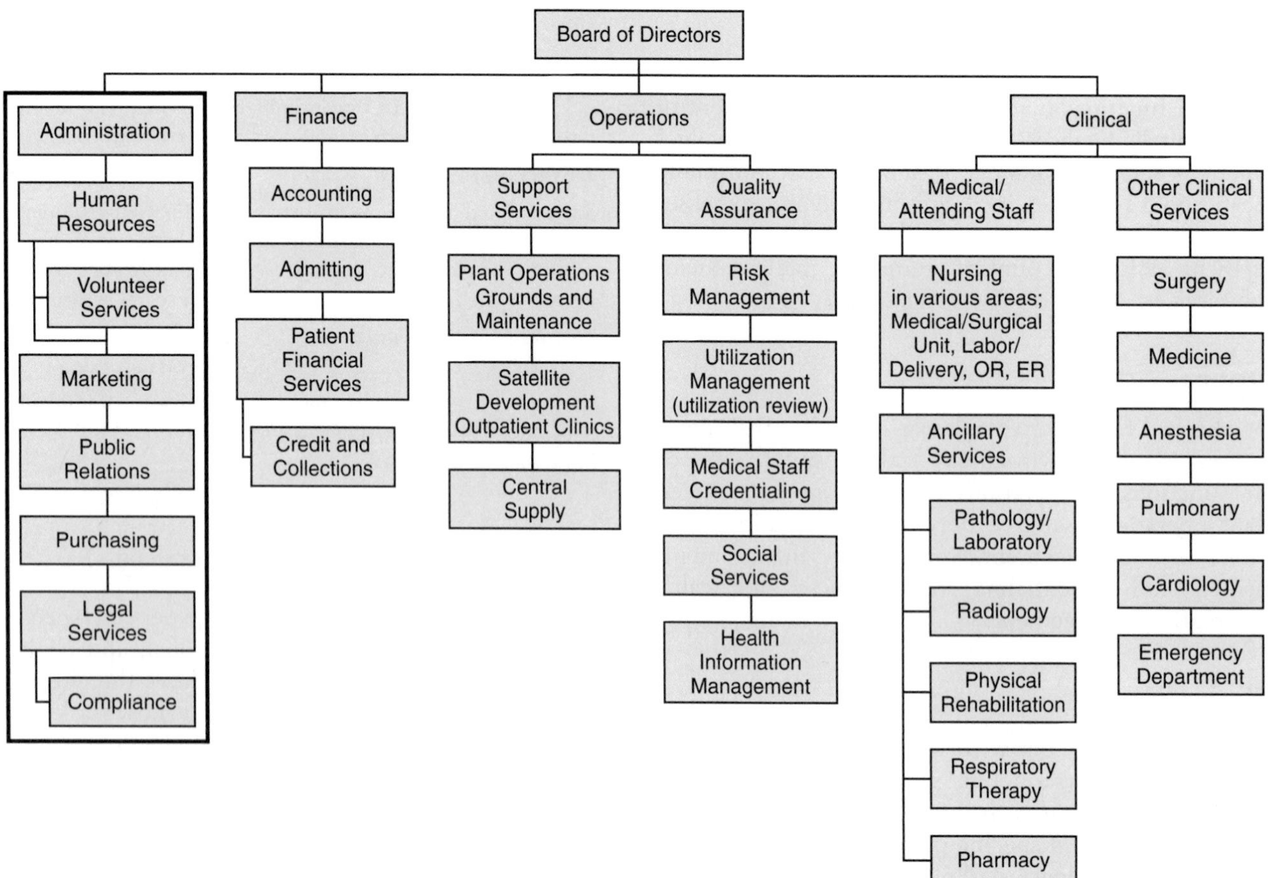

Figure 3-5 Administrative departments.

TEST YOUR *Knowledge* BOX 3-1

HOSPITAL ORGANIZATIONAL STRUCTURE; HOSPITAL FUNCTIONS CATEGORIZED

1. Explain the relationship between a hospital's organizational structure and its ability to achieve its mission.

2. List two reasons why hospital organizational structures may vary.

3. Financial functions are critical to the hospital's maintenance of a sound financial base. Discuss the role that billing and coding professionals play in maintaining a sound financial base.

4. Hospital billing and coding professionals also play an important role in ensuring ______________ with ______________ , ______________, and ______________ guidelines.

5. Provide an outline of the four categories of hospital functions.

6. List the category of functions that relates to the direction and management of services to support the provision of patient care.

7. An efficient organizational design typically groups functions into like categories. This is referred to as ______________.

8. State which function category relates to planning, organizing, and controlling finances.

9. Describe clinical functions within a hospital.

10. Legal functions may be found under what functional category on an organizational chart?

administrative, financial, operational, and clinical functions required for the hospital to provide patient care services and maintain financial stability.

Administrative Functions

Administrative functions involve the coordination and management of various tasks required to provide patient care services such as recruitment and management of personnel and volunteer services, advertising and public relations, purchasing and inventory of supplies, materials, and equipment, and various legal tasks including compliance. The following administrative departments are assigned responsibility for such functions: Human Resources, Marketing, Public Relations, Purchasing, and Legal Services (Figure 3-5).

Human Resources Department

The Human Resources Department is responsible for the overall management of personnel. This department develops policies and procedures regarding all aspects of personnel management, including recruitment, training, and evaluation of personnel. It is also responsible for staff development, benefit and compensation management, and development of performance appraisal systems.

Volunteer Services

Hospitals very often have individuals who volunteer within the hospital. Functions performed by volunteers may include greeting patients, escorting patients, and other supportive tasks. The Human Resources Department is responsible for the volunteer services function, which involves recruiting, training, and coordinating volunteer staff.

Marketing Department

The Marketing Department is responsible for the marketing efforts required to maintain visibility of the hospital in the community. Hospitals that are more visible will generally receive more patient referrals from individuals, medical professionals, and businesses. Marketing efforts may include advertising, planning, and coordinating community events such as a health fair or a workshop on diabetes.

Public Relations Department

The Public Relations Department is responsible for presenting and maintaining a positive image of the hospital within the community. Public relations personnel are involved in planning and organizing various community events sponsored by the hospital.

Purchasing Department

The Purchasing Department is responsible for the purchase and inventory of all items and services required by the hospital. Scheduled maintenance of equipment is often a function of purchasing as well. The Purchasing Department is sometimes referred to as Material Management.

Legal Department

The Legal Department is responsible for all legal issues that arise within the hospital. Legal issues include malpractice, contracts, and compliance with all federal and state regulations. To ensure compliance with guidelines, many hospitals have a Compliance Department to oversee the compliance program.

Compliance

As discussed in Chapter 2, hospitals are required to comply with various federal and state regulations. To ensure compliance with all regulations, many hospitals develop and implement a compliance program, which contains details regarding how the hospital will ensure compliance. Compliance will be discussed at length in Chapter 14.

Financial Functions

Hospital financial functions involve the overall management of the hospital's finances. The development and monitoring of budgets, monitoring of income and expenses, analyzing financial reports, and negotiating contracts are a few of the functions required. The departments responsible for the financial aspects of the hospital include Accounting, Admitting, Patient Financial Services, and Credit and Collections (Figure 3-6).

Accounting Department

The Accounting Department is responsible for recording, monitoring, and analyzing financial transactions. Accounting includes posting to the general ledger, accounts payable, payroll, cost accounting, and preparation of cost reports.

Admitting Department

The Admitting Department is responsible for the admission process. The **admission process** involves all tasks required to receive a patient in the hospital, including obtaining demographic, insurance, and medical information and entering the data into the computer system (Figure 3-7). Appropriate consents, authorizations, and other required information such as an advance beneficiary notice are also obtained during the admission process. Personnel in the admitting department perform other functions such as preparing the patient's chart, assigning a room and bed, and updating the hospital census. **Census** is an inventory of rooms available in the hospital and the patients assigned to those rooms (Figure 3-8).

Patient Financial Services (PFS) Department

PFS is commonly referred to as Patient Accounts or the Business Office. The PFS Department is responsible for recording patient transactions such as charges, payments, adjustments, and write-offs. The business office prepares insurance claim forms and patient statements. Personnel in this department also assist patients in understanding their account and resolving billing issues.

BOX 3-3 ■ KEY POINTS

Functions of Patient Financial Services

Record Patient Transactions

- Charges, payments, adjustments, and write-offs

Prepare Charges for Submission

- Patient statements
- Claim form CMS-1450 (UB-04)
- Claim form CMS-1500

Credit and Collections Department

The Credit and Collections Department is responsible for the follow-up on outstanding accounts. The term commonly used to describe these accounts is accounts

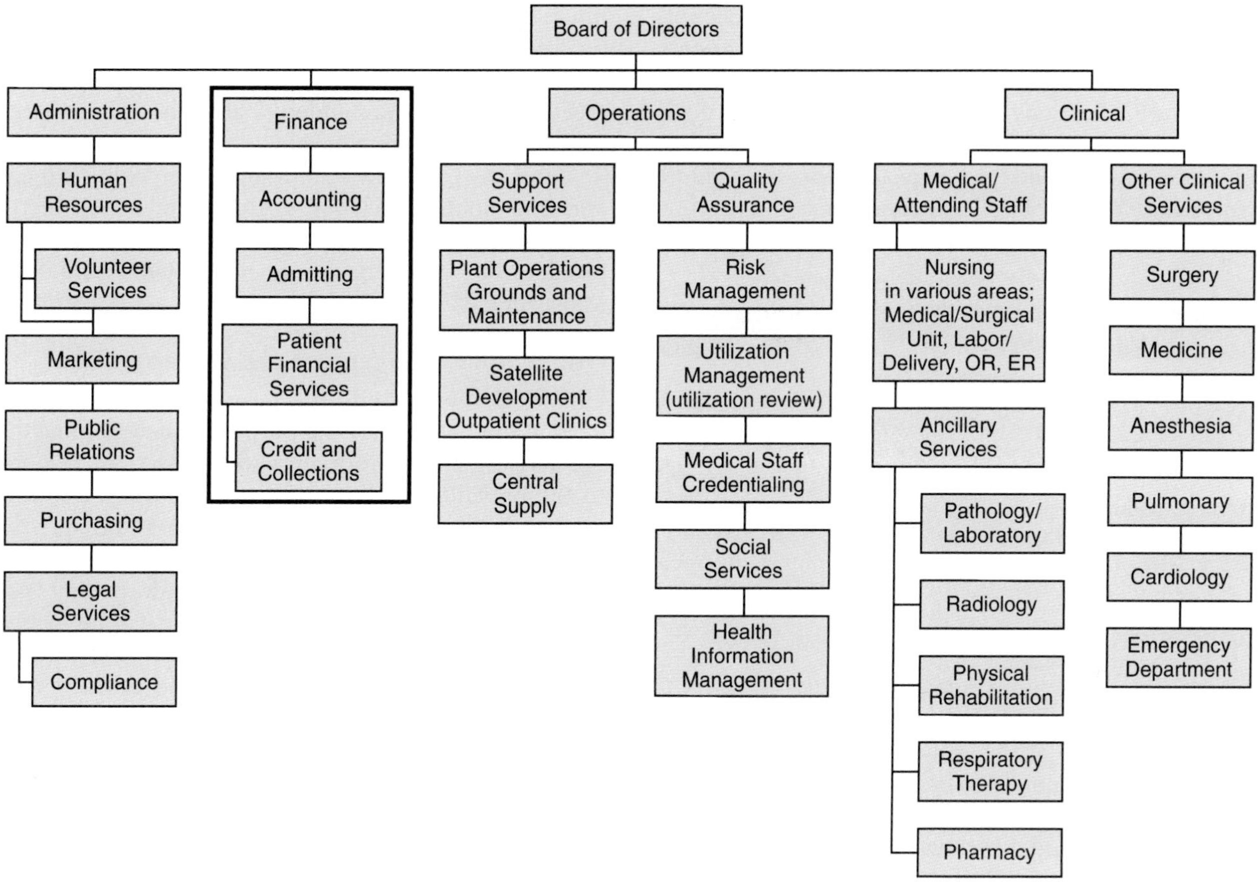

- Board of Directors
  - Administration
    - Human Resources
      - Volunteer Services
    - Marketing
    - Public Relations
    - Purchasing
    - Legal Services
      - Compliance
  - Finance
    - Accounting
    - Admitting
    - Patient Financial Services
      - Credit and Collections
  - Operations
    - Support Services
      - Plant Operations Grounds and Maintenance
      - Satellite Development Outpatient Clinics
      - Central Supply
    - Quality Assurance
      - Risk Management
      - Utilization Management (utilization review)
      - Medical Staff Credentialing
      - Social Services
      - Health Information Management
  - Clinical
    - Medical/ Attending Staff
      - Nursing in various areas; Medical/Surgical Unit, Labor/ Delivery, OR, ER
      - Ancillary Services
        - Pathology/ Laboratory
        - Radiology
        - Physical Rehabilitation
        - Respiratory Therapy
        - Pharmacy
    - Other Clinical Services
      - Surgery
      - Medicine
      - Anesthesia
      - Pulmonary
      - Cardiology
      - Emergency Department

Figure 3-6 Finance departments.

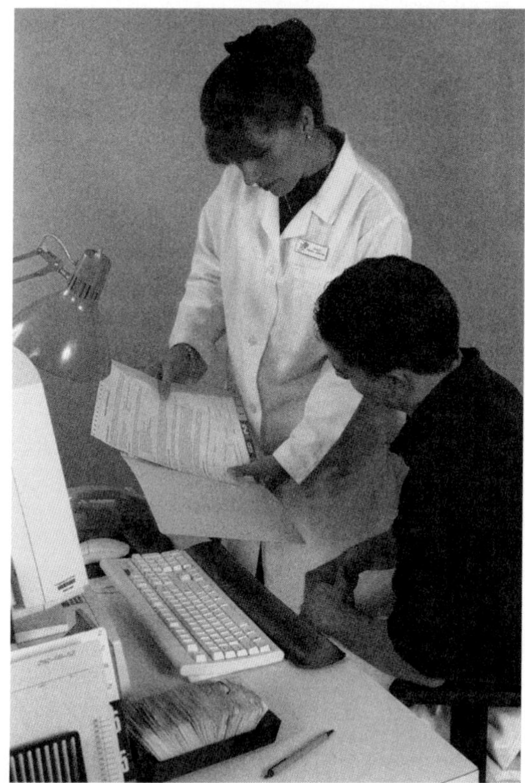

Figure 3-7 The admission process includes obtaining information and registration and involves entering the data into the computer system.

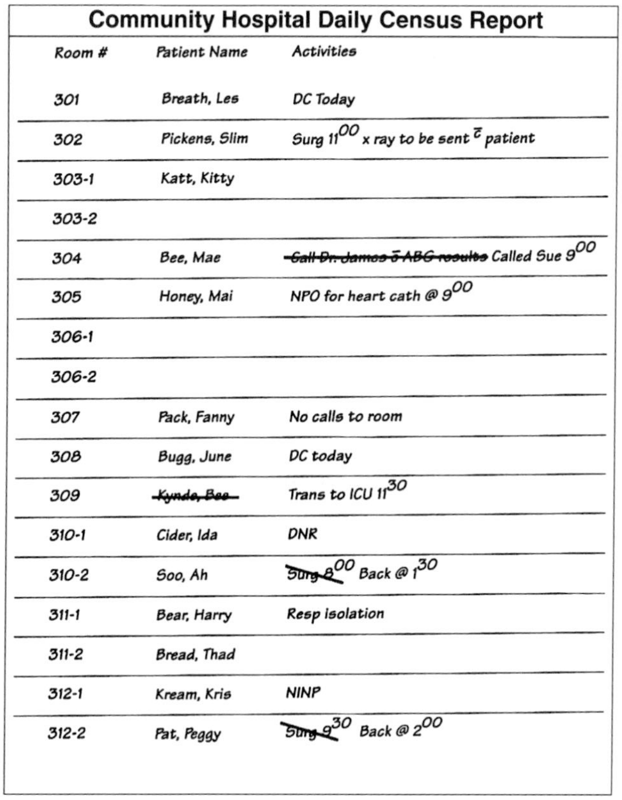

Community Hospital Daily Census Report

Room #	Patient Name	Activities
301	Breath, Les	DC Today
302	Pickens, Slim	Surg 11^{00} x ray to be sent c̄ patient
303-1	Katt, Kitty	
303-2		
304	Bee, Mae	~~Call Dr. James c̄ ABG results~~ Called Sue 9^{00}
305	Honey, Mai	NPO for heart cath @ 9^{00}
306-1		
306-2		
307	Pack, Fanny	No calls to room
308	Bugg, June	DC today
309	~~Kynde, Bee~~	Trans to ICU 11^{30}
310-1	Cider, Ida	DNR
310-2	Soo, Ah	~~Surg 8^{00}~~ Back @ 1^{30}
311-1	Bear, Harry	Resp isolation
311-2	Bread, Thad	
312-1	Kream, Kris	NINP
312-2	Pat, Peggy	~~Surg 9^{30}~~ Back @ 2^{00}

Figure 3-8 Hospital daily census report. *(Modified from Brooks ML, Gillingham ET:* Health unit coordinating, *ed 5, St Louis, 2004, Saunders.)*

receivable. **Accounts receivable** are outstanding accounts in which money is owed to the hospital by patients, insurance companies, or government programs. The Credit and Collections Department is also involved in resolving billing issues through research, communication with payers, and the appeals process. A more involved discussion of collections and accounts receivable management will follow later in Chapter 6.

BOX 3-4 ■ KEY POINTS

Functions of Credit and Collections

Follow up on accounts receivable (outstanding accounts in which money is owed to the hospital by patients, insurance companies, and other payers)

Resolve billing issues through research, communications with payers, and the appeals process

Operational Functions

Operational functions include various tasks necessary to maintain consistent and efficient operations of the hospital by ensuring that the grounds, building, and equipment are maintained. Departments that perform operational functions are Support Services, Plant Operations, Grounds and Maintenance, Satellite Development Outpatient Clinics, Central Supply, Quality Assurance, Risk Management, Utilization Management, Medical Staff Credentialing, Social Services, and Health Information Management (Figure 3-9).

Plant Operations Department

The Plant Operations Department is responsible for maintenance of the hospital building, equipment, and grounds to ensure that the working environment is clean and safe. Plant operations functions may include repairs to the building, air conditioning, heating, or other systems.

Satellite Development Department

The Satellite Development Department identifies and develops areas for various types of outpatient services to be performed off the facility's main campus. Many hospitals have satellite campuses that include primary care offices, urgent care center, walk-in clinic, imaging center, or ambulatory surgery center.

Central Supply Department

The Central Supply Department is responsible for the inventory and distribution of various clinical supplies and instruments required throughout the hospital.

Quality Assurance (QA) Department

The QA Department is designed to monitor and improve the quality of service, product, or process. QA functions help hospitals identify areas that do not meet specified standards and implement actions to improve standards in those areas. QA measures are required to meet accreditation standards and the participation requirements of many payers.

The QA, UM, and Risk Management Departments perform functions relative to quality of care, effective resource utilization, and risk management. Table 3-1 provides a comparison of QA, UM, and Risk Management.

Utilization Management (UM) Department

UM focuses on monitoring health care resources utilized in the hospital for the purpose of determining that the services are appropriate and necessary in response to the patient's condition, thereby ensuring maximum resource utilization. The hospital's goal is to ensure that facilities and resources, both human and nonhuman, are used maximally but consistently with patient care needs. UM is a planned, systematic review of the patient in a health care facility against patient criteria for admission, interval stays, and discharge. The primary functions of UM are utilization review, case management, and discharge planning (Table 3-1).

BOX 3-5 ■ KEY POINTS

Functions of Quality Assurance

Designed to monitor and improve the quality of patient care services, products, or processes

Helps hospitals to identify areas that do not meet specified standards and to implement actions to improve standards in those areas

BOX 3-6 ■ KEY POINTS

Functions of UM

Focus on monitoring health care resources utilized in the hospital for the purpose of ensuring maximum resource utilization

Functions

- Utilization review (UR)
- Case management
- Discharge planning

Utilization Review (UR)

UR involves activities intended to ensure that all health services provided to a patient are medically necessary and are provided in the most appropriate setting. The UR process requires assessment of medical necessity for a patient case at the time of admission, during the

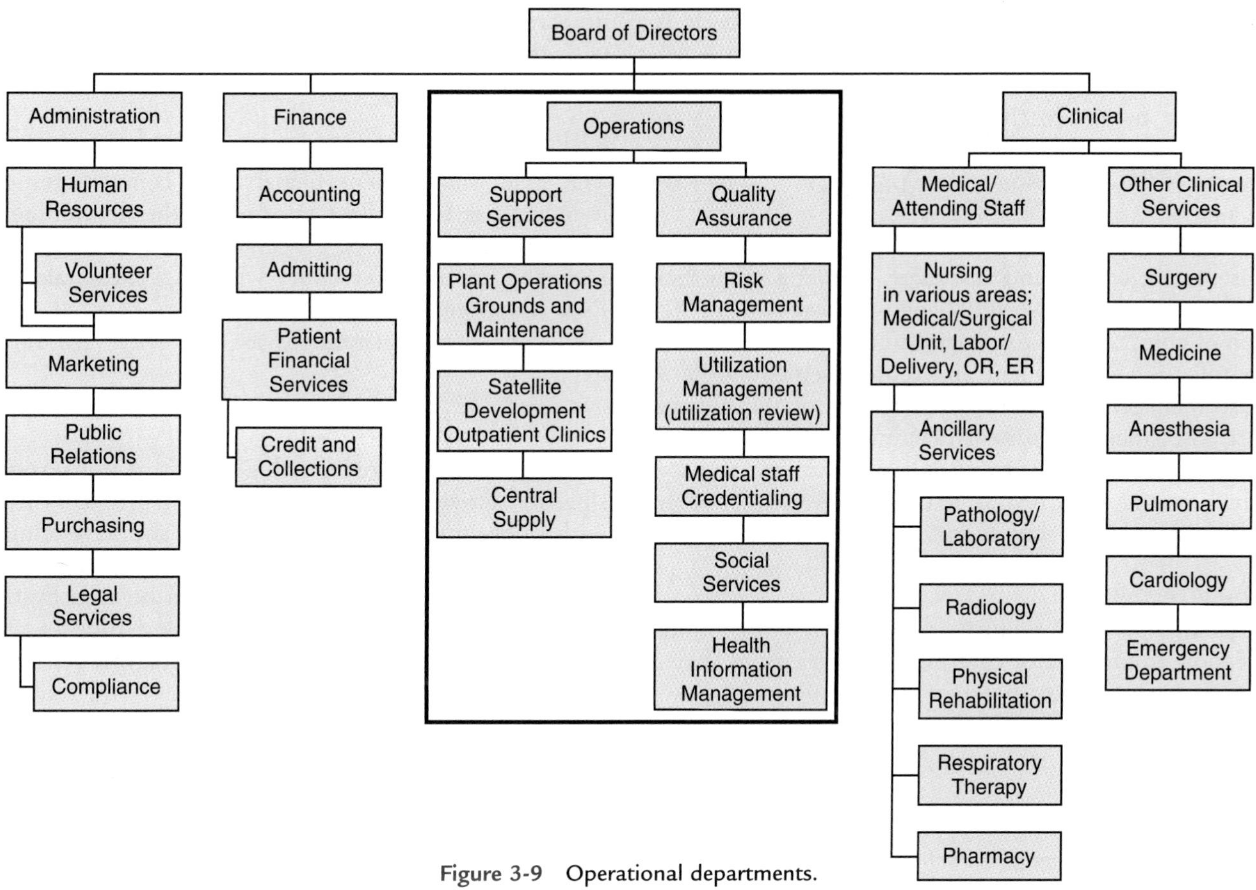

Figure 3-9 Operational departments.

TABLE 3-1 Comparison of the QA, UM, and Risk Management Departments

	Quality Assurance	Utilization Management	Risk Management
Purpose	Improve quality of care and services	Efficient and effective use of resources	Avoid or manage financial liability
Reference population	Groups of similar cases	Individual patients	Individual patients, employees, visitors, and professional staff
Time frame/ process employed	Retrospective/criterion-referenced documentation review	Concurrent individual patient needs/characteristics compared with criteria to determine need for health care services	Concurrent/review causes of single events or occurrences and patterns of events
Tools/techniques	Statistical analysis	Discharge planning, case management	Occurrence screening
Primary question(s)	Can the outcome of care or service be improved?	Can the necessary treatment or service be provided elsewhere more cost effectively or equally effectively using a less invasive approach?	Could the occurrence have been prevented? Can we minimize the loss?
Actions	Revise policies, procedures, or processes	Approve or deny patient access to or payment for diagnostic services and clinical treatments	Revise processes, change environment, allocate financial resources
Key external driver	Accrediting and regulatory agencies, managed care organizations, and other payers	Managed care organizations and other payers	Liability insurers

From Abdelhak M, Grostick S, Hanken MA, Jacobs E (editors): Health information: management of a strategic resource, *ed 2, St Louis, 2001, Saunders.*

patient stay, or when the patient is discharged. It is critical for the hospital to have a UR process in order to meet payer requirements, such as preadmission certifications to ensure that the appropriate reimbursement is received for the patient case. Figure 3-10 illustrates the utilization review process.

Case Management

Case management and discharge planning are other primary functions of UM designed to ensure the provision of comprehensive and continuous services and the coordination of payment and reimbursement of care. Case management involves the review of the patient care assessment, treatment planning, referral, and follow-up. Case management is a concurrent activity, which means that review is conducted at admission, during the patient stay, and at discharge.

Discharge Planning

Discharge planning requires coordination and communication among health care providers to ensure that a patient has a planned program of continuing or follow-up care at discharge. Hospital discharge planners work with the patient and family to ensure that all postdischarge needs are met.

Risk Management Department

The Risk Management Department concentrates on reducing risk to the hospital through the development and implementation of procedures designed to minimize the potential for injury within the hospital. The Risk Management Department is also charged with addressing liability situations as they arise (see Table 3-1).

Medical Staff Credentialing Department

The Medical Staff Credentialing Department is responsible for activities required to evaluate providers who wish to become a part of the hospital and have admitting privileges. Privileges define the scope of patient services and types of patients that can be seen by the health care provider. The credentialing process and required documentation vary by hospital but generally include a review of licensing, education and training,

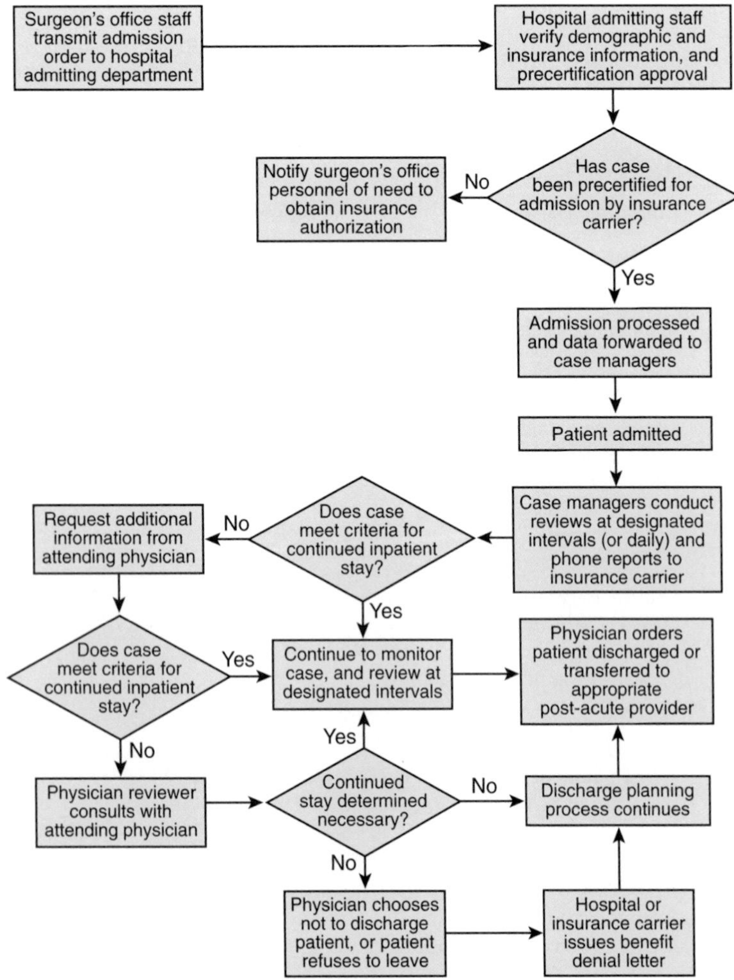

Figure 3-10 Utilization review process. *(Courtesy Patrice Spath, B.A., RHIT, Healthcare Quality Specialist, Forest Grove, Ore. Used with permission.)*

clinical competence, the individual's health status, and liability insurance coverage. The process is very involved, as it requires verification of all the information submitted.

BOX 3-7 ■ KEY POINTS

Risk Management

Concentration on reducing risk to the hospital
Develop and implement procedures designed to minimize the potential for injury within the hospital
Address liability situations as they arise

BOX 3-8 ■ KEY POINTS

Medical Staff Credentialing

Process required to evaluate providers who wish to become part of the hospital and/or have admitting privileges
Privileges define the scope of patient services and types of patients that can be seen by the health care provider
Required documentation includes information regarding licensing, education, and training, clinical competence, an individual's health status, and liability insurance coverage

Social Services Department

The Social Services Department consists of licensed social workers and other personnel involved with helping patients and family members understand their illness, treatment, and recovery from a social and economic perspective. Social Services are generally involved in the discharge planning process. They are responsible for coordinating the medical and financial resources required for the patient when discharged.

Health Information Management (HIM) Department

The **HIM**, or Medical Records Department, is responsible for the organization, maintenance, production, storage, retention, dissemination, and security of patient health information. Patient records include various documents relative to the patient's diagnosis and treatment. Patient records are legal documents, and the confidentiality and security of these records is a critical function of HIM. This department also monitors documentation to ensure that documentation standards are met throughout the hospital. To achieve this goal, HIM may be involved in the development and revision of hospital forms. Health information is stored in the patient's medical record and on a computer system designed for hospital patient, medical, and billing information and is called **health information systems**.

The medical record contains information regarding the patient's condition, treatment, and progress required to support charges submitted to various payers. This information is referred to as **medical record documentation**. Documentation is maintained in a chart called the medical record. An electronic version of the patient medical record is called the electronic health record (EHR). The chart is organized in sections that contain relative forms and notes. The forms and notes found in a patient chart are illustrated in Figure 3-11.

HIM functions also include transcribing medical and surgical notes, coding diagnoses, procedures, and items, releasing health information, retrieving and storing medical information, managing databases, and filing information. These functions are vital to the provision of effective and efficient patient care services and to preparing charges for submission to payers for reimbursement. Personnel in HIM include certified coders whose responsibilities include coding of patient medical records, charge description master maintenance, and auditing.

All the administrative, financial, and operational functions outlined above are a necessary part of providing patient care in a hospital setting. These functions are not directly billed to patients or third-party payers.

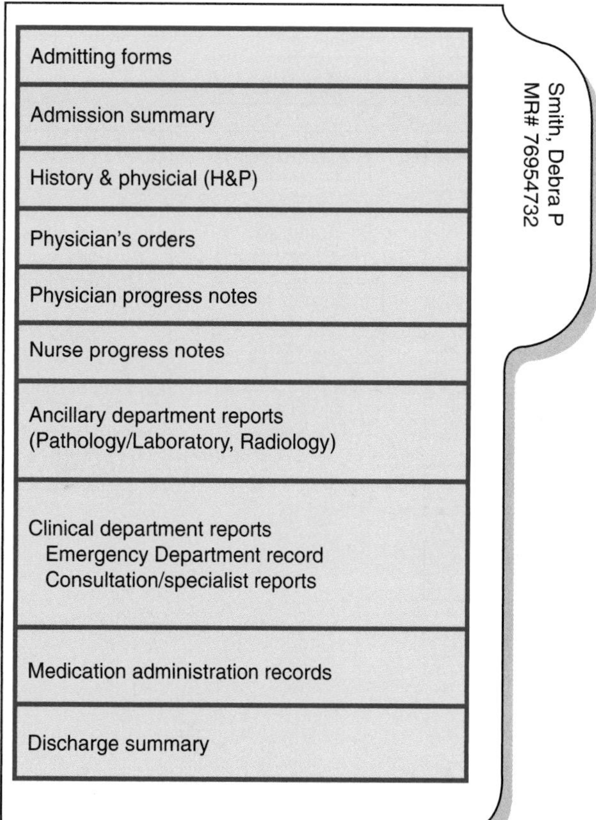

Figure 3-11 Various forms and reports found in the patient's medical record.

The hospital pricing structure for billable patient care services is determined by taking into account the cost of overhead for the above functions.

> **BOX 3-9 ■ KEY POINTS**
>
> **Functions of Health Information Management (HIM)**
>
> Tasks required for the organization, maintenance, production, storage, retention, dissemination, and security of patient health information, including:
> - Transcribing medical and surgical notes
> - Coding diagnoses, procedures, and items
> - Releasing health information
> - Retrieving and storing medical information
> - Managing databases
> - Filing information

Clinical Functions

Clinical functions include various tasks related to patient care services that are provided with the assistance of clinical departments such as nursing, ancillary, and other clinical departments (Figure 3-12).

Nursing Department

The Nursing Department is responsible for the provision of nursing services. Nursing services are provided to patients in a variety of clinical settings in the hospital such as the Medical/Surgical Unit, Labor and Delivery, Operating Room, and Emergency Department. Patient care services provided by nursing staff include a variety of tasks, such as assessment and monitoring of patients and administering various clinical therapies. Nurses are trained and licensed according to specific educational and competence standards. Nursing services within a hospital are considered part of the inpatient or outpatient services provided by the hospital and therefore are not separately billable to patients or third-party payers.

Ancillary Departments

Various departments within the hospital provide ancillary services. **Ancillary services** are supportive services required to diagnose and treat patients. These services

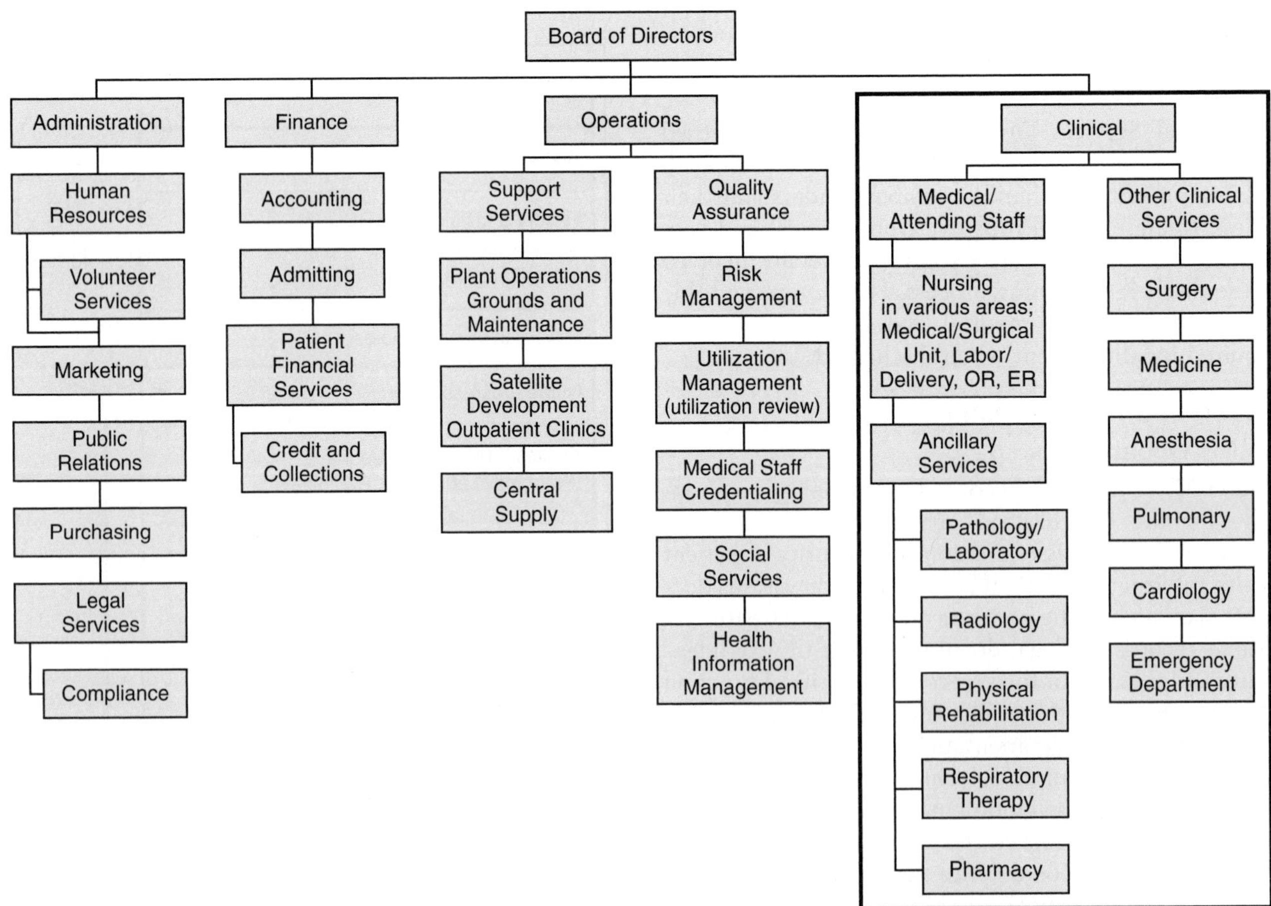

Figure 3-12 Clinical departments.

are the income-producing services of the hospital and they are billed to patients and third party payers. Departments that provide ancillary services are Pathology/Laboratory, Radiology, Physical Rehabilitation, Respiratory Therapy, and Pharmacy, and they are referred to as ancillary departments.

Pathology/Laboratory Department

The Pathology/Laboratory Department provides diagnostic and therapeutic services that are performed utilizing various techniques to study body fluids and tissue. Clinical professionals who are trained to utilize medical laboratory technology under the supervision of a pathologist provide these services. Specimens can be collected at the hospital or at various provider locations in the community. The specimens collected by providers in the community may be sent to the hospital for processing.

BOX 3-10 ■ KEY POINTS

Clinical Department Functions

Tasks required to provide patient care services:

- Nursing services
- Ancillary services: Pathology/Laboratory, Radiology, Physical Rehabilitation, Respiratory Therapy, Pharmacy
- Other clinical services: Medicine, Surgery, Anesthesia, Pulmonary, Cardiology, Emergency

Radiology Department

Radiology is commonly referred to as diagnostic and therapeutic imaging. Radiology procedures are diagnostic and therapeutic services usually performed by technicians using various radiology equipment and techniques (Figure 3-13). The hospital can bill for the **technical component** of a radiology procedure, which represents the overhead utilized in performing the service, such as the technician, supplies, materials, and equipment. The **professional component** of a radiology procedure represents the physician's work in performing the service, such as reading and interpretation of a radiology film. The reading and interpretation of a radiology procedure is not billed by the hospital unless the radiologist is employed by or under contract with the hospital.

Physical Rehabilitation Department

Physical rehabilitation services involve diagnosis and treatment of conditions requiring restoration of certain functions or training to assist the patient in dealing with certain disabilities. Physical rehabilitation includes physical therapy, occupational therapy, and speech therapy. Licensed therapists perform services in these areas (Figure 3-14).

BOX 3-11 ■ KEY POINTS

Technical versus Professional Components

Technical Component

The portion of a procedure that represents the overhead utilized in performing the service, such as the technician, supplies, materials, and equipment

- Billed by the facility where the procedure was performed

Professional Component

The portion of a procedure that represents the physician's work in performing the service, such as reading and interpretation of a radiology film

- Billed by the physician who performed the procedure

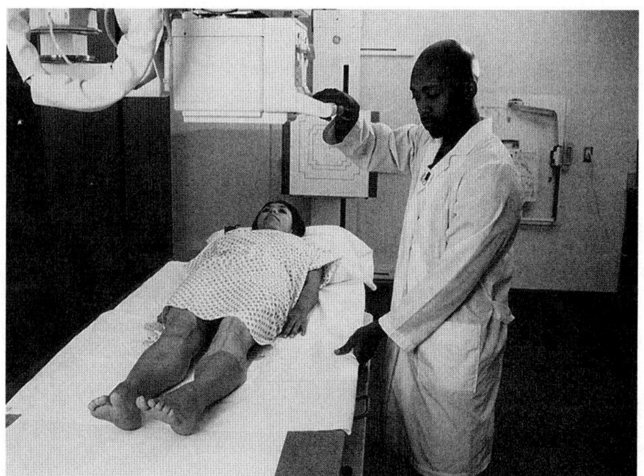

Figure 3-13 Radiology procedures are performed utilizing various equipment and techniques. *(From Bontrager KL, Lampignano JP: Textbook of radiographic positioning and related anatomy, ed 6, St Louis, 2005, Mosby.)*

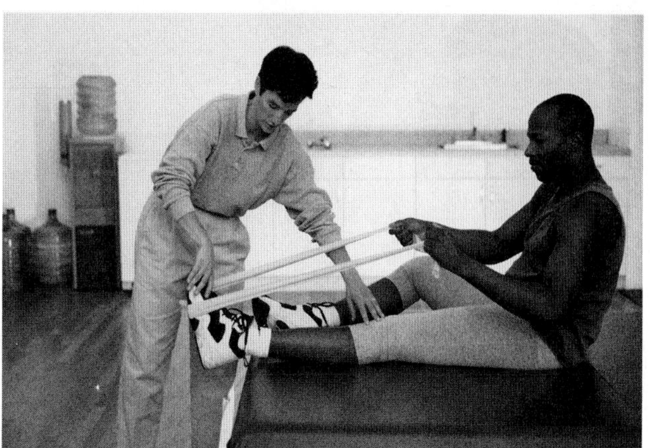

Figure 3-14 Physical rehabilitation includes physical, occupational, and speech therapy.

- *Physical therapy* involves various treatments to assist the patient in restoring range of motion, flexibility, and strength.
- *Occupational therapy* provides a patient with retraining for activities of daily living such as bathing and dressing.
- *Speech therapy* assists the patient with communication deficiencies.

Respiratory Therapy Department

The Respiratory Therapy Department provides various services to patients who have difficulty breathing because of illness. Services involve both diagnosis and treatment and are performed by licensed respiratory therapists.

Pharmacy Department

Pharmacy Department services involve maintaining, preparing and dispensing medications (Figure 3-15). Medications are distributed to various nursing units within the hospital for administration to patients. Documentation regarding dose and route of administration is provided. Pharmacy services are provided under the supervision of a licensed pharmacist.

Clinical Departments

Various clinical departments within the hospital perform diagnostic, therapeutic, palliative, and preventive services to patients.

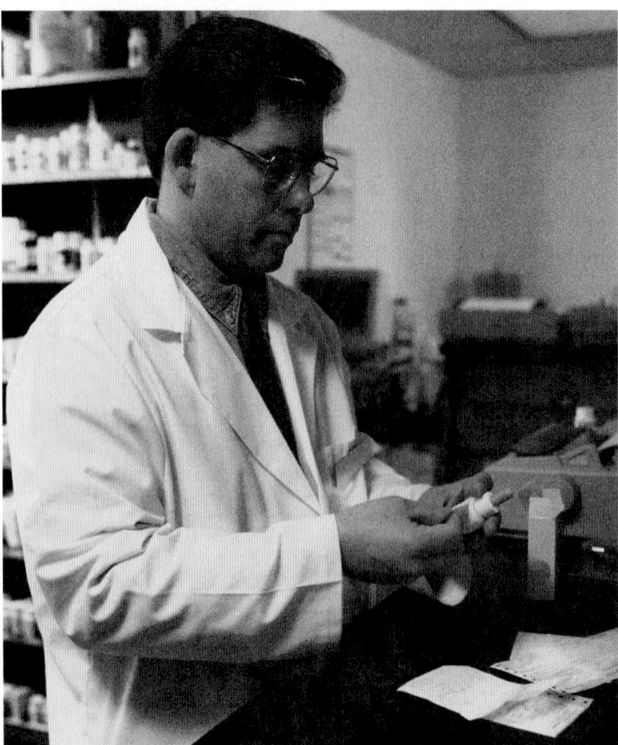

Figure 3-15 The hospital pharmacy maintains medications that are distributed to patient care areas for administration.

Medicine Department

The Department of Medicine is responsible for the coordination and monitoring of all medical services provided to patients within the hospital.

Surgery Department

The Surgery Department coordinates diagnostic and therapeutic surgical procedures to be performed for various medical conditions (Figure 3-16). The department also performs necessary tasks required to set up the operating room or other areas where surgical procedures are performed in the hospital.

Anesthesia Department

The Anesthesia Department is commonly referred to as Anesthesiology. This department performs the required tasks in preparation for anesthesia services to be provided to patients undergoing surgical procedures.

Pulmonary Department

The Pulmonary Department coordinates various procedures required to diagnose and treat pulmonary conditions such as bronchoscopy and tracheotomy.

Cardiology Department

The Cardiology Department coordinates various procedures required to diagnose and treat cardiac conditions, for example, cardiac catheterizations and bypass procedures.

Emergency Department (ED)

The **ED** is responsible for the coordination of patient care services provided in the emergency room (ER) to patients who present with conditions that require immediate attention (Figure 3-17). Patients seen in the ER usually present with acute conditions such as myocardial infarction or closed head injury, or they have developed a complication of a chronic condition such

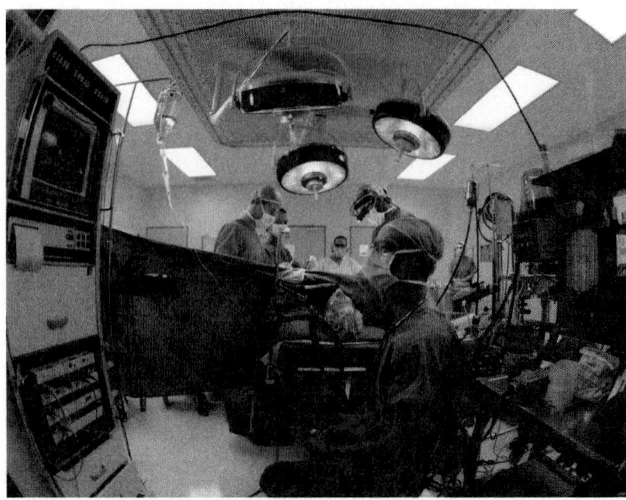

Figure 3-16 Surgical services are coordinated by the Surgery Department.

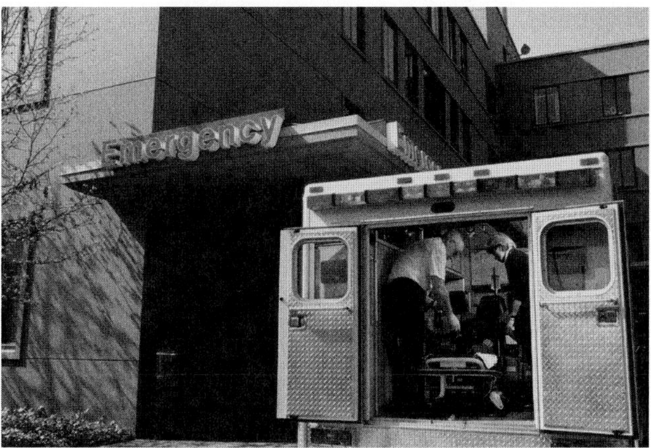

Figure 3-17 The Emergency Department provides services to patients who present with a condition that requires immediate attention. *(From McSwain NE, Patus JL: The basic EMT 2003, ed 3, St Louis, 2002, Mosby.)*

as ketoacidosis, which may occur with diabetes. **Acute** refers to the sudden onset of a condition or symptom.

The departments outlined above perform services at the request of a physician. The admitting or attending physician prepares written orders describing services required from these departments. Physician's orders may also be communicated verbally. On receipt of the order, the department performs the service and records pertinent information regarding the service in the patient's medical record. The admitting or attending physician will monitor the patient's condition and revise orders as required.

All of the administrative, financial, and operational functions outlined above are a necessary part of providing patient care in a hospital setting. These functions are not directly billed to patients or third-party payers. The hospital pricing structure for billable patient care services is determined by taking into account the cost of overhead for the above functions.

LEVELS FOR PROVISION OF SERVICES

Hospitals provide diagnostic, therapeutic, palliative, and preventive services to patients at various levels, as discussed in Chapter 1. It is important for coding and billing professionals to understand each of these levels because the guidelines vary for each level. Services can be provided on an outpatient, inpatient, or non-patient basis, as illustrated in Figure 3-18.

Outpatient

Outpatient services are procedures or services performed at the hospital, and the patient is released from the hospital the same day. Various departments such as Pathology/Laboratory, Radiology, and Physical Rehabilitation provide outpatient services. Service areas within a hospital designed specifically for the provision of outpatient services are the Ambulatory Surgery Center, Observation, Emergency Department, Outpatient Clinic, or Primary Care Network.

Ambulatory Surgery Center (ASC)

Hospitals generally have an ambulatory surgery area where outpatient surgeries can be performed. The area may be a surgery unit or an ASC. An ASC can be free-standing or located within the hospital. Ambulatory surgery is performed on the same day the patient is released.

The hospital provides space, nursing and technical staff, supplies, instruments, drugs, equipment, and other materials required for the surgery. Various clinical professionals may be involved in an ambulatory surgery, such as a surgeon, anesthesiologist, assistant surgeon, certified registered nurse anesthetist (CRNA), or physician assistant (PA).

Observation

An attending physician may see the need to monitor a patient closely for 24 hours or more based on the severity of the patient's illness. The patient may be admitted for observation in these cases. Observation care is considered an outpatient service. Generally the decision to discharge or admit a patient is made within 24 hours; however, some payers may allow observation services for up to 72 hours when medically necessary.

Emergency Room (ER)

The ER is an area in the hospital where services are provided to patients presenting with a condition or illness that requires immediate attention. The patient is treated and released on the same day unless further medical care is required; then the patient is admitted as an inpatient. The ER physician performs an evaluation and management (E/M) service to determine the patient's condition and the treatment required. Diagnostic studies may be required to diagnose a patient. Ancillary departments within the hospital may provide services to an ER patient, such as Pathology/Laboratory or Radiology. Once a diagnosis is determined, the patient is treated and released. If the ER physician determines that the patient requires further care, arrangements may be made to admit the patient as an inpatient.

Outpatient Clinic

Many hospitals have hospital-based clinics throughout the community such as a walk-in or urgent care clinics. Patients present for diagnosis and treatment at the clinics. The hospital submits charges to the patient or third-party payer for all services rendered within the clinic. Hospitals may bill for the professional and technical components of services performed when the physician is employed by or under contract with the hospital.

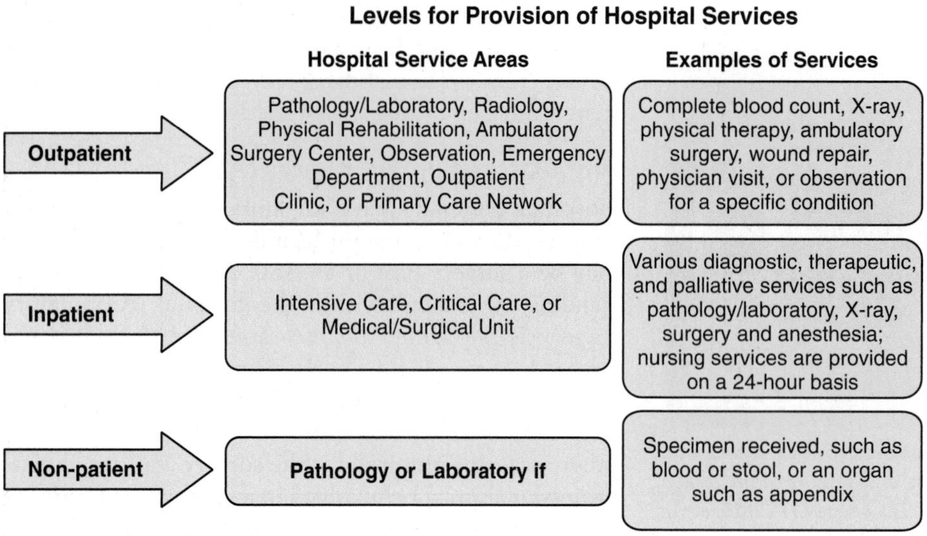

Levels for Provision of Hospital Services

	Hospital Service Areas	Examples of Services
Outpatient	Pathology/Laboratory, Radiology, Physical Rehabilitation, Ambulatory Surgery Center, Observation, Emergency Department, Outpatient Clinic, or Primary Care Network	Complete blood count, X-ray, physical therapy, ambulatory surgery, wound repair, physician visit, or observation for a specific condition
Inpatient	Intensive Care, Critical Care, or Medical/Surgical Unit	Various diagnostic, therapeutic, and palliative services such as pathology/laboratory, X-ray, surgery and anesthesia; nursing services are provided on a 24-hour basis
Non-patient	**Pathology or Laboratory if**	Specimen received, such as blood or stool, or an organ such as appendix

Figure 3-18 Levels for provision of hospital services. Note that professional services are not billed by the hospital unless the provider is employed by the hospital.

TEST YOUR *Knowledge* BOX 3-2

DEPARTMENTAL FUNCTIONS

1. Name two departments involved in performing administrative functions.
2. Discuss why it is important to have a Compliance Department in the hospital.
3. Name two departments involved in performing financial functions.
4. Explain how the Accounting, Patient Financial Services, and Credit and Collection Departments contribute to maintaining financial stability.
5. Name two departments involved in performing operational functions.
6. Provide a description of functions performed by the Health Information Management Department.
7. Name two departments involved in performing clinical functions.
8. Explain how the functions of the Health Information Management Department relate to charge submission.
9. Explain the importance of medical record documentation.
10. List vital functions performed by the Health Information Management Department.

Primary Care Network

Many hospitals have hospital-based primary care networks throughout the community. Patients present for primary care services, and the primary care physician provides diagnostic or therapeutic services as required. The physician providing primary care services is generally employed by the hospital. Hospitals may bill for the professional and technical components of services performed when the physician is employed by or under contract with the hospital.

BOX 3-12 ■ KEY POINTS

Levels for Provision of Hospital Services

Outpatient

- Patient receives care and is released from the hospital on the same day.

Inpatient

- Patient is admitted with the expectation that he or she will be in the hospital for more than 24 hours.

Non-Patient

- Specimen is received for processing and the patient is not present.

Inpatient

A patient who requires care on an ongoing basis, for more than 24 hours, is admitted to the hospital as an inpatient. **Inpatient** is when a patient is admitted with the expectation that he or she will be in the hospital for more than 24 hours. The patient can be admitted from various locations—home, clinic, nursing home, ER, other facility. The attending physician determines what type of admission is required. After a history and physical is performed, the admitting physician prepares orders that outline the diagnostic, therapeutic, or palliative services are required. **History and physical (H&P)** is a detailed accounting of the history, physical examination, and decision making involved regarding the patient's condition on admission. Inpatient admissions require assignment of a room (bed). The hospital provides 24-hour nursing care during the stay, and various departments contribute to the patient's care and treatment. Other physicians may be called in to see the patient, such as a cardiologist or endocrinologist. The attending physician determines when to discharge the patient. The discharge orders are prepared by the attending physician, and the patient is discharged.

Non-Patient Care

Non-patient care is provided when the Pathology/Laboratory department receives a specimen for processing. The specimen can be delivered from somewhere within the hospital, such as the operating room, or it can be received from an outside physician office. The specimen is processed and the patient is not present. The results are forwarded to the requesting physician.

CHAPTER SUMMARY

The functional design of the hospital groups various tasks into administrative, financial, operational, and clinical categories. Departments are developed to carry out the tasks required for each category. Administrative departments are responsible for personnel, public relations, marketing, and purchasing. Financial departments handle all the issues related to monetary transactions. Patient transactions and related financial tasks are performed by accounting, admitting, business office, and credit and collections. Operational departments are responsible for various tasks involving the physical setting, quality of services, risk, credentialing, medical records, and health information systems. Clinical departments focus on patient care services. It is important to have knowledge of hospital departments and their functions to gain a complete understanding of how they relate to patient accounts, data flow, and the billing process, which will be discussed in the following chapters.

TEST YOUR *Knowledge* BOX 3-3

LEVELS FOR PROVISION OF SERVICES

1. List three service areas where patients can be treated in the hospital.
2. Provide a definition for inpatient.
3. Explain the difference between outpatient and non-patient services.
4. Describe observation services.
5. Provide an overview of Emergency Department services.

CHAPTER REVIEW 3-1

True/False

1. Hospitals bill for all services, items, and professional work done by physicians. T F
2. Observation services are considered inpatient services. T F
3. Hospitals can bill nursing services separately in addition to other services. T F
4. The admitting process includes obtaining demographic, insurance, and medical information. T F
5. Utilization management monitors health care services to determine the level of malpractice risk. T F

Fill in the Blank

6. A ____________________ ____________________ contains details regarding how the hospital will ensure ____________________ with all ____________________.
7. To ensure that the hospital is in compliance with federal and state regulations a ____________________ may be created to oversee the compliance program.
8. A hospital mission statement outlines the hospital's purpose. The most significant portion of the mission statement is ____________________.
9. Patient records include various documents outlining details regarding the patient's ____________________ and ____________________.
10. A computer system designed for hospital patient medical and billing information is called ____________________.

Match the Following Definitions With the Terms at Right

11. ___ The portion of a procedure that includes use of a technician, supplies, materials, and equipment to perform the services.
12. ___ An area in the hospital where services are provided to patients presenting with a condition or illness that requires immediate attention.
13. ___ Supportive services provided by various departments, such as Radiology.
14. ___ Outstanding accounts in which money is owed to the hospital by patients, third-party payers, and government payers.
15. ___ HIM coding professionals are responsible for this.

A. Ancillary services
B. Coding patient records, chargemaster maintenance, and auditing
C. Accounts receivable
D. Emergency Department
E. Technical component

Research Project

Obtain a hospital organizational chart either through Internet research or contact with a local hospital. Compare the organizational chart obtained to that in Figure 3-1, discuss how the charts differ, and provide an explanation as to why they might differ.

GLOSSARY

Accounts receivable Outstanding accounts in which money is owed by the patient, insurance company, or government program.

Acute Sudden onset of a condition or symptoms.

Admission process Tasks required to receive a patient in the hospital including obtaining demographic, insurance, and medical information, and entering the data into the computer system.

Ancillary services Supportive services provided by various departments, such as radiology.

Census Inventory of rooms available in the hospital and the patients assigned to those rooms.

Clinical Refers to tasks related to medical practice.

Electronic Health Record (EHR) An electronic version of the patient's medical record that contains information regarding the patient's condition, treatment, and progress.

Emergency Department (ED) An area in the hospital where services are provided to patients presenting with a condition or illness that requires immediate attention.

Health Information Management (HIM) Hospital department responsible for the organization, maintenance, production, storage, retention, dissemination, and security of patient health information. HIM is sometimes referred to as Medical Records.

Health information system Computer system designed for hospital patient medical and billing information.

History and Physical (H&P) A detailed accounting of the history, physical examination, and decision making involved regarding the patient's condition on admission.

Inpatient Patient who is admitted with the expectation that he or she will be in the hospital for more than 24 hours.

Medical record documentation Information regarding the patient's condition, treatment, and progress, required to support charges submitted to various payers. Documentation is maintained in a chart, called the medical record.

Outpatient Services are performed at the hospital and the patient is released from the hospital the same day.

Professional component The portion of a procedure that represents the physician's work in performing the service, such as the reading and interpretation of a radiology film.

Technical component The portion of a procedure that represents the overhead utilized in performing the service, such as the technician, supplies, materials, and equipment.

Utilization Management (UM) Focuses on monitoring health care resources utilized in the hospital for the purpose of determining whether the services are appropriate and necessary in response to the patient's condition, thereby ensuring maximum resource utilization.

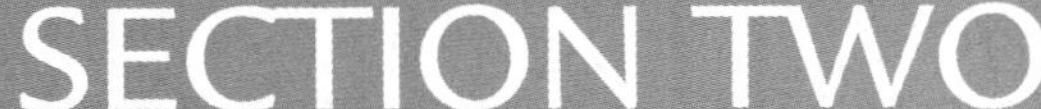

SECTION TWO

Hospital Billing and Coding Process

Patient Accounts and Data Flow in the Hospital

Hospital Billing Process

Accounts Receivable (A/R) Management

Chapter 4

Patient Accounts and Data Flow in the Hospital

The purpose of this chapter is to provide a basic understanding of the patient care process and how data flow within a hospital from the time a patient is admitted to when charges are submitted for patient care services. The flow of information is a critical factor in providing efficient patient care and billing for services rendered during the patient visit. The process of admitting, treating, discharging, and billing patient care services requires various departments to perform specific functions simultaneously. One function is to document all information regarding patient care services including the patient's condition, disease, injury, illness, or other reason for treatment. Designated personnel within each department are responsible for documenting patient care services in the patient's medical record. Patient care services are coded and charges are entered by specified personnel in various clinical departments and by the Health Information Management (HIM) Department. Patient charges are submitted to patients and third-party payers after the patient is discharged. The concepts presented in this chapter are critical to understanding the hospital billing and claims process, which will be discussed in the next chapter.

Chapter Objectives

- Define terms, phrases, abbreviations, and acronyms related to patient accounts and data flow.
- Demonstrate an understanding of patient accounts and data flow for outpatient, ambulatory surgery, and inpatient services.
- Define patient admission and discuss procedures required to ensure quality of patient care.
- Outline the patient care process and provide an explanation of each phase.
- Demonstrate an understanding of the admission process and forms utilized during the process.
- Provide an explanation of the insurance verification process.
- Describe the relationship between the admission process and billing for patient services.
- Discuss the purpose of medical record documentation and various forms and documents used in the medical record.

(*Continued*)

Outline

- Demonstrate an understanding of patient care services provided by a hospital.
- Provide an explanation of how charges are captured in the hospital.
- State the role of Health Information Management (HIM) in billing patient services.
- Demonstrate an understanding of the hospital billing process, including denied, pended, and paid claims, and posting patient transactions.
- Demonstrate an understanding of the importance of accounts receivable (A/R) management and reports utilized.

Key Terms

Accounts receivable (A/R) aging report
Admission
Admission Evaluation Protocol (AEP)
Admission summary
Advance Beneficiary Notice (ABN)
Advance directives
Ambulatory Payment Classification (APC)
Assignment of Benefits
Charge capture
Charge Description Master (CDM)
CMS-1450 (UB-04)
CMS-1500
Co-insurance
Co-payment
Concurrent review
Deductible
Explanation of Benefits (EOB)
Explanation of Medicare Benefits (EOMB)
Encounter form
Facility charges
Financial class
Guarantor
Informed Consent for Treatment
Insurance verification
Medical necessity
Medical record
Medical record number (MRN)
Medicare Severity Diagnosis Related Groups (MS-DRG)
Patient registration form
Professional charges
Prospective review
Quality Improvement Organization (QIO)
Remittance advice (RA)
Retrospective review
Written Authorization for Release of Medical Information

Acronyms and Abbreviations

AEP—Admission Evaluation Protocol
ABN—Advance Beneficiary Notice
APC—Ambulatory Payment Classification
A/R—Accounts receivable
ASC—ambulatory surgery center
CCS—Certified Coding Specialist
CDM—Charge Description Master
CPC—Certified Professional Coder
DME—durable medical equipment
EMC—electronic medical claim
EOB—Explanation of Benefits
EOMB—Explanation of Medicare Benefits
ED—Emergency Department
ER—emergency room
H&P—history and physical
HIM—Health Information Management
MAR—Medication administration record
MRN—Medical record number
MS-DRG—Medicare Severity Diagnosis Related Groups
OR—operating room
PFS—Patient Financial Services
PPS—Prospective Payment System
QIO—Quality Improvement Organization
RA—Remittance advice
RHIT—Registered Health Information Technician
TJC—The Joint Commission
UB-04—CMS-1450 Universal Bill implemented in 2007.
UM—Utilization Management
UR—Utilization Review

PATIENT ACCOUNTS AND DATA FLOW

The flow of information in the hospital includes the patient's demographic, insurance, and medical information. The flow of data begins when the patient reports to the hospital for patient care services. The type of data and flow vary based on the type of service the patient requires. As discussed in the previous chapter, various administrative, financial, operational, and clinical departments perform functions required to provide efficient patient care and submit charges to patients and third-party payers for services rendered. Clinical departments provide patient care services. Various administrative and operational departments perform other critical functions such as human resource management, com-

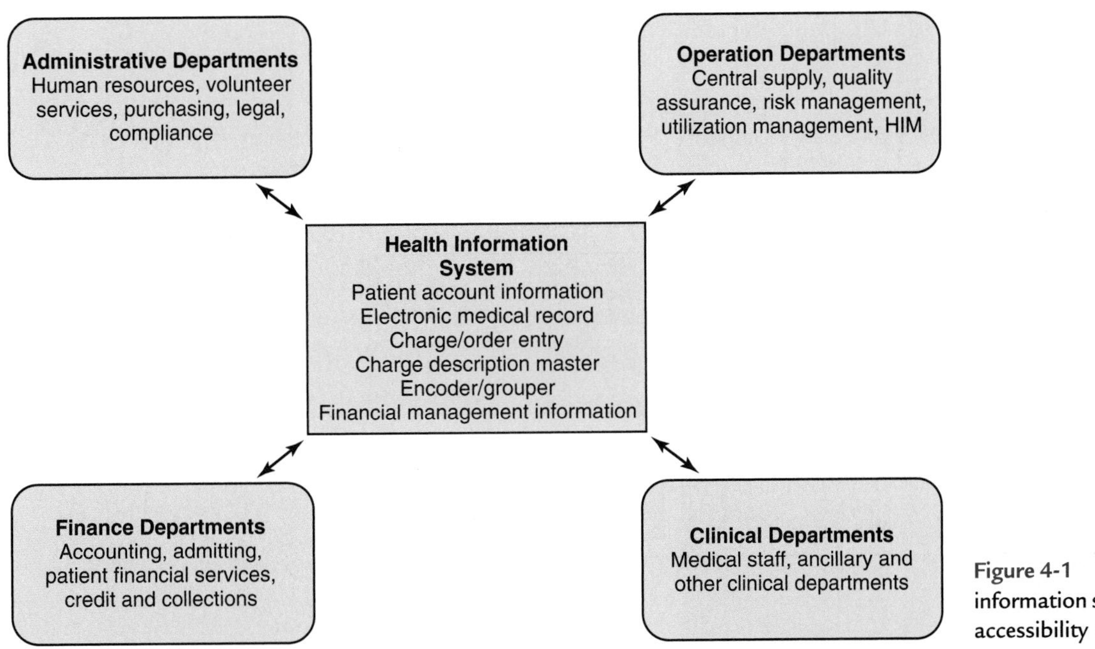

Figure 4-1 The hospital's health information system enhances data accessibility and use.

pliance, health information management, and utilization management. Financial departments are responsible for preparing charges for submission and accounts receivable management. The data flow in a hospital is designed to ensure that required data are accessible for personnel to perform various functions. Automation of the patient's accounts, order entry, charge capture, billing, and accounts receivable allow greater access to patient information by various individuals within the hospital, as illustrated in Figure 4-1.

The hospital's health information system allows the recording, storage, processing, and access of data by various departments simultaneously. Departments that perform specific functions may use data entered by another department. This level of automation enhances the flow and use of information throughout the hospital.

The flow of information begins when the patient is received during the admission process. Variations in the flow of information occur based on whether the patient presents for outpatient services, ambulatory surgery, or inpatient services. The flow of data is similar in each scenario; however, there are some variations in the data and its flow, as illustrated in this chapter.

BOX 4-1 ■ KEY POINTS

Flow of Information

Flow of information includes the following patient information:
- Demographic information
- Insurance information
- Medical information

BOX 4-2 ■ KEY POINTS

Hospital Information System

The information system allows the simultaneous recording, storage, processing, and access of data by various departments:
- Patient's account
- Patient medical record
- Order entry/charge capture
- Coding
- Billing process
- Accounts receivable management

Outpatient

Outpatient services are those that are provided on the same day that the patient is released. The patient is received in various outpatient areas such as the Emergency Department, laboratory, radiology, clinic, or primary care office. Admission tasks required to receive the patient are performed. Patient care services are rendered. Pharmaceuticals and other items such as supplies and equipment may be required. All patient care services are recorded in the medical record. Charges for hospital outpatient services are entered through the **Charge Description Master (CDM)**, commonly referred to as the chargemaster, which is a computerized system used by the hospital to inventory and record services and items provided by the hospital. Charges for services provided in a clinic or primary care office are posted to the patient account. The patient is released and the billing process begins. Accounts are monitored for follow-up to ensure that payment is collected in a timely manner. The flow of data for outpatient services is illustrated in Figure 4-2, *A*.

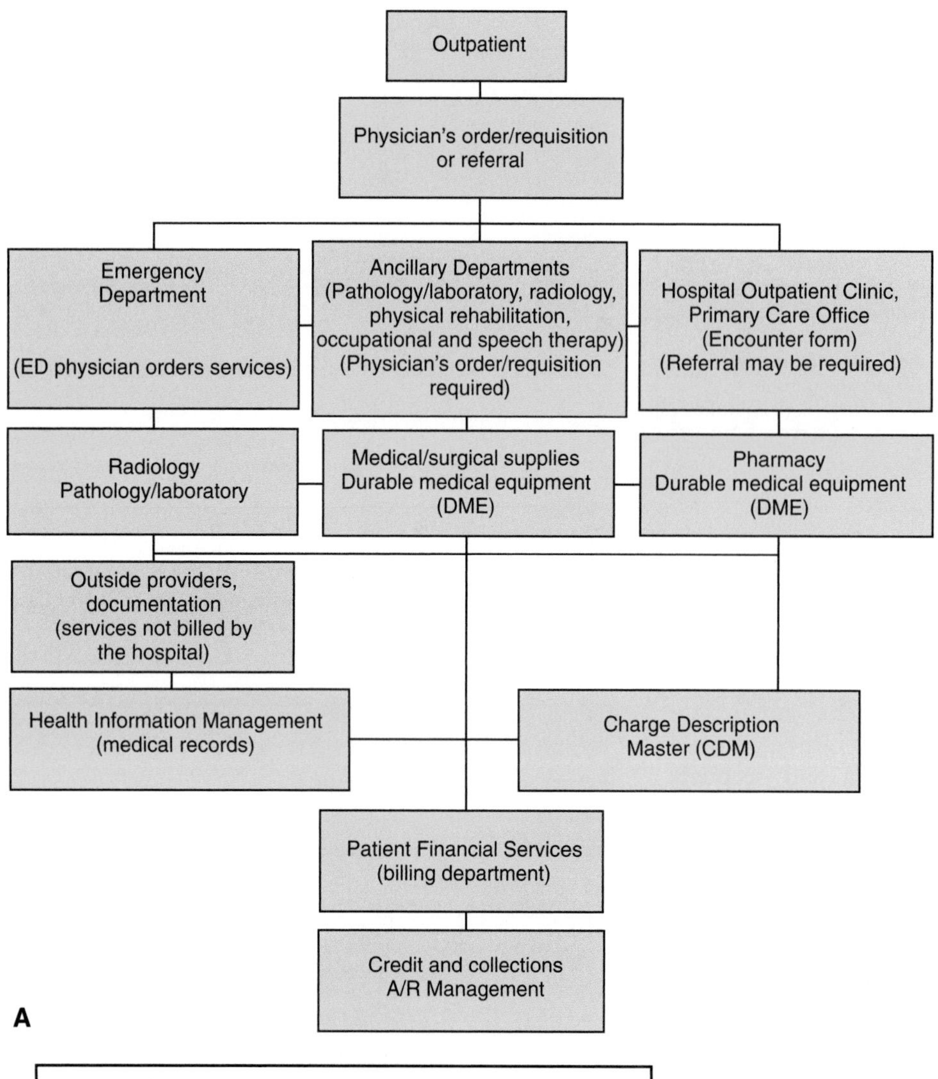

RADIOLOGY REQUISITION

PATIENT NAME:	ORDERING PHYSICIAN:
DOB:	ACCOUNT #
PHYSICIAN SIGNATURE:	DATE:
INDICATIONS:	

PLEASE FAX SCRIPT PRIOR TO PATIENTS SCEHDUELD APPOINTMENT

PLEASE CHECK

GENERAL X-RAY
- ☐ 74415 IVP D
- ☐ 74000 KUB
- ☐ 74020 Abdominal Series (2V)
- ☐ 74022 Acute Abdominal Series (3V)
- ☐ 73610 Ankle L/R
- ☐ 72050 C-Spine (min 4V)
- ☐ 72040 C-Spine (max 3V)
- ☑ _____ Chest (2V)
- ☐ 73080 Elbow L/R
- ☐ 73550 Femur L/R
- ☐ 73630 Foot L/R
- ☐ 73090 Forearm L/R
- ☐ 73130 Hand L/R
- ☐ 73500 Hip L/R
- ☐ 73060 Humerus L/R
- ☐ 73564 Knee L/R
- ☐ 72110 L Spine (min. 4V)
- ☐ 72170 Pelvis
- ☐ 71100 Ribs - Unilat L/R
- ☐ 71110 Ribs-Bilat
- ☐ Other_______________

MRI
- ☐ 74181 Abd wo/contrast
- ☐ 74182 Abd w/contrast
- ☐ 74183 Abd w/wo contrast
- ☐ 70551 Brain wo/contrast
- ☐ 70552 Brain w/contrast
- ☐ 70553 Brain w/wo contrast
- ☐ 72141 C-Spine w/o contrast
- ☐ 72156 C-Spine w/wo contrast
- ☐ 71550 Chest wo/contrast
- ☐ 71551 Chest w/contrast
- ☐ 71552 Chest w/wo contrast
- ☐ 73721 Lower Extremity (jt.) R/L
- ☐ 73718 Lower Extremity (no jt.) R/L
- ☐ 72148 L-Spine wo/contrast
- ☐ 72158 L-Spine w/wo contrast

MRA ☐ MRV ☐
- ☐ 74185 Abd w/wo contrast
- ☐ 71555 Chest w/wo contrast (Exc Myocardium)
- ☐ 70544 Head wo/contrast
- ☐ 70546 Head w/wo contrast
- ☐ 70545 Head w/contrast
- ☐ 73725 Lower Ext. w/wo contrast
- ☐ 70547 Neck wo/contrast
- ☐ 70548 Neck w/contrast
- ☐ 70549 Neck w/wo contrast
- ☐ 73225 Upr. Ext. w/wo contrast
- ☐ Other_______________

CT SCAN
- ☐ _____ Abd wo/contrast
- ☑ _____ Abd w/wo contrast
- ☐ 70450 Brain wo/contrast
- ☐ 70470 Brain w/wo contrast
- ☐ 72125 C-Spine wo/contrast
- ☐ 71250 Chest wo/contrast
- ☐ 71260 Chest w/contrast
- ☐ 71270 Chest w/wo contrast
- ☐ 70482 IAC's, Orbits, Pituitary w/wo cont. ☐ 72131 L-Spine wo/contrast
- ☐ 70486 Maxiofacial (Sinus) wo/contrast
- ☐ 72192 Pelvis wo/contrast
- ☐ 72193 Pelvis w/contrast
- ☐ 72194 Pelvis w/wo contrast
- ☐ 70491 Soft Tissue Neck w/contrast
- ☐ 72128 T-Spine wo/contrast
- ☐ 74150/72192 Urogram

ULTRASOUND
- ☐ 76700 Abd Total
- ☐ 76705 Abd, Single Organ/Quadrant
- ☐ 93925 Arterial Lower Ext.-Bilat.
- ☐ 93926 Arterial Lower Ext.-Unilat. L/R
- ☐ 93930 Arterial Upper Ext. - Bilat.
- ☐ 93931 Arterial Upper Ext. - Unilat. L/R
- ☐ 76645 Breast L/R
- ☐ 93880 Carotid
- ☐ 76880 Extremity, Non Vascular L/R
- ☐ 76801 OB - 1st Trimester
- ☐ Other_______________

MAMMOGRAPHY
- ☐ 76092 Screening mammography
- ☐ 76091 Diagnostic mammography - Bilat
- ☐ 76090 Diagnostic mammography - Unil L/R

DEXA SCAN
- ☐ 76075 Bone Density, DEXA

ECHOCARDIOGRAM
- ☐ 93307/93320/93325 Echo, Dop. Echo w/pulsect wave and color flow

PET SCAN

Specify Area_______________

STRESS TEST
- ☐ 78465 Dual Isotope Nuclear Stress Test
- ___ Adenosine/Dubutamine

☐ CORRELATION or ☐ COMPARISON:
Please compare with exam done on
________ ______ ______

B

Figure 4-2 **A,** Patient account data flow for outpatient services. **B,** Sample ancillary depardment requisition form for Radiology. *(From Ingenix coding lab: facilities and ancillary services 2004, Eden Prairie, Minn., 2004, Ingenix.)*

COMMUNITY GENERAL HOSPITAL

Primary Care Associates
Bernardo Linquinti, M.D.
Sandra Balcomanter, M.D.

8192 South Street
Mars, Florida 37373
(747) 722-1800

X	DESCRIPTION	CODE	AMOUNT
	PATIENT VISITS		
	NEW PATIENT		
	Problem focused Hx	99201	
	Expanded prob/Focused Hx	99202	
	Detailed Hx	99203	
	Comp Hx/Moderate complex	99204	
	Comp Hx/High complex	99205	
	ESTABLISHED PATIENT		
	Minimal	99211	
	Problem focused Hx	99212	
	Expanded prob/Focused Hx	99213	
	Detailed Hx	99214	
	Comprehensive Hx	99215	
	CONSULTATION		
	Problem focused Hx	99241	
	Expanded prob/Focused Hx	99242	
	Detailed Hx	99243	
	Comp Hx/Moderate complex	99244	
	Comp Hx/High complex	99245	
	NURSE SPECIALIST		
	Computer analysis	99090	
	Group health ed	99078	
	Skills management (15 min.)	97535	
	PROCEDURES		
	Accucheck/One Touch	7182948	
	EKG w/interpretation	93000	
	IV infusion, up to 1 hr.	90780	
	IV infusion, each add'l hr.	90781	
	Immunization administration	90471	
	Two or more vaccines/toxoids	90472	
	Therapeutic/diagnostic injection Specify: med/dose	90782	
	Injection of antibiotic Specify: med/dose	90788	
	Occult blood (guaiac)	82270	
	ANS	95937	
	24 hour cardiac monitor	93230	
	Pap smear	88150	
	Thyroid fine needle asp. (proc.)	7190357	
	Group counseling, 30 min.	99411	
	Group counseling, 60 min.	99412	

X	DESCRIPTION	CODE	ALPHA	AMOUNT
	PROCEDURES cont.			
	Preventive counseling, 15 min.	99401		
	Preventive counseling, 30 min.	99402		
	Preventive counseling, 45 min.	99403		
	Preventive counseling, 60 min.	99404		
	DIABETES/LIPID			
X	DESCRIPTION	CODE	ALPHA	AMOUNT
	Cholesterol, HDL	7190053	HDL	
	C-peptide	7190219	CPEP	
	Glucose serum	7182947	GLU	
	HGB A1 C	7190057	HA1	
	Insulin	7190343	INS	
	Lipoprotein panel A	7175004		
	Micral, random	7190335	MLBU	
	Protein, urine 24 hr.	7195011	PROU	
	GONADAL			
	Estradiol	7190044	ESD	
	FSH	7190048	FSH	
	LH	7190069	LH	
	Progesterone	7190078	PROG	
	PSA	7190079	PSA	
	SHBG	7190622	SHBG	
	Testosterone	7190086	TEST	
	Testosterone, Free	7190322	FTES	
	PSA, Free	7184999		
	PROFILES			
	Basic metabolic panel	7180049	CH7	
	Comp. metabolic panel	7180054	CMP	
	Electrolyte panel	7180051	ELEC	
	Hepatic function panel	7180058	HFPA	
	Hepatitis panel	7180059		
	Lipid profile 2	7190257	LPP2	
	THYROID			
	Antimicrosomal antibody	7190213	TM	
	TSI	7190476	TSIG	
	Thyroglobulin	7190584	THY	
	T4 - Thyroxine	7190047	FT4	
	T3 uptake	7190292	TU	
	Total T3	7190095	T3 C	
	T3-Free	7190595	FT3	
	TSH (Thyroid stim hormone)	7190253	TSH	

X	DESCRIPTION	CODE	ALPHA	AMOUNT
	CALCIUM/BONE/KIDNEY			
	Calcium, ionized	7190821	ICAL	
	Calcium, serum	7190311	CAL	
	Calcium, urine 24 hr.	7190222	CALU	
	Creatinine, clearance ht. __ wt.___	7194754	CRCP	
	Microalbumin, urine 24 hr.	7190335	MLBT	
	Magnesium, serum	7190317	MAG	
	Parathyroid hormo	7190387	PTH	
	ADRENAL/PITUITARY			
X	DESCRIPTION	CODE	ALPHA	AMOUNT
	ACTH	7190005	ACTH	
	Aldosterone, serum	7190204	ALD	
	Androstenedione	7190336	AND	
	Cortisol, serum	7190032	COR	
	DHEA	7190341	DHEA	
	DHEA S serum	7190312	DHES	
	Human growth hormone	7190379	HGH	
	Prolactin	7190316	PRL	
	17OH Progesterone	7190479	HY17	
	17OH Pregnegalone	7190480	LONE	
	Urine catecholimine 24 hr.	7190021	CATU	
	Urine cortisol 24 hr.	7190033	CORU	
	Urine metanephrines 24 hr.	7190475	METU	
	Urine potassium 24 hr.	7190077	POTU	
	Urine sodium 24 hr.	7190261	SODU	
	Urine VMA 24 hr.	7190534	VMAU	
	CHEMISTRY/HEMATOLOGY			
	CBC w/diff & platelets	7190327	CBC1	
	Erthrocyte sed rate	7190330	ESR	
	Potassium, serum	7184813	POT	
	Urine culture	7190041	BACTI	
	Urinalysis, routine	7190334	URTN	
	Urinalysis, dipstick	7190384	URCH	
	Venipuncture	7190323	VENI	
	GGI	7184773		
	HCE	7190329		

AUTHORIZATION #
DIAGNOSIS
SPECIAL INSTRUCTIONS

REFERRING MD

Tax ID #	62-1162462
Previous bal.	
Amount paid	
Today's chrg	
Amount paid	
Total rec'd	
Balance due	

Physician signature: Date:

I authorize release of any medical information necessary to process this claim. I also authorize the direct payment of any benefits due me for the described services to I understand I am financially responsible for paying any unpaid balance and will be responsible for the entire bill if this claim is not covered. **Medicare Patients:** The Medicare program requires that all diagnosis be ICD 9 coded. We are unable to provide this service to you at the time of your visit, and therefore, require that you permit us to file an insurance claim with your Medicare carrier.

Patient (Beneficiary) signature: Date:

Check one:
☐ Cash
☐ Check, M.O.# ____________
☐ MC ☐ VISA
☐ Care Card # ____________

98381 7/99

C

Figure 4-2, *cont'd* **C,** Sample encounter form. *(C Modified from Abdelhak M, Grostick S, Hanken MA, Jacobs E (editors):* Health information: management of a strategic resource, *ed 2, St Louis, 2001, Saunders.)*

Outpatient Data and Flow Variations

Some variations in the type of data collected and how it flows involve the physician's orders, requisitions, and referrals, Emergency Department services, and physician service charges.

Orders, Requisitions, Encounter Forms, and Referrals

A physician's order or requisition is required for services provided by hospital ancillary departments such as cardiovascular, laboratory, radiology, or physical rehabilitation. These documents provide information to the department regarding the services required. Figure 4-2, *B,* illustrates an ancillary department requisition for radiology.

Hospital-based physician clinics or offices do not require an order when the patient presents for services. Hospital-based physician services are recorded in the patient's medical record. An **encounter form** is utilized as a charge tracking document to record services, procedures, and items provided during the visit and the medical reason for the services provided (Figure 4-2, C).

A physician referral may be required as outlined in the patient's insurance plan. If services are required from other departments within the hospital, the clinic or primary care physician will prepare an order or requisition.

Emergency Department Services

Emergency Department visits do not require an order when the patient presents for service. If services are required from other departments within the hospital, the emergency room (ER) physician will prepare an order or requisition.

If the patient is admitted to the hospital, all charges related to the Emergency Department visit are included on the inpatient bill.

Physician Services

Various physicians are part of the patient care team within the hospital. They provide services to patients and document those services in the patient's medical record. Each physician bills charges for his or her service to the patient and third-party payers. Physician services are not billed by the hospital unless the physician is employed by or under contract with the hospital.

BOX 4-3 ■ KEY POINTS

Outpatient Services

Services are provided in accordance with physician's orders, requisition, or referral. Services are performed and the patient is released on the same day. The following areas are involved:

- Emergency Department
- Laboratory
- Radiology
- Clinic
- Primary care office

Ambulatory Surgery

Ambulatory surgery is a surgical procedure that is performed on a patient on the same day the patient is released (sent home). It is considered an outpatient service. Ambulatory surgeries can be performed in a hospital-based ambulatory surgery center (ASC) or in a designated area within the hospital. Physician's orders are prepared by the surgeon and submitted to the ambulatory surgery unit. The patient is received in the ambulatory surgery unit or the preadmission testing area. Admission tasks required to receive the patient are performed. The appropriate clinical departments render patient care services. Pharmaceuticals, supplies, equipment, and other items may be required. All patient care services are recorded in the medical record. Hospital charges for services and items are posted through the chargemaster. The patient is discharged and the billing process begins. Accounts are monitored for follow-up to ensure that payment is collected in a timely manner. The flow of data for ambulatory surgery services is illustrated in Figure 4-3.

Ambulatory Surgery Data and Flow Variations

Some variations in the type of data collected and how it flows involve the physician services.

Physician Services

Ambulatory surgery involves a team of physicians such as a surgeon and anesthesiologist. Similar to the process for outpatient services, physician services performed for an ambulatory surgery are recorded in the patient's medical record. Each physician submits charges for services performed. Professional charges for physician services are not billed by the hospital unless the physician is employed by or under contract with the hospital.

BOX 4-4 ■ KEY POINTS

Ambulatory Surgery

Ambulatory surgery services are provided in accordance with physician's orders. Ambulatory surgery is performed in a hospital-based ambulatory surgery center (ASC) or other designated area within the hospital.

Surgery is performed on the patient on the same day the patient is released.

Ambulatory surgery is an outpatient service.

Inpatient

In an inpatient admission, the patient is admitted to the hospital with the expectation that he or she will be there for longer than 24 hours. A room/bed is assigned, and 24-hour nursing care is provided. There are several ways a patient can be referred to the hospital for an inpatient admission: through the ER, by outside physician referral, or from another facility.

Physician's orders are prepared by the admitting physician and provided to the hospital. Admission tasks required to receive the patient are performed. The appropriate clinical departments render patient care services. Pharmaceuticals, supplies, equipment, and other items may be required. All patient care services are recorded in the medical record. Hospital charges for services and items are posted through the chargemaster. The patient is discharged and the billing process begins. Accounts are monitored for follow-up to ensure that payment is collected in a timely manner. The flow of data for inpatient services is illustrated in Figure 4-4.

Inpatient Data and Flow Variations

Variation in the data and flow of information for an inpatient case varies based on where the patient is admitted. For example, if the patient is admitted through the ER, much of the admission process is performed there. Another variation in the process involves physician service charges.

Physician Services

As discussed previously, physician services are documented in the patient's medical record. Each provider submits charges for his or her services. They are not billed by the hospital. Professional charges for physi-

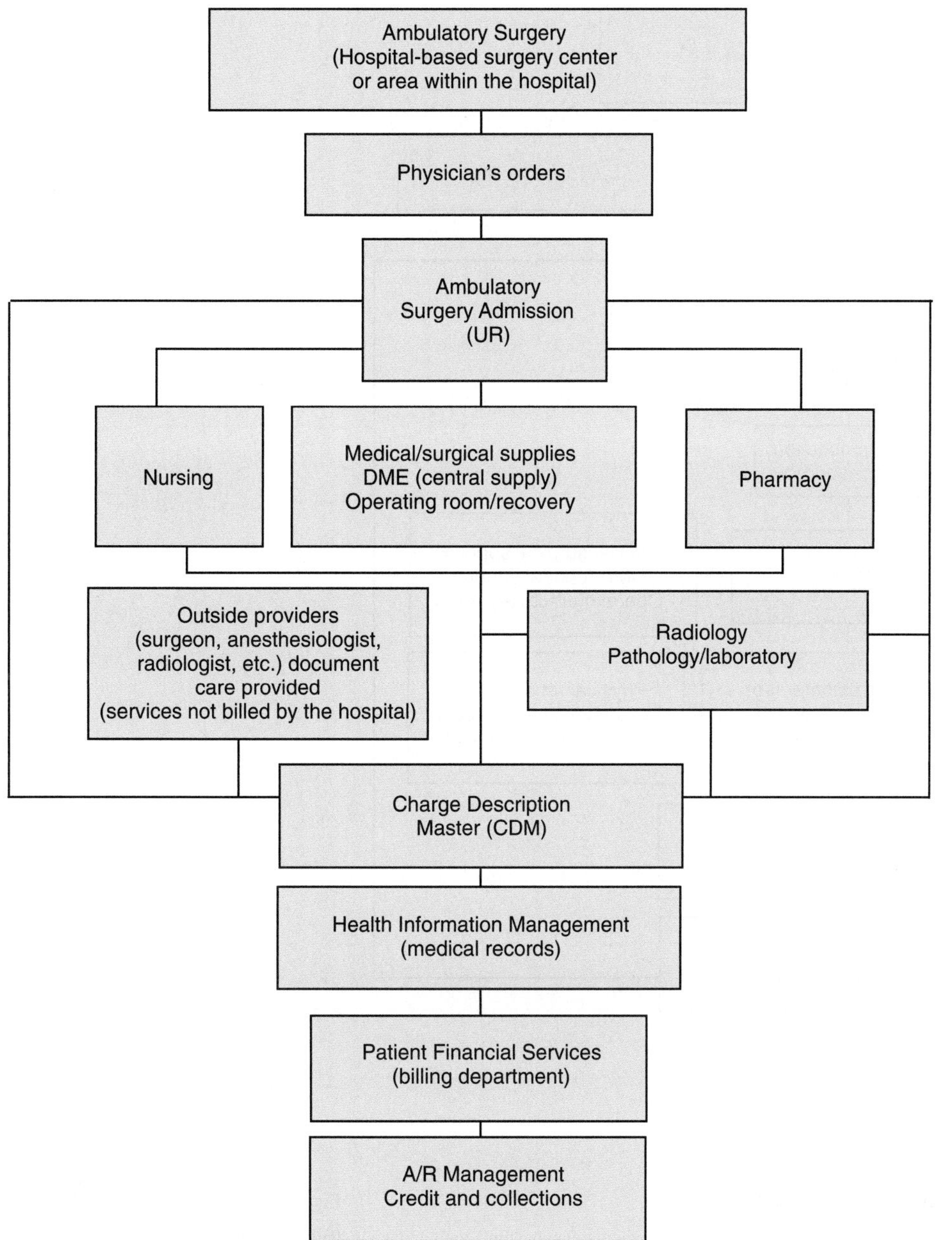

Figure 4-3 Patient account data flow for ambulatory surgery.

cians such the radiologist, cardiologist, surgeon, or anesthesiologist are not billed by the hospital unless the physician is employed by or under contract with the hospital.

BOX 4-5 ■ KEY POINTS

Inpatient Services

A patient is admitted with the expectation that he or she will be in the hospital for more than 24 hours. Services are provided in accordance with physician's orders.

The patient is assigned a room/bed.

Nursing care is provided on a 24-hour basis.

Diagnostic and therapeutic services are provided by various clinical departments.

BOX 4-6 ■ KEY POINTS

Admission Process Variations

Variations in the process and in the information obtained are based on the type of admission, as follows:

- Outpatient
  - Emergency Department
  - Ancillary departments (Radiology, Pathology/Laboratory, etc.)
  - Clinic
  - Primary care office
- Ambulatory surgery
- Inpatient

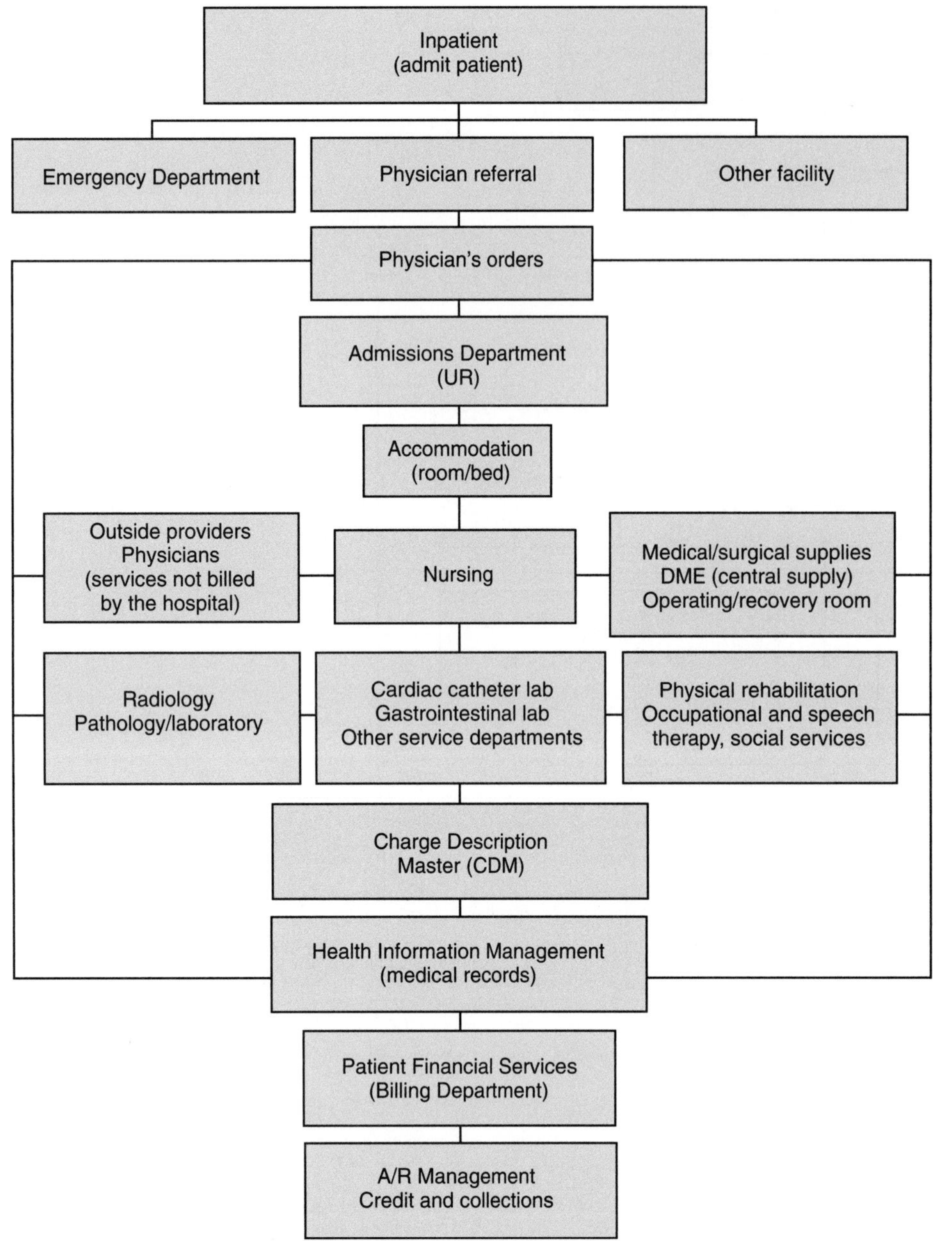

Figure 4-4 Patient account data flow for inpatient services.

Regardless of where the patient is received, the data collected at admission flows to various clinical departments that are involved in the patient's care. Each department involved in patient care, directly or indirectly, records pertinent information regarding patient care services in the patient's medical record. Hospital charges are posted to the patient's account through the chargemaster. The chargemaster is reviewed and updated continually by the HIM Department. When the patient is discharged, the medical record is forwarded to the HIM Department for review, coding, and assignment of the appropriate Prospective Payment System group such as the Medicare Severity Diagnosis Related Groups (MS-DRG) for inpatient cases or Ambulatory Payment Classification (APC) for outpatient surgical cases.

The Utilization Management (UM) Department is responsible for case management and utilization review of patient cases, as discussed in previous chapters. UM conducts reviews of patient cases to determine the appropriateness of services provided based on the patient's condition. The initial review performed by UM is done when the patient is admitted.

The billing process utilizes all information that has accumulated during the patient care process to submit charges to the patient and/or third-party payers. Outstanding accounts are monitored for follow-up by the Patient Financial Services (PFS) Department, commonly referred to as Credit and Collections. The chargemaster and prospective payment systems will be discussed in detail in future chapters.

BOX 4-7 ■ KEY POINTS

Patient Account Data Flow

Information collected at admission
Clinical departments render patient care services
Medical record documentation
Charge capture
Patient discharge, medical record forwarded to HIM
PFS prepares charges for submission
Accounts receivable management monitors and follows-up on outstanding accounts

BOX 4-8 ■ KEY POINTS

Admission

Admission is defined as "the act of being received into a place" or "patient accepted for inpatient services in a hospital."
Patients can be received at the Emergency Department, an ancillary department, a clinic, a primary care office, ambulatory surgery, or inpatient admission.
The admission process includes various functions required to receive a patient at the hospital facility for the purpose of obtaining required information to address patient care needs and bill for services rendered.

To provide a better understanding of the flow of patient account data and the patient care process, we will first discuss the concept of patient admission.

PATIENT ADMISSION

The definition of **admission** is "the act of being received into a place" or "patient accepted for inpatient services in a hospital." The admission process consists of various functions required to receive a patient at the hospital facility. Admission functions must be performed regardless of whether the patient presents to the hospital for outpatient services, ambulatory surgery, or inpatient admission. The purpose of the process is to obtain required information, determine patient care needs, and put a system into place to address patient care needs. A patient can be received in various areas in the hospital such as at the Emergency Department, ambulatory surgery, or inpatient hospital level.

A patient admission requires the hospital to follow specific procedures to ensure that quality patient care services are provided such as preadmission testing. Hospitals must meet Admission Evaluation Protocols (AEPs) for admission. Utilization review (UR) is performed to evaluate compliance with AEPs and other standards. Payers also conduct reviews to ensure that services provided are medically necessary, such as those conducted by a Quality Improvement Organization (QIO).

Preadmission Testing

Preadmission testing is required when a patient is admitted on an inpatient basis or for ambulatory surgery. The admitting physician prepares orders outlining preadmission testing requirements. Preadmission testing will vary based on the reason the patient is being admitted and the patient's condition. Preadmission testing can include but is not limited to blood tests, EKG, X-ray, urinalysis, ultrasound, and echocardiograms. The purpose of preadmission testing is to identify potential medical problems prior to surgery and to obtain a baseline of health care information on the patient's body system functions. The tests are done prior to admission to allow time for the results to be reviewed before the patient is admitted. It is important to remember that preadmission diagnostic services provided by the hospital within 3 days prior to the admission of a Medicare patient are included in the inpatient payment.

Utilization Review (UR)

The purpose of the UR process, as discussed in the previous chapter, is to ensure that the care provided is medically necessary and that the level where care is provided is appropriate based on the patient's condition. **Medical necessity** refers to services or procedures that are reasonable and medically necessary in response to the patient's symptoms, according to accepted standards of medical practice. The definition of medical necessity varies from payer to payer. Hospitals have implemented utilization management measures to ensure that patient care standards are met as required by:

- Federal and state licensing requirements
- The Joint Commission (TJC)
- Participating provider agreements with various payers and government programs
- Peer review organizations that have the authority to deny payment for services that do not meet stated requirements

The hospital's UM Department performs various functions to ensure that all guidelines for utilization are met and that hospital services are reimbursed appropriately. The UM Department monitors health care resources utilized at the facility by conducting URs of patient cases to determine whether:

- Services are medically necessary as defined in participating provider agreements
- The level of service for provision of health care is appropriate according to the patient's condition
- Quality patient care services are provided in accordance with standards of medical care
- The hospital length of stay is appropriate

The UM Department will determine whether documentation provides explanation and support for medical necessity, level of care, length of stay, and quality of care. If the documentation is not sufficient, a request for additional information is submitted to the provider. Discharge planning is another function performed by the UM Department; it includes an evaluation of the patient to determine whether discharge is appropriate and to identify patient needs after discharge. The department assists in developing a discharge plan that addresses patient care needs after discharge and coordinates various medical and financial resources in the community to meet patient care needs.

The UM Department is involved in resource utilization prior to the admission process, during the patient stay, and after the discharge process. URs can be conducted before, during, and after services are rendered.

BOX 4-9 ■ KEY POINTS

Utilization Review (UR)

Review patient care services to ensure that:

- Services are medically necessary
- Level of service is appropriate
- Quality patient care services are provided
- Hospital length of stay is appropriate

Admission Evaluation Protocol (AEP)

As discussed previously, a function of the UM Department is to conduct URs. Requirements for URs implemented under the Prospective Payment System (PPS) mandate that organizations follow specific criteria for the admission of Medicare patients. Other health care payers such as Blue Cross/Blue Shield (BC/BS), Aetna, and Cigna have also implemented UR measures in their plans. UR criteria will vary from payer to payer. Most payer requirements for appropriateness of hospital cases are based on the patient's condition. The purpose of the UR requirements is to ensure that hospital services provided are appropriate and medically necessary.

The review of hospital admissions for Medicare patients is designed to determine the appropriateness of an admission, based on the patient's condition. Appropriateness of admission is determined utilizing the **AEP** that outlines appropriate conditions for a hospital admission based on standards referred to as the IS/SI criteria. IS refers to the intensity of service criteria. SI refers to the severity of illness criteria.

BOX 4-10 ■ KEY POINTS

Admission Evaluation Protocols (AEPs)

As mandated under Prospective Payment Systems (PPS), hospitals must follow specific criteria for the admission of a Medicare patient.

The appropriateness of an admission is determined utilizing AEP criteria, which outline appropriate conditions for a hospital admission based on the following criteria:

- Intensity of service (IS)
- Severity of illness (SI)

Hospitals conduct a UR for each patient admission to determine whether the AEP criteria for each specific payer are met. As outlined in Tables 4-1 and 4-2, an admission can be certified if one of the SI or IS criteria is met. Contact is generally made with the payer within 24 hours to obtain admission certification. The purpose of obtaining admission certification is to ensure that the hospital is reimbursed for the hospital stay. Health care payers also conduct URs to determine the appropriateness of admission. Medicare, for example, utilizes a QIO to perform this function.

Quality Improvement Organization (QIO)

A QIO is an organization that contracts with Medicare and other payers to review patient cases to assess appropriateness and medical necessity. Medicare provides information on an admission to the QIO for evaluation. The QIO has a direct impact on reimbursement because it has the authority to deny payment for a hospital admission if it is determined that the AEP criteria are not met. The QIO may conduct reviews before the patient is admitted, at the time of admission, or at some point during the inpatient stay. The various reviews based on time are referred to as prospective, concurrent, or retrospective reviews, as defined below:

Prospective Review

A prospective review is performed prior to the patient's admission. Information regarding the patient's condition is reviewed to determine appropriateness for the admission and length of stay.

Concurrent Review

A concurrent review is generally ongoing throughout the hospital stay; it begins at admission. A review is performed to determine appropriateness of admission and care provided.

BOX 4-11 ■ KEY POINTS

Quality Improvement Organization (QIO)

QIOs contract with Medicare and other payers to review patient cases to ensure that:

- Services are medically necessary
- Admission Evaluation Protocol (AEP) criteria are met

QIOs have a direct impact on reimbursement because they have the authority to deny payment if AEP criteria are not met. The types of reviews are as follows:

- Prospective
- Concurrent
- Retrospective

TABLE 4-1 Screening Criteria Designed for Non-Physician Use

Severity of Illness	Notes/Examples
1. Oral temperature ≥101°F (rectal temperature ≥102°F)	
a. Culture/smear positive for pathogens (culture may be ordered and unreported at time of first review), or	
b. WBC ≥15,000/cu.mm	
2. Hemoglobin of <8 grams or >18 grams	Newly discovered
3. Hematocrit of <25% or >55%	Newly discovered
4. WBC >15,000/cu.mm	Newly discovered
5. Serum sodium <120 mEq/L or >156 mEq/L	
6. Serum potassium <3 mEq/L or >6 mEq/L	
7. Blood pH <7.3 or >7.5	Newly discovered
8. PO_2 <60 mm Hg and PCO_2 >50 mm Hg	Newly discovered
9. Blood culture positive for pathogens	
10. Sudden onset of functional impairment evidenced by one of the following: Loss of sight/hearing Loss of speech Loss of sensation or movement of body part Unconsciousness Disorientation/confusion/neurobehavioral changes Severe, incapacitating pain	
11. Uncontrolled active bleeding at present time	
12. Wound disruption (after major surgical procedure) requiring reclosure	
13. History of vomiting or diarrhea and any one of the following: Serum Na >156 mEq/L HCT >55 or Hgb >16 Urine specific gravity >1.026 Creatinine >2 mg% (recent onset) BUN >35mg%	Findings indicative of dehydration as a in any body system and requiring in-hospital care
14. Acute onset of chest pain/pressure; dyspnea/cyanosis	
15. Malignancy or recent history of surgey for malignancy	Scheduled for IV chemotherapy or radiation

From Abdelhak M, Grostick S, Hanken MA, Jacobs E (editors): Health information: management of a strategic resource, *ed 2, St Louis, 2001, Saunders.*
BUN, Blood urea nitrogen; *HCT,* hematocrit; *IV,* intravenous; *WBC,* white blood count.

Retrospective Review

A retrospective review is performed after the patient is discharged. The review is performed to determine appropriateness of admission and care provided.

PATIENT CARE PROCESS

The patient care process is complex, as it involves many departments simultaneously performing various tasks related to patient care services. The process of providing patient care begins when a patient arrives at the hospital for care and continues until the patient is discharged. To provide effective and efficient patient care services and maintain financial stability, it is necessary to obtain all information required to evaluate and treat the patient and to bill for patient care services. All patient care activities must be recorded in the patient's medical record to ensure that appropriate care is provided based on the patient's condition. It is critical to capture all charges for submission to patients and third-party payers. Outstanding accounts must be monitored to obtain reimbursement in a timely manner. To achieve high standards of patient care and maintain financial stability, the hospital must have an efficient flow of information through the patient care process. Figure 4-5 illustrates the phases of the patient care process: patient admission, patient care services, medical record documentation, charge capture, coding, patient discharge, billing, and accounts receivable management.

TABLE 4-2 **Screening Criteria Designed for Non-Physician Use**

Intensity of Service	Notes/Examples
1. Special monitoring every 2 hours or more often as necessary/appropriate for patient's condition	TPR, B/P, CVP, ABG, pulmonary artery pressure (Swan-Ganz), arterial lines
2. Observation and monitoring of neurological status every 2 hours or more often as necessary/appropriate for patient's condition	Documented in medical record
3. Intravenous fluids (except KVO) and requiring at least 2000 cc in 24 hours	
4. IV or IM medications every 12 hours or more frequently	If applicable to severity of illness
5. IV or IM analgesics 3 or more times daily	Pain not controlled as an outpatient
6. Respiratory assistance	Ventilator, O_2
7. Surgery performed (excluding outpatient surgery procedures list)	On admission or scheduled within 24 hours in continued stay
8. IV chemotherapy: antineoplastic agent	
9. Radiation	
Discharge Indicators	
1. Continued care and services could be rendered safely and effectively in an alternate setting	
2. Oral temperature <101°F for at least 24 hours without antipyretics	
3. Type and/or dosage of major drug unchanged for past 24 hours	
4. No parental analgesics/narcotics for last 12 hours	Exception: chronic pain from terminal illness or appropriate transfers to other facility
5. Voiding or draining urine (at least 800 cc) for last 24 hours or catheter removed and voiding sufficiently	
6. Passing flatus/fecal matter	
7. Diet tolerated for 24 hours without nausea or vomiting	
8. Wound(s) healing; no evidence of infection without documented, appropriate plan of outpatient treatment	
9. Discharged to SNF but refuses available SNF bed	
10. Stable hemoglobin/hematocrit	

From Abdelhak M, Grostick S, Hanken MA, Jacobs E (editors): Health information: management of a strategic resource, *ed 2, St Louis, 2001, Saunders.*
ABG, Arterial blood gas; *B/P*, blood pressure; *CVP*, central venous pressure; *IM*, intramuscular; *IV*, intravenous; *KVO*, keep vein open; *SNF*, skilled nursing facility; *TPR*, temperature, pulse, and respiration; *WBC*, white blood count.

BOX 4-12 ■ KEY POINTS

Patient Care Process

Admission
Patient care services
Medical record documentation
Charge capture and coding
Patient discharge
Billing
Accounts receivable management

ADMISSIONS PROCESS

The admissions process refers to the various tasks performed when a patient is received at the hospital or admitted as an inpatient. The purpose of the process is to obtain all required information to evaluate and treat the patient. The phases in the process are standard; however, there are variations based on the type of admission. Variations may involve the forms used and some of the functions. The Admissions Department

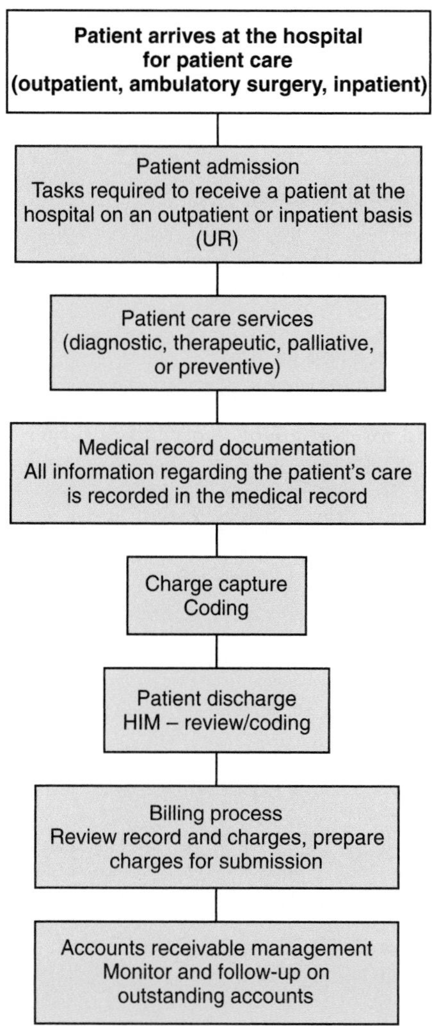

Figure 4-5 Phases of the patient care process.

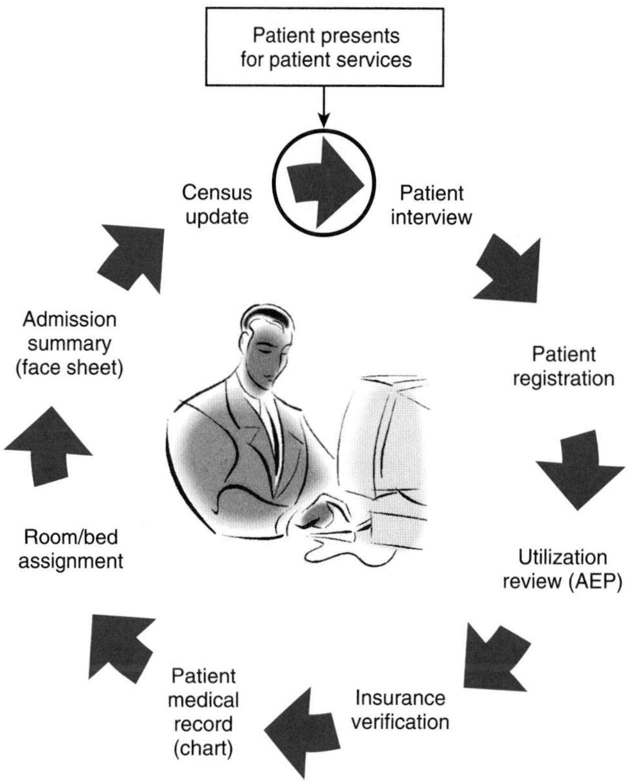

Figure 4-6 The admissions process.

performs functions required to receive the patient, which involves obtaining all required information. The UR Department conducts a review of the admission to ensure that AEP criteria are met. This process begins with the patient interview and it includes registration of patient information, utilization review, insurance verification, preparation of the patient chart, assignment of a room/bed, preparation of an admission summary (face sheet), and updating the hospital's census (Figure 4-6).

Patient Interview

The patient interview is conducted for the purpose of obtaining information regarding the patient and his or her insurance. Required consents and authorizations are also obtained during the patient interview, including a signed Informed Consent for Treatment, Written Authorization for Release of Information, signed Assignment of Benefits, the patient's advance directives, and an Advance Beneficiary Notice when appropriate. The information obtained from the patient is entered into the patient's computer account and placed in the patient's medical record. It may also be necessary to obtain financial information from the patient to assist the patient in finding alternative resources for payment of health care services.

BOX 4-13 ■ KEY POINTS

Admissions Process

Patient interview
Patient registration
Utilization review
Insurance verification
Patient's medical record(chart)
Room/bed assignment
Admissions summary (face sheet)
Census update

Patient and Insurance Information

Patient information is obtained by the hospital through the use of a **patient registration form**. The patient registration form varies by hospital. The form generally contains fields for information regarding the patient, insurance carrier, guarantor, diagnosis, and physician, as illustrated in Figure 4-7. The patient registration form

TEST YOUR *Knowledge* BOX 4-1

PATIENT ACCOUNTS AND DATA FLOW; PATIENT ADMISSION

1. List three types of information included in the flow of information in a hospital.
2. Explain how the hospital's health information system enhances the access and flow of data.
3. Discuss three service types that result in variations of the type of data and its flow.
4. Explain when a physician order, requisition, or referral is required for outpatient, ambulatory surgery, or inpatient services.
5. How does the type of data and flow vary for inpatient services?
6. List five outpatient areas where a patient may be seen in the hospital.
7. List three areas where data and flow of information varies for outpatient services.
8. Define ambulatory surgery.
9. Explain when physician services are billed by the hospital.
10. Explain what an inpatient admission is and list three areas from which a patient can be admitted.
11. Provide a definition of admission.
12. Discuss the purpose of preadmission testing.
13. Provide a brief explanation of the purpose of utilization review.
14. How does utilization review relate to medical necessity?
15. Hospitals are required to follow specific admission criteria for Medicare patients as outlined under what regulations?
16. State the purpose of AEP protocols and list two standards that hospitals follow.
17. Explain what department within the hospital is involved in AEP protocol reviews.
18. What is a QIO?
19. Discuss the impact QIO reviews can have on reimbursement.
20. List and provide a brief explanation of three types of reviews conducted by a QIO.

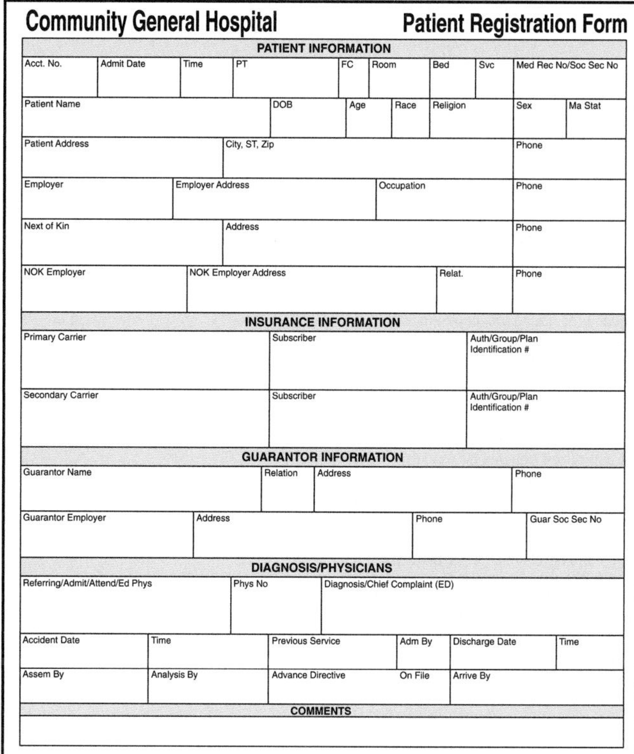

Community General Hospital **Patient Registration Form**

PATIENT INFORMATION

Acct. No. | Admit Date | Time | PT | FC | Room | Bed | Svc | Med Rec No/Soc Sec No

Patient Name | DOB | Age | Race | Religion | Sex | Ma Stat

Patient Address | City, ST, Zip | Phone

Employer | Employer Address | Occupation | Phone

Next of Kin | Address | Phone

NOK Employer | NOK Employer Address | Relat. | Phone

INSURANCE INFORMATION

Primary Carrier | Subscriber | Auth/Group/Plan Identification #

Secondary Carrier | Subscriber | Auth/Group/Plan Identification #

GUARANTOR INFORMATION

Guarantor Name | Relation | Address | Phone

Guarantor Employer | Address | Phone | Guar Soc Sec No

DIAGNOSIS/PHYSICIANS

Referring/Admit/Attend/Ed Phys | Phys No | Diagnosis/Chief Complaint (ED)

Accident Date | Time | Previous Service | Adm By | Discharge Date | Time

Assem By | Analysis By | Advance Directive | On File | Arrive By

COMMENTS

Figure 4-7 Sample patient registration form.

is completed by the patient and reviewed by the admission representative.

Patient Information

This section is utilized for recording the patient's demographic information. Demographic information is data about the patient such as the patient's name, address, phone number, date of birth, sex, religion, and employer. A copy of the patient's driver's license is generally obtained for identification purposes.

Insurance Information

This section is utilized to record information regarding the insurance carrier or government program under which the patient has coverage. Insurance information includes the name, address, and phone number of the primary and secondary carrier. The plan information is also required, such as plan and group number and patient identification number. The subscriber name is required if the patient is not the policyholder.

Insurance card(s) contain information regarding the insurance plan or government program under which the patient has coverage. A copy of the insurance card is made (front and back) and maintained in the patient's medical record. It is important to copy both sides of the card since they contain information regarding the patient's co-payments, the authorization phone numbers, and the insurance company address.

Guarantor Information

This section is utilized to record the name, address, phone number, and Social Security number of the guarantor. The **guarantor** is the individual who is responsible for paying for services rendered. The patient is the guarantor unless he or she is a minor or incapable. In these situations the patient's guardian or person holding the power of attorney may be the guarantor, for example, when a power of attorney is designated for an elderly patient who is unable to handle his or her affairs.

Diagnosis and Physician Information

Information regarding the patient's condition and the referring or admitting physician is recorded in this section. It is important to obtain information regarding the patient's condition as it provides an explanation of the reason for the hospital visit. This information is utilized to determine compliance with AEP criteria, verify insurance, and obtain an Advance Beneficiary Notice (ABN).

Financial Information

It may be necessary to obtain information regarding the patient's financial status, such as income, expenses, and assets. When the patient does not have insurance coverage, the PFS Department may utilize this information to provide assistance in finding other funding resources for health care services.

BOX 4-14 ■ KEY POINTS

Patient and Insurance Information

The following information is obtained during the admission process:

- Patient information (demographic)
- Insurance information
- Guarantor information
- Diagnosis and physician information
- Financial information

Consents and Authorizations

Hospitals utilize a variety of forms to obtain consents and authorizations. A facility may use one form that contains the informed consent, authorization, and assignment of benefits (Figure 4-8). Other facilities may have separate forms for such benefit information.

Informed Consent for Treatment

The Informed Consent for Treatment form is utilized by the hospital to obtain the patient's authorization for treatment. The form must be signed by the patient before treatment can be provided. The patient usually signs the Informed Consent for Treatment unless the patient is a minor or incapable. When the patient is

COMMUNITY GENERAL HOSPITAL
PATIENT CONSENT AND AUTHORIZATION

PATIENT AGREEMENT and CONSENT

As a condition of my or my child's admission or treatment to the Hospital/Facility I hereby agree to the following:

1. **CONSENT TO TREATMENT:** I hereby authorize the physicians in charge of my care and the Hospital/Facility to provide services including, but not limited to, emergency medical services, routine diagnostic procedures, and medical procedures as their judgment may deem necessary or advisable. I understand that, under the direction of my treating Physician, a Physician's Assistant, Advanced Registered Nurse Practitioner, students or residents affiliated with the Hospital/Facility may be utilized in my care and treatment.

2. **CONSENT TO TRANSFER TO 24 HOUR FACILITY:** I hereby consent to be transferred to a 24 hour facility for further medical treatment when my medical condition indicates that level of care is appropriate in the judgment of my treating physician.

3. **AUTHORIZATION TO RELEASE MEDICAL INFORMATION:** I hereby authorize the Hospital/Facility and/or any treating physician(s) to release to any third party payor (such as an insurance company, its designated review agency or a government agency) only such diagnostic and therapeutic information (including psychiatric, drug abuse, alcohol, or HFV status) as may be necessary to determine benefits entitlement and to process payment claims for health care services provided to me, commencing on this date. The Hospital/Facility and any physician(s) rendering service at the Hospital/Facility are authorized to release information from my medical records to any skilled nursing facility or other health care facility to which I may be transferred for continuing care or research purposes.

4. **MEDICARE/MEDIGAP/MEDICAID/PATIENT CERTIFICATION/RELEASE OF INFORMATION & PAYMENT REQUEST:** I certify that the information given to apply for payment under Title XVIII and/or Title XIX, of the Social Security Act is correct. I authorize any holder of medical or other information about me to release to the Social Security Administration or its intermediaries or carriers any information needed for this or a related Medicare claim. I request that payment of authorized benefits be made on my behalf. I assign the benefits payable for physician services to the physician or organization furnishing the services or authorize such physician or organization to submit a claim to Medicare, Medigap or Medicaid for payment to me. I understand that I am responsible for any health insurance deductibles and co-payments.

5. **ASSIGNMENT OF INSURANCE BENEFITS:** I hereby authorize, request and direct any and all assigned insurance companies to pay directly to the Hospital/Facility and/or any treating physician(s) the amount due me in my pending claims for hospital/facility benefits under the respective policies. I agree that should the amount be insufficient to cover the entire Hospital/Facility expense, including the co-payment and the deductible, I will be responsible for payment of the difference, and that if the nature of the services rendered are not covered by said policy, I will be responsible to the Hospital/Facility and/or any treating physician for payment of the entire bill.

6. **GUARANTEE OF PAYMENT:** For value received, including but not limited to the services rendered, I agree to guarantee and promise to pay the Hospital/Facility and/or any treating physician(s), all charges and expenses incurred in my treatment, including those expenses not covered by any insurance policy presently in force, including any co-payment and/or deductible. Unless specifically agreed in writing, all charges shall be paid at discharge. Unpaid accounts shall bear interest at the rate provided by law, whether suit is brought or appeal taken. If any action at law or in equity is brought to enforce this agreement, the Hospital/Facility and/or any treating physician(s) shall be entitled to recover reasonable attorney's fees, court costs, and any other costs of collection incurred.

7. **RELEASE OF RESPONSIBILITY AND LIABILITY FOR PERSONAL VALUABLES:** I understand and agree that the Hospital/Facility is not responsible for personal valuables or belongings brought into the health system, or claimed to have been brought into the health system by me or my agent. Personal valuables or belongings include, but are not limited to, clothing, personal hygiene products, toiletries, dentures, glasses, prosthetic devises (such as hearing aides, artificial limbs, or assist devices such as: canes, walkers, or wheelchairs), credit cards, jewelry and money. I understand that the Hospital/Facility discourages retaining personal valuables at bedside and that a locked area is available for securing my personal valuables small enough to fit in a security envelope. Valuables not claimed within 90 days of discharge will be discarded.

8. **RECEIPT OF "AN IMPORTANT MESSAGE FROM MEDICARE/ CHAMPUS":** I understand that after my discharge from the Hospital/Facility, an individual from the State of Florida's Peer Review Organization (PRO) may review my records of care. I understand that the purpose of this review is to determine whether or not admission to the Hospital/Facility was necessary and to review the quality of care given to me during the time I was hospitalized. My signature only acknowledges my receipt of "An Important Message from Medicare" and does not waive any of my rights to request a review or make me liable for my payment.

9. **RECEIPT OF PATIENT'S BILL OF RIGHTS AND RESPONSIBILITIES BROCHURE AND NOTICE OF PRIVACY PRACTICES:** By my signature on this document, I acknowledge receipt of a Patient's Bill of Rights and Responsibilities brochure pursuant to Florida Statute 381.026, prior to or at the time of admission and the Notice of Privacy Practices.

I CERTIFY THAT THE INFORMATION CONTAINED IN THIS DOCUMENT HAS BEEN READ BY OR EXPLAINED TO ME AND I UNDERSTAND THIS INFORMATION. I WILL RECEIVE A COPY OF THIS DOCUMENT UPON REQUEST. I ACKNOWLEDGE THAT A COPY OF THIS DOCUMENT SHALL BE AS EFFECTIVE AS THE ORIGINAL.

Patient Signature____________ Date______ Patient unable to sign because____________

Signature of Patient's Authorized Representative________ Relationship to Patient____________

Figure 4-8 Sample combined patient consent, authorization, and assignment of benefits.

unable to sign, a parent, guardian, health surrogate, or an individual with a power of attorney may sign.

Written Authorization for Release of Medical Information

The Written Authorization for Release of Medical Information provides the hospital with the authorization to release personal health information when required for treatment and to obtain payment for services. A breach of confidentiality will occur if information is released without authorization from the patient.

Assignment of Benefits

The patient signs the Assignment of Benefits form to instruct the insurance company or government plan to forward benefits (payments for services) to the hospital.

Advance Directives

The patient's **advance directives** provide instructions regarding measures that should or should not be taken in the event that medical treatment is required to prolong life. The hospital can provide a patient with advance directive forms for completion if the patient has no advance directives.

An advance directive can be either a living will or a durable power of attorney. A living will is a written document that allows a competent adult to indicate his or her wishes regarding life-prolonging medical treatment. A durable power of attorney for health care is a

ADVANCE DIRECTIVE CHECKLIST

Patient Name: ______________________

❑ Advance Directives Brochure Provided ❑ Advance Directives Brochure Refused

The Following Information Was Obtained From: ❑ Patient ❑ Other: ______

❑ **Patient HAS executed the following Advance Directive(s):**	**COPY RECEIVED THIS ADMIT**	**COPY RECEIVED PRIOR ADMIT**	**COPY REQUESTED**
❑ Declaration for Health Care Decisions (Living Will)	❑	❑	❑
❑ Medical Power of Attorney (MPOA) Name: ______ Relationship: ______	❑	❑	❑
❑ Mental Healthcare Power of Attorney (MHPOA) Name: ______ Relationship: ______	❑	❑	❑
❑ Combination Power of Attorney (that includes MPOA language)	❑	❑	❑
❑ Other: (specify)	❑	❑	❑

❑ Patient **HAS NOT** executed Advance Directive(s). (Check items below **ONLY** when talking with patient.)	**PATIENT Was Advised On** ______ (date).
❑ **PATIENT** requests more information.	❑ of the *right to accept or refuse medical treatment.*
❑ Social Services notified.	❑ of the *right to formulate Advance Directives.*
❑ **PATIENT** chooses not to execute Advance Directives at this time.	❑ of the *right to receive medical treatment whether or not there is an Advance Directive.*

For Home Health/Hospice Use Only:

❑ Patient **HAS** EXECUTED Prehospital Medical Care (Arizona's Orange Card).

❑ Patient was advised of the *right to have Advance Directives followed by the health care facility and caregivers to the extent permitted by law.*

Signature of Facility Representative:	Department:	Date:

IF ADVANCED DIRECTIVE IS UNAVAILABLE, *the patient indicates that the substance of the directive is as follows: (see reverse for script)*

Living Will: ______

Medical Power of Attorney: ______

❑ Patient signature (legal representative if applicable): ______

❑ Witness signature (if patient physically unable to sign): ______ Reason: ______

Verification Upon Admit/Re-Admit or Transfer:

Verified with patient/legal representative that Advance Directives in medical record are current.	Verified with patient/legal representative that Advance Directives in medical record are current.	Verified with patient/legal representative that Advance Directives in medical record are current.
Signature:	Signature:	Signature:
Date:	Date:	Date:

PATIENT IDENTIFICATION

Figure 4-9 Sample advance directive checklist. *(From Brooks ML, Gillingham ET:* Health unit coordinating, *ed 5, St Louis, 2004, Saunders.)*

written document that is used to appoint a competent adult to make any medical decisions on his or her behalf in the event the person becomes incapacitated.*

Many hospitals use an advance directives checklist to document that a patient was informed about advance directives (Figure 4-9).

Advance Beneficiary Notice (ABN)

An ABN informs the patient that there is reason to believe the admission will not be covered by Medicare. The patient's signature is required on this form to acknowledge that he or she will be financially responsible if Medicare does not cover the service (Figure 4-10).

*From Abdelhak M, Grostick S, Hanken MA, Jacobs E (eds): *Health information: management of a strategic resource*, ed 2, Philadelphia, 2001,WB Saunders.

BOX 4-15 ■ KEY POINTS

Consents and Authorizations

The following consents and authorizations are obtained during the admission process:

- Informed Consent for Treatment
- Written Authorization for Release of Medical Information
- Assignment of Benefits
- Advance directives
- Advance Beneficiary Notice (ABN)

(A) **Notifier(s):**
(B) **Patient Name:** *(C)* **Identification Number:**

ADVANCE BENEFICIARY NOTICE OF NONCOVERAGE (ABN)

NOTE: If Medicare doesn't pay for ***(D)***_____________ below, you may have to pay.

Medicare does not pay for everything, even some care that you or your health care provider have good reason to think you need. We expect Medicare may not pay for the ***(D)***____________ below.

*(D)*______________	*(E)* Reason Medicare May Not Pay:	*(F)* Estimated Cost:

WHAT YOU NEED TO DO NOW:

- Read this notice, so you can make an informed decision about your care.
- Ask us any questions that you may have after you finish reading.
- Choose an option below about whether to receive the ***(D)***____________listed above.
  Note: If you choose Option 1 or 2, we may help you to use any other insurance that you might have, but Medicare cannot require us to do this.

(G) **OPTIONS:** **Check only one box. We cannot choose a box for you.**

❑ **OPTION 1.** I want the ***(D)***__________ listed above. You may ask to be paid now, but I also want Medicare billed for an official decision on payment, which is sent to me on a Medicare Summary Notice (MSN). I understand that if Medicare doesn't pay, I am responsible for payment, but **I can appeal to Medicare** by following the directions on the MSN. If Medicare does pay, you will refund any payments I made to you, less co-pays or deductibles.

❑ **OPTION 2.** I want the ***(D)***__________ listed above, but do not bill Medicare. You may ask to be paid now as I am responsible for payment. **I cannot appeal if Medicare is not billed.**

❑ **OPTION 3.** I don't want the ***(D)***__________listed above. I understand with this choice I am **not** responsible for payment, and **I cannot appeal to see if Medicare would pay.**

(H) **Additional Information:**

This notice gives our opinion, not an official Medicare decision. If you have other questions on this notice or Medicare billing, call **1-800-MEDICARE** (1-800-633-4227/**TTY**: 1-877-486-2048).

Signing below means that you have received and understand this notice. You also receive a copy.

(I) **Signature:**	*(J)* **Date:**

According to the Paperwork Reduction Act of 1995, no persons are required to respond to a collection of information unless it displays a valid OMB control number. The valid OMB control number for this information collection is 0938-0566. The time required to complete this information collection is estimated to average 7 minutes per response, including the time to review instructions, search existing data resources, gather the data needed, and complete and review the information collection. If you have comments concerning the accuracy of the time estimate or suggestions for improving this form, please write to: CMS, 7500 Security Boulevard, Attn: PRA Reports Clearance Officer, Baltimore, Maryland 21244-1850.

Form CMS-R-131 (03/08) Form Approved OMB No. 0938-0566

Figure 4-10 Advance Beneficiary Notice (ABN). *(From www.cms.hhs.gov.)*

Patient Registration

The patient registration process consists of creating a patient account on the hospital's computer system and entering patient information obtained during the patient interview. The patient's account is the computerized record by which the patient information is recorded and maintained. An account and medical record number are assigned to each patient either by the system or by the person entering the information. The account is updated when required to reflect new information or changes in current information. Financial activity is also entered on the patient's account. Financial activity is discussed in detail in Chapter 5.

Utilization Review (UR)

As discussed previously, the UM Department performs a UR to ensure that AEP criteria are met and that patient care services are appropriate and medically necessary.

Insurance Verification

Insurance verification is the process of contacting the patient's insurance plan to determine various aspects of coverage such as whether the patient's coverage is active, what services are covered, authorization requirements, and patient responsibility. Insurance verification is required to ensure that the hospital will receive payment for services rendered and to determine the patient's share of the hospital's charges, referred to as the patient's responsibility. The individual responsible for verifying insurance contacts the insurance company or government program to:

- Verify that the patient's insurance coverage is active
- Determine what services will be covered
- Ensure that AEP criteria are met
- Obtain prior authorization or precertification
- Determine the amount for which the patient is responsible (deductible, co-insurance, or co-payment).

BOX 4-16 ■ KEY POINTS

Insurance Verification

Contact is made with the patient's insurance plan to:

- Verify that the patient's insurance is active
- Ascertain what services will be covered
- Ensure that Admission Evaluation Protocol (AEP) criteria are met
- Obtain prior authorization or precertification
- Determine the patient's responsibility

BOX 4-17 ■ KEY POINTS

Patient Responsibility

The patient is required to pay the following in accordance with his or her health care plan:

- Deductible. An annual amount determined by the payer that the patient must pay before the plan pays benefits
- Co-insurance. A percentage of the approved amount that the patient is required to pay
- Co-payment. A fixed amount determined per service that the patient must pay

The **deductible** is an annual amount determined by each payer that the patient must pay before the plan pays benefits for services. For example, the patient may be required to meet a $500 deductible annually before the payer will provide reimbursement for services.

Co-insurance is an amount the patient is responsible to pay that is calculated based on a percentage of approved charges. An example of co-insurance may be a plan that requires the patient to pay 20% of the approved amount for health care services.

A **co-payment** is a set amount that is paid by the patient for specific services. Co-payment amounts vary by service. For example, the patient's plan may require the patient to pay a $300 co-payment for an ambulatory surgery procedure. Co-payment is commonly referred to as co-pay.

The insurance verification process can be performed during the preadmission process or on the date of admission. A representative from the Admissions Department or the PFS Department may perform verification.

Patient's Medical Record (Chart)

The patient's **medical record** is a chart or folder where the patient's information is stored, including demographic, insurance, financial, and medical information. An electronic version of the patient medical record is called the electronic heath record (EHR). Each patient seen in the hospital has a medical record. Medical records are assigned a medical record number. The **medical record number (MRN)** is a unique identification number assigned by the hospital to each patient's medical record. The MRN assigned by the hospital generally remains the patient's medical record number indefinitely. Many hospitals have an electronic medical record system where the patient's medical information is maintained on a computer system. A bracelet is prepared with the patient's name, room number, medical record number, and admitting physician's name. The patient is required to wear the bracelet for the purpose of identification while in the hospital.

Room/Bed Assignment

A patient who is admitted on an inpatient basis is assigned a room and/or a bed. Semiprivate rooms have two beds in each room; therefore the patient would be assigned a room and a bed. Room assignment is also performed in outpatient areas such as Ambulatory Surgery, the Emergency Department, or Observation. The room assignment is recorded on the patient's record.

Admission Summary (Face Sheet)

An **admission summary** is also known as a face sheet; it is a summary of information about the patient's admission, such as the patient's name and address, insurance company name, reason(s) for admission, attending physician's name, and referring physician's name. The admission summary is prepared and distributed to the appropriate individuals (Figure 4-11).

Census Update

The hospital's census is a daily listing of rooms available for assignment (Figure 4-12). To update the hospital's census list, admissions personnel must record the patient's name next to the room/bed that was assigned. Room assignments are also recorded on the computer system for reporting purposes. The census is maintained

1 PATIENT HOSP.NO.(M.R.#) 987-654 | INFO STATUS | ACCOUNT NO. (BUS. OFF.) 123-456

2 PATIENT NAME LAST Andrews / FIRST Iver | MIDDLE S. | ADM. DATE MO. DAY YR. 8 / 7 / XX | ADM. TIME 1345 | HOW BROUGHT TO HOSPITAL Amb.

3 PATIENT'S CURRENT ADDRESS STREET, P.O. BOX, APT. NO. 701 East Danish Lane | CITY Carpenterville, | STATE AZ | ZIP CODE 85013 | TELEPHONE NO. 246-XXXX

4 PATIENT'S PERMANENT ADDRESS STREET, P.O. BOX, APT. NO. Same | CITY | STATE | ZIP CODE | TELEPHONE NO.

5 SEX 1. MALE 2. FEMALE [1] | MARITAL STATUS 1. SINGLE 2. MARRIED 3. SEPARATED 4. DIVORCED 5. WIDOWED [5] | RACE 1. WHITE 2. BLACK 3. INDIAN 4. ORIENTAL 5. OTHER [1] | RELIGION 1. CATHOLIC 2. JEWISH 3. PROTESTANT 4. OTHER 5. LDS [3] | AREA OF RESIDENCE

6 BIRTHDATE 10/6/XX | AGE 69 | PLACE OF BIRTH N.J. | MAIDEN NAME | SOC. SEC. NO./MEDICARE NO. 151-18-XXXX

7 PATIENT'S OCCUPATION Retired | UNION & LOCAL NO. | PATIENT'S EMPLOYER | ADDRESS | TELEPHONE NO.

8 PREVIOUSLY TREATED HERE? ☒ YES ☐ NO NAME USED Same | PREV. ADM. DATE MO. DA. YR. 2/3/XX | PREV. ADMISSION 1. INPATIENT 2. OUTPATIENT [1] | IF NEWBORN, MOTHER'S HOSP. NO.

9 UNIT A5 | ROOM NO. | ACCOM. CODES 1. PRI 2. SEMI 3. NURSERY 4. PREMIE 5. ICU 6. RCU 7. CCU 8. VIP [2] | ROOM RATE | PAY STATUS | CLASS OF ADMISSION 1. EMERGENCY 2. ELECTIVE 3. URGENT 4. OTHER [3]

10 ADMITTING DIAGNOSIS Cerebrovascular accident

11 PHYSICIAN NAME I.M. Human | PHYSICIAN NO. 432 | ADM. SERVICE Med. | INFORMATION OBTAINED FROM: daughter

12 SPOUSE OR NEAREST RELATIVE (NEXT OF KIN) Kay Ellis | RELATIONSHIP daugh | ADDRESS 301 West Restful Dr. Phoenix | TELEPHONE NO. 258-XXXX

13 SECOND RELATIVE OR FRIEND Marie Darrow | RELATIONSHIP sister | ADDRESS 12 Center St. Danstown, CA | TELEPHONE NO. 837-XXXX

14 RESPONSIBLE PARTY NAME Self | RELATIONSHIP | SOC. SEC. NO.

15 RESP. PARTY ADDRESS STREET P.O. BOX APT. NO. | CITY | STATE | ZIP CODE | TELEPHONE NO.

16 RESP. PARTY OCCUPATION | NO. YRS. IN THIS EMPLOY | RESP. PARTY EMPLOYER | ADDRESS | TELEPHONE NO.

17 LENGTH OF TIME IN ARIZ. 10 yrs. | 1. OWN HOME 2. RENT HOME [1] | TYPE OF HOME Single | BANK NAME & BRANCH Desert National - Camelhead | 1. SAVINGS 2. CHECKING [1]

18 CREDIT REFERENCES 1. NAME Deep River S&L | ADDRESS 9832 N. LasVegas Pl. Phoenix | TELEPHONE NO. 943-XXXX

19 2. NAME Yucca Federal | ADDRESS 1903 W. Bottletree Ave. Phoenix | TELEPHONE NO. 246-XXXX

20 INDUSTRIAL INJURY DATE: MO. DA. YR. | CLAIM NO. | EMPLOYER'S NAME AND ADDRESS AT TIME OF INJURY

21 BLUE CROSS NAME OF PLAN | GROUP NO. | IDENTIFICATION | EFFECTIVE DATE MO. DA. YR. | CITY | STATE

22 CHAMPUS DATA PATIENT'S ID NO. | CARD EFFECTIVE MO. DA. YR. | CARD EXPIRES MO. DA. YR. | PATIENT OR SPONSORS BRANCH OF SERVICE | SERVICE CARD NO.

23 SPONSORS NAME | RANK-SERVICE NO. | DUTY STATION

24 OTHER INSURANCE (INC. BLOOD BANK & BLUE SHIELD) INS. CO. NO. 1000 | COMPANY NAME Desert State | POLICY HOLDER NAME Iver Andrews | POLICY NO. A657483 | DATE ISSUED MO. DA. YR. 2/17/XX | CITY | STATE AZ

25 INS. CO. NO. | COMPANY NAME | POLICY HOLDER NAME | POLICY NO. | DATE ISSUED MO. DA. YR. | CITY | STATE

26 NAME OF HEALTH FACILITY DISCHARGED FROM WITHIN LAST 60 DAYS None | ADDRESS

27 OTHER INFO. V.A. ☐ | COORDINATION OF BENEFITS ☐ | INTERVIEWED BY G. Talker | TYPED BY W.K.S.

28 REMARKS:

Figure 4-11 Sample admission summary (face sheet). *(From Brooks ML, Gillingham ET:* Health unit coordinating, ed 5, *St Louis, 2004, Saunders.)*

daily, and census statistics are frequently reviewed to monitor the hospital's admissions.

MEDICAL RECORD DOCUMENTATION

Medical record documentation is critical to the provision of patient care services and for billing patient care services. The HIM Department is involved in both areas as it is responsible for the patient's medical record and performs many important functions related to reimbursement for patient care services.

As discussed previously, all pertinent information regarding patient care services is recorded in the patient's medical record. Patient records include various documents gathered throughout the patient stay from admission to after discharge. They are legal documents, and ensuring the confidentiality and security of these records is a critical function of HIM. As discussed previously, HIM is responsible for the organization, maintenance, production, storage, retention, dissemination, and security of patient information. The HIM Department also monitors documentation to ensure that documentation standards are met throughout the hospital. To achieve this goal, HIM may be involved in the development and revision of hospital forms. Two important functions performed by HIM that have a direct impact on the reimbursement process are:

1. Maintenance of the chargemaster.
2. Coding of clinical data for claim submission.

HIM personnel include certified coders whose responsibilities include coding procedures, items, and patient conditions recorded in the patient's medical record. The codes selected by HIM are recorded in the computer system, and they are utilized for MS-DRG/APC assignment and to describe what services were performed and patient conditions (why) on the claim form.

To understand the significance of the medical record and HIM responsibilities, it is necessary to understand the purpose and content of medical record documentation.

Community Hospital Daily Census Report

Room #	Patient Name	Activities
301	Breath, Les	DC Today
302	Pickens, Slim	Surg 11^{00} x ray to be sent c̄ patient
303-1	Katt, Kitty	
303-2		
304	Bee, Mae	~~Call Dr. James c̄ ABG results~~ Called Sue 9^{00}
305	Honey, Mai	NPO for heart cath @ 9^{00}
306-1		
306-2		
307	Pack, Fanny	No calls to room
308	Bugg, June	DC today
309	~~Kynde, Bee~~	Trans to ICU 11^{30}
310-1	Cider, Ida	DNR
310-2	Soo, Ah	~~Surg 8~~^{00} Back @ 1^{30}
311-1	Bear, Harry	Resp isolation
311-2	Bread, Thad	
312-1	Kream, Kris	NINP
312-2	Pat, Peggy	~~Surg 9~~^{30} Back @ 2^{00}

Figure 4-12 Hospital daily census report. *(Modified from Brooks ML, Gillingham ET:* Health unit coordinating, *ed 5, St Louis, 2004, Saunders.)*

BOX 4-18 ■ KEY POINTS

The Role of HIM in Medical Record Documentation

HIM is responsible for the following areas of medical record documentation and reimbursement:

- Organization, maintenance, production, storage, retention, dissemination, and security of patient information
- Maintenance of the chargemaster

Purpose of Documentation

The purpose of medical record documentation is to have a detailed accounting of all patient care activities. Medical record documentation serves many purposes in a health care facility, such as enhancing communications, supporting charges billed, improving utilization review, and providing protection from liability.

Communication

A detailed recording of all information regarding the patient's condition and patient care services enhances communication between providers involved with the patient's care. Review of complete and detailed documentation can assist providers in gaining a better understanding of all aspects of the patient case. This knowledge is critical to the provider's ability to assess the patient's condition and develop an effective treatment plan.

Support Charges Billed

The Golden Rule in coding and billing is "***IF IT IS NOT DOCUMENTED, DO NOT CODE IT OR BILL IT.***" Comprehensive documentation that includes all services and items provided is necessary for submission of charges to payers. Payers do not provide reimbursement for services that are not medically necessary. A detailed recording of all information regarding the patient's condition provides an explanation of the medical necessity for services provided.

Utilization Review

Documentation is utilized for UR conducted within the hospital to determine the appropriateness of care. Documentation is also utilized for payer reviews such as those conducted by the QIO.

Liability

Thorough and complete documentation is considered the best defense in a liability case. Medical records are reviewed in liability cases to determine negligence with regard to the provision of patient care services.

It is because documentation serves so many purposes that the content of a medical record is very detailed. To provide an understanding of how documentation relates to each of the purposes discussed above, it is necessary to look at the content of a medical record.

BOX 4-19 ■ KEY POINTS

Purpose of Documentation

Documentation provides a detailed accounting of all patient care activity, which serves the following purposes:

- Enhancement of communications among providers
- Support for charges billed
- Improvement of utilization review
- Protection in liability review

BOX 4-20 ■ KEY POINTS

The Golden Rule in Coding and Billing

IF IT IS NOT DOCUMENTED, DO NOT CODE IT OR BILL IT.

Content of the Patient's Medical Record

Documentation is a chronological recording of a patient's assessment, diagnosis, treatment plan, and outcomes of treatments. Specific elements are required in documentation:

TEST YOUR *Knowledge* BOX 4-2

PATIENT CARE PROCESS; ADMISSION PROCESS

1. Explain the relationship between UR and AEP protocols.
2. Discuss why the patient care process is complex in the hospital.
3. When does the patient care process begin?
4. Explain why it is important to obtain all required information to treat the patient and bill for services.
5. List seven phases in the patient care process.
6. How does the admission process relate to the patient care process?
7. Provide a brief explanation of what the admission process is and its purpose.
8. Outline the major functions performed during the admission process.
9. State the purpose of the patient interview.
10. Describe three types of information obtained during the patient interview.
11. Define guarantor and discuss what guarantor information is required.
12. Discuss four reasons why information regarding the patient's diagnosis must be obtained.
13. Indicate the purpose of the Assignment of Benefits form.
14. Identify the form required to prevent breach of confidentiality.
15. State the purpose of an ABN.
16. Provide a brief explanation of the patient registration process.
17. State the purpose of insurance verification and provide a brief overview.
18. What is the purpose of the patient's medical record?
19. Discuss how room/bed assignment affects census updating.
20. Provide a brief explanation of an admission summary.

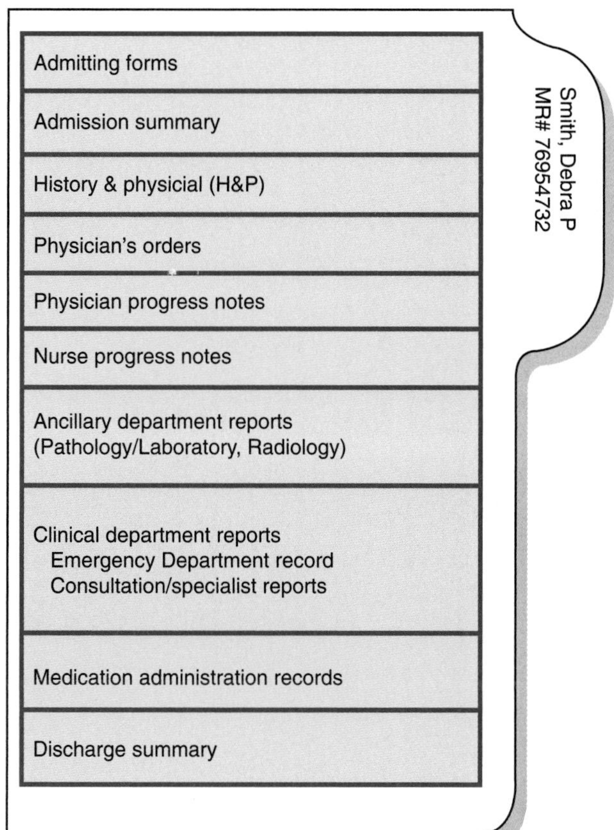

Figure 4-13 Content of the patient's medical record.

- All conditions, diagnosis, injury, illness, disease, and/or other reasons for the visit
- Plan of care for treatment of the patient's condition
- All diagnostic and therapeutic procedures performed
- Outcomes of diagnostic and therapeutic procedures

Documentation is maintained in a chart called the medical record. The chart is organized in sections that contain relative forms and notes. The medical record contains the following documents: admission forms, admission summary, history and physical, physician orders, progress notes, ancillary and other clinical department reports, medication administration records, and a discharge summary. Figure 4-13 provides an outline of the medical record documents.

Admitting Forms

Various forms are obtained when the patient is admitted, including patient registration, authorizations, release of information, Written Consent for Treatment, Assignment of Benefits, advance directives, and an ABN when required.

Admission Summary (Face Sheet)

As discussed earlier, the face sheet is an outline of information regarding the patient's admission, such as date of admission, admitting diagnosis, admitting physician, referring physician, and insurance. This summary is maintained in the patient's chart (see Figure 4-11).

History and Physical (H&P)

The H & P is a detailed accounting of the history, physical examination, and decision making regarding the patient's condition at the time of admission. The H&P is performed when the patient is admitted and is dictated or written by the admitting physician (Figure 4-14).

BOX 4-21 ■ KEY POINTS

Content of Documentation

A chronological recording of the patient's assessment, diagnosis, and treatment includes the following elements:

- Every condition, diagnosis, injury, illness, disease, and/or other reason for the visit
- Plan of care for the treatment of the patient's condition
- All diagnostic and therapeutic procedures performed
- Outcomes of diagnostic and therapeutic procedures

Physician's Orders

Physician's orders outline instructions provided by the admitting physician regarding diagnostic and therapeutic care that the patient is to receive according to the treatment plan, such as lab tests, X-ray procedures, diet, and physical restrictions. Physician's orders can be written or they can be given verbally (Figure 4-15). Physician's orders and instructions are entered into an order entry system and distributed to the appropriate department(s) to render patient care services.

Physician Progress Notes

Progress notes outline the patient's status, results of diagnostic studies, and response to treatments. The physician completes progress notes each time the patient is seen (Figure 4-16).

BOX 4-22 ■ KEY POINTS

Physician's Orders

Services provided in the hospital are performed in accordance with a physician's order:

- Outlines instructions provided by the admitting physician regarding the diagnostic and therapeutic care the patient is to receive in accordance with the treatment plan

Patient Number: 765 466
Patient Name Marcia Clerk
Physician Name Joan Simone

HISTORY AND PHYSICAL EXAMINATION

Patient is a 56-year-old female admitted with the chief complaint of severe upper cervical spine pain The patient has rheumatoid spondylitis and has a fusion of most of the cervical spine, but the upper two vertebra still have motion in their joints, and the patient is experiencing considerable pain because of the progressive arthritis at this level.

PAST HISTORY: Reveals the patient to have some elevated blood pressure problems. She is currently taking Hygroton, aspirin, and Indocin. Patient has had an appendectomy, a hysterectomy, and a bilateral salpingo-oophorectomy.

REVIEW OF SYSTEMS: No auditory or visual symptoms.
CARDIORESPIRATORY: No orthopnea, dyspnea, hemoptysis.
G.I. TRACT: No weight gain, weight loss, or change in bowel habits.
G.U. TRACT: No pyuria, dysuria or frequency.
NEUROMUSCULAR: See present complaints.

PHYSICAL EXAMINATION: A somewhat frail female in no acute distress. Patient walks about room with neck flexed. She is unable to extend neck.

CHEST: Expansion is limited. The lungs are clear to auscultation. Heart tones are regular. No murmurs. No cardiomegaly.

ABDOMEN: Soft. LKS not palpable.

BACK: Marked limitations of lumbodorsal motion. No paraspinous muscle spasm noted.

EXTREMITY: The patient has limitations of right shoulder motion, active and passive motion cause her significant discomfort, and crepitation is noted. The neurovascular status of all extremities is intact.

Dr. Joan Simone

Joan Simone, D. O.

Figure 4-14 History and physical (H & P). *(From Brooks ML, Gillingham ET:* Health unit coordinating, *ed 5, St Louis, 2004, Saunders.)*

Nurse Progress Notes

The nurse records notes during each shift. The nurse's progress notes indicate the patient status, responses from the patient regarding their condition, and vital signs such as blood pressure, pulse, and temperature (Figure 4-17).

Ancillary Department Reports

Various reports prepared by ancillary departments such as Radiology, Laboratory/Pathology, and Respiratory Therapy are also maintained in the patient record. Ancillary services are those that are considered supportive, such as X-rays, blood tests, or respiratory therapy. The report indicates the diagnostic and therapeutic care provided to the patient and the patient's response to care.

Clinical Department Reports

Health care personnel from other clinical departments such as the ED perform various patient care services that are documented in the patient's medical record. Consultation and specialist's reports are also maintained in the medical record.

Emergency Department Record

When a patient is seen in the ER, information is obtained and an ED record is prepared with information regarding the patient and insurance. Clinical personnel in the ER who record information regarding the patient's condition and patient care services provided utilize this form. The ER physician documents orders for services and items required on the ED record (Figure 4-18).

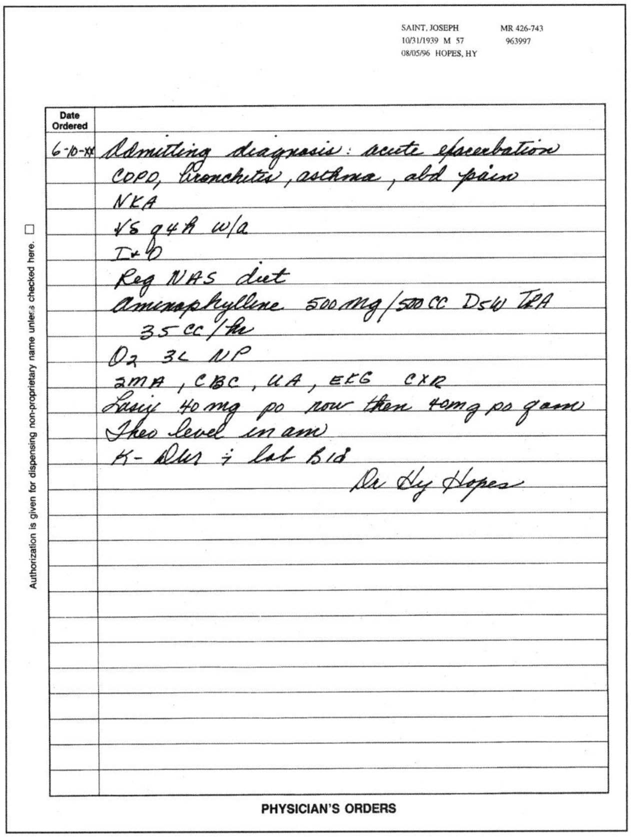
SAINT, JOSEPH MR 426-743
10/31/1939 M 57 963997
08/05/96 HOPES, HY

Date Ordered	
6-10-xx	Admitting diagnosis: acute exacerbation COPD, bronchitis, asthma, abd pain
	NKA
	VS q4h w/a
	I+O
	Reg NAS diet
	Aminophylline 500 mg/500 cc D5W IPA 35 cc/hr
	O2 3L NP
	SMA, CBC, UA, EEG, CXR
	Lasix 40 mg po now then 40 mg po qam
	Theo level in am
	K-Dur ī tab BID
	Dr Hy Hopes

Authorization is given for dispensing non-proprietary name unless checked here. ☐

PHYSICIAN'S ORDERS

Figure 4-15 Physician's orders. *(From Brooks ML, Gillingham ET: Health unit coordinating, ed 5, St Louis, 2004, Saunders.)*

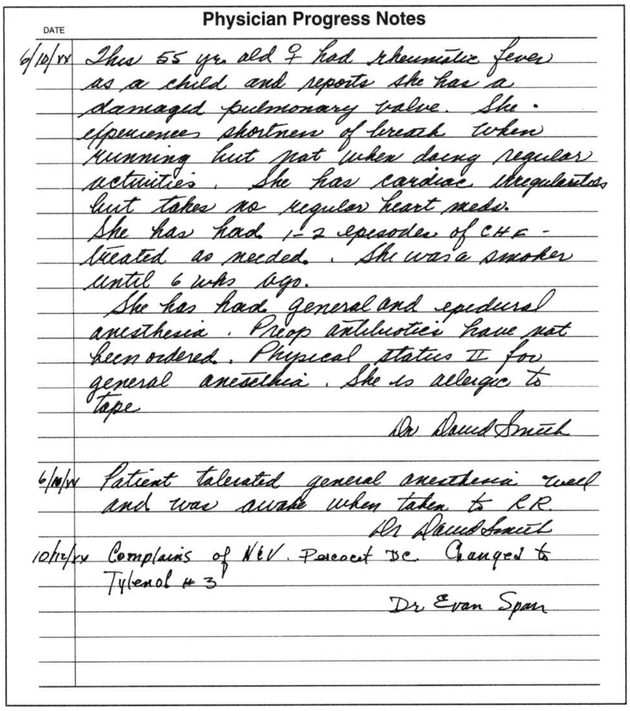
Physician Progress Notes

DATE	
6/10/xx	This 55 yr. old ♀ had rheumatic fever as a child and reports she has a damaged pulmonary valve. She experiences shortness of breath when running but not when doing regular activities. She has cardiac irregularities but takes no regular heart meds. She has had 1-2 episodes of CHF treated as needed. She was a smoker until 6 wks ago. She has had general and epidural anesthesia. Preop antibiotics have not been ordered. Physical status II for general anesthesia. She is allergic to tape.
	Dr David Smith
6/10/xx	Patient tolerated general anesthesia well and was awake when taken to RR.
	Dr David Smith
10/12/xx	Complains of N&V. Percocet DC. Changed to Tylenol #3
	Dr. Evan Span

Figure 4-16 Physician progress notes. *(Modified from Brooks ML, Gillingham ET: Health unit coordinating, ed 5, St Louis, 2004, Saunders.)*

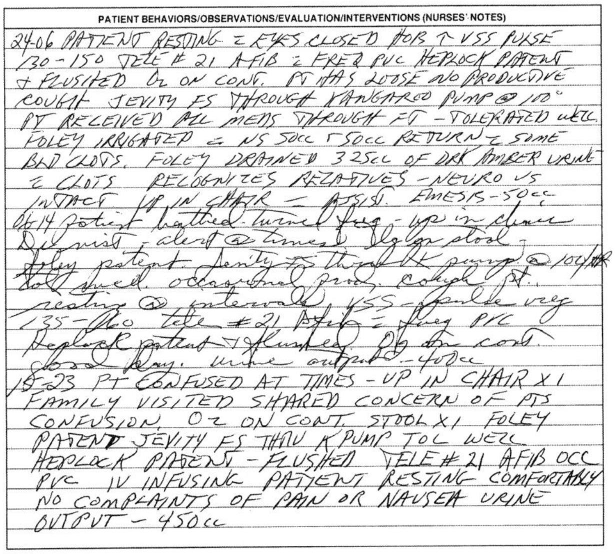
PATIENT BEHAVIORS/OBSERVATIONS/EVALUATION/INTERVENTIONS (NURSES' NOTES)

2406 PATIENT RESTING ē EYES CLOSED HOB ↑ VSS PULSE 130-150 TELE # 21 AFIB ē FREQ PVC HEPLOCK PATENT & FLUSHED O2 ON CONT. PT HAS LOOSE NO PRODUCTIVE COUGH JEVITY FS THROUGH KANGAROO PUMP @ 100° PT RECEIVED ALL MEDS THROUGH FT - TOLERATED WELL FOLEY IRRIGATED ē NS 50CC ↑ 50CC RETURN ē SOME BLD CLOTS. FOLEY DRAINED 325CC OF DRK AMBER URINE ē CLOTS RECOGNIZES RELATIVES - NEURO VS INTACT UP IN CHAIR — ASSIST. EMESIS-50CC

0614 Patient bathed, turned freq - up in chair ... alert @ times ... stool ... Foley patent. Jevity FS thru K pump @ 100/hr ... occasional ... resting @ intervals. VSS - pulse ... 135-150 tele #21 Afib ... PVC Heplock patent & flushed O2 on cont. ... urine output - 400cc

1523 PT CONFUSED AT TIMES - UP IN CHAIR X1 FAMILY VISITED SHARED CONCERN OF PTS CONFUSION. O2 ON CONT. STOOL X1 FOLEY PATENT JEVITY FS THRU K PUMP TOL WELL HEPLOCK PATENT - FLUSHED TELE # 21 AFIB OCC PVC IV INFUSING PATIENT RESTING COMFORTABLY NO COMPLAINTS OF PAIN OR NAUSEA URINE OUTPUT - 450cc

PATIENT RECORD - 4

Figure 4-17 Nurse progress notes. *(From Brooks ML, Gillingham ET: Health unit coordinating, ed 5, St Louis, 2004, Saunders.)*

Consultations and Specialist Reports

All physician consultants and specialists record information regarding the patient visit in the patient's medical record.

Medication Administration Records (MARs)

MARs are used to record medications administered to the patient. The record contains the name of the medication ordered, the dose, and the route of administration. Clinical personnel, such as a nurse, record administration of a medication. The nurse also places his or her initials, the date, and the time on the record. If medication is refused, the nurse will note this on the record. The medication administration record is sometimes referred to as Med Mars (Figure 4-19).

Discharge Summary

The discharge summary provides an overview of patient care activity during the patient stay, including the patient's condition at admission, care provided during the course of the hospital stay, and the patient's history and physical status prior to discharge. Elements of a discharge summary include the admitting diagnosis, history of present illness, hospital course, discharge diagnosis, and medications. The admitting physician dictates the discharge summary after a detailed history and physical is performed to determine if the patient is ready to be discharged. The admitting physician completes the discharge summary when the patient is discharged (Figure 4-20).

Hospital-Based Clinic/Primary Care Office

A patient medical record is also maintained by hospital-based clinics and primary care offices. The record con-

EMERGENCY ROOM

Medical Record No	567-435
Med Service	Orth
Date	5/23/XX
Soc Sec No/Medicare No	527-48-XXXX
Patient Name (Last, First, Middle)	Lowrey, Holly, Elinor
Hospitalization Insurance - 1	Sunstate
Policy/Group No	100-0000
Patient's Permanent Address	10001 North Mountain, Sky, AZ 85000
Tel	942-XXXX
Address	2222 N.Tower Pl. Sky, AZ
Birthdate	5/3/XX
Age	22
Effective Date - 1	1/06/XX
Sex	Female
Marital Status	Married
Race	Black
Religion	Other
Industrial - Patient's Employer	No
Responsible Party Name	SELF
Spouse or Nearest Relative	Iris Lowrey
Relationship	Mother
Tel	943-XXXX
Relative Notified	Time 1800, By whom M. Loor
Address	211 E. Sun Dr. Sky, AZ 85000
Police Notified	Time 1730, By whom M. Loor
E R Physician	Thomas V. Riggs
Attending Physician	B. Urself

Events and care given prior to arrival / Chief complaint: Pt. states she was involved in an auto accident 10am to-day – no loss of consciousness – Complaint of pain Right shoulder – right knee – 3 inch lac. to left cheek area – abrasion (R) hand

Vital signs: Temp 98⁴ Oral P 88 R 24 BP 130/80

Allergies: Codeine

Last Tetanus: July 1971

Time: 5pm; Physician's name: B. Urself; Called 5:45p, 5:55p; Contacted 6:10p; Arrived 7pm; X-ray 5:30p

Brought in by: Associated ambulance

Disposition of valuables: to husband

Nurse's signature: Mable Jones RN

ORDERS

1. CERVICAL - XTABLE 1ST
2. SKULL
3. R SHOULDER
   R KNEE
   R HAND
4. 1% LIDOCAINE
   4-0 - NYLON WHITE
   6-0 NYLON - BLACK

abrasions, laceration cleansed c̄ betadine soln, dressed c̄ neosporin, dry dressing.

HISTORY: PHYSICAL FINDINGS & TREATMENT

S. ↓ ROM R SHOULDER 2° TO PAIN

Obj 1. VS - STABLE
2. HEAD ① PERLA, EOM'S, disc NORMAL
② EAR'S - NO BLOOD
③ Ⅱ CRANIAL NERVE SENSATION L=R
4. 3" LAC FACE
3. NECK - SUPPLE
4 CHEST - GOOD EXPANSION LUNGS CLEAR
5. ABD - GOOD BS, NO HS MEGLY, NO TENDERNESS, REBOUND OR REFERRED PAIN.
6 EXT - R SHOULDER - ECHYMOSIS, ↓ ROM
R KNEE - CONTUSION + ABRASION
R - HAND - ABRASION
7 XRAYS - SKULL, CERVICAL, R SHOULDER - NEG

Ass A/A, LACERATION, ABRASION + CONTUSION

PLAN HEAD SHEET / STITCHES OUT - 4DAYS / ICE

Signature of ER Physician: Thomas V. Riggs MD

MEDICAL RECORDS

Figure 4-18 Emergency Department record. *(From Brooks ML, Gillingham ET:* Health unit coordinating, *ed 5, St Louis, 2004, Saunders.)*

tains all information regarding patient care provided in the clinic or physician office, including patient demographic and insurance information, initial visit and progress notes, and medication information. The record also contains reports from other providers, such as pathology/laboratory, radiology, consultations, and the hospital. As discussed previously, physician services provided in the clinic or primary care office are recorded on the encounter form and used to post charges to the patient's account for each visit (see Figure 4-2, C).

PATIENT CARE SERVICES

The admitting physician directs all services provided within the hospital. The physician's orders provide instructions detailing patient care services to be provided during the patient stay. The admitting physician reviews the patient status and updates the orders as needed. Outpatient services are directed by the referring physician or, in the case of an ED visit, the ER physician. In accordance with the physician's orders, various clinical departments are involved in providing patient care services such Nursing, Pharmacy, Pathology/Laboratory, and Radiology. The Central Supply or Sterile Supply Department provides medical supplies and instruments required to perform patient care services. It is important for hospital coding and billing professionals to understand the categories of patient care services provided in a hospital in order to ensure that charges are billed appropriately. A review of cat-

SAINT, JOSEPH MR 426-743
10/31/1939 M 57 963997
08/05/96 HOPES, HY

MEDICATION RECORD

						ROOM NO. 224-2			ROOM NO. 224-2			ROOM NO. 224-2		
						LAST NAME Smyth			LAST NAME Smyth			LAST NAME Smyth		
	DATE	DRUG DOSE	ROUTE	DATE DC	SCHEDULE	11-7	7-3	3-11	11-7	7-3	3-11	11-7	7-3	3-11
1	8/11	Dilantin 100mg	I.V. P.O. R. I.M.		tid		10 2	10						
2	8/11	Indocin 25mg	I.V. P.O. R. I.M.		bid		10	10						
3	8/11	Premarin 1.25mg	I.V. P.O. R. I.M.		qd		10							
4			I.V. P.O. R. I.M.											
5			I.V. P.O. R. I.M.											
6			I.V. P.O. R. I.M.											
7			I.V. P.O. R. I.M.											
8			I.V. P.O. R. I.M.											
9			I.V. P.O. R. I.M.											
10			I.V. P.O. R. I.M.											
11			I.V. P.O. R. I.M.											
12			I.V. P.O. R. I.M.											
13			I.V. P.O. R. I.M.											
14			I.V. P.O. R. I.M.											
15			I.V. P.O. R. I.M.											
16			I.V. P.O. R. I.M.											
17			I.V. P.O. R. I.M.											
18			I.V. P.O. R. I.M.											
19			I.V. P.O. R. I.M.											
20			I.V. P.O. R. I.M.											
21			I.V. P.O. R. I.M.											
22			I.V. P.O. R. I.M.											
23			I.V. P.O. R. I.M.											
24			I.V. P.O. R. I.M.											
25			I.V. P.O. R. I.M.											
26			I.V. P.O. R. I.M.											
27			I.V. P.O. R. I.M.											
28	8/13	Compazine 10mg	I.V. P.O. R. I.M.	8/16	q4h prn n/v	2 30 RT								
29	8/13	Ambien 5mg	I.V. P.O. R. I.M.	8/16	hs prn			10						
30	8/13	Demerol 50mg	I.V. P.O. R. I.M.	8/16	q4h prn		8 30 LT							
						MN	MN	MN	MN	MN	MN	MN	MN	MN

CODES
LU - LUQ
RU - RUQ
OD - RT. EYE
O - NOT GIVEN
LT - LT. THIGH
RT - RT. THIGH
OS - LT. EYE
ABD - ABDOMEN
LA - LT. ARM
RA - RT. ARM
OU - BOTH EYES
IVPB - IV PIGGYBACK
SQ - SUBCUTANEOUS

IDIOSYNCRACIES: Morphine
DIAGNOSIS: Cholecystitis

MR-1012 REV. 12/84 MEDICATION RECORD

Figure 4-19 Medication administration record (MAR). *(From Brooks ML, Gillingham ET:* Health unit coordinating, *ed 5, St Louis, 2004, Saunders.)*

DISCHARGE SUMMARY

PATIENT NAME: Sonia Sample
MR NUMBER: 12-34-56
ADMISSION DATE: 04/19/00
DISCHARGE DATE: 04/27/00

ADMITTING IMPRESSION: Acute abdominal pain, rule out diverticulitis.

HISTORY OF PRESENT ILLNESS:
The patient is a 57-year-old white female who has history of hypertension, valvular heart disease, and cardiomyopathy, who was seen in the emergency room with complaints of acute abdominal pain. On evaluation, she was found to be very tender in the abdomen. She had white blood cell count of 19,000 and was admitted with a diagnosis of rule out diverticulitis.

HOSPITAL COURSE:
CT scan of the abdomen was consistent with cholecystitis and ultrasound of the gallbladder was consistent with cholelithiasis. She was cleared for surgery by cardiologist Dr. Chen and was treated preoperatively with intravenous antibiotics, intravenous fluids, and pain medication. On 4/22/00, the patient underwent laparoscopic cholecystectomy. On 4/26/00, she underwent an endoscopic retrograde cholangiopancreatography. The postoperative course was remarkable for some shortness of breath, otherwise the patient was doing well. She remained very stable, afebrile, and was discharged home.

DISCHARGE DIAGNOSES
1. Cholelithiasis with acute cholecystitis; status post laparoscopic cholecystectomy
2. Mitral valve disorder
3. Hypertensive heart disease with history of angiopathic cardiomyopathy

MEDICATIONS
1. Cozaar
2. Hytrin
3. Lasix
4. Potassium
5. Lanoxin

Figure 4-20 Discharge summary. *(From Abdelhak M, Grostick S, Hanken MA, Jacobs E (editors):* Health information: management of a strategic resource, *ed 2, St Louis, 2001, Saunders.)*

egories of hospital services will provide an understanding of the type of patient care services provided by the hospital.

Common Categories of Hospital Services and Items

The patient account data flow includes information regarding patient care services provided and supplies or items required to provide those services. Hospital patient care services and items can be categorized as accommodations, medical surgical supplies, pharmacy, and clinical services. Table 4-3 illustrates common categories of services and items required for an inpatient admission as outlined.

Accommodations

Patients who are admitted on an inpatient basis are assigned a room/bed. The patient may be assigned a private room or a semiprivate room. Semiprivate rooms generally have two beds; however, some may have up to four beds. Accommodation services include the room and overhead for nursing coverage during the patient stay.

Operating Room (OR)

Patients requiring surgery are generally placed in an OR suite prior to surgery. Surgery is performed in the OR. The patient is generally moved to the recovery room after surgery. Hospital OR services include the amount of time in each room, which includes the setup and overhead for OR staff such as the OR technician and the circulator nurse. Some procedures are performed in other areas of the hospital such as the catheterization laboratory or endoscopy suite.

Medical/Surgical Supplies

Various departments supply materials, supplies, instruments, and durable medical equipment in accordance with physician's orders. As outlined in the Central Supply requisition in Figure 4-21, medical and surgical supply items may include adult disposable diapers, pressure pads, feeding pumps, and various kits or sterile trays. This department may also supply durable medical equipment.

Pharmacy

Medications and other pharmaceuticals required during the patient stay are provided by the Pharmacy Department in accordance with the physician's orders. Figure 4-22 illustrates physician's orders outlining medications to be supplied by the pharmacy including Keflex, Theragram, Monopril, and Dalmane. Medications are prepared, labeled, and forwarded to the nursing unit for administration. The Pharmacy Department also

TEST YOUR *Knowledge* BOX 4-3

MEDICAL RECORD DOCUMENTATION

1. What is medical record documentation?
2. Provide a brief explanation of Health Information Management's responsibilities related to patient information.
3. List four specific purposes of medical record documents.
4. Discuss how medical record documentation is utilized to support charges submitted to payers.
5. Provide a brief outline of how documentation is utilized for utilization review.
6. State four elements of information required in the patient's medical record.
7. Outline the types of admitting forms that are found in the patient's medical record.
8. Discuss physician orders and what purpose they serve in the patient care process.
9. How is the emergency room record utilized?
10. Explain the difference between an admission summary and a discharge summary.

TABLE 4-3 **Categories of Services and Items Required for Admission**

Service Category	Description
Accommodations (room and board) Inpatient	Admission—Room/bed assigned to the patient on admission. Rooms may be private or semiprivate (more than one bed). Rooms are assigned on various units or wards: medical, surgical, OB/GYN, oncology, psychiatric, intensive care, coronary care, or nursery. Nursing services are included in overhead charges.
Operating room (OR) suite, operating room, recovery room	Patients requiring surgery are placed in an OR suite before surgery. Surgery is performed in the OR. The patient is generally moved to the recovery room after surgery. Some procedures are performed in other areas of the hospital such as the catheterization laboratory or the endoscopy suite.
Medical/surgical supplies	Materials, supplies, and instruments supplied by various departments such as Central Supply; items include bandages, splints, instruments, and bed pans.
Pharmacy	Medications ordered by the physician are supplied by the Pharmacy Department.
Ancillary services	Diagnostic and therapeutic services ordered by the physician are provided by various clinical departments such as Pathology/Laboratory, Radiology, Physical Rehabilitation, and Respiratory Therapy.
Other clinical services	Various medical departments coordinate and provide services required as outlined in the physician's orders such as Surgery, Medicine, Anesthesia, Pulmonology, and Cardiology.

Doctor Ordering ______________ ☐ Stat
Today's Date ______________ ☐ Routine
Requested by ______________

CSD (Central Service Department)

☐ Adult disposable diapers
☐ Alternating pressure pad
☐ Colostomy kit
☐ Colostomy irrigation bag
☐ Egg-crate mattress
☐ Elastic abdominal binder size ______
☐ Footboard
☐ Feeding pump with bag and tubing
☐ Feeding bag and tubing
☐ Footboard
☐ Foot cradle
☐ Hypothermia machine
☐ Isolation pack
☐ IV infusion pump with tubing
☐ K-pad with motor
☐ Nasal gastric tube type ______ size ______
☐ Pleur-evac
☐ Pneumatic hose
☐ Restraints type ______
☐ Sitz bath, disposable
☐ Stomal bags type ______ size ______
☐ Suction canister and tubing
☐ Suction catheter type ______ size ______
☐ Ted hose size ______
☐ Vaginal irrigation kit

Sterile Trays:

☐ Bone marrow
☐ Central line
☐ Lumbar puncture (spinal tap)
☐ Paracentesis
☐ Thoracentesis
☐ Tracheostomy

☐ Write in item ______________

Figure 4-21 Central Supply requisition. *(From Brooks ML, Gillingham ET:* Health unit coordinating, *ed 5, St Louis, 2004, Saunders.)*

Community Hospital

Smith, Johnathan
ID #354792

DOCTOR'S ORDERS

	Orders		
Date 1/20/00 Time 120 pm	CBC U/A CXR F Rose	Date 1-20-00 Time 130 pm	[signature]
Date 1/21/00 Time 830 AM	KEFLEX 500mg F Rose	Date Time	
Date Time	THERAGRAM TABSQD	Date Time	
Date Time	Monopril 10 mg P.O. bid Dlamane 15 mg P.O. qh.s.	Date Time	

Figure 4-22 Physician orders for medications. *(From Davis N, Lacour M:* Introduction to health information technology, *ed 1, St Louis, 2002, Saunders.)*

supplies pharmaceuticals and other biologicals that are required to perform various therapeutic and diagnostic procedures such as saline solution or contrast material. Some durable medical equipment (DME) items are supplied by the pharmacy as well.

Ancillary Services

Various ancillary departments such as Pathology/Laboratory, Radiology, Physical Rehabilitation, and Respiratory Therapy provide diagnostic and therapeutic services ordered by the physician. Figure 4-23 illustrates computerized order screens that highlight examples of the types of services provided by these departments, such as CBC, chest X-ray, training on crutches, and oxygen or other breathing treatments.

Other Clinical Services

Various clinical departments, such as Cardiology, coordinate and provide patient services as outlined in the physician's orders. For example, the Cardiology Department is involved in the performance of cardiac catheterizations, and charges related to performing these procedures are posted by the Cardiology Department.

BOX 4-23 ■ KEY POINTS

Common Categories of Patient Care Services

Accommodations
Operating room
Medical/surgical supplies
Pharmacy
Ancillary services
Other clinical services

CHARGE CAPTURE

A hospital cannot maintain financial stability if the cost of providing care is not reimbursed appropriately. From the time a patient is received at the hospital to discharge, services and items are provided. The complexity of providing patient care services and capturing charges within a hospital setting requires efficient systems that can capture all data required. It is important to remember that the access to and flow of patient care data are enhanced by the automation of the patient's account and other functions. Information collected at registration is utilized throughout the patient stay for order entry, rendering of patient care services, and capturing charges.

Charge Capture Procedures

Charge capture is the term commonly used to describe the process of gathering charge information and recording it on the patient's account. The process of capturing

LABORATORY ORDER SCREEN

Doctor Ordering ______ ☐ Stat
Today's Date ______ ☐ Routine
Collection Date ______ Time ______
Collected by ______
Requested by ______

Hematology	Serology	Urinalysis/Urine Chemistry
☐ Bleeding Time, Ivy	☐ ANA	☐ Routine Ua
☐ CBC c̄ Diff	☐ ASO Titer	☐ Amylase (2hr)
☐ CBC c̄ Manual Diff	☐ CEA	☐ Bilirubin
☐ Factor VIII	☐ CMV	☐ Calcium
☐ Fibrinogen	☐ IgG	☐ Chloride
☐ HCT	☐ IgM	☐ Creatinine Clearance
☐ HGB	☐ Cocci Screen	☐ Glucose Tolerance
☐ H & H	☐ EBV Panel	☐ Nitrogen
☐ Eosinophil Ct Absolute	☐ Enterovirus Ab Panel 1	☐ Occult Blood
☐ Eosinophil Smear	☐ Enterovirus Ab Panel 2	☐ Osmolality

PHYSICAL REHABILITATION ORDER SCREEN

Doctor Ordering ______
Date to be done ______ Time to be done ______
Today's Date ______ Requested by ______
Clinical Indication ______
Transportation ☐ portable ☐ stretcher ☐ wheelchair ☐ ambulatory

O_2 ☐ yes ☐ no   Diabetic ☐ yes ☐ no   Hearing deficit ☐ yes
IV ☐ yes ☐ no   Seizure disorder ☐ yes ☐ no   Sight deficit ☐ yes ☐
Isolation ☐ yes ☐ no   Non-English speaking ☐ yes ☐ no

Comments: ______
☐ CMP ______
☐ Crutch training ______
☐ ES ______
☐ Exercises ______
☐ Evaluation ______
☐ Hot packs ______
☐ Hubbard tank ______
☐ ROM ______
☐ Shortwave diathermy ______

RADIOLOGY ORDER SCREEN

Doctor Ordering ______
Date to be done ______ ☐ Stat ☐ Routine ☐ ASAP
Today's Date ______ Requested by ______

Diagnostic Imaging - X-Ray Procedures

Clinical Indication ______
Transportation ☐ portable ☐ stretcher ☐ wheelchair ☐ ambulatory

O_2 ☐ yes ☐ no   Diabetic ☐ yes ☐ no   Hearing deficit ☐ yes
IV ☐ yes ☐ no   Seizure disorder ☐ yes ☐ no   Sight deficit ☐ yes ☐
Isolation ☐ yes ☐ no   Non-English speaking ☐ yes ☐ no

Comments: ______
☐ Abdomen ______
☐ Bone x-ray order: ______
☐ Chest order: ______
☐ KUB order: ______
☐ Mammogram ______

RESPIRATORY THERAPY ORDER SCREEN

Doctor Ordering ______
Date to be done ______ Time to be done ______
Today's Date ______ Requested by ______

Comments: ______
☐ O_2 ______ L/M   ☐ NP   ☐ Mask   ☐ Tent   ☐ Other ______
☐ SVN ______
☐ CPT ______
☐ IPPB ______
☐ Incentive spirometry ______
☐ USN ______
☐ HA ______
☐ Bi PAP ______
☐ CPAP ______
Write-in order ______

Ventilator orders
IMV mode ______ TV ______ FIO_2 ______ PO_2 ______ PS ______

Figure 4-23 Computer order screens for laboratory, radiology, physical rehabilitation, and respiratory therapy ancillary services. *(Modified from Brooks ML, Gillingham ET:* Health unit coordinating, *ed 5, St Louis, 2004, Saunders.)*

charges begins with physician's orders and is completed when charges are entered on the patient's account, as illustrated in Figure 4-24.

Order Entry

Patient care services are provided in accordance with physician's orders. Orders are entered into the computer order entry system. Services and items to be provided are communicated to the appropriate departments by computer or by requisition.

Patient Care Services Rendered

Physician's orders are communicated to various clinical departments involved in the patient's care. When the department receives the order, the required diagnostic and therapeutic procedures are performed.

Documentation

All patient care services are documented in the patient's medical record, including a detailed description of the service, results, and other information about the service. Items utilized to perform the service are also documented.

Charge Capture Process

I
Physician orders a complete blood count (CBC) → Order entered via the computer order entry system
Order communicated to the Laboratory Department by computer or requisition / Order communicated to the Nursing Department → Blood specimen is obtained by nursing staff or by laboratory personnel and forwarded to the laboratory

II CBC performed by the laboratory → III Results filed in the patient's medical record → IV Charge posted by laboratory personnel

Figure 4-24 *I*, Physician's orders; *II*, patient care services rendered; *III*, documentation; *IV*, charge posted. *(Modified from Brooks ML, Gillingham ET:* Health unit coordinating, *ed 5, St Louis, 2004, Saunders.)*

Charge Posted

The department providing the service or item is generally responsible for posting appropriate charges to the patient's account through the chargemaster. In addition to the medical record, other documents are utilized to capture charges such as requisitions and encounter forms. As discussed previously, requisitions provide instructions regarding services to be rendered. The encounter form is utilized by hospital-based clinics or physicians' offices to record services, procedures, and items provided during the visit. The medical reason for services is also recorded on the encounter form.

BOX 4-24 ■ KEY POINTS

Charge Capture

Charge capture is the process of gathering charge information and recording it on the patient's account, including the following:

- Order entry
- Patient care services rendered
- Documentation
- Charge posted

Hospital Charges

Hospital charges are referred to as facility charges, as they represent the technical component of patient care services. The professional component of patient care services is recorded in the patient's medical record; however, the hospital only bills professional services when the physician is employed by or under contract with the hospital. Figure 4-25 illustrates examples of hospital facility charges. To bill hospital services accurately, it is important for hospital professionals to understand the difference between the technical and professional component of services.

Facility Charges—Technical Component

Hospitals bill facility charges for patient care services provided such as laboratory tests, X-rays, or ambulatory surgery. **Facility charges** represent the cost and overhead for the technical component of services, including space, equipment, supplies, drugs and biologicals, and technical staff. Facility charges are posted to the patient's account by various departments through the chargemaster.

Professional Charges—Professional Component

Professional charges represent physician and other nonphysician clinical services, the professional component of services performed. As discussed previously, the hospital can bill professional services when the physician is employed by or under contract with the hospital. An example of this situation is a hospital-based primary care office or clinic. Charges for professional services provided by a hospital physician, in a hospital-based primary care office, are posted to the patient account utilizing an encounter form.

BOX 4-25 ■ KEY POINTS

Hospital Facility Charges

The facility charge is determined based on the cost and overhead of providing services and items in the hospital.

Facility charges represent the cost and overhead for the technical component of patient care services, which includes space, equipment, supplies, drugs and biologicals, and technical staff

PATIENT DISCHARGE

Prior to discharge, the admitting physician performs an H&P and prepares discharge orders so the patient can

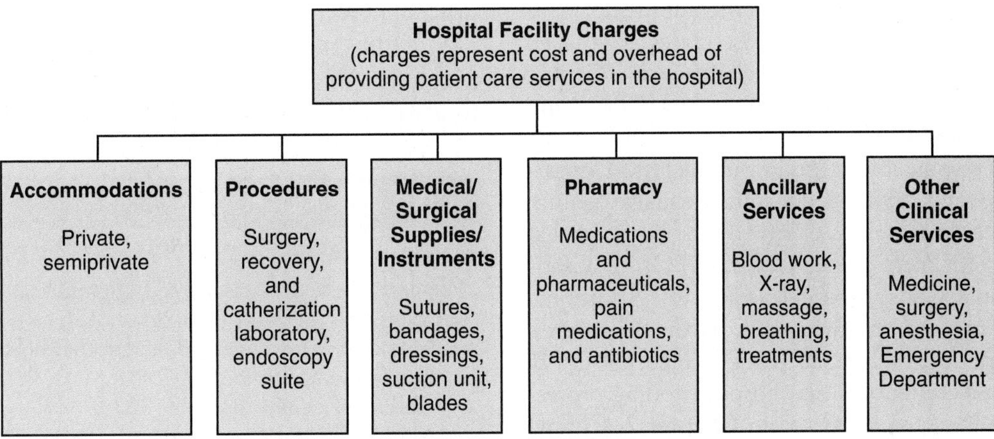

Figure 4-25 Examples of hospital facility charges.

be processed for discharge. Patients may be discharged to home or they may be discharged to other facilities such as a rehabilitation center or nursing home. After the patient is discharged, the patient's record is forwarded to the HIM Department for review and coding of clinical information.

Health Information Management (HIM) Procedures

The functions of the HIM Department were discussed previously. In addition to data maintenance, security, and management of medical records, HIM plays a vital role in the reimbursement process. The HIM Department is responsible for maintenance of the chargemaster. The HIM Department performs periodic reviews of the chargemaster to ensure that codes and various payer edits corresponding to services and items are current. Other functions performed by HIM related to the reimbursement process include review of the patient's medical record, coding of clinical data, and MS-DRG or APC assignment.

Medical Record Review

Patient medical records are sent to the HIM Department after the patient is discharged. HIM performs a detailed review of the medical record to ensure that all documentation requirements are met.

Coding of Clinical Data

The HIM Department is also responsible for coding clinical data required for submission of claim forms to various third-party payers. An HIM coding worksheet sheet is often utilized to abstract information regarding the patient's diagnosis(es) and procedure(s) (Figure 4-26). The coding worksheet is then utilized to enter codes into the computer. Most hospitals utilize a software program called an encoder that assists HIM personnel with code assignment. Data coded by the HIM Department generally include the principal procedure and other procedures in addition to the admitting, principal, and secondary diagnoses. These codes are placed in the appropriate fields of the claim form. Coding systems utilized in the hospital include HCPCS and ICD-9-CM, as outlined in Figure 4-27, *A*.

Individuals responsible for coding in the HIM Department are generally certified. Hospitals usually require coding certifications such as Certified Coding Specialist (CCS), Certified Professional Coder (CPC), or Certified Professional Coder-Hospital (CPC-H). Additional certifications may be required such as the Registered Health Information Technician (RHIT). Figure 4-27, *B*, outlines various credentials that hospital coding professionals may pursue, as discussed in Chapter 2. Coding Systems will be discussed in future chapters.

HEALTH INFORMATION MANAGEMENT
CODING WORKSHEET

DEMOGRAPHICS
Medical Record Number: **Bill Type#:**
Patient Name: Last, First, Middle Init: | Admit Hour Code: | Discharge Hour Code:
Admit Type Code: | Discharge Status Code:
Admit Source Code:
Condition Code (s) | Occurrence Span Code and Date | Value Code and Amount

ADMISSION INFORMATION
Type of Admission: **ER** **Facility** **Physician Referral** **Other** **Unknown**
Admitting Diagnosis | **HIM Code(s)**
Principal Diagnosis (Including complications and co-morbidities if applicable) | **HIM Code**
Other Secondary Diagnoses (Including complications and co-morbidities if applicable) | **HIM Code(s)**
Principal Procedure (Significant procedure performed for definitive treatment or that most closely relates to the principal diagnosis) **Date:** | **HIM Code**
Other Significant Procedure(s) **Date:** | **HIM Code(s)**
Medications, supplies, equipment or other item (s) **Date:** | **HIM Code(s)**

DISCHARGE INFORMATION
Home Facility AMA Deceased Other

DRG ASSIGNMENT | **APC ASSIGNMENT**
MDC: | Surgical/Medical:
CONTRIBUTING FACTORS:
Age | Sex | Discharge Status | Complications/Comorbidities | Birthweight
Questions/Need Clarification:

Figure 4-26 HIM coding worksheet.

Medicare Severity Diagnosis Related Groups (MS-DRG) or Ambulatory Payment Classification (APC) Assignments

Hospitals are reimbursed utilizing various payment methods including the MS-DRG and APC. These payment systems are utilized for reimbursement of services provided to Medicare patients. MS-DRG is a PPS implemented to provide reimbursement for hospital inpatient services. Under MS-DRG, the facility is paid a fixed fee based on the patient's condition and relative treatments. APC is a PPS implemented to provide reimbursement for hospital outpatient services. Under APC, the facility is paid a fixed fee based on the resources utilized to provide the service or procedure. The appropriate MS-DRG or APC group must be assigned to hospital claims. HIM utilizes a program called a grouper to assist with the assignment of the MS-DRG or APC

BOX 4-26 ■ KEY POINTS

Patient Discharge and HIM Procedures

When the patient is discharged, the medical record is forwarded to the HIM Department for:

- Medical record review to ensure that documentation requirements are met
- Coding of clinical data
- MS-DRG or APC assignments

A

Procedure Coding Systems
(Services or Items)

HCPCS Level I
Current Procedural Terminology (CPT)

HCPCS Level II
Medicare National Codes

International Classification of Diseases, 9th Revision, Clinical Modification (ICD-9-CM)
Volume III (Alphabetical and numerical listing of procedures)

Diagnosis Coding Systems
(Conditions, disease, illness, injury, or other)

International Classification of Diseases, 9th Revision, Clinical Modification (ICD-9-CM) – Volume I & II (alphabetical and numerical listing of diseases, signs and symptoms, encounters and external causes of injury)

B

Organization	Credentials
American Academy of Professional Coders (AAPC)	Certified Professional Coder (CPC) Certified Professional Coder-Hospital (CPC-H)
American Health Information Management Association (AHIMA)	Registered Health Information Technician (RHIT) Certified Coding Associate (CCA) Certified Coding Specialist (CCS) Certified Coding Specialist Physician (CCS-P)
American Association of Healthcare Administration Management (AAHAM)	Certified Patient Account Technician (CPAT) Certified Account Technician (CCAT) Certified Patient Accounts Manager (CPAM)

Figure 4-27 **A,** Coding systems utilized in the hospital. **B,** Various credentials obtained by hospital coding and billing professionals. *(B From Davis N, Lacour M:* Introduction to health information technology, *ed 1, St Louis, 2002, Saunders.)*

BOX 4-27 ■ KEY POINTS

Computer Software Utilized by HIM

Encoder software allows the HIM professional to enter specified information regarding patient care services and the patient's condition. The program utilizes the data entered to identify potential codes.

Grouper software allows the HIM professional to enter specified information that the program utilizes to assign an MS-DRG or APC group.

group(s). Information required for MS-DRG or APC assignment includes diagnosis and procedure codes and other information regarding the patient. Prospective Payment Systems will be discussed further in later chapters.

HOSPITAL BILLING PROCESS

To maintain financial stability the hospital must have an efficient process for obtaining reimbursement from patients and third-party payers. The hospital billing process begins when orders are submitted for patient care services, and it ends when the account balance is paid (Figure 4-28). As illustrated previously, automation of the registration, order entry, and charge capture process allows for the gathering of data required for billing throughout the patient stay. These data are utilized by the PFS Department to perform billing functions, which include charge submission and posting of patient transactions. The billing process includes preparation and submission of claim forms to third-party payers, preparation and submission of patient statements, and posting patient transactions such as payments and adjustments. This section will provide a brief overview of the billing process to illustrate the flow of information. The billing process is discussed in detail in Chapter 5.

Charge Submission

Hospitals submit charges after the patient is discharged. On discharge the HIM Department receives the patient's medical record for review, coding, and MS-DRG or APC assignment. When the HIM Department functions are complete, the PFS Department prepares insurance claim forms and/or patient statements for submission of charges.

Insurance Claim Forms

Insurance claim forms are prepared and submitted to third-party payers. The goal is to submit a claim that contains accurate information and is completed in accordance with payer specifications so that it is paid on the first submission. Prior to submission of a claim, an editing process is performed to ensure that the claim is complete and accurate. Hospitals utilize computer software referred to as a claim scrubber to perform this function. The claim scrubber software is programmed to perform various checks to ensure that required fields contain data and also to check codes to make sure they are valid. Common problems identified include:

- Facility information is not complete or missing
- Patient name and identification number are not complete or missing
- Diagnosis or procedure codes are invalid.

The appropriate claim form is prepared. The **CMS-1450 (UB-04)** is the universally accepted claim form used to submit facility charges for inpatient, ambulatory surgery, emergency room, and ancillary department services (Figure 4-29). The universally accepted claim form for submission of physician and outpatient services and charges for durable medical equipment (DME) is

TEST YOUR *Knowledge* BOX 4-4

PATIENT CARE SERVICES; CHARGE CAPTURE AND PATIENT DISCHARGE

1. Explain the relationship between the physician's orders and patient care services rendered in the hospital.
2. Provide an explanation of how outpatient services are directed.
3. Categories of services provided in the hospital include accommodations. Explain this category.
4. Provide an explanation of patient care services that may be provided by ancillary departments.
5. Discuss the relationship between patient accounts data flow and charge capture.
6. List the automated systems that enhance the flow and access of data related to charge capture.
7. Explain the relationship between charge capture and order entry.
8. State the relationship between documentation and hospital charges.
9. What department is generally responsible for posting charges to the patient's account?
10. Explain the difference between facility charges and professional service charges.
11. Provide a brief overview of the patient discharge process.
12. List two reasons why the HIM Department reviews patient medical records.
13. What type of document is utilized to abstract information from the patient record regarding the patient's diagnosis(es) and procedure(s) performed during the patient stay?
14. List the coding systems utilized in the hospital.
15. Discuss why HIM utilizes grouper software.

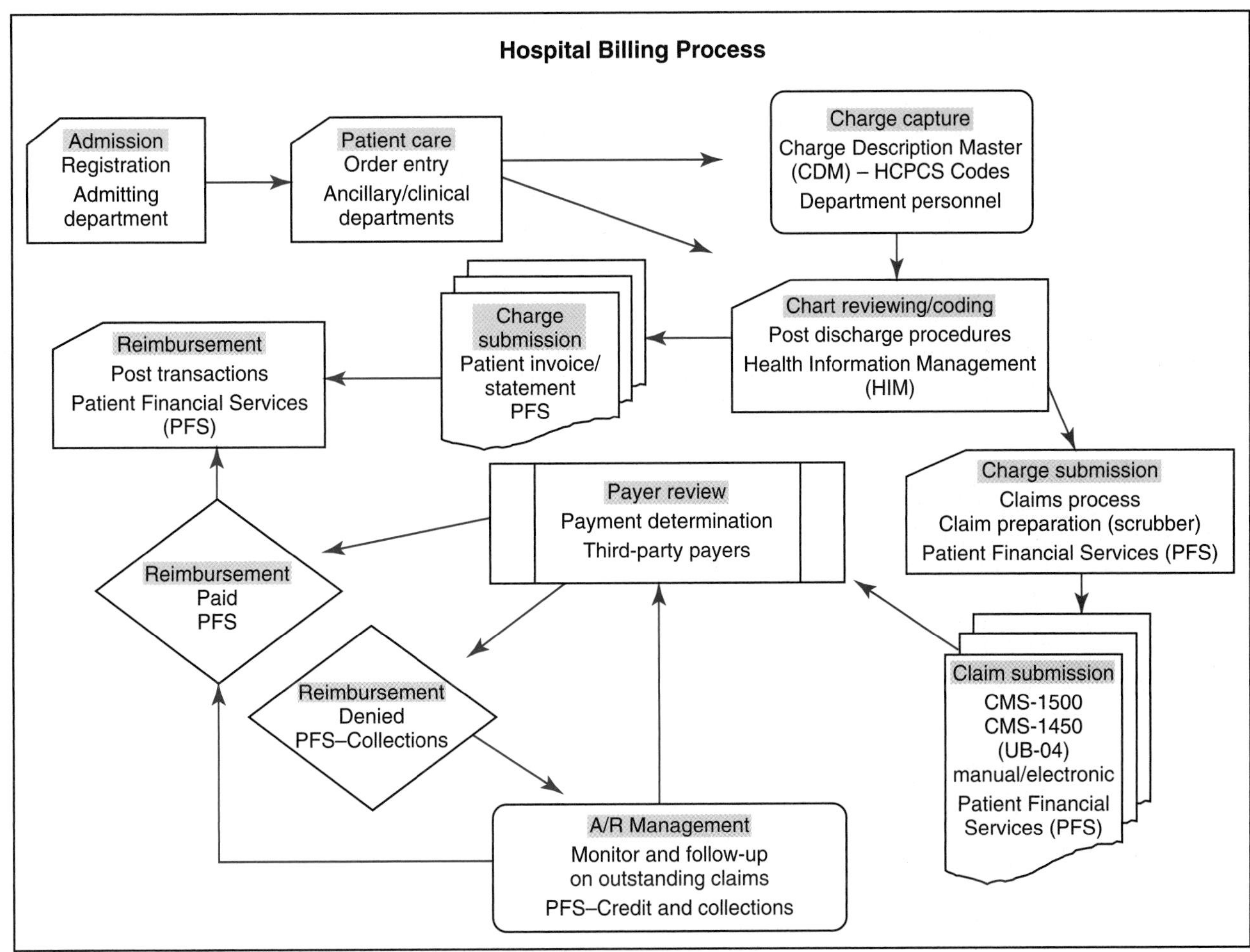

Figure 4-28 The hospital billing process: key functions and the primary departments involved in performing those functions. *(Revision of illustration courtesy Sandra Giangreco.)*

the **CMS-1500** (Figure 4-30). Claim forms are discussed in detail in Chapter 10.

The claim forms are submitted to payers electronically or manually. Claim forms submitted electronically are referred to as electronic medical claims (EMCs). Manual claims are printed on paper and mailed. Payers may require a detailed itemized statement be included with paper claims. Payers receiving electronic claims may request a detailed itemized statement after initial review of the claim. Copies of insurance claim forms are filed for follow-up.

Patient Statements

Patient statements list dates of service, description of services, charges, payments, and balance due. They are printed and mailed to patients. Patient statements generally include messages regarding outstanding balances.

Patient Transactions

Payers review claims submitted to determine payment on the claim. When payment determination is made, the payer communicates how the claim was processed and the payment status to the hospital utilizing a **remittance advice** (RA), which is a document prepared by payers to communicate payment determination to hospitals and patients. The RA includes detailed information about the charges submitted and an explanation of how the claim was processed. Payers utilize different names to describe this document, such as an **Explanation of Medicare Benefits (EOMB)** or **Explanation of Benefits (EOB)**. Patient transactions are posted to the patient's account when the RA is received (Figure 4-31).

Third-Party Payer Transactions

Third-party payers forward an RA to the hospital, which includes detailed information about the charges submitted and an explanation of how the claim was processed. Payer actions on a claim may include:

- Denial or rejection of the claim and reason
- Payment of the claim (covered and noncovered charges)
- Request for additional information

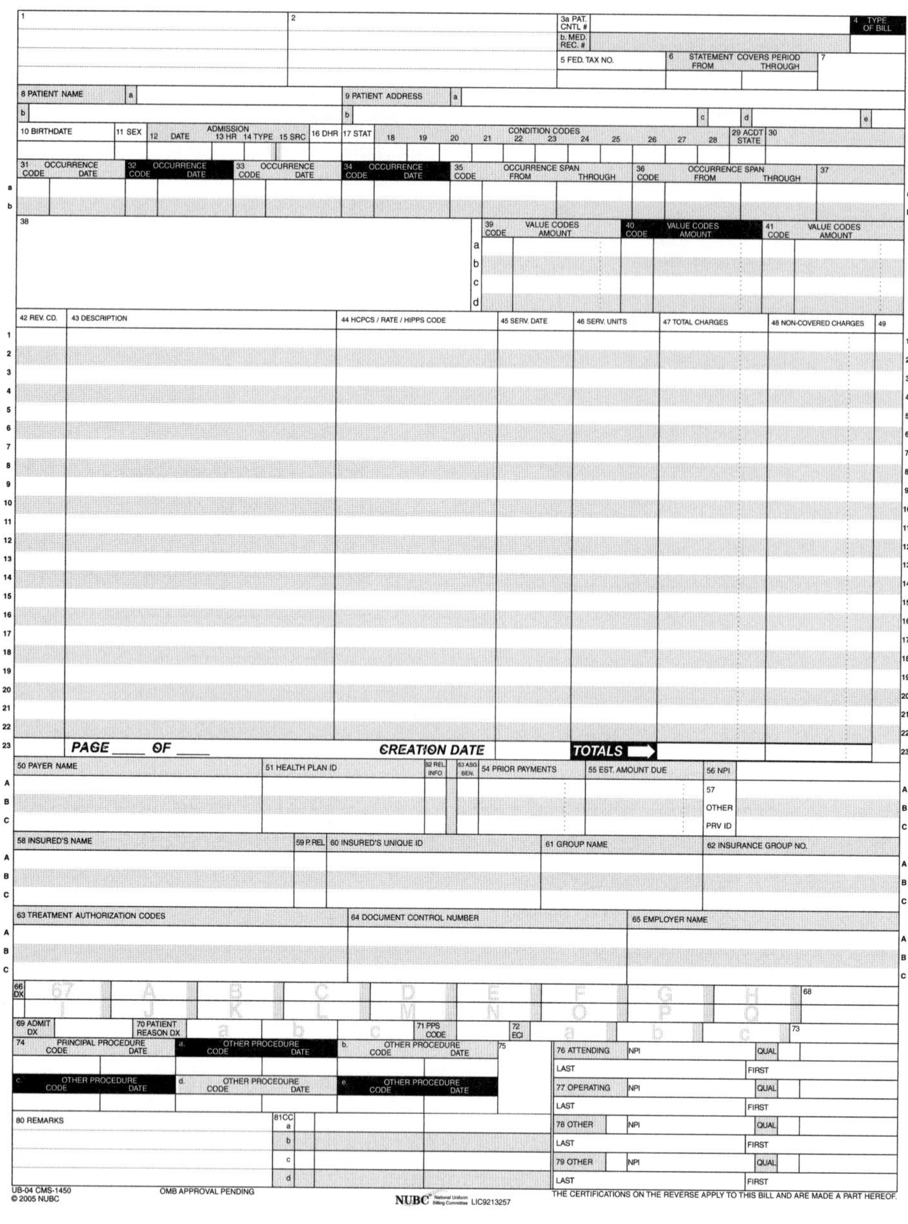

1 | 2 | 3a PAT. CNTL # | b. MED. REC. # | 4 TYPE OF BILL
5 FED. TAX NO. | 6 STATEMENT COVERS PERIOD FROM THROUGH | 7
8 PATIENT NAME a | b
9 PATIENT ADDRESS a | b | c | d | e
10 BIRTHDATE | 11 SEX | ADMISSION 12 DATE 13 HR 14 TYPE 15 SRC | 16 DHR | 17 STAT | CONDITION CODES 18 19 20 21 22 23 24 25 26 27 28 | 29 ACDT STATE | 30
31 OCCURRENCE CODE DATE | 32 OCCURRENCE CODE DATE | 33 OCCURRENCE CODE DATE | 34 OCCURRENCE CODE DATE | 35 OCCURRENCE SPAN CODE FROM THROUGH | 36 OCCURRENCE SPAN CODE FROM THROUGH | 37
38 | 39 VALUE CODES CODE AMOUNT | 40 VALUE CODES CODE AMOUNT | 41 VALUE CODES CODE AMOUNT
42 REV. CD. | 43 DESCRIPTION | 44 HCPCS / RATE / HIPPS CODE | 45 SERV. DATE | 46 SERV. UNITS | 47 TOTAL CHARGES | 48 NON-COVERED CHARGES | 49
PAGE ___ OF ___ | CREATION DATE | TOTALS
50 PAYER NAME | 51 HEALTH PLAN ID | 52 REL. INFO | 53 ASG. BEN. | 54 PRIOR PAYMENTS | 55 EST. AMOUNT DUE | 56 NPI | 57 OTHER PRV ID
58 INSURED'S NAME | 59 P.REL | 60 INSURED'S UNIQUE ID | 61 GROUP NAME | 62 INSURANCE GROUP NO.
63 TREATMENT AUTHORIZATION CODES | 64 DOCUMENT CONTROL NUMBER | 65 EMPLOYER NAME
66 DX | 67 | A B C D E F G H | I J K L M N O P Q | 68
69 ADMIT DX | 70 PATIENT REASON DX | a b c | 71 PPS CODE | 72 ECI | a b c | 73
74 PRINCIPAL PROCEDURE CODE DATE | a. OTHER PROCEDURE CODE DATE | b. OTHER PROCEDURE CODE DATE | 75
c. OTHER PROCEDURE CODE DATE | d. OTHER PROCEDURE CODE DATE | e. OTHER PROCEDURE CODE DATE
76 ATTENDING NPI QUAL LAST FIRST
77 OPERATING NPI QUAL LAST FIRST
78 OTHER NPI QUAL LAST FIRST
79 OTHER NPI QUAL LAST FIRST
80 REMARKS | 81CC a b c d
UB-04 CMS-1450 © 2005 NUBC | OMB APPROVAL PENDING | NUBC National Uniform Billing Committee LIC9213257
THE CERTIFICATIONS ON THE REVERSE APPLY TO THIS BILL AND ARE MADE A PART HEREOF.

Figure 4-29 CMS-1450 (UB-04).

The process of posting transactions to a patient's account is as follows:

1. Third-party payer payments are posted to the patient's account.
2. A contractual adjustment is applied where applicable.
3. The balance is billed to the patient or forwarded to a secondary or tertiary payer when applicable.
4. Claim denials require research to determine whether the denial is appropriate.

Patient Payments

Patient payments are posted to the patient's account. Patient statements are generally mailed monthly when the patient account has a remaining balance.

BOX 4-28 ■ KEY POINTS

Billing Process

Charge Submission

- Insurance claim forms
- Patient statements

Patient Transactions

- Third-party payer transactions
- Patient payments

1500

HEALTH INSURANCE CLAIM FORM

APPROVED BY NATIONAL UNIFORM CLAIM COMMITTEE 08/05

PICA | PICA | CARRIER

1. MEDICARE (Medicare #) MEDICAID (Medicaid #) TRICARE CHAMPUS (Sponsor's SSN) CHAMPVA (Member ID#) GROUP HEALTH PLAN (SSN or ID) FECA BLK LUNG (SSN) OTHER (ID)

1a. INSURED'S I.D. NUMBER (For Program in Item 1)

2. PATIENT'S NAME (Last Name, First Name, Middle Initial)

3. PATIENT'S BIRTH DATE MM DD YY SEX M F

4. INSURED'S NAME (Last Name, First Name, Middle Initial)

5. PATIENT'S ADDRESS (No., Street)

6. PATIENT RELATIONSHIP TO INSURED Self Spouse Child Other

7. INSURED'S ADDRESS (No., Street)

CITY STATE

8. PATIENT STATUS Single Married Other

CITY STATE

ZIP CODE TELEPHONE (Include Area Code) ( )

Employed Full-Time Student Part-Time Student

ZIP CODE TELEPHONE (Include Area Code) ( )

9. OTHER INSURED'S NAME (Last Name, First Name, Middle Initial)

10. IS PATIENT'S CONDITION RELATED TO:

11. INSURED'S POLICY GROUP OR FECA NUMBER

a. OTHER INSURED'S POLICY OR GROUP NUMBER

a. EMPLOYMENT? (Current or Previous) YES NO

a. INSURED'S DATE OF BIRTH MM DD YY SEX M F

b. OTHER INSURED'S DATE OF BIRTH MM DD YY SEX M F

b. AUTO ACCIDENT? YES NO PLACE (State)

b. EMPLOYER'S NAME OR SCHOOL NAME

c. EMPLOYER'S NAME OR SCHOOL NAME

c. OTHER ACCIDENT? YES NO

c. INSURANCE PLAN NAME OR PROGRAM NAME

d. INSURANCE PLAN NAME OR PROGRAM NAME

10d. RESERVED FOR LOCAL USE

d. IS THERE ANOTHER HEALTH BENEFIT PLAN? YES NO *If yes*, return to and complete item 9 a-d.

READ BACK OF FORM BEFORE COMPLETING & SIGNING THIS FORM.

12. PATIENT'S OR AUTHORIZED PERSON'S SIGNATURE I authorize the release of any medical or other information necessary to process this claim. I also request payment of government benefits either to myself or to the party who accepts assignment below.

SIGNED ____ DATE ____

13. INSURED'S OR AUTHORIZED PERSON'S SIGNATURE I authorize payment of medical benefits to the undersigned physician or supplier for services described below.

SIGNED ____

PATIENT AND INSURED INFORMATION

14. DATE OF CURRENT: MM DD YY ILLNESS (First symptom) OR INJURY (Accident) OR PREGNANCY(LMP)

15. IF PATIENT HAS HAD SAME OR SIMILAR ILLNESS. GIVE FIRST DATE MM DD YY

16. DATES PATIENT UNABLE TO WORK IN CURRENT OCCUPATION MM DD YY FROM TO MM DD YY

17. NAME OF REFERRING PROVIDER OR OTHER SOURCE

17a.

17b. NPI

18. HOSPITALIZATION DATES RELATED TO CURRENT SERVICES MM DD YY FROM TO MM DD YY

19. RESERVED FOR LOCAL USE

20. OUTSIDE LAB? YES NO $ CHARGES

21. DIAGNOSIS OR NATURE OF ILLNESS OR INJURY (Relate Items 1, 2, 3 or 4 to Item 24E by Line)

1. ___ . ___

2. ___ . ___

3. ___ . ___

4. ___ . ___

22. MEDICAID RESUBMISSION CODE ORIGINAL REF. NO.

23. PRIOR AUTHORIZATION NUMBER

	24. A. DATE(S) OF SERVICE From MM DD YY	To MM DD YY	B. PLACE OF SERVICE	C. EMG	D. PROCEDURES, SERVICES, OR SUPPLIES (Explain Unusual Circumstances) CPT/HCPCS	MODIFIER	E. DIAGNOSIS POINTER	F. $ CHARGES	G. DAYS OR UNITS	H. EPSDT Family Plan	I. ID. QUAL.	J. RENDERING PROVIDER ID. #
1											NPI	
2											NPI	
3											NPI	
4											NPI	
5											NPI	
6											NPI	

25. FEDERAL TAX I.D. NUMBER SSN EIN

26. PATIENT'S ACCOUNT NO.

27. ACCEPT ASSIGNMENT? (For govt. claims, see back) YES NO

28. TOTAL CHARGE $

29. AMOUNT PAID $

30. BALANCE DUE $

31. SIGNATURE OF PHYSICIAN OR SUPPLIER INCLUDING DEGREES OR CREDENTIALS (I certify that the statements on the reverse apply to this bill and are made a part thereof.)

SIGNED DATE

32. SERVICE FACILITY LOCATION INFORMATION

a. NPI b.

33. BILLING PROVIDER INFO & PH # ( )

a. NPI b.

PHYSICIAN OR SUPPLIER INFORMATION

NUCC Instruction Manual available at: www.nucc.org

APPROVED OMB-0938-0999 FORM CMS-1500 (08-05)

Figure 4-30 CMS-1500.

MEDICARE PART A

P.O. BOX 167953

TEMPE AR 72207 TEL# 800 660 4235 VER# 4010-A1

PROV #69542A PROVIDER NAME: Dr. Martin Samerston PART A PAID DATE: 06/26/2006 REMIT#: 7654 PAGE:1

PATIENT NAME HIC NUMBER FROM DT THRU DT CLM STATUS	PATIENT CNTRL NUMBER ICN NUMBER NACHG HICHG TOB COST COVDY NCOVDY	RC REM DRG# RC REM OUTCD CAPCD RC REM PROF COMP RC REM DRG AMT	DRG OUT AMT NEW TECH MSP PAYMT DEDUCTIBLES	COINSURANCE COVD CHGS NCOVD CHGS DENIED CHGS	PAT REFUND ESRD NET ADJ INTEREST PRE PAY ADJ	CONTRACT ADJ PER DIEM RTE PROC CD AMT NET REIMB
Smith John 109876543210 06/01/2006 06/05/2006 6	7 9 407692738872 084327777A 00 3 111	149	6,895.72	1,463.72	.00	4556.00
		M 45	.00	.00	.00	.00
SUBTOTAL FISCAL YEAR - $000		M 138	.00	.00	.00	.00
		45.03	876.00	5,432.00	.00	4,556.00
			.00	.00	.00	.00
			.00	.00	.00	.00
SUBTOTAL PART A		.00	.00	.00	.00	.00
TOTAL PART A			876.00	5,432.00	.00	4556.00

Figure 4-31 Sample Medicare remittance advice (RA). *(Data from Centers for Medicare & Medicaid Services: Sample Medicare remittance advice, www.cms.hhs.gov.)*

ACCOUNTS RECEIVABLE (A/R) MANAGEMENT

Hospitals monitor outstanding accounts for the purpose of ensuring that payments are received in a timely manner. The term used to describe outstanding accounts is accounts receivable. A division of the PFS Department, Credit and Collections, is responsible for monitoring outstanding claims to determine accounts that require follow-up. Data required to monitor outstanding accounts are provided through the automated billing system. The billing system generally groups accounts based on financial classes. Accounts are also monitored based on the number of days the account is outstanding, which is referred to as aging. Two reports utilized to monitor outstanding accounts are the financial class report and the accounts receivable report.

BOX 4-29 ■ KEY POINTS

Accounts Receivable (A/R) Management

The follow-up on outstanding accounts is monitored as follows:

- **Financial class report:** outlines claim information such as charges, payments, and outstanding balances grouped according to type of payer.
- **Accounts receivable aging report (A/R):** outstanding accounts are categorized based on the number of days the balance has been outstanding.

Financial Class Report

A **financial class** is a classification of patient accounts and information such as charges, payments, and outstanding balances, grouped according to payer types. All payers are assigned to a financial class. An example of a financial class might be the category "Commercial," in which data on all commercial carriers may be grouped. Common financial classes are Commercial, Blue Cross/Blue Shield, Medicaid, Medicare, TRICARE, Auto, and Worker's Compensation. Managed care plans may also have a separate financial class assigned to them. Designation of financial classes allows detailed tracking and reporting of charges, payments, and outstanding balances per payer type. A financial class report can be generated from the computer system to analyze outstanding charges by payer type. A payer financial class report is illustrated in Figure 4-32.

Accounts Receivable Aging Report (A/R Report)

Accounts are also categorized based on the number of days the balance is outstanding. Outstanding balances are referred to as accounts receivable, and the report outlining categories of claims based on the age of the account is referred to as an **accounts receivable report**,

COMMUNITY GENERAL HOSPITAL
Payer Financial Class Report
02/01/06–06/30/06

Financial Class	Patient Name	Service Date	Total Charges	Payment	Contractual Adjustment	Balance
01 BC/BS	Adams, Harold	02/02/2006	$1,356.50	$868.16	$271.30	$217.04
	Boyter, Susan	03/17/2006	$27,865.00	$17,833.60	$5,573.00	$4,458.40
	Johns, Tina	06/22/2006	$42,677.97	$27,313.90	$8,535.59	$6,828.48
	Xavier, George	02/25/2006	$18,433.56	$11,797.48	$3,686.71	$2,949.37
	Yohanson, Phil	05/31/2006	$879.97	$563.18	$175.99	$140.80
02 Commercial	Beard, Bobby	06/22/2006	$42,677.97	$27,313.90	$8,535.59	$6,828.48
	Baxter, Morris	03/17/2006	$27,865.00	$17,833.60	$5,573.00	$4,458.40
	James, John	02/25/2006	$18,433.56	$11,797.48	$3,686.71	$2,949.37
	Hatley, Hanna	02/02/2006	$1,356.50	$868.16	$271.30	$217.04
	Mannie, Minnie	05/31/2006	$879.97	$563.18	$175.99	$140.80
03 Medicaid	Harold, Adam	02/02/2006	$572.00	$171.60	$400.40	$0.00
	Harpo, Harold	03/17/2006	$877.97	$0.00	$614.58	$263.39
	Morris, Baxter	06/22/2006	$256.34	$76.90	$179.44	$0.00
	Polo, Marco	02/25/2006	$72.82	$0.00	$50.97	$21.85
	Smith, Ima	05/31/2006	$10,423.00	$0.00	$7,296.10	$3,126.90
04 Medicare	Anson, Annie	02/02/2006	$1,356.50	$868.16	$271.30	$217.04
	Chan, William	02/25/2006	$18,433.56	$11,797.48	$3,686.71	$2,949.37
	Cater, Cody	03/17/2006	$27,865.00	$17,833.60	$5,573.00	$4,458.40
	Janson, Jonnie	05/31/2006	$879.97	$563.18	$175.99	$140.80
	Williams, Meta	06/22/2006	$42,677.97	$27,313.90	$8,535.59	$6,828.48

Figure 4-32 Sample payer financial class report.

COMMUNITY GENERAL HOSPITAL
PATIENT A/R REPORT
December 30, 2006

Account #	Name	Phone	Current	31-60	61-90	91-120	121-150	151-180	180+	Total Balance
05962	Applebee, Carla	(813) 797-4545							724.45	724.45
23456	Borden, Andrew	(813) 423-9678		200.00			47.52			247.52
16955	Cox, Anthony	(813) 233-7794	175.00		695.00		199.53			1069.53
14355	Freeman, Tina	(727) 665-7878					592.14			592.14
00876	Holtsaver, Marshall	(727) 874-2945	485.72		400.00				1583.66	2469.38
00023	James, John	(813) 201-2054			350.00		963.68			1313.68
10245	Marcus, Xavier	(727) 779-3325		2745.21						2745.21
19457	Peters, Samantha	(413) 544-2243			1545.23		1022.69			2567.92
99645	Snowton, Michael	(941) 333-4325			1314.00	3254.00				4568.00
	Report Totals		**660.72**	**2945.21**	**4304.23**	**3254**	**2825.56**	**0**	**2308.11**	**16297.83**
	% Aged		4.05%	18.07%	26.41%	19.97%	17.34%	0.00%	14.16%	

Figure 4-33 Sample patient A/R report.

or **A/R report** (Figure 4-33). Common aging report categories are over 30 days, 31 to 60 days, 61 to 90 days, 91 to 120 days, and over 120 days.

A/R reports are generated for the purpose of identifying accounts that require follow-up. Hospitals establish policies regarding collection of outstanding accounts that include priorities for collection efforts based on the age of the account. For example, the hospital policy may indicate that collection personnel should concentrate on accounts that are in the 91- to 120-day aging category. The hospital policy may also provide criteria for accounts that should be sent to an outside collection agency or an attorney. A/R management is discussed in detail in Chapter 6.

TEST YOUR *Knowledge* BOX 4-5

BILLING PROCESS; ACCOUNTS RECEIVABLE MANAGEMENT

1. Why is the billing process important?
2. Explain when the billing process begins in a hospital.
3. Explain what department performs billing functions and how automation assists with those functions.
4. List functions included in the billing process.
5. When does a hospital bill third-party payers and patients?
6. List two documents used to submit charges to patients and third-party payers.
7. What computer software is utilized to edit third-party payer claims?
8. Describe two claim forms utilized to submit charges to third-party payers.
9. State the difference between the CMS-1450 and the CMS-1500.
10. Outline the information on a patient statement.
11. List three actions a payer can take on a claim.
12. Provide an outline of the process of posting transactions to a patient's account.
13. State the purpose of accounts receivable management.
14. Define financial class and provide examples.
15. Discuss the purpose and content of an A/R report.

CHAPTER SUMMARY

The patient account and data flow is a critical element in the hospital's ability to effectively access and utilize data collected throughout the hospital. Automated systems for registration, order entry, charge capture, billing, and accounts receivable management enhance the ability of various departmental personnel to access and utilize data simultaneously. Data collected are utilized through the patient care process for admissions, rendering patient care services, and billing for those services. The patient care process from admission to discharge involves capturing and recording information regarding the patient and care provided. Patient information is stored in the hospital's health information system and in the patient's medical record. Services and items provided are recorded in the patient's record and on the patient's account. The coding and billing process begins at discharge. The HIM Department receives the medical record for review, coding, and assignment of MS-DRG or APC. The PFS Department prepares claim forms for submission and patient statements to be sent. The Credit and Collections Department monitors outstanding accounts and works to collect outstanding balances from patients, insurance companies, and government payers. It is critical for coding and billing professionals to have complete and accurate information for billing payers and patients.

CHAPTER REVIEW 4-1

True/False

1. Information obtained during the patient admission process is utilized for billing. T F
2. The admission process consists of functions required to discharge a patient. T F
3. Quality Improvement Organization (QIO) reviews have a direct impact on reimbursement. T F
4. Written Authorization for Release of Medical Information is required before patient information can be released. T F
5. Verification of insurance is required to ensure that appropriate reimbursement for services is received. T F

Fill in the Blank

6. A form used to provide authorization for a payer to make payment to the hospital is called ____________________.
7. Services that are considered appropriate and necessary in response to the patient's condition are ____________________.
8. A room/bed is assigned to patients who are admitted on an ____________________ basis.
9. Health Information Management (HIM) procedures performed after the patient is discharged include: ____________________, ____________________, and ____________________.
10. Testing performed prior to an inpatient or surgical admission is called ____________________.

Match the Following Definitions With the Terms at Right

11. ___ Specific criteria used to determine whether a patient admission is appropriate and necessary.
12. ___ Universally accepted claim form used to submit charges for hospital inpatient and ambulatory surgery charges.
13. ___ Classification of outstanding claims according to payer.
14. ___ A software program utilized by HIM personnel to assist with the assignment of an MS-DRG or APC group.
15. ___ A listing of categories of outstanding accounts by days outstanding.

A. Financial class
B. CMS-1450 (UB-04)
C. Grouper
D. A/R report (aging report)
E. Admission Evaluation Protocols (AEPs)

Research Project

Refer to the CMS Web site at www.cms.gov.

Find information on general admission procedures in the hospital manual.

Discuss the procedures discussed in Section 300 of the hospital manual.

Discuss how to handle situations where you cannot obtain information in Section 301 of the hospital manual.

GLOSSARY

Accounts receivable (A/R) Aging Report A report outlining categories of claims based on the age of the account.

Admission The act of being received into a place or a patient accepted for inpatient services in a hospital.

Admission Evaluation Protocols (AEP) Outlines appropriate conditions for a hospital admission based on standards referred to as the IS/SI criteria. IS refers to the intensity of service criteria. SI refers to the severity of illness criteria.

Admission summary A summary of information about the patient's admission, such as the patient's name and address, insurance company name, reason(s) for admission, attending physician's name, and referring physician's name. The admission summary is also known as a face sheet.

Advance Beneficiary Notice (ABN) A notice informing the patient that there is reason to believe the admission will not be covered by Medicare. The patient's signature is required on this form to acknowledge that he or she will be financially responsible if Medicare does not cover the service.

Advance directives Provide instructions regarding measures that should or should not be taken in the event medical treatment is required to prolong life.

Ambulatory Payment Classification (APC) A Prospective Payment System (PPS) implemented to provide reimbursement for hospital outpatient services. Under APC, the facility is paid a fixed fee based on the resources utilized to provide the service or procedure.

Assignment of Benefits Instructs the insurance company or government plan to forward benefits (payments for services) to the hospital.

Charge capture The process of gathering charge information and recording it on the patient's account.

Charge Description Master (CDM) A computerized system used by the hospital to inventory and record services and items provided by the hospital. CDM is commonly referred to as the chargemaster.

CMS-1450 (UB-04) Universally accepted claim form used to submit facility charges for hospital inpatient and outpatient services.

CMS-1500 Universally accepted claim form for submission of physician and outpatient services and Durable Medical Equipment (DME).

Co-insurance An amount the patient is responsible to pay that is calculated based on a percentage of approved charges.

Co-payment A set amount that is paid by the patient for specific services. Co-payment is commonly referred to as a copay.

Concurrent review Ongoing review throughout the hospital stay to determine appropriateness of the admission and care provided.

Deductible An annual set amount determined by each payer that the patient must pay before the plan pays benefits for services.

Encounter form A charge tracking document utilized to record services, procedures, and items provided during the visit and the medical reason for the services provided.

Explanation of Benefits (EOB) Another term used for remittance advice.

Explanation of Medicare Benefits (EOMB) Another term used for remittance advice.

Facility charges Charges that represent the cost and overhead for the technical component of patient care services, which include space, equipment, supplies, drugs and biologicals, and technical staff.

Financial class A classification of patient accounts and information such as charges, payments, and outstanding balances, grouped according to payer types.

Guarantor The individual who is responsible to pay for services provided.

Informed Consent for Treatment A form utilized by the hospital to obtain the patient's authorization for treatment. The form must be signed by the patient before treatment can be provided.

Insurance verification The process of contacting the patient's insurance plan to determine various aspects of coverage such as whether the patient's coverage is active, what services are covered, authorization requirements, and patient responsibility.

Medical necessity Services or procedures that are reasonable and medically necessary in response to the patient's symptoms according to accepted standards of medical practice.

Medical record A chart or folder where patient's information is stored, including demographic, insurance, financial, and medical information.

Medical record number (MRN) A unique identification number assigned by the hospital to each patient's medical record. The MRN remains the patient's medical record number indefinitely.

Medicare Severity Diagnosis Related Groups (MS-DRG) A reimbursement method implemented under PPS that pays hospitals a fixed amount for a hospital stay based on the patient's diagnosis and the severity of that condition.

Patient registration form A form utilized by the hospital to obtain patient information including demographic, insurance, and financial information.

Professional charges Charges that represent physician and other non-physician clinical services, the professional component of patient care services.

Prospective review A review performed prior to the patient admission to determine appropriateness of the admission and length of stay.

Remittance advice (RA) A document prepared by payers to communicate payment determination to hospitals and patients. The RA includes detailed information about the charges submitted and an explanation of how the claim was processed.

Retrospective review A review conducted after the patient is discharged to determine appropriateness of admission and care provided.

Written Authorization for Release of Medical Information Provides authorization for the hospital to release personal health information when required for treatment and to obtain payment for services.

Chapter 5

Hospital Billing Process

The purpose of this chapter is to provide an overview of the hospital billing process. The billing process includes submitting charges to third-party payers and patients, posting patient transactions, and following-up on outstanding accounts. As discussed in previous chapters, information collected during the patient visit is utilized to complete the tasks required to bill for services rendered. A review of the purpose of the billing process will provide an understanding of how vital billing functions are for the hospital to maintain a sound financial base.

The role of hospital billing and coding professionals is complicated because of the ever-changing health insurance environment and variations in payer guidelines. It is essential for billing and coding professionals to understand payer guidelines in order to ensure that proper reimbursement is obtained and to be compliant with payer guidelines. A review of several elements of the participating provider agreement "payer contract" will illustrate how payer guidelines vary and the significant impact they have on the billing process. A discussion of how charges are captured, coding systems, and claim forms will provide a basis for an understanding of the billing process. The chapter will close with an overview of the hospital billing process from patient admission to collections. Many of the concepts presented in this chapter are described briefly. More detailed discussion will be provided in later chapters.

Chapter Objectives

- Define terms, phrases, abbreviations, and acronyms related to the hospital billing and claims process.
- Demonstrate an understanding of the billing process and its purpose.
- Discuss the relationship among participating provider agreements, claim forms, reimbursement methods, and the billing process.
- Explain the significance of submitting a clean claim.
- Demonstrate understanding of the variations in claim requirements by payer type and type of service.
- Explain the purpose of the chargemaster and its relationship to billing.
- List and explain data elements in the chargemaster and discuss maintenance of the chargemaster.
- Provide an overview of categories of services and items billed by the hospital.

(Continued)

Outline

- Differentiate between coding systems utilized for outpatient services versus those used for inpatient services.
- Discuss the purpose of the detailed itemized statement.
- Briefly discuss the purpose of a claim form and provide a brief outline of information recorded on a claim form.
- Demonstrate an understanding of all elements and phases in the hospital billing process.
- Explain the significance of A/R management.
- Discuss claims that do not meet clean claim status.

Key Terms

Accounts receivable (A/R) management
Ambulatory Payment Classifications (APC)
Ambulatory surgery
Batch
Billing process
Capitation
Case mix
Case rate
Charge Description Master (CDM)
Claims process
Clean claim
Clearinghouse
CMS-1450 (UB-92)
CMS-1500
Collections
Contract rate
Detailed itemized statement
Electronic data interchange (EDI)
Electronic media claim (EMC)
Encoder
Facility charges
Fee-for-service (FFS)
Fee schedule
Flat rate
Form locator (FL)
Grouper
Health Care Common Procedure Coding System (HCPCS)
Inpatient Prospective Payment System (IPPS)
Medicare Severity Diagnosis Related Groups (MS-DRG)
Outpatient Prospective Payment System (OPPS)
Participating provider agreement
Patient invoice
Patient statement
Per diem
Percentage of accrued charges
Professional charges
Prospective Payment System (PPS)
Reimbursement
Relative value scale (RVS)
Resource-based relative value scale (RBRVS)
Revenue code
Third-party payer
Usual, customary, and reasonable (UCR)

Acronyms and Abbreviations

APC—Ambulatory Payment Classification
CMS—Centers for Medicare and Medicaid Services
CDM—Charge Description Master
EDI—electronic data interchange
EMC—electronic media claim
FL—form locator
HCPCS—Health Care Common Procedure Coding System
IPPS—Inpatient Prospective Payment System
MS-DRG—Medicare Severity Diagnosis Related Groups
NUBC—National Uniform Billing Committee
OPPS—Outpatient Prospective Payment System (OPPS)
RBRVS—resource-based relative value scale
RVS—Relative value scale
UCR—Usual, Customary, and Reasonable.
UB-04—CMS-1450 Universal Bill implemented in 2007.

PURPOSE OF THE BILLING PROCESS

The purpose of the hospital billing process is to obtain reimbursement for services and items rendered by the hospital. Reimbursement is received from patients, insurance carriers, and government programs. The hospital billing process begins when a patient arrives at the hospital for diagnosis and treatment of an injury, illness, disease, or condition. The patient's demographic and insurance information is obtained and registered in the hospital's information system. Physician's orders or a requisition outlines the patient care services required. Patient care services and items provided during the patient's stay are recorded on the patient's account. Charges are posted to the patient's account by various departments. When the patient leaves the hospital, all information and charges are prepared for billing. The **billing process** involves all the functions required to prepare charges for submission to patients and third-party payers in order for the hospital to obtain reimbursement. It includes patient registration, posting charges to the patient's account, chart review and coding, preparing claim forms and patient invoices or statements for charge submission, and monitoring and follow-up of outstanding accounts. The term **claims process** refers to the portion of billing that involves preparing claims for submission to payers. An extension of the billing process is **collections**, also known as A/R management, which involves monitoring accounts that are outstanding and pursuing collection of those balances from patients and third-party payers. The hospital billing process is illustrated in Figure 5-1.

The complexity of the hospital billing process is a result of the health care industry's evolution. The history of hospitals explains how medicine changed over the years and how hospitals evolved as a result of that change. It also shows the relationship among advances in medicine, hospital evolution, and rising health care costs. Health insurance and government-funded health care benefit programs were born. Over the years, more insurance companies and government programs came into existence. Regulation of the health care industry was enhanced. Contracts between providers and payers were initiated. The process of submitting charges became more involved than providing services and collecting a fee from the patient. It now involves authorizations and certifications, medical record documentation, coding, participating provider agreements, various payer guidelines, and different reimbursement systems (Figure 5-2). Because of the complexity of this

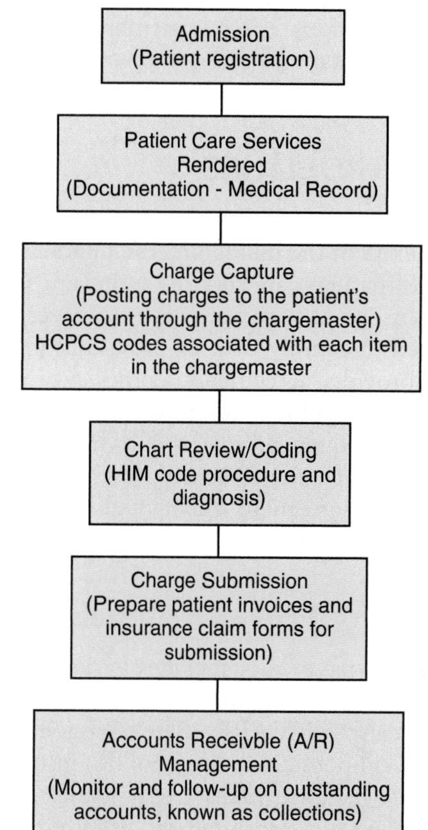

Figure 5-1 The hospital billing process involves all the functions required to prepare charges for submission to patients and third-party payers to obtain reimbursement.

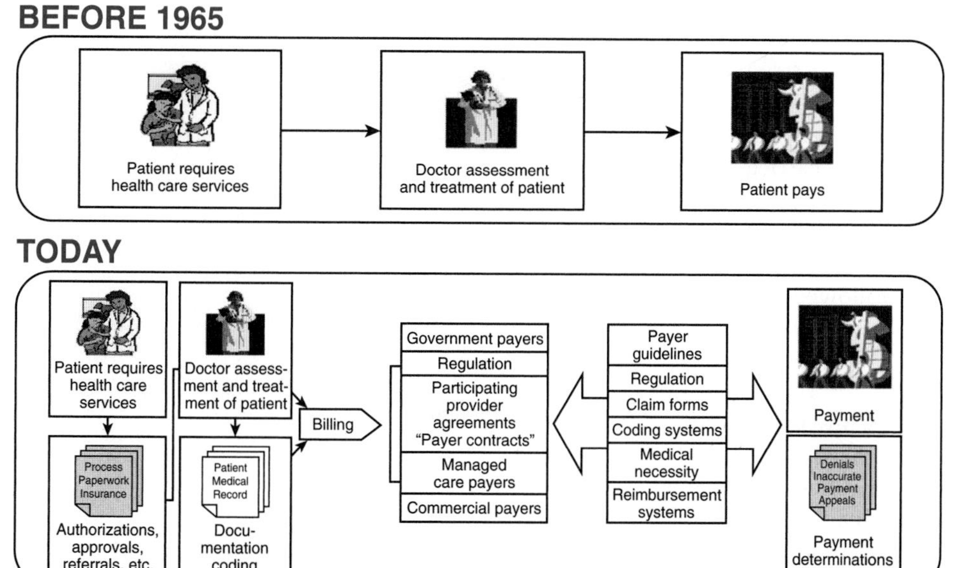

Figure 5-2 The evolution and complexity of the billing process from 1965 to today.

system, hospital billing and coding professionals are required to have knowledge of all these elements to ensure that appropriate reimbursement is obtained and that the hospital is in compliance with payer guidelines.

PAYER GUIDELINES

Variations in payer guidelines contribute significantly to the complexity of the billing process. Guidelines for the provision of patient care services and claim submission and reimbursement vary from payer to payer. Hospitals are required to comply with all provisions in their participating provider agreements. Compliance with these guidelines is a condition for receiving reimbursement, and legal consequences may result from noncompliance. A review of some common provisions in a participating provider agreement will highlight the relationship between the agreements and the billing process.

Participating Provider Agreements

The hospital's payer mix includes various payers that provide coverage to patients seen at the hospital. Medicare, Medicaid, TRICARE, Blue Cross/Blue Shield, Worker's Compensation, automobile insurance, and various managed care plans are generally part of the hospital's payer mix. Hospitals and other providers may elect to enter into a written agreement to participate with several different payers, known as the participating provider agreement. A **participating provider agreement** is a written agreement between the hospital and a payer that outlines the terms and specifications of participation for the hospital and the payer. The next section provides a brief overview of some of the key elements of a participating provider agreement. Figures 5-3 and 5-4 highlight common provisions related to patient care services, patient financial responsibility, billing requirements, and reimbursement.

Patient Care Services

The participating provider agreement outlines the services that are covered for plan members. Participating providers are encouraged to refer patients to providers within the network for the plan. All payers include provisions regarding medical necessity and utilization management protocols that must be followed to ensure that the appropriate reimbursement is received.

Medical Necessity

Providers are statutorily obligated to provide patient care services that are considered medically necessary. All payers have medical necessity guidelines that must be met as a condition of receiving payment for those services. Medically necessary services are those that are considered reasonable and medically necessary to address the patient's condition based on standards of medical practice. Interpretations of medical necessity based on standards of medical practice vary by payer.

BOX 5-1 ■ KEY POINTS

Medical Necessity

Medically necessary services are those that are considered reasonable and medically necessary in order to address the patient's condition based on standards of medical practice.

Utilization Management

Utilization management involves monitoring and managing health care resources for the purpose of controlling cost and ensuring that quality care is provided. In accordance with the participating provider agreement, providers are required to follow utilization management requirements outlined in the payer contract. Precertification, prior authorization, and second surgical opinions are examples of utilization management requirements.

Patient Financial Responsibility

Participating provider agreements include information regarding the patient's financial responsibility under the plan. The patient's responsibility is the amount that the patient is required to pay in accordance with his or her health care plan. All health care plans require the patient to pay some portion of the charges for services rendered. As outlined in the patient's plan, the patient's responsibility amount may represent a deductible, coinsurance, or a co-payment amount. The agreement further specifies the participating provider's contractual obligation to collect a specified amount from the patient and the consequences if the provider does not make every attempt to collect the patient's share.

BOX 5-2 ■ KEY POINTS

Patient Responsibility

The amount the patient is required to pay in accordance with their health care plan:

- Deductible—Annual amount determined by the payer that the patient must pay before the plan pays benefits
- Co-insurance—A percentage of the approved amount that the patient is required to pay
- Co-payment—A fixed amount determined per service that the patient must pay

Billing Requirements

Billing requirements are outlined in each participating provider agreement. Billing requirements vary accord-

Participating Provider Agreement

This Agreement is entered into by and between **Community Hospital,** contracting on behalf of itself, **ABC Health Insurance,** Inc. and the other entities that are ABC Affiliates (collectively referred to as "ABC") and Community ("Hospital").

This Agreement is effective on the later of the following dates (the "Effective Date"):
i) December 31, 2006 or the first day of the first calendar month that begins at least thirty days after the date when this Agreement has been executed by all parties. Through contracts with physicians and other providers of health care services, ABC maintains one or more networks of providers that are available to Customers. Hospital is a provider of health care services. ABC wishes to arrange to make Hospital's services available to Customers. Hospital wishes to provide such services, under the terms and conditions set forth in this Agreement. The parties therefore enter into this Agreement.

Article I. Definitions

The following terms when used in this Agreement have the meanings set forth below:

1.1 "Benefit Plan" means a certificate of coverage or summary plan description, under which a Payer is obligated to provide coverage of Covered Services for a Customer.

1.2 "Covered Service" is a health care service or product for which a Customer is entitled to receive coverage from a Payer, pursuant to the terms of the Customer's Benefit Plan with that Payer.

1.3 "Customary Charge" is the fee for health care services charged by Hospital that does not exceed the fee Hospitals would ordinarily charge another person regardless of whether the person is a Customer.

1.4 "Customer" is a person eligible and enrolled to receive coverage from a Payer for Covered Services.

1.5 "Hospital" is a duly licensed and qualified under the laws of the jurisdiction in which Covered Services are provided, who practices as a shareholder, partner, or employee of Hospital, or who practices as a subcontractor of Hospital.

Article II. Representations and Warranties

2.1 Representations and Warranties of Hospital. Hospital, by virtue of its execution and delivery of this Agreement, represents and warrants as follows:

(a) Hospital is a duly organized and validly existing legal entity in good standing under the laws of its jurisdiction of organization.

(b) Hospital has all requisite corporate power and authority to conduct its business as presently conducted, and to execute, deliver and perform its obligations under this Agreement.

(c) The execution, delivery and performance of this Agreement by acknowledges the **Hospital do not and will not violate or conflict with** (i) the organizational documents of Hospital, (ii) any material agreement or instrument to which Hospital is a party or by which Hospital or any material part of its property is bound, or (iii) **applicable law.**

(d) Hospital has reviewed the Protocols and Payment Policies and acknowledges it is bound by the Protocols and that claims under this Agreement will be paid in accordance with the Payment Policies.

(f) **Each submission of a claim** by Hospital pursuant to this Agreement shall be deemed to constitute the representation and warranty by it to ABC that (i) the representations and warranties of it set forth in this section 2.1 and elsewhere in this Agreement are true and correct as of the date the claim is submitted, (ii) it has complied with the requirements of this Agreement with respect to the Covered Services involved and the submission of such claim, (iii) the charge amount set forth on the claim is the Customary Charge and (iv) the claim is a valid claim.

Article III. Applicability of this Agreement

3.1 Hospital's Services. This Agreement applies to services that are medically necessary and reasonable to diagnose and treat customer's condition.

3.2 Services not covered under a Benefit Plan. This Agreement does not apply to services not covered under the applicable Benefit Plan. Hospital may seek and collect payment from a Customer for such services, provided that the Hospital first obtains the Customer's written consent. This section does not authorize Hospital to bill or collect from Customers for Covered Services for which claims are denied or otherwise not paid. That issue is addressed in section 7 of this Agreement.

–1–

Figure 5-3 A participating provider agreement, highlighting provisions regarding patient care services, patient responsibility, billing, and reimbursement.

ing to plan. Most plans outline provisions in the participating provider agreement regarding documentation, coding, claim form requirements, timely filing, and the appeals process.

Reimbursement

Participating provider agreements contain provisions regarding timely processing of claims and reimbursement. Reimbursement is provided for services covered under the patient's plan that are considered medically necessary. The agreement also explains how payment determinations are made and what reimbursement method will be utilized to calculate payment for covered services.

It is important to remember that reimbursement for services provided to plan members is contingent on the provider's compliance with plan terms and specifications. It is critical for hospital personnel involved in the billing process to have an understanding of the terms in the provider agreement to ensure compliance with program specifications and to optimize reimbursement. Participating provider agreements will be discussed further in Chapters 11 to 13. To enhance our understanding of the complexity of the billing process, the following section provides a basic review of payer variations in claim form requirements and reimbursement methods utilized to determine payments to the hospital.

Participating Provider Agreement

3.4 Health Care. Hospital acknowledges that this Agreement does not dictate the health care provided by Hospital or Hospital Professionals, or govern Hospital's or Hospital Professional's determination of what care to provide their patients, even if those patients are Customers. The decision regarding what care is to be provided remains with Hospital and Hospital Professionals and with Customers, and not with ABC or any Payer. Hospital will not allow coverage decisions to determine or influence treatment decisions.

Article V. Duties of Hospital

5.1 Provide Covered Services. Hospital will provide Covered Services that are considered Medically Necessary to Customers at the location specified in section 3.1.

5.2 Cooperation with Protocols. Hospital will cooperate with and be bound by ABC's and Payers' Protocols. The Protocols include but are not limited to all of the following:

1. Hospital will use reasonable commercial efforts to direct Customers only to other providers that participate in ABC's network, except as otherwise authorized by ABC or Payer.
2. Hospital will follow Utilization Management protocols and provide notification for certain Covered Services as defined by ABC or Payer, including the following requirements:
   (a) Provide notification, as further described in the Protocols, prior to a scheduled inpatient admission of a Customer, by telephone, at least five (5) business days prior to the admission; in cases in which the admission is scheduled less than five business days in advance, Hospital will give notice at the time the admission is scheduled.
   (b) With regard to the inpatient admission of a Customer, provide notification, as further described in the Protocols, no later than the next business day, by telephone, if a Customer is admitted on an emergency basis or for observation.
   (c) Obtain required authorizations and certifications and authorizations as outlined in Appendix B.
3. Hospital will obtain customer consent to release Medical Record information.
4. Hospital will follow ABC protocols and fulfill responsibility for the collection of deductible, co-payment or co-insurance amounts outlined in Appendix C as the customer's responsibility.

Article VII. Submission, Processing and Payment of Claims

7.1 Form and content of claims. Hospital must submit claims for Covered Services in a manner and format prescribed by ABC, as further described in the Protocols. Unless otherwise directed by ABC, Hospital shall submit claims using current CMS-1500 or CMS-1450 (UB-04) forms, whichever is appropriate, with applicable coding including, but not limited to, ICD, CPT, Revenue and HCPCS coding. Hospital shall comply with all claim form completion guidelines as outlined in Appendix C.

7.2 Electronic filing of claims. Within six months after the Effective Date of this Agreement, Hospital will use electronic submission for all of its claims under this Agreement that ABC is able to accept electronically

7.3 Time to file claims. All information necessary to process a claim must be received by ABC no more than 90 days from the date that Covered Services are rendered. Payment to the hospital may be denied if the Hospital does not comply with Timely Filing Protocols in Appendix D and does not file a timely claim

7.4 Denial of Claims. Hospitals may appeal claim denials in accordance with Protocols outlined in Appendix E.

7.5 Reimbursement - Payment of claims. **ABC** will pay claims for Covered Services according to the lesser of, the Hospital's Customary Charge or the applicable fee schedule, as provided in Appendix F. Payment determinations are subject to the Payment Policies, and minus any co-payment, deductible, or coinsurance as applicable under the Customer's Benefit Plan. The obligation for payment under this Agreement is solely that of ABC.

7.6 Timely payment. In accordance with provisions in this agreement and legal statutes, ABC is obligated to process claims and remit payment or explanation of non-payment within 30 days of the date the claim is received.

–2–

Figure 5-4 A participating provider agreement, highlighting provisions regarding patient care services, patient responsibility, billing, and reimbursement.

Claim Forms

The purpose of the claim form is to submit charges to third-party payers. A **third-party payer** is an organization or other entity that provides coverage for medical services, such as insurance companies, managed care plans, Medicare, and other government programs. All the information collected and recorded on the patient account and in the patient record is utilized to complete the claim form.

There are two universally accepted claim forms utilized for submission of charges to various payers—the CMS-1500 and the CMS-1450 (UB-04). These forms were formerly called the HCFA-1500 and the HCFA-1450 (UB-92). The Health Care Financing Administration (HCFA) changed their name to the Centers for Medicare and Medicaid Services (CMS), and the forms are now referred to as the CMS-1500 and CMS-1450.

The CMS-1450 (UB-92) was replaced by the UB-04 on May 23, 2007. The National Uniform Billing Committee (NUBC) announced the period for public comment, the process that will be followed after all comments are in, and finally the scheduled implementation dates (Figure 5-5). The release indicates that

> Following the close of a public comment period and careful review of comments received, the National Uniform Billing Committee approved the UB-04 as the replacement for the UB-92. Receivers (health plans and clearinghouses) need to be ready to receive the new UB-04 by March 1, 2007. Submitters (health care providers such as hospitals) can use the UB-04 beginning March 1, 2007; however, they will have a transitional period between March 1, 2007 and May 22, 2007 where they can use the UB-04 or the UB-92.*

---

*From NUBC Web page: http://www.nubc.org.

FOR IMMEDIATE RELEASE—UB-04 scheduled to replace CMS-1450 (UB-92)

NUBC Announces 45-day Public Comment Period, ending February 1, 2005, for the New UB-04 Data Set and Form

December 17, 2004

The National Uniform Billing Committee (NUBC) announced today the opening of a 45-day public comment period, ending February 1, 2005, for the new UB-04 data set and form to replace the UB-92. The UB-04 contains a number of improvements and enhancements that resulted from nearly four years of research. The NUBC is conducting this final survey to better understand the timelines and transition issues surrounding the implementation of the UB-04. Those wishing to comment on the UB-04 are encouraged to visit the NUBC website http://www.nubc.org/ for further information.

NUBC ANNOUNCES APPROVAL OF UB-04

Following the close of a public comment period and careful review of comments received, the National Uniform Billing Committee approved the UB-04 as the replacement for the UB-92 at its February 2005 meeting.

Receivers (health plans and clearinghouses) need to be ready to receive the new UB-04 by March 1, 2007.

Submitters (health care providers such as hospitals, skilled nursing facilities, hospice, and other institutional claim filers) can use the UB-04 **beginning March 1, 2007,** however, they will have a transitional period between March 1, 2007 and May 22, 2007 where they can use the UB-04 or the UB-92.

Starting May 23, 2007 all institutional paper claims must use the UB-04; the UB-92 will no longer be acceptable after this date.

The final image of the UB-04 form, a summary of the public comments/NUBC responses, and information on how to obtain a beta version of the UB-04 Data Specifications Manual can be found on the NUBC website.

Figure 5-5 The National Uniform Billing Committee announces replacement of the CMS-1450 (UB-92) with the UB-04 in 2007. *(Modified from National Uniform Billing Committee: UB-04 Proofs, www.nubc.org.)*

BOX 5-3 ■ KEY POINTS

NUBC Announces UB-04 Scheduled to Replace the CMS-1450 (UB-92)

Receivers

Health plans and clearinghouses need to be ready to receive the new UB-04 by March 1, 2007

Submitters

Health care providers such as hospitals can use the UB-04 beginning March 1, 2004; however, they will have a transitional period between March 1, 2007 and May 23, 2007 in which they can use the UB-04 or the UB-92

This chapter will discuss the CMS-1450 (UB-04) as it relates to the hospital billing process. Claim forms will be discussed further in Chapter 10.

Claim form requirements vary by payer, and the participating provider agreement defines what claim form should be used to submit charges. The CMS-1500 is generally required for submission of charges related to physician and outpatient services (Figure 5-6). The CMS-1450 (UB-04) is generally used to submit facility charges for services provided in the hospital. This form is commonly referred to as the UB-04 or just UB (Figure 5-7). Payers specify the claim form required for submission of charges based on the following service categories: outpatient, inpatient, and non-patient. The following section provides an overview of which claim form is required for these service categories, as shown in Table 5-1.

Outpatient

Hospital outpatient services are generally submitted to payers utilizing the UB-04; however, some payers may require the CMS-1500. Outpatient services include Ambulatory Surgery, Emergency Department, other outpatient department services, and clinic services.

Ambulatory Surgery

Ambulatory surgery may be performed in a hospital Ambulatory Surgery Department or in a hospital-based certified ambulatory surgery center (ASC). Ambulatory surgery is considered an outpatient service because the patient is released the same day the procedure is performed. Hospital-based ambulatory surgery services are generally submitted utilizing the UB-04. Some payers may require ambulatory surgery services performed in a certified ASC to be submitted utilizing the CMS-1500.

Emergency Department

Facility charges for Emergency Department visits are generally submitted utilizing the UB-04. Again, some payers may require the CMS-1500. Emergency Room (ER) physician charges are not billed by the hospital. The ER physician will submit charges for services he or she provides on the CMS-1500. Emergency Department charges are included on the inpatient claim utilizing the UB-04 when the patient is admitted as an inpatient from the ER.

Ancillary Departments

Charges for services provided by ancillary departments such as Radiology, Laboratory, or Physical, Occupational, and Speech Therapy on an outpatient basis are generally submitted utilizing the UB-04. Infusion therapy and observation services are also submitted on the UB-04.

Hospital-Based Primary Care Office or Hospital-Based Clinic

Charges for services provided in a hospital-based primary care office are generally submitted on the CMS-1500. These charges will include the physician services if the physician is an employee of or under contract with the hospital. Charges for services provided in a hospital-based clinic are generally submitted on the CMS-1450. These charges do not include the physician services unless the physician is an employee of the hospital.

1500

HEALTH INSURANCE CLAIM FORM

APPROVED BY NATIONAL UNIFORM CLAIM COMMITTEE 08/05

PICA | PICA | CARRIER

1. MEDICARE (Medicare #) MEDICAID (Medicaid #) TRICARE CHAMPUS (Sponsor's SSN) CHAMPVA (Member ID#) GROUP HEALTH PLAN (SSN or ID) FECA BLK LUNG (SSN) OTHER (ID)

1a. INSURED'S I.D. NUMBER (For Program in Item 1)

2. PATIENT'S NAME (Last Name, First Name, Middle Initial)

3. PATIENT'S BIRTH DATE MM DD YY SEX M F

4. INSURED'S NAME (Last Name, First Name, Middle Initial)

5. PATIENT'S ADDRESS (No., Street)

6. PATIENT RELATIONSHIP TO INSURED Self Spouse Child Other

7. INSURED'S ADDRESS (No., Street)

CITY STATE

8. PATIENT STATUS Single Married Other

CITY STATE

ZIP CODE TELEPHONE (Include Area Code) ( )

Employed Full-Time Student Part-Time Student

ZIP CODE TELEPHONE (Include Area Code) ( )

9. OTHER INSURED'S NAME (Last Name, First Name, Middle Initial)

10. IS PATIENT'S CONDITION RELATED TO:

11. INSURED'S POLICY GROUP OR FECA NUMBER

a. OTHER INSURED'S POLICY OR GROUP NUMBER

a. EMPLOYMENT? (Current or Previous) YES NO

a. INSURED'S DATE OF BIRTH MM DD YY SEX M F

b. OTHER INSURED'S DATE OF BIRTH MM DD YY SEX M F

b. AUTO ACCIDENT? PLACE (State) YES NO

b. EMPLOYER'S NAME OR SCHOOL NAME

c. EMPLOYER'S NAME OR SCHOOL NAME

c. OTHER ACCIDENT? YES NO

c. INSURANCE PLAN NAME OR PROGRAM NAME

d. INSURANCE PLAN NAME OR PROGRAM NAME

10d. RESERVED FOR LOCAL USE

d. IS THERE ANOTHER HEALTH BENEFIT PLAN? YES NO *If yes*, return to and complete item 9 a-d.

READ BACK OF FORM BEFORE COMPLETING & SIGNING THIS FORM.

12. PATIENT'S OR AUTHORIZED PERSON'S SIGNATURE I authorize the release of any medical or other information necessary to process this claim. I also request payment of government benefits either to myself or to the party who accepts assignment below.

SIGNED DATE

13. INSURED'S OR AUTHORIZED PERSON'S SIGNATURE I authorize payment of medical benefits to the undersigned physician or supplier for services described below.

SIGNED

PATIENT AND INSURED INFORMATION

14. DATE OF CURRENT: MM DD YY ILLNESS (First symptom) OR INJURY (Accident) OR PREGNANCY(LMP)

15. IF PATIENT HAS HAD SAME OR SIMILAR ILLNESS. GIVE FIRST DATE MM DD YY

16. DATES PATIENT UNABLE TO WORK IN CURRENT OCCUPATION FROM MM DD YY TO MM DD YY

17. NAME OF REFERRING PROVIDER OR OTHER SOURCE 17a. 17b. NPI

18. HOSPITALIZATION DATES RELATED TO CURRENT SERVICES FROM MM DD YY TO MM DD YY

19. RESERVED FOR LOCAL USE

20. OUTSIDE LAB? YES NO $ CHARGES

21. DIAGNOSIS OR NATURE OF ILLNESS OR INJURY (Relate Items 1, 2, 3 or 4 to Item 24E by Line)

1. ___ . ___ 3. ___ . ___

2. ___ . ___ 4. ___ . ___

22. MEDICAID RESUBMISSION CODE ORIGINAL REF. NO.

23. PRIOR AUTHORIZATION NUMBER

24. A. DATE(S) OF SERVICE From MM DD YY To MM DD YY	B. PLACE OF SERVICE	C. EMG	D. PROCEDURES, SERVICES, OR SUPPLIES (Explain Unusual Circumstances) CPT/HCPCS MODIFIER	E. DIAGNOSIS POINTER	F. $ CHARGES	G. DAYS OR UNITS	H. EPSDT Family Plan	I. ID. QUAL.	J. RENDERING PROVIDER ID. #
1								NPI	
2								NPI	
3								NPI	
4								NPI	
5								NPI	
6								NPI	

25. FEDERAL TAX I.D. NUMBER SSN EIN

26. PATIENT'S ACCOUNT NO.

27. ACCEPT ASSIGNMENT? (For govt. claims, see back) YES NO

28. TOTAL CHARGE $

29. AMOUNT PAID $

30. BALANCE DUE $

31. SIGNATURE OF PHYSICIAN OR SUPPLIER INCLUDING DEGREES OR CREDENTIALS (I certify that the statements on the reverse apply to this bill and are made a part thereof.)

SIGNED DATE

32. SERVICE FACILITY LOCATION INFORMATION a. NPI b.

33. BILLING PROVIDER INFO & PH # ( ) a. NPI b.

PHYSICIAN OR SUPPLIER INFORMATION

NUCC Instruction Manual available at: www.nucc.org

APPROVED OMB-0938-0999 FORM CMS-1500 (08-05)

Figure 5-6 CMS-1500 is the universally accepted claim form utilized for submission of charges for physician and outpatient services.

Inpatient

Inpatient charges are submitted on a UB-04. It is important to remember that if the patient is seen in the Emergency Department and later admitted to the hospital as an inpatient, the Emergency Department charges will be included on the UB-04 for the inpatient claim.

Non-patient

Non-patient services are those required by a laboratory when a specimen is received and processed when the patient is not present. Non-patient services are generally submitted on a UB-04.

Some payers define claim form requirements based on the part of the plan that covers specific services. For example, the UB-04 is used to submit charges covered under Medicare Part A. The CMS-1500 is used to submit charges covered under Medicare Part B. Durable medical equipment is covered under Medicare Part B; therefore, charges for these items are submitted on the CMS-1500.

Payer guidelines also dictate required methods of submission and claim completion requirements. Claims can be submitted manually by sending a paper claim or via electronic data interchange (EDI). Claim form elements will be discussed later in this chapter. The purpose of this section is to show the relationship between payer guidelines and the billing process.

Clean Claim

The hospital's major goal when submitting claims to third-party payers is to submit a clean claim the first time. A **clean claim** is one that does not need to be

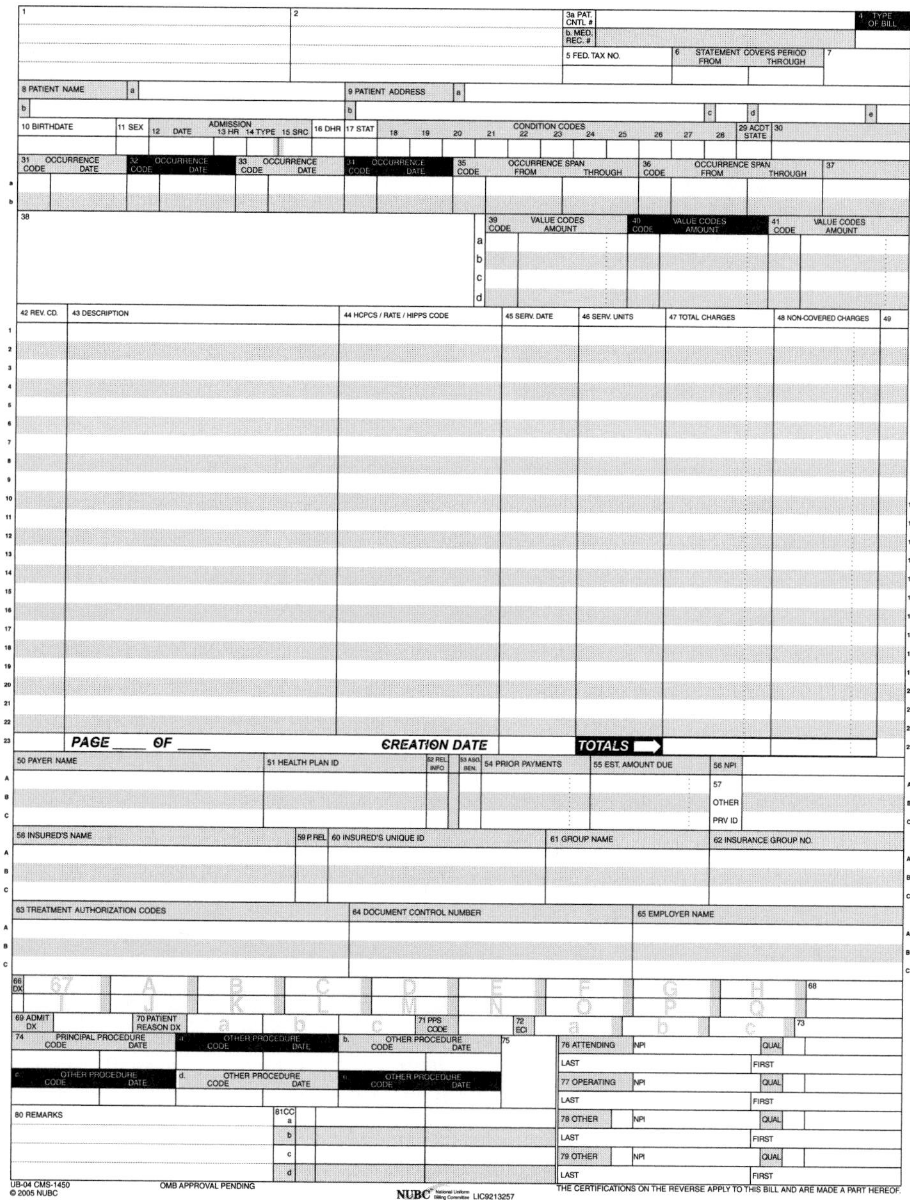

1 2 3a PAT. CNTL # b. MED. REC. # 4 TYPE OF BILL
5 FED. TAX NO. 6 STATEMENT COVERS PERIOD FROM THROUGH 7
8 PATIENT NAME a b 9 PATIENT ADDRESS a b c d e
10 BIRTHDATE 11 SEX ADMISSION 12 DATE 13 HR 14 TYPE 15 SRC 16 DHR 17 STAT CONDITION CODES 18 19 20 21 22 23 24 25 26 27 28 29 ACDT STATE 30
31 OCCURRENCE CODE DATE 32 OCCURRENCE CODE DATE 33 OCCURRENCE CODE DATE 34 OCCURRENCE CODE DATE 35 OCCURRENCE SPAN CODE FROM THROUGH 36 OCCURRENCE SPAN CODE FROM THROUGH 37
38 39 VALUE CODES CODE AMOUNT 40 VALUE CODES CODE AMOUNT 41 VALUE CODES CODE AMOUNT a b c d
42 REV. CD. 43 DESCRIPTION 44 HCPCS / RATE / HIPPS CODE 45 SERV. DATE 46 SERV. UNITS 47 TOTAL CHARGES 48 NON-COVERED CHARGES 49
PAGE ___ OF ___ CREATION DATE TOTALS
50 PAYER NAME 51 HEALTH PLAN ID 52 REL. INFO 53 ASG. BEN. 54 PRIOR PAYMENTS 55 EST. AMOUNT DUE 56 NPI 57 OTHER PRV ID
58 INSURED'S NAME 59 P. REL 60 INSURED'S UNIQUE ID 61 GROUP NAME 62 INSURANCE GROUP NO.
63 TREATMENT AUTHORIZATION CODES 64 DOCUMENT CONTROL NUMBER 65 EMPLOYER NAME
66 DX 67 A B C D E F G H I J K L M N O P Q 68
69 ADMIT DX 70 PATIENT REASON DX a b c 71 PPS CODE 72 ECI a b c 73
74 PRINCIPAL PROCEDURE CODE DATE a. OTHER PROCEDURE CODE DATE b. OTHER PROCEDURE CODE DATE 75 76 ATTENDING NPI QUAL LAST FIRST
c. OTHER PROCEDURE CODE DATE d. OTHER PROCEDURE CODE DATE e. OTHER PROCEDURE CODE DATE 77 OPERATING NPI QUAL LAST FIRST
80 REMARKS 81CC a b c d 78 OTHER NPI QUAL LAST FIRST 79 OTHER NPI QUAL LAST FIRST
UB-04 CMS-1450 © 2005 NUBC OMB APPROVAL PENDING NUBC National Uniform Billing Committee LIC9213257 THE CERTIFICATIONS ON THE REVERSE APPLY TO THIS BILL AND ARE MADE A PART HEREOF.

Figure 5-7 UB-04 is the universally accepted claim form utilized for submission of facility charges.

investigated by the payer. A clean claim passes all internal billing edits and payer-specific edits, and is paid without need for additional intervention.

Examples of claims that do not meet the clean claim status include:

- Claims that need additional information
- Claims that need Medicare secondary payer (MSP) screening information
- Claims that need information to determine coverage
- Claims that do not pass payer edits

Hospital billing and coding professionals carefully review claim information to ensure submission of a clean claim. It is necessary for hospital billing and coding professionals to have an understanding of payer guidelines in order to ensure compliance and prevent delay in payments. Payer guidelines outline the reimbursement method utilized to determine payment for services.

> **BOX 5-4 ■ KEY POINTS**
>
> **Clean Claim**
>
> A claim that does not need to be investigated by the payer. A clean claim passes all internal billing edits and payer-specific edits and is paid without need for additional intervention.

Reimbursement Methods

Reimbursement is the term used to describe the amount paid to the hospital by patients and third-party payers

TABLE 5-1 Claim Form Variations

Hospital Service Categories of "Facility Charges"	CMS-1500	CMS-1450 UB-04	Variations
Outpatient			
Ambulatory surgery—performed in a hospital outpatient surgery department		X	Some payers require ambulatory surgery charges to be submitted on the CMS-1500
Ambulatory surgery—performed in a certified Ambulatory Surgery Center (ASC)	X		
Emergency Department		X	Some payers require outpatient department charges to be submitted on the CMS-1500
Ancillary departments: Radiology; Laboratory; Physical, Occupational and Speech Therapy		X	Some payers require outpatient department charges to be submitted on the CMS-1500
Other Outpatient Services: Infusion Therapy and Observation		X	Some payers require outpatient department charges to be submitted on the CMS-1500.
Hospital-based Primary Care Office	X		Physician services may be included if employed by the hospital
Other hospital-based clinic	X		
Inpatient			
All services and items provided by the hospital during the inpatient stay		X	**Emergency Department charges are included on the inpatient claim when the patient is admitted from the ER
Non-patient		X	
A specimen received and processed; the patient is not present		X	Some payers require outpatient department charges to be submitted on the CMS-1500

CMS-1450 (UB-04) is utilized to submit charges to Medicare Part A.
CMS-1500 is utilized to submit charges to Medicare Part B.

for services rendered. The purpose of the billing process is to obtain the appropriate reimbursement within a reasonable period after the services are rendered. Most reimbursement for hospital services is received from third-party payers. Payers utilize various reimbursement methods to determine the payment amount for a service or item. Reimbursement methods can be categorized as traditional methods, fixed payment methods, and Prospective Payment Systems (PPS). Table 5-2 provides definitions for the various payment methods.

Traditional Payment Methods

Historically, payments for health care services were primarily based on charges submitted. Insurance companies and government programs processed payments for services utilizing four reimbursement methods—fee-for-service, fee schedule, percentage of accrued charges, and usual, customary, and reasonable.

Fee-for-Service (FFS)

Fee-for-service is a reimbursement method that provides payment for hospital services based on an established fee schedule for each service.

Fee Schedule

Fee schedule is a listing of established, allowed amounts for specific medical services and procedures.

Percentage of Accrued Charges

Percentage of accrued charges is a reimbursement method that calculates payment for charges accrued during a hospital stay based on a percentage of accrued charges.

Usual, Customary, and Reasonable (UCR)

Reimbursement is based on a review of the usual and customary fee to determine the fee that is considered reasonable.

1. Usual fee—the fee usually submitted by the provider for a service or item
2. Customary fee—the fee that providers of the same specialty in the same geographic area charge for a service or item
3. Reasonable fee—the fee that is considered reasonable

Figure 5-8 illustrates examples of payment calculations utilizing traditional payment methods—fee-for-service, percentage of accrued charges, fee schedule, and UCR.

BOX 5-5 ■ KEY POINTS

Traditional Payment Methods

Fee-for-service
Fee schedule
Percentage of accrued charges
Usual, customary, and reasonable (UCR)

Fixed Payment Methods

Efforts to control the rising costs of health care changed reimbursement methods to systems involving predetermined amounts paid to hospitals. The advent of managed care also brought with it fixed payment methods. The following are reimbursement methods in which the payment is a fixed amount: capitation, case

TABLE 5-2 Reimbursement Methods Defined

Traditional	
Fee-for-service	A reimbursement method where hospitals are paid for each service provided, based on an established fee schedule.
Fee schedule	A listing of established allowed amounts for specific medical services and procedures.
Percentage of accrued charges	A reimbursement method that calculates payment for charges accrued during a hospital stay. Payment is based on a percentage of approved charges.
Usual, Customary, and Reasonable (UCR)	Reimbursement is based on review of 3 fees: (1) usual fee, the fee usually submitted by the provider a service or item; (2) customary fee, fees that providers of the same specialty in the same geographic area charge for a service or item; (3) reasonable fee, the fee that is considered reasonable.
Fixed Payment	
Capitation	Reimbursement method where payment is a fixed amount paid per member per month. Capitation methods are generally utilized to provide reimbursement for primary care physician services and other specified outpatient services provided to managed care plan members.
Case rate	A set rate is paid to the hospital for the case. The payment rate is based on the type of case and resources utilized to treat the patient.
Contract rate	Reimbursement to the hospital is a set rate as agreed to in the contract between the hospital and the payer.
Flat rate	Reimbursement is a set rate for a hospital admission regardless of charges accrued.
Per diem	The hospital is paid a set rate per day rather than payment based on total accrued charges.
Relative value scale (RVS)	A relative value that represents work, practice expense, and cost malpractice insurance assigned to professional services.
Prospective Payment System (PPS)	
Ambulatory payment classification (APC)	An Outpatient Prospective Payment System (OPPS) that is utilized by Medicare and other government programs to provide reimbursement for hospital outpatient services including ambulatory surgery performed in a hospital outpatient department. The hospital is paid a fixed fee based on the procedure(s) performed.
Medicare Severity Diagnosis Related Groups (MS-DRG)	An Inpatient Prospective Payment System (IPPS) that is utilized by Medicare and other government programs to provide reimbursement for hospital inpatient services. The hospital is paid a fixed fee based on the severity of the patient's condition and relative treatment.
Resource-based relative value scale (RBRVS)	A reimbursement method implemented under PPS for Medicare and other government programs to provide reimbursement for physician and outpatient services. A unit value is assigned to each procedure. The unit value represents physician time, skill, practice overhead, and malpractice.

Fee-for-Service

	Charges Submitted	Established Fee (Reimbursement)
Level IV ER Visit	$575.00	$475.00
Chest X-Ray	$135.00	$110.00
CBC	$95.00	$95.00

Payer determines payment for each charge

Fee Schedule

	Charges Submitted	Allowed Amount (Reimbursement)
Level IV ER Visit	$575.00	$500.00
Chest X-Ray	$135.00	$120.00
CBC	$95.00	$65.00

Payer determines payment for services based on a fee schedule

Percentage of Accrued Charges

Accrued Charges Submitted		Approved/ Eligible Amount	Payment 80%
Level IV ER Visit	$575.00	$475.00	$380.00
Chest X-Ray	$135.00	$110.00	$88.00
CBC	$95.00	$95.00	$76.00

Payer determines payment based on a percentage of approved amounts for charges accrued

Usual, Customary, and Reasonable (UCR)

Charges Submitted		Usual	Customary
MRI	$575.00	$475.00	$380.00
	Payment Amount (Reasonable Fee)		$380.00

Payer formula for reasonable amount varies (in this case the reasonable amount is the lower of the amount charged, the usual and customary charge)

Figure 5-8 Examples of traditional payment methods.

rate, contract rate, flat rate, per diem, and relative value scale.

Capitation

Capitation is a reimbursement method utilized that provides payment of a fixed amount, paid per member per month. Capitation methods are generally utilized to provide reimbursement for primary care physician services and other specified outpatient services provided to managed care plan members.

Case Rate

Case rate reimbursement is a set rate paid to the hospital for the case. The payment rate is based on the type of case and resources utilized for the case.

Contract Rate

Contract rate reimbursement is a set rate as agreed to in a contract between the hospital and the payer.

Flat Rate

Flat rate reimbursement is a set rate for the hospital admission regardless of charges accrued.

Per Diem

Per diem reimbursement is a set rate per day rather than payment based on the total of accrued charges.

Relative Value Scale (RVS)

RVS is a relative value that represents work, practice expense, and the cost of malpractice insurance that is assigned to professional services.

Figure 5-9 illustrates examples of some of the most common fixed payment methods utilized to reimburse hospitals for services (case rate, contract rate, flat rate, and per diem).

BOX 5-6 ■ KEY POINTS

Fixed Payment Methods

Capitation
Case rate
Contract rate
Flat rate
Per diem
Relative value scale (RVS)

The government became one of the largest payers of health care services with the establishment of the Medicare and Medicaid programs in 1965. Over the following 30 years, due to the continued growth in the aged population and the rising cost of health care, the government found it necessary to devise reimbursement methods that provided fixed payment amounts for health care services. **Prospective Payment Systems (PPS)** were implemented to provide reimbursement for inpatient, outpatient, and professional services provided to members of government health care programs. A PPS is a method of determining reimbursement to health care providers based on predetermined factors, not on individual services. Today, members of government sponsored plans who are provided with hospital services are paid based on different Prospective Payment Systems.

BOX 5-7 ■ KEY POINTS

Prospective Payment Systems (PPS)

Medicare Severity Diagnosis Related Groups (MS-DRG)
Resource-based relative value scale (RBRVS)
Ambulatory payment classification (APC)

BOX 5-8 ■ KEY POINTS

Inpatient Prospective Payment System (IPPS)

Implemented in 1983 to provide reimbursement for hospital inpatient services

- Diagnosis Related Group (DRG), now MS-DRG

Other Prospective Payment Systems

Implemented over a 5-year period beginning January 1992 to provide reimbursement for physician and outpatient services

- Resource-based relative value scale (RBRVS)

Outpatient Prospective Payment System (OPPS)

Implemented in 2000 to provide reimbursement for hospital outpatient services

- Ambulatory payment classification (APC)

Case Rate			Contract Rate		
Charges Submitted		Case Rate (Reimbursement)	Charges Submitted		Contract Rate (Reimbursement)
Arthroscopic Surgery	$3,913.23	$2,500.00	Hospital Inpatient Stay 3 days Peripheral Vascular Shunt	$27,780.19	$23,613.16
Payer reimbursement based on a rate for the arthroscopy case			**Payer determines payment for services based on a fee schedule**		
Flat Rate			**Per Diem**		
Charges Submitted		Flat Rate (Reimbursement)	Charges Submitted		Per Diem Rate $5,450 per day (Reimbursement)
Hospital Inpatient Inpatient Days 9 Respiratory Failure Obstructive Chronic Bronchitis	$22,548.11	$19,750.00	Hospital Inpatient Stay 3 days Peripheral Vascular Shunt	$27,780.19	$16,350.00
Payer determines payment based on flat rate			**Payer determines payment based on a per diem rate of $5,450.00 per day**		

Figure 5-9 Examples of fixed payment methods.

Prospective Payment Systems (PPS)

The Inpatient Prospective Payment System (IPPS) was established as mandated by the Tax Equity and Fiscal Responsibility Act (TEFRA) in 1983 to provide reimbursement for acute hospital inpatient services. The system implemented under IPPS is known as Diagnosis Related Groups (DRG). The DRG reimbursement method was replaced with Medicare Severity Diagnosis Related Groups (MS-DRG) effective 10/1/07.

Medicare Severity Diagnosis Related Groups (MS-DRG)

MS-DRG is the IPPS payment system utilized by Medicare and other government programs to provide reimbursement for hospital inpatient services. Under the MS-DRG system, the hospital is paid a fixed fee based on the severity of the patient's condition and relative treatment. MS-DRG assignment is determined based on the principal diagnosis, secondary diagnosis, significant procedures, complications and co-morbidities, age and sex of the patient, and discharge status of the patient.

Resource-Based Relative Value Scale (RBRVS)

Resource-based relative value scales (RBRVS) were implemented over a 5-year period beginning January 1992 to provide reimbursement for services provided by physicians.

RBRVS is a payment method utilized by Medicare and other government programs to provide reimbursement for physician and some outpatient services. The RBRVS system consists of a fee schedule of approved amounts calculated based on relative values. A relative value unit (RVU) is assigned to each procedure. The RVU represents physician time and skill, practice overhead, and malpractice insurance. The RVU is used in a formula that multiplies the RVU by a geographic adjustment factor (GAF) and a monetary conversion factor (CF).

CMS implemented the Outpatient Prospective Payment System (OPPS), effective August 2000. The OPPS provides reimbursement for hospital outpatient services. The system implemented under OPPS is known as Ambulatory Payment Classification (APC).

Ambulatory Payment Classification (APC)

APC is the OPPS utilized by Medicare and other government programs to provide reimbursement for hospital outpatient services. Under the APC system, the hospital is paid a fixed fee based on the procedure(s) performed. Services reimbursed under APC include ambulatory surgical procedures, chemotherapy, clinic visits, diagnostic services and tests, Emergency Department visits, implants, and other outpatient services.

PPS methods were implemented to provide preestablished payment amounts for reimbursement to providers for services rendered to members of government health care programs. Figure 5-10 illustrates payment determination utilizing the MS-DRG and APC reimbursement systems. PPSs will be discussed further in Chapter 13.

As discussed previously, hospitals provide various services including outpatient, inpatient, non-patient, and professional services, as illustrated in Figure 5-11. Reimbursement methods vary based on many factors, such as payer category and the type of services provided. Hospital billing professionals strive to achieve an understanding of the various reimbursement methods utilized to ensure that appropriate payment is provided for services rendered. It is also important to understand guidelines relating to each of the different payment methods. Three major categories of third-party payers are government programs, commercial payers, and

<table>
<tr><th colspan="3">Ambulatory Payment Classification (APC)</th><th colspan="2">Medicare Severity Diagnosis Related Group (MS-DRG)</th></tr>
<tr><td>Procedures Reported</td><td>APC Group</td><td>Payment Rate</td><td colspan="2">Inpatient admission
Principal diagnosis Skull Fracture
Secondary diagnosis None
Principal procedure Craniotomy
Age 18
Gender Male
Length of stay 3 days
Charges submitted $9,684.32</td></tr>
<tr><td>#1 Cystourethroscopy</td><td>0160</td><td>$375.39</td><td>MS-DRG</td><td>Payment Rate</td></tr>
<tr><td>#2 MRA, Neck with contrast</td><td>0284</td><td>$388.28</td><td>26</td><td>$6,782.45</td></tr>
<tr><td>#3 Emergency Department Visit Complex</td><td>0612</td><td>$226.30</td><td></td><td></td></tr>
<tr><td colspan="3">Payer determines reimbursement based on payment rate for APC Group assigned to each procedure</td><td colspan="2">Payer determines reimbursement based on the payment rate for MS-DRG Group assigned</td></tr>
</table>

Figure 5-10 Examples of APC and MS-DRG, both of which are PPS reimbursement methods.

Levels of Provision of Hospital Services

	Hospital Service Areas	Examples of Services
Outpatient	Pathology/Laboratory, Radiology, Physical Rehabilitation, Ambulatory Surgery Center, Observation, Emergency Department, Outpatient Clinic, or Primary Care Network	Complete blood count, X-ray, physical therapy, ambulatory surgery, wound repair, physician visit, or observation for a specific condition
Inpatient	Intensive Care, Critical Care, or Medical/Surgical Unit	Various diagnostic, therapeutic, and palliative services such as pathology/laboratory, X-ray, surgery and anesthesia; nursing services are provided on a 24-hour basis
Non-patient	*Pathology or Laboratory*	Specimen received, such as blood, stool, or an organ such as appendix

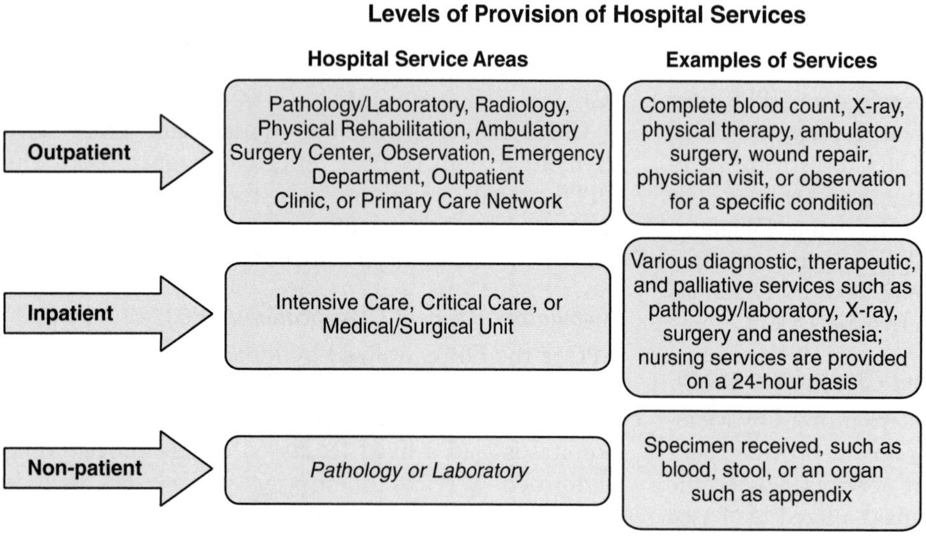

Figure 5-11 Hospital services are provided on an outpatient, inpatient, or non-patient basis. Note that professional services are not billed by the hospital unless the provider is employed by the hospital.

managed care plans. Each of the payer types listed utilizes various methods of reimbursement for outpatient, inpatient, non-patient, and professional services.

Reimbursement Methods by Service Category

Outpatient Services

Outpatient services are those that are performed on the same day the patient is released (sent home). Examples of outpatient services are ambulatory surgery and various diagnostic and therapeutic procedures performed by hospital departments such as Radiology and Laboratory.

Ambulatory Surgery

Ambulatory surgery services can be performed in a hospital outpatient surgery department or in a certified ambulatory surgery center (ASC). The surgery is performed and the patient is released the same day. Ambulatory surgery services are provided in accordance with the physician's orders. Charges related to the ambulatory surgery are submitted to the payers for reimbursement. Ambulatory surgery services are reimbursed utilizing various methods including APC, case rate, contract rate, fee-for-service, fee schedule, and percentage of accrued charges.

Inpatient Services

Inpatient services are provided when a patient is admitted to the hospital with the expectation that he or she will be in the hospital for more than 24 hours. Inpatient admissions and services required are provided in accordance with the admitting physician's orders. All charges incurred during the hospital stay are submitted to the payers for reimbursement. Inpatient

TABLE 5-3 Reimbursement Methods by Payer Category*

	SERVICE LEVEL AND REIMBURSEMENT METHODS		
Payer Category	**Hospital Outpatient Services**	**Hospital Inpatient Services**	**Hospital Professional and Non-Patient Services**
Government programs Medicare, TRICARE, Medicaid (implemented under Prospective Payment	Ambulatory payment classification (APC).	Medicare Severity Diagnosis Related Groups (MS-DRG).	Resource-based relative value scale (RBRVS).
PPS method basis	Hospital is reimbursed a set fee based on the APC payment rate for the procedure performed.	Hospital is reimbursed a set fee based on the MS-DRG payment rate for the patient's condition and related treatment.	A relative value is assigned to each CPT code, which represents physician time, skill, and overhead.
Commercial and other third-party payers	Case rate Contract rate	Case rate Contract rate	Fee-for-service Fee schedule
Blue Cross/Blue Shield, Aetna, Humana, Worker's compensation	Fee-for-service Fee schedule Percentage of accrued charges	Fee-for-service Flat rate Percentage of accrued charges Per diem	Relative value scale (RVU) Usual, customary, and reasonable (UCR)
Managed care plans	Case rate Contract rate	Case rate Contract rate	Capitation Contract Fee schedule

*Many commercial and managed care payers are adopting prospective payment–type reimbursement methods, such as APC and MS-DRG.

services are reimbursed utilizing various methods including MS-DRG, case rate, contract rate, fee-for-service, flat rate, percentage of accrued charges, or per diem.

Non-Patient Services

Non-patient services are provided when a specimen is received by the Laboratory or Pathology Department for processing. Specimens from within the hospital as well as provider offices are received for testing. A specimen may be blood or other body fluid, stool, or tissue. Non-patient services are reimbursed utilizing various methods including RBRVS, fee-for-service, fee schedule, relative value scale, UCR, capitation, or a contract rate.

Professional Services

Professional services are patient care services provided by physicians and other non-physician clinical providers such as a physician assistant. Evaluation and management, surgery, and the professional component of a radiology procedure are examples of professional services. Hospitals do not bill professional services unless the physician providing the service is employed by the hospital. Professional services are reimbursed utilizing various methods including RBRVS, fee-for-service, fee schedule, relative value scale, UCR, capitation, or a contract rate.

Some of the most common reimbursement methods utilized by government programs, commercial payers, and managed care plans are outlined in Table 5-3 for outpatient, inpatient, non-patient, and professional services. Reimbursement methods will be discussed further as they relate to each of the payer categories later in this text.

Reimbursement Methods by Payer Category

Government Programs

Medicare, TRICARE, Medicaid, and other government payers utilize reimbursement methods implemented under PPS: RBRVS, APC, and MS-DRG. The following is an outline of common reimbursement methods used by government payers for outpatient, inpatient, professional, and non-patient services.

Outpatient Services

The APC system provides payment for outpatient services performed in the hospital, such as ambulatory surgery performed in a hospital outpatient surgery department, X-rays, and laboratory procedures.

Inpatient Services

The MS-DRG system is utilized to reimburse hospitals for inpatient cases.

Professional and Non-Patient Services

RBRVS is a reimbursement method to pay for professional services performed by physicians and non-patient services.

Commercial Payers

Blue Cross/Blue Shield, Aetna, Metropolitan, Cigna, and other payers with whom the providers are not participating are considered commercial payers. Commercial payers utilize various reimbursement methods, including fee schedule, UCR, case rate, per diem, and contract rate. The following is an outline of common reimbursement methods used by commercial payers for outpatient, inpatient, professional, and non-patient services.

Outpatient Services

Outpatient services performed in a hospital are reimbursed utilizing one of the following reimbursement methods—case rate, contract rate, fee-for-service, fee schedule, or percentage of accrued charges.

Inpatient Services

All charges accrued during the inpatient hospital stay are submitted to payers, and reimbursement is determined utilizing various reimbursement methods such as case rate, contract rate, fee-for-service, flat rate, percentage of accrued charges, and per diem.

Professional and Non-Patient Services

Services performed by physicians, other health care professionals, and non-patient services are reimbursed using a fee-for-service, fee schedule, relative value scale, or UCR. Two of the most common are fee schedule and UCR.

Managed Care Plans

Government programs and many insurance carriers offer managed care plans. Managed care plans are designed to provide health care services efficiently through the application of utilization management techniques to monitor and control the utilization of health care services by their members. Utilization management techniques will be discussed in later chapters. Managed care plans utilize various reimbursement methods such as contract rate and capitation. The managed care contract between the payer and the provider will outline the method of payment utilized to determined reimbursement for services or items.

Outpatient Services

Services provided on an outpatient basis such as ambulatory surgery, X-rays, and laboratory services are also reimbursed utilizing case rate or contract rate methods to determine payment.

Inpatient Services

Inpatient services are often reimbursed utilizing case rate and contract rate reimbursement methods.

Professional and Non-Patient Services

Professional and non-patient services may be reimbursed by managed care plans utilizing a capitation, contract rate, or fee schedule method for reimbursement.

BOX 5-9 ■ KEY POINTS

Payer Types

Government Programs

Medicare, TRICARE, and Medicaid

Commercial Payers

BC/BS, Aetna, Cigna, and other insurance plans that do not have a contract with the provider

Managed Care Plans

Plans offered by various payers

CHARGE DESCRIPTION MASTER (CDM)

A critical component of the entire billing process in the hospital environment is the CDM. Hospitals provide a wide range of services and items to patients on an outpatient, inpatient, and non-patient basis in various areas of the hospital such as the Radiology or Laboratory Department or on the floor or unit. From the time a patient arrives at the hospital, a complex network of highly specialized personnel within the hospital becomes involved in the patient's stay in a clinical and/or administrative capacity.

As discussed in Chapter 4, the collection of information, assessment of the patient's condition, and provision of diagnostic and therapeutic services require a system designed to allow storage, maintenance, and access to the data. The data collected include services and items provided to the patient during the visit. The system must also accommodate an inventory of charges for procedures, services, items, and drugs provided during the patient's stay. Information regarding the patient's condition, diagnostic and therapeutic treatments, and responses are recorded in the patient record. Services and items are also recorded in the patient record.

The CDM, also known as the chargemaster, is the computerized system utilized by hospitals to inventory and record services and items provided in various locations in the hospital during a patient stay. The chargemaster is designed to capture charges for all services and items provided for the purpose of posting charges to the patient's account and billing those charges on the claim form. The chargemaster is usually automated and linked with the billing system. Items in the chargemaster are generally organized by department. Each item in the chargemaster is associated with the appropriate procedure code, revenue code, service or item description, charge, and other information required for the submission of the hospital's facility charges. To provide a better understanding of items in the chargemaster, we will first explore categories of service provided in the hospital.

Services and Items Billed by the Hospital

The hospital provides a variety of services and items during a patient's visit. It is critical for the hospital's financial stability to capture charges for services and items provided during the patient stay. An outline of hospital facility charges that are captured through the chargemaster is provided in Figure 5-12. It is important for hospital personnel to understand the difference between facility and professional charges.

Facility Charges

Hospitals submit facility charges for patient care services provided on an outpatient basis such as laboratory tests, X-rays, or ambulatory surgery. **Facility charges** represent cost and overhead for providing patient care services, which include space, equipment, supplies, drugs and biologicals, and technical staff. Facility charges represent the technical component of the services. They are captured through the chargemaster and submitted on the UB-04.

TEST YOUR *Knowledge* BOX 5-1

PURPOSE OF THE BILLING PROCESS

1. Provide a definition of the hospital billing process and explain the purpose of the process.
2. List the functions involved in the billing process.
3. Discuss the claims process and its relationship to the billing process.
4. Participating provider agreements outline the terms and specifications of participation for hospitals and payers. List four common provisions covered in these agreements that relate to the billing process.
5. Define medical necessity.
6. List three amounts that may represent the patient's responsibility.
7. What is the purpose of a claim form?
8. Identify two claim forms that are currently utilized by hospitals to submit charges to various payers.
9. Provide an explanation of what claim form is generally used to submit facility charges for services provided in the hospital.

TEST YOUR *Knowledge* BOX 5-1

PURPOSE OF THE BILLING PROCESS—*cont'd*

10. Outline four examples of claims that do not meet clean claim status.

11. Define reimbursement.

12. List four examples of traditional reimbursement methods.

13. Describe the percentage of accrued charges reimbursement method.

14. Explain the difference between traditional and fixed-payment methods.

15. Discuss what IPPS is, when it was implemented, and why.

16. State what OPPS is, when it was implemented, and why.

17. Explain the difference between the APC and MS-DRG reimbursement methods.

18. Provide a listing of the reimbursement methods utilized by government programs to pay hospitals for outpatient and inpatient services.

19. Identify six reimbursement methods commonly used by commercial payers for inpatient services.

20. Outline four reimbursement methods commonly utilized by managed care plans for outpatient and inpatient hospital services.

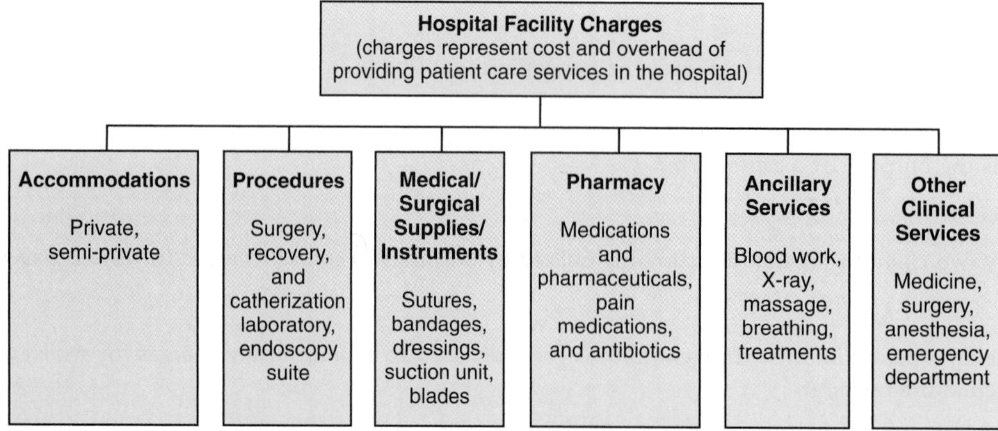

Figure 5-12 Categories of hospital facility charges.

Professional Charges

Professional charges represent the professional component of patient care services performed by physicians and other non-physician clinical providers. The professional component of surgery, anesthesia administration, interpretation of an X-ray, or office visit is billed by the physician. Professional services may be billed by the hospital if the physician is an employee or under contract with the hospital. Professional charges are submitted on the CMS-1500.

Hospital Categories of Services and Items

As discussed in the previous chapter, hospital services and items can be categorized as follows: accommodations; operating and recovery room; medical surgical supplies; pharmacy; ancillary services; and other clinical services. Charges for services and items provided are captured at various points in the patient care process, as outlined below (Table 5-4).

Accommodations (Room and Board)

An inpatient admission requires the assignment of a room/bed to accommodate the patient overnight. The admitting physician orders the patient admission and room assignment is performed in accordance with the physician's orders. Rooms are available on various units or wards in the hospital such as the medical, surgical, OB/GYN, oncology, intensive care, coronary care, or nursery unit. The patient is charged for the accommodations, commonly referred to as room and board. Hospital personnel take a census around 12:00 P.M. each evening to identify which patients occupy specific rooms and beds. Charges for room and board are posted to the patient's account daily.

Operating and Recovery Room

When a patient is scheduled for a surgical procedure, an operating and recovery room is assigned for use during the patient's surgery. The rooms are furnished with highly specialized equipment required for the surgery. Surgical services are performed in accordance with the physician's orders. Specially trained nursing personnel are available to perform required functions related to the surgery and recovery of the patient. Charges are captured for operating and recovery room services based on the amount of time the patient occupied the room. Various forms are utilized by hospitals to capture these charges such as the operating room records, illustrated in Figure 5-13. Charges are posted to the patient's account after the procedure is performed.

Medical/Surgical Supplies

The Central Supply Department or other similar department posts charges for medical and surgical supplies

TABLE 5-4 Hospital Service Categories

Service Category	Description
Accommodations (room and board)	Inpatient admission—Room/bed assigned to the patient on admission. Rooms may be private or semi-private (more than one bed). Rooms are assigned on various units or wards: medical, surgical, OB/GYN, oncology, psychiatric, intensive care, coronary care, or nursery. **Nursing services are included in overhead charges.**
Operating room (OR) suite, operating room, recovery room	Patients requiring surgery are placed in an OR suite before surgery. Surgery is performed in the operating room. The patient is generally moved to the recovery room after surgery. Some procedures are performed in other areas such as the catheterization laboratory or the endoscopy suite.
Medical surgical supplies	Materials, supplies, and instruments supplied by various departments such as Central Supply. Items include bandages, splints, instruments, and bed pans.
Pharmacy	Medications ordered by the physician are supplied by the Pharmacy Department.
Ancillary services	Diagnostic and therapeutic services ordered by the physician are provided by various clinical departments such as Pathology/Laboratory,
Other clinical services	Various medical departments coordinate and provide services required as outlined in the physician's orders such as Surgery, Medicine, Anesthesia, Pulmonology, and Cardiology.

OPERATING ROOM NURSES NOTES

967 801
CHAIR MORRIS
DR C SCOFE
M 68 SURG INS

Date: 11/06/XX (Mo. Day Yr.)

Operating Room # 4

Anesthesia Method: ☒ General ☐ Caudal ☐ Local Infiltrate ☐ Regional Blk. ☐ Spinal ☐ Epidural

Begin Anesthesia 0740
Begin Surgery 0810
End Surgery 0910
Leave Room 0925

Administered By: Gerald Sleep, M.D.

Surgeon: Robert Cutt, M.D. Assistant: Rufus Strung, M.D.

Perfusionist: ____ Observers: ____

Scrub Nurse: L. Smythe O.R.T. Circulating Nurse: P. Bridge, RN

Relief: ____ @ ____ Relief: ____ @ ____

Pre-Operative Diagnosis: Left Rotator Cuff Tendonitis

Post-Operative Diagnosis: Same

Operation: Exploratory arthrotomy left shoulder, Bristow procedure

Radiopaque Sponges 4x4	Laparotomy Sponges	No Sponge Count Taken ☐	
	5 5	Sponge Count Correct (Yes / No)	
		Before Incision Made	☑ ☐
		Cavity Closure	☐ ☐
		Skin Closure	☑ ☐
Rondic	Laminectomy	Cottoniods	Wound Classificaiton A ☑ B ☐ C ☐ D ☐ E ☐
Dissect.			

Tissue: ____ To Path Lab By: ____
Culture: ____ To Bacteriology By: ____
Implants: Manufacturer: Zimmer Serial # ____ Size: 1 inch
Type: Bone screw

Date	Time	Comments/Complications
		T+C 3PC.
		Adhesive for closure caused skin reaction near incision

RN Signature: Phoebe Bridge, RN

A OPERATING ROOM NURSE'S NOTES

Figure 5-13 Sample operating room record used to capture OR charges. *(From Brooks ML, Gillingham ET:* Health unit coordinating, *ed 5, St Louis, 2004, Saunders.)*

RADIOLOGY REQUISITION

PATIENT NAME:	ORDERING PHYSICIAN:
DOB:	ACCOUNT #
PHYSICIAN SIGNATURE:	DATE:
INDICATIONS:	

PLEASE FAX SCRIPT PRIOR TO PATIENTS SCEHDUELD APPOINTMENT

PLEASE CHECK

GENERAL X-RAY
☐ 74415 IVP D
☐ 74000 KUB
☐ 74020 Abdominal Series (2V)
☐ 74022 Acute Abdominal Series (3V)
☐ 73610 Ankle L/R
☐ 72050 C-Spine (min 4V)
☐ 72040 C-Spine (max 3V)
☑ ____ Chest (2V)
☐ 73080 Elbow L/R
☐ 73550 Femur L/R
☐ 73630 Foot L/R
☐ 73090 Forearm L/R
☐ 73130 Hand L/R
☐ 73500 Hip L/R
☐ 73060 Humerus L/R
☐ 73564 Knee L/R
☐ 72110 L Spine (min. 4V)
☐ 72170 Pelvis
☐ 71100 Ribs - Unilat L/R
☐ 71110 Ribs-Bilat
☐ Other____

MRI
☐ 74181 Abd wo/contrast
☐ 74182 Abd w/contrast
☐ 74183 Abd w/wo contrast
☐ 70551 Brain wo/contrast
☐ 70552 Brain w/contrast
☐ 70553 Brain w/wo contrast
☐ 72141 C-Spine w/o contrast
☐ 72156 C-Spine w/wo contrast
☐ 71550 Chest wo/contrast
☐ 71551 Chest w/contrast
☐ 71552 Chest w/wo contrast
☐ 73721 Lower Extremity (jt.) R/L
☐ 73718 Lower Extremity (no jt.) R/L
☐ 72148 L-Spine wo/contrast
☐ 72158 L-Spine w/wo contrast

MRA ☐ MRV ☐
☐ 74185 Abd w/wo contrast
☐ 71555 Chest w/wo contrast (Exc Myocardium)
☐ 70544 Head wo/contrast
☐ 70546 Head w/wo contrast
☐ 70545 Head w/contrast
☐ 73725 Lower Ext. w/wo contrast
☐ 70547 Neck wo/contrast
☐ 70548 Neck w/contrast
☐ 70549 Neck w/wo contrast
☐ 73225 Upr. Ext. w/wo contrast
☐ Other____

CT SCAN
☐ ____ Abd wo/contrast
☑ ____ Abd w/wo contrast
☐ 70450 Brain wo/contrast
☐ 70470 Brain w/wo contrast
☐ 72125 C-Spine wo/contrast
☐ 71250 Chest wo/contrast
☐ 71260 Chest w/contrast
☐ 71270 Chest w/wo contrast
☐ 70482 IAC's, Orbits, Pituitary w/wo cont. ☐ 72131 L-Spine wo/contrast
☐ 70486 Maxiofacial (Sinus) wo/contrast
☐ 72192 Pelvis wo/contrast
☐ 72193 Pelvis w/contrast
☐ 72194 Pelvis w/wo contrast
☐ 70491 Soft Tissue Neck w/contrast
☐ 72128 T-Spine wo/contrast
☐ 74150/72192 Urogram

ULTRASOUND
☐ 76700 Abd Total
☐ 76705 Abd, Single Organ/Quadrant
☐ 93925 Arterial Lower Ext.-Bilat.
☐ 93926 Arterial Lower Ext.-Unilat. L/R
☐ 93930 Arterial Upper Ext. - Bilat.
☐ 93931 Arterial Upper Ext. - Unilat. L/R
☐ 76645 Breast L/R
☐ 93880 Carotid
☐ 76880 Extremity, Non Vascular L/R
☐ 76801 OB - 1st Trimester
☐ Other____

MAMMOGRAPHY
☐ 76092 Screening mammography
☐ 76091 Diagnostic mammography - Bilat
☐ 76090 Diagnostic mammography - Unil L/R

DEXA SCAN
☐ 76075 Bone Density, DEXA

ECHOCARDIOGRAM
☐ 93307/93320/93325 Echo, Dop. Echo w/pulsect wave and color flow

PET SCAN
Specify Area____

STRESS TEST
☐ 78465 Dual Isotope Nuclear Stress Test
____ Adenosine/Dubutamine

☐ CORRELATION or ☐ COMPARISON:
Please compare with exam done on
____ ____ ____

Figure 5-14 Sample Radiology Department requisition used to indicate patient care services required. *(From Ingenix:* Ingenix coding lab: facilities and ancillary services 2004, *Eden Prairie, Minn., 2004, Ingenix.)*

required during the hospital stay. Medical and surgical supplies and instruments are provided in accordance with providing patient care services as outlined in the physician's orders. Supplies and items are issued to the respective patient care area. Departmental personnel post charges for the items through the chargemaster.

Pharmacy

Drugs and biologicals required during the hospital stay are issued by the Pharmacy Department in accordance with providing patient care services as outlined in the physician's orders. Drugs and biologicals are issued to the appropriate patient care area. Departmental personnel post charges for pharmacy items through the chargemaster.

Ancillary Services

Various ancillary services are provided to patients during the hospital stay. Hospital departments such as Radiology, Pathology/Laboratory, and Physical Rehabilitation provide services in accordance with the physician's orders or a requisition. As discussed in the previous chapter, the physician's orders are entered into the hospital's information systems and distributed to various departments. Outpatient services are provided in accordance with the physician's orders or a requisition. A sample radiology requisition is illustrated in Figure 5-14. Charges for ancillary services are posted through the chargemaster by the department performing the services.

Other Clinical Services

Services provided by various clinical departments within the hospital such as the Emergency Department are provided in accordance with the ER physician's orders. Department personnel post charges through the chargemaster. Emergency Department charges do not represent the professional services performed by the Emergency Department physician. The ER physician will submit charges for his or her professional services separately.

Hospital-Based Clinic or Primary Care Office

Many hospitals provide patient care services in a clinic or primary care office. Physician services provided in the clinic or primary care office are recorded on the encounter form. Charges are posted to the patient's account for each visit. The hospital submits professional charges for these services when the physician is employed by or is under contract with the hospital. Professional charges are submitted on the CMS-1500, as discussed previously.

Services and items provided by a hospital are determined by the hospital's specialization and case mix. **Case mix** is a term used to describe the type of patient cases treated by the hospital. For example, a trauma center will treat different types of patient cases than those treated by a burn center. Chargemasters vary by hospital as a result of the variation in the type of cases seen by the hospital. Because of the wide variety of services and items provided by the hospital, a chargemaster will typically have thousands of entries.

Content of the Charge Description Master (CDM)

Services, procedures, and items provided by the hospital are listed in the chargemaster with various data elements required for charging patient accounts and billing services and items on the claim form. Chargemaster data elements vary by hospital; however, basic information will include the chargemaster number, department number, item and service description, HCPCS and modifier, general ledger codes, quantity or dose and the charge as outlined in Figure 5-15.

Chargemaster Number

The chargemaster number is an internal control number assigned to each service or item provided by the hospital. This number may be referred to by other names, such as charge description number, internal control number, or service code number. Many hospitals also include a general ledger number for accounting purposes.

Community General Hospital

Charge Description Master (CDM)

Chargemaster Number/ Department #/ General Ledger #	Item/Service Description	Procedure/ Item Code HCPCS/ NDC and Modifier	Revenue Code	Quantity/ Dose	Charge
100/977	Room C532		0110	1	1042
200/164	Cefepime inj 2 G	J0692	0250	2 g	133
300/116	Tray hyperal dre	A4550	0270	1	33
300/169	ABD/KUB flatplat	74470	0320	1	148
400/137	Oximeter	S8105	0410	1	49
700/138	Prothrombin time	85210	0300	1	57
700/138	CBC with diff	85025	0300	1	68
700/139	Blood culture	87040	0300	1	121
700/140	Basic metabolic	80048	0300	1	53
700/167	Dopp-venous lowe	93303	0400	1	583
700/169	X-ray chest	71020	0320	1	185
700/169	X-ray chest fluoroscopy	71090	0320	1	185

Figure 5-15 Sample hospital Charge Description Master (CDM) illustrating common data elements of a CDM.

Department Number

Each service and item in the chargemaster is assigned a number representing the department that provides the service or item. Many departments further categorize services. For example, the Radiology Department may be department number 700. Within the Radiology Department, nuclear medicine and radiation oncology services may be assigned numbers such as 710 and 720. Department numbers are utilized to track procedures and items provided by that department.

Item or Service Description

All services and items are given a written statement that describes the service or item within the chargemaster. Descriptions vary by hospital. Some hospitals assign a clinical description, and others may utilize a billing description. The billing description appears on the detailed itemized statement. Many hospitals use the HCPCS or NDC code descriptions.

Procedure or Item Code

Each item in the chargemaster is assigned the appropriate code from the HCPCS coding system or a National Drug Code (NDC). The appropriate HCPCS Level I CPT or HCPCS Level II Medicare National Code is assigned according to payer specifications. Modifiers are also recorded in the chargemaster where appropriate. The NDC may be assigned to various drugs provided by the hospital in accordance with payer specifications.

Revenue Code

A **revenue code** is a four-digit number assigned to each service or item provided by the hospital that designates the type of service or where the service was performed. For example, general pharmacy charges are assigned revenue code number 0250, and ER services are assigned revenue code number 0450. Figure 5-16 provides a listing of some of the most common general revenue codes.

The National Uniform Billing Committee (NUBC) defines revenue code categories, and they are required for completion of the UB-04. Information regarding revenue codes can be obtained from many sources such as the CMS Web site at www.cms.gov or the NUBC Web site at www.nubc.org.

Quantity or Dose

A quantity, unit, or dose is assigned to each service or item in the chargemaster. HCPCS Level I CPT and Level II Medicare National codes represent a specific

SERVICE	REVENUE CODES
Room and Board	0110
Nursery	0170
Intensive Care	0200
Coronary Care	0210
Pharmacy	0250
IV Therapy	0260
Medical Surgical Supplies	0270
Laboratory, Clinical	0300
Radiological Services	0320
Operating Room	0360
Anesthesia	0370
Blood	0380
Respiratory Services	0410
Physical Therapy	0420
Occupational Therapy	0430
Speech/Language Therapy	0440
Emergency Room	0450
Cardiology	0480
Recovery Room	0710
Labor/Delivery Room	0720
EKG/ECG and EEG	0730
Gastrointestinal Services	0750
Treatment or Observation Room	0760
Lithotripsy	0790
Inpatient Renal Dialysis Services	0800
Organ Acquisition	0810
Professional Fees	0960

Figure 5-16 Sample revenue code list for various categories of services. *(Data from NUBC, National Billing Committee.)*

quantity that indicates the number of times the service was performed or the number of items that were provided. Codes for drugs have an associated quantity that represents the specific dose or quantity of the drug provided.

Charge

The amount charged for each service or item is listed on the chargemaster. Some hospitals may designate a different charge for services or items based on whether the service was provided on an inpatient versus outpatient basis. However, many hospitals assign the same charge regardless of whether the service or item was provided on an inpatient or outpatient basis.

BOX 5-10 ▪ KEY POINTS

Charge Description Master (CDM) Data Elements

Chargemaster number
Department number
Item or service description
Procedure or item code
Revenue code
Quantity or dose
Charge

Chargemaster Maintenance

The challenge for hospitals is to develop and maintain a chargemaster that incorporates required information for claim preparation, for monitoring of resource utilization, and obtaining appropriate reimbursement. The HIM Department is generally responsible for the maintenance and updating of the chargemaster, which involves changes, revisions and deletions of codes, and incorporation of changes in payer guidelines. The appropriate revenue codes must be assigned to each HCPCS code utilized. As a result, hospital billing and coding professionals are becoming more involved in chargemaster functions. Many hospitals assign a committee to perform updating and auditing functions to identify discrepancies in the chargemaster.

CODING SYSTEMS

Historically, providers submitted a written description of conditions, services, and items on claims. Coding systems were developed to standardize descriptions of conditions, services, and items for the purpose of consistent reporting and tracking of conditions and procedures. Coding systems consist of numeric and alphanumeric codes that represent a translation of the written descriptions of conditions, services, or items provided as documented in the patient's medical record. Services and items provided are submitted to third-party payers utilizing two distinct coding systems—a procedure coding system and a diagnosis coding system.

BOX 5-11 ▪ KEY POINTS

Procedure Coding Systems

Health Care Common Procedure Coding System (HCPCS)
- Level I: CPT-4
- Level II: Medicare National Codes

International Classification of Diseases, 9th revision, Clinical Modification (ICD-9-CM), Volume III, Procedures

Diagnosis Coding Systems

International Classification of Diseases, 9th revision, Clinical Modification (ICD-9-CM), Volume I and II

TEST YOUR *Knowledge* BOX 5-2

CHARGE DESCRIPTION MASTER (CDM)

1. What is a CDM?
2. Explain the purpose of the chargemaster.
3. How is the chargemaster utilized within the hospital?
4. List six categories of services for which hospitals submit facility charges.
5. List seven data elements generally contained in a CDM.
6. What description on the chargemaster is used by hospitals for services and items?
7. Name the procedure or item codes that are utilized on the chargemaster.
8. Explain the purpose of revenue codes.
9. State the role of the National Uniform Billing Committee (NUBC) with regard to revenue codes.
10. What does updating the chargemaster involve and what department is generally responsible for chargemaster maintenance?

Procedure Coding Systems

Procedure coding systems are utilized to provide descriptions of procedures, services, and items provided. Procedure codes are listed on the claim form to describe the charges submitted. Payer guidelines regarding procedure codes vary. The standard procedure coding system utilized today to submit charges to payers is referred to as the **Health Care Common Procedure Coding System (HCPCS)**, which consists of two levels of codes—Level I CPT Codes and Level II Medicare National Codes (Figure 5-17).

Another coding system utilized for report procedures is ICD-9-CM Volume III Procedure Codes. The ICD-9-CM Volume III procedure coding system is commonly referred to as the ICD-9-PC. This coding system is utilized for reporting significant procedures on the claim form.

Procedure Coding Systems
(Services or Items)

HCPCS Level I
Current Procedural Terminology (CPT)

HCPCS Level II
Medicare National Codes

International Classification of Diseases, 9th Revision, Clinical Modification (ICD-9-CM)
Volume III (Alphabetical and numerical listing of procedures)

Diagnosis Coding Systems
(Conditions, disease, illness, injury, or other)

International Classification of Diseases, 9th Revision, Clinical Modification (ICD-9-CM) – Volume I & II (alphabetical and numerical listing of diseases, signs and symptoms, encounters and external causes of injury)

Figure 5-17 Coding systems utilized by hospital for submission of charges.

Diagnosis Coding Systems

Diagnosis coding systems are utilized to describe the patient's injury, illness, condition, disease, or other reason for hospital visit. They are used describe the reason why services or items were provided. ICD-9-CM Volume I and II is the diagnosis coding system currently utilized for coding the reason for services or items that were provided. An explanation of the patient's condition or other reason for the service is essential to establishing medical necessity.

Coding Systems for Outpatients and Inpatients

Coding systems utilized vary by payer according to whether the services are provided on an outpatient or inpatient basis, as illustrated in Table 5-5.

Outpatient

Outpatient is the term used to describe patient care services or items provided on the same day the patient is released. Hospitals perform various services on an outpatient basis, such as radiology, laboratory, physical and occupational therapy, ER, observation, and ambulatory surgery services. Coding systems utilized for outpatient services are HCPCS and ICD-9-CM. HCPCS and ICD-9-CM Volume I and II codes are reported on the CMS-1500 to report patient conditions and services provided to evaluate and treat those conditions. HCPCS and ICD-9-CM procedures codes will be discussed further in Chapters 7 and 8.

Inpatient

Hospitals perform a variety of services on patients who are admitted as inpatients. Inpatient services are performed on patients who are admitted to the hospital for

TABLE 5-5 Coding System Variations

Hospital Service Categories of Facility Charges	Procedures HCPCS Level		Procedures ICD-9-CM	Diagnosis ICD-9-CM Volume I & II	Variations
	I CPT	II Medicare National			
Outpatient					
Ambulatory surgery	X	*	†	X	Some payers may require ICD-9-CM Volume III procedures for ambulatory surgery claims submitted on the UB-04.
Emergency Department	X	*	†	X	
Ancillary departments: Radiology; Laboratory; Physical, Occupational, and Speech Therapy	X	*	†	X	
Other outpatient services: Infusion; Therapy and Observation	X	*	†	X	
Durable medical equipment: provided on an outpatient or inpatient basis	X	*	†	X	
Hospital-based primary care office	X	*	†	X	
Other hospital-based clinic	X	*	†	X	
Inpatient					
Inpatient services	X	*	†	X	
Non-Patient					
A specimen received and processed—the patient is not present	X	*	†	X	

*CPT codes are generally utilized to describe services and some items. Medicare National codes are utilized when a CPT code cannot be found that adequately describes the service or item or when the payer requires a Level II code.
†Varies by payer; generally required to report significant procedures on the UB-04 claim form.

more than 24 hours. A wide range of services and items are provided during the patient's hospital visit. They are coded utilizing the HCPCS and the ICD-9-CM Volume III procedure coding systems. Conditions, diseases, illnesses, injuries, and other reasons for the hospital stay are coded utilizing the ICD-9-CM Volume I and II diagnosis coding system. The codes are listed on the claim form to describe services and items provided and the medical reason why they were provided. ICD-9-CM Volume I and II codes are utilized to report diagnoses on the UB-04. ICD-9-CM Volume III codes are required to report significant procedures on the UB-04. Some payers require the Volume III codes when the UB-04 is required for submission of ambulatory surgery services. HCPCS codes are utilized to post charges for services, procedures, and items through the chargemaster for inpatient claims.

Hospital billing and coding professionals are involved in the coding process and submission of charges for payment to patients and payers. It is essential for hospital billing and coding professionals to understand coding system requirements in order to ensure coding compliance and to obtain the proper reimbursement. Billing professionals are required to understand coding and related guidelines for various payers to ensure that the claim form is completed accurately and that proper reimbursement is obtained. Coding professionals are required to understand and apply coding principals and guidelines outlined by payers to ensure that accurate descriptions of services, items, and reasons for the hospital stay are submitted. A detailed discussion of each of these coding systems follows in later chapters.

TEST YOUR *Knowledge* BOX 5-3

CODING SYSTEMS

1. Why were coding systems developed?
2. What are coding systems?
3. Explain the relationship between coding systems and the claim form.
4. Name two types of coding systems utilized to code services rendered and the reasons why they were rendered.
5. Explain what coding system is utilized to describe the reason why services were rendered.
6. Outline and describe coding systems utilized for outpatient claims.
7. Describe coding systems utilized for inpatient claims.
8. State two levels of the HCPCS coding system.
9. Explain how coding systems vary by payer.
10. Provide an explanation of the relationship between diagnosis codes and medical necessity.

UNIVERSALLY ACCEPTED CLAIM FORMS

Claim forms are utilized to submit charges for services and items rendered to third-party payers. There are two universally accepted claim forms used for submission of charges to payers—CMS-1500 and CMS-1450 (UB-04). A detailed discussion of claim form completion will be provided in Chapter 10. The following section provides an outline of the claim form information required for the CMS-1500 and the UB-04. It is important to remember that payer guidelines define what claim form is required for outpatient, inpatient, and non-patient services.

CMS-1500

The CMS-1500 is used to submit charges to payers for professional and specified outpatient services provided by physicians and other providers to payers. As discussed previously, hospitals do not submit charges for physician services unless the physician is employed by or under contract with the hospital. The CMS-1500 consists of 33 fields, referred to as blocks, utilized to record information regarding the patient visit. The payer requires four areas of information—patient and insurance information, diagnosis, and charge information including appropriate code(s), and provider information. Figure 5-18 highlights the four sections of information on the CMS-1500.

CMS-1450 (UB-04)

The CMS-1450 is also referred to as the UB-04 because it is the universal bill accepted by most payers. The UB-04 is used to submit hospital facility charges for patient care services rendered during a patient visit. The UB-04 consists of 81 fields, which are referred to as **form locators (FLs)**. As illustrated in Figure 5-19, the claim form can be viewed in four sections in which information regarding the facility, patient, charges, and payer is recorded.

BOX 5-12 ■ KEY POINTS

Universally Accepted Claim Forms

CMS-1500

Charges for physician and outpatient services

UB-04

Hospital facility charges for inpatient and outpatient services

Detailed Itemized Statement

The detailed itemized statement includes information collected and posted to the patient's account throughout the patient's stay. The **detailed itemized statement** is a listing of all charges incurred during the patient visit. The statement and its content vary from hospital to hospital. The basic information included on a detailed itemized statement is patient's name and address, hospital name and address, patient account and medical record number, admit and discharge date, and all information describing the services and items charged. The data outlined on the detailed itemized statement are obtained throughout the patient care process. Charges are posted and maintained through the chargemaster during the patient's visit. Figure 5-20 on page 157 illustrates a detailed itemized statement highlighting the following four parts of information outlined:

1. Facility, patient, and insurance information.
2. Detailed information for each charge.
3. Revenue code for each charge.
4. Procedure code, description, quantity, dose, and total for each charge.

Detailed Itemized Statement Part 1

Section 1 of the detailed itemized statement contains information regarding the facility, patient, and insurance, including hospital name, address, phone number, and tax identification number, patient and medical record number, bill date, admission and discharge dates, and bill type. The patient and insurance information is obtained during the admission process. This information is registered on the hospital's system, and a patient account number and medical record number is assigned.

Detailed Itemized Statement Part 2

Section 2 is utilized to record charge detail for services and items provided during the patient stay, including date of service, chargemaster number, and department number. This information is captured throughout the patient visit as charges are posted through the chargemaster by various departments. Services and items listed on the detailed itemized statement are documented in the patient's medical record and are provided in accordance with physician's orders.

Detailed Itemized Statement Part 3

Section 3 highlights the revenue code column. A revenue code is assigned to each service or item provided by the hospital. Revenue codes are associated with HCPCS codes listed in the chargemaster. When hospital departments post charges to the patient's account, all the assoiated data such as revenue codes are recorded on the patient's account with the charge.

1500

HEALTH INSURANCE CLAIM FORM

APPROVED BY NATIONAL UNIFORM CLAIM COMMITTEE 08/05

PICA | PICA | CARRIER

1. MEDICARE (Medicare #) | MEDICAID (Medicaid #) | TRICARE CHAMPUS (Sponsor's SSN) | CHAMPVA (Member ID#) | GROUP HEALTH PLAN (SSN or ID) | FECA BLK LUNG (SSN) | OTHER (ID)

1a. INSURED'S I.D. NUMBER (For Program in Item 1)

2. PATIENT'S NAME (Last Name, First Name, Middle Initial)

3. PATIENT'S BIRTH DATE MM DD YY SEX M F

4. INSURED'S NAME (Last Name, First Name, Middle Initial)

5. PATIENT'S ADDRESS (No., Street)

6. PATIENT RELATIONSHIP TO INSURED Self Spouse Child Other

7. INSURED'S ADDRESS (No., Street)

CITY STATE

8. PATIENT STATUS

CITY STATE

PART I PATIENT AND INSURANCE INFORMATION]

ZIP CODE TELEPHONE (Include Area Code) ( )

Employed | Full-Time Student | Part-Time Student

ZIP CODE TELEPHONE (Include Area Code) ( )

9. OTHER INSURED'S NAME (Last Name, First Name, Middle Initial)

10. IS PATIENT'S CONDITION RELATED TO:

11. INSURED'S POLICY GROUP OR FECA NUMBER

a. OTHER INSURED'S POLICY OR GROUP NUMBER

a. EMPLOYMENT? (Current or Previous) YES NO

a. INSURED'S DATE OF BIRTH MM DD YY SEX M F

b. OTHER INSURED'S DATE OF BIRTH MM DD YY SEX M F

b. AUTO ACCIDENT? YES NO PLACE (State)

b. EMPLOYER'S NAME OR SCHOOL NAME

c. EMPLOYER'S NAME OR SCHOOL NAME

c. OTHER ACCIDENT? YES NO

c. INSURANCE PLAN NAME OR PROGRAM NAME

d. INSURANCE PLAN NAME OR PROGRAM NAME

10d. RESERVED FOR LOCAL USE

d. IS THERE ANOTHER HEALTH BENEFIT PLAN? YES NO *If yes,* return to and complete item 9 a-d.

READ BACK OF FORM BEFORE COMPLETING & SIGNING THIS FORM.

12. PATIENT'S OR AUTHORIZED PERSON'S SIGNATURE I authorize the release of any medical or other information necessary to process this claim. I also request payment of government benefits either to myself or to the party who accepts assignment below.

SIGNED DATE

13. INSURED'S OR AUTHORIZED PERSON'S SIGNATURE I authorize payment of medical benefits to the undersigned physician or supplier for services described below.

SIGNED

PATIENT AND INSURED INFORMATION

14. DATE OF CURRENT: MM DD YY ILLNESS (First symptom) OR INJURY (Accident) OR PREGNANCY(LMP)

15. IF PATIENT HAS HAD SAME OR SIMILAR ILLNESS. GIVE FIRST DATE MM DD YY

16. DATES PATIENT UNABLE TO WORK IN CURRENT OCCUPATION FROM MM DD YY TO MM DD YY

17. NAME OF REFERRING PROVIDER OR OTHER SOURCE 17a. 17b. NPI

18. HOSPITALIZATION DATES RELATED TO CURRENT SERVICES FROM MM DD YY TO MM DD YY

19. RESERVED FOR LOCAL USE

20. OUTSIDE LAB? YES NO $ CHARGES

PART II PATIENT DIAGNOSIS INFORMATION

21. DIAGNOSIS OR NATURE OF ILLNESS OR INJURY (Relate Items 1, 2, 3 or 4 to Item 24E by Line)

1. ___ . ___ 3. ___ . ___

2. ___ . ___ 4. ___ . ___

22. MEDICAID RESUBMISSION CODE ORIGINAL REF. NO.

23. PRIOR AUTHORIZATION NUMBER

24. A. DATE(S) OF SERVICE From MM DD YY To MM DD YY	B. PLACE OF SERVICE	C. EMG	D. PROCEDURES, SERVICES, OR SUPPLIES (Explain Unusual Circumstances) CPT/HCPCS MODIFIER	E. DIAGNOSIS POINTER	F. $ CHARGES	G. DAYS OR UNITS	H. EPSDT Family Plan	I. ID. QUAL.	J. RENDERING PROVIDER ID. #
1								NPI	
2								NPI	
3			PART III CHARGE INFORMATION					NPI	
4								NPI	
5								NPI	
6								NPI	

PHYSICIAN OR SUPPLIER INFORMATION

25. FEDERAL TAX I.D. NUMBER SSN EIN

26. PATIENT'S ACCOUNT NO.

27. ACCEPT ASSIGNMENT? (For govt. claims, see back) YES NO

28. TOTAL CHARGE $

29. AMOUNT PAID $

30. BALANCE DUE $

31. SIGNATURE OF PHYSICIAN OR SUPPLIER INCLUDING DEGREES OR CREDENTIALS (I certify that the statements on the reverse apply to this bill and are made a part thereof.)

32. SERVICE FACILITY LOCATION INFORMATION

33. BILLING PROVIDER INFO & PH # ( )

PART IV PROVIDER INFORMATION

SIGNED DATE a. NPI b. a. NPI b.

NUCC Instruction Manual available at: www.nucc.org APPROVED OMB-0938-0999 FORM CMS-1500 (08-05)

Figure 5-18 CMS-1500 highlighting sections of required information.

Detailed Itemized Statement Part 4

Section 4 contains a procedure or item code, description, quantity, and total charge for each service or item. All services and items provided by the hospital are assigned a numerical or alphanumerical procedure or item code and a charge. As discussed previously, coding systems utilized for procedures and items are HCPCS Level I CPT or HCPCS Level II Medicare National code. Some payers require that a National Drug Code (NDC) be used to identify drugs and biologicals. A written description of the item or service is listed in the description line. The quantity or dose and total amount charged is listed in the next columns for each code.

Many payers require submission of a detailed itemized statement with the claim. Payers that do not require submission of the detailed itemized statement with the claim form may request one after initial review of the claim. A patient may also request a detailed itemized statement after review of the summary statement or invoice.

Manual versus Electronic Claim Submission

Claim forms can be submitted manually or via electronic media. Manual claim form submission involves

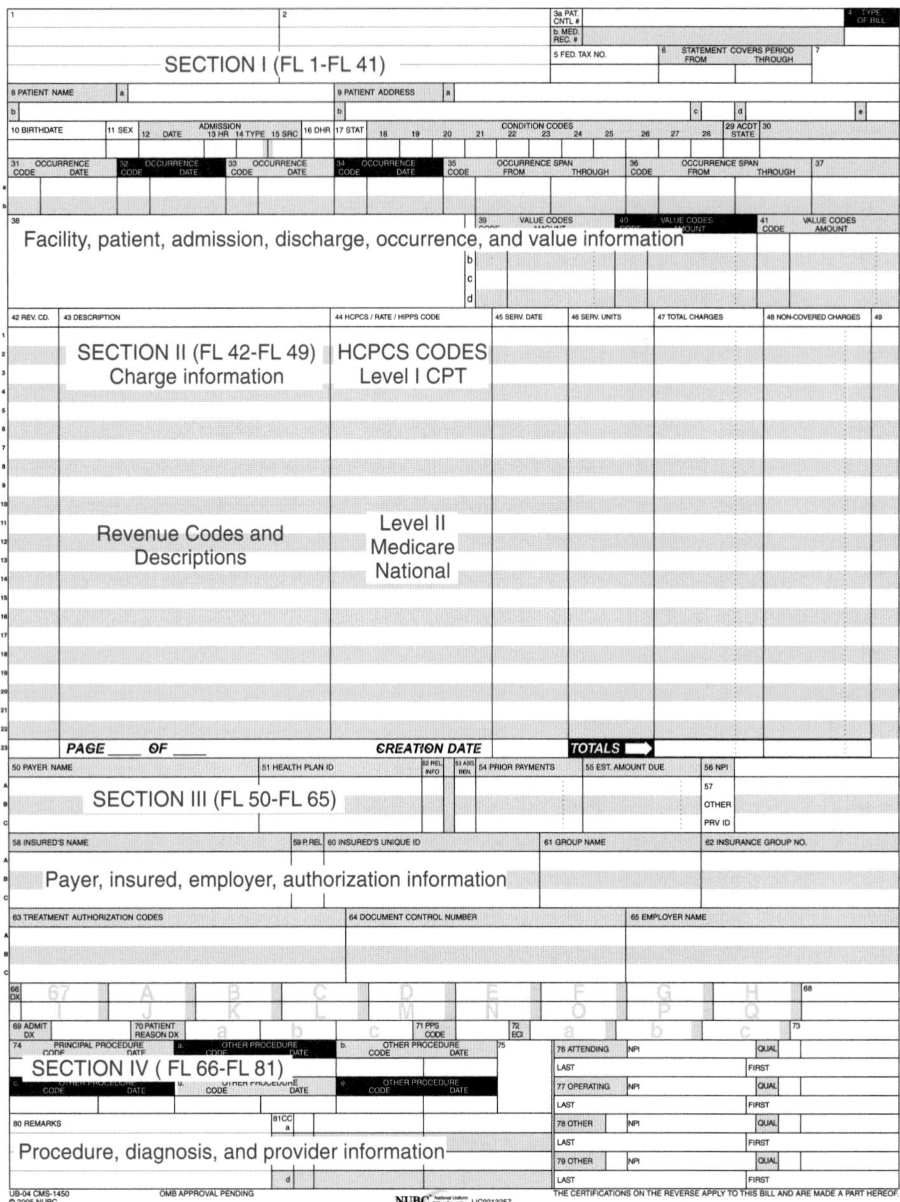

Figure 5-19 UB-04 highlighting sections of required information.

printing a paper claim and detailed itemized statement when required. Both are reviewed for accuracy and submitted to the appropriate third-party payer via mail or fax transmission when the claim must be resubmitted. Electronic claims are submitted via **electronic data interchange (EDI),** which is the term used to describe the process of sending information from one place to another via computer. The claim form sent via EDI is called an **electronic media claim (EMC)**. EMCs are submitted to payers electronically. Many hospitals utilize a clearinghouse to submit claims electronically. The **clearinghouse** receives claim form information from hospitals and other providers in various formats. The clearinghouse also reviews the claim for completeness and verification of accuracy. The claim is converted to the required format for each specific payer and submitted electronically.

CMS-1500 and UB-04 claim form requirements vary by payer. Payers receiving the UB-04 have specific requirements based on the type of facility submitting the claim and whether service was provided on an outpatient or inpatient basis. A detailed discussion of the UB-04 and completion instructions is provided later in the text.

The complex process of billing is difficult to understand without knowledge of the purpose of billing, the chargemaster, coding systems, claim forms, and the detailed itemized statement. The process is similar to a puzzle, and hospital billing and coding professionals need to know all the pieces of the puzzle in order to fit

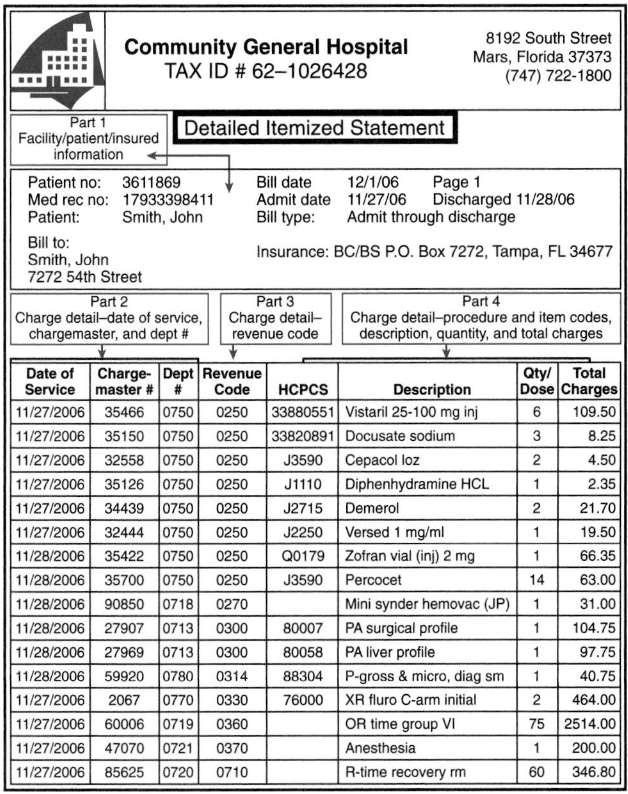

Community General Hospital
TAX ID # 62–1026428

8192 South Street
Mars, Florida 37373
(747) 722-1800

Part 1
Facility/patient/insured information

Detailed Itemized Statement

Patient no: 3611869
Med rec no: 17933398411
Patient: Smith, John

Bill date 12/1/06 Page 1
Admit date 11/27/06 Discharged 11/28/06
Bill type: Admit through discharge

Bill to:
Smith, John
7272 54th Street

Insurance: BC/BS P.O. Box 7272, Tampa, FL 34677

Part 2
Charge detail–date of service, chargemaster, and dept #

Part 3
Charge detail–revenue code

Part 4
Charge detail–procedure and item codes, description, quantity, and total charges

Date of Service	Charge-master #	Dept #	Revenue Code	HCPCS	Description	Qty/ Dose	Total Charges
11/27/2006	35466	0750	0250	33880551	Vistaril 25-100 mg inj	6	109.50
11/27/2006	35150	0750	0250	33820891	Docusate sodium	3	8.25
11/27/2006	32558	0750	0250	J3590	Cepacol loz	2	4.50
11/27/2006	35126	0750	0250	J1110	Diphenhydramine HCL	1	2.35
11/27/2006	34439	0750	0250	J2715	Demerol	2	21.70
11/27/2006	32444	0750	0250	J2250	Versed 1 mg/ml	1	19.50
11/28/2006	35422	0750	0250	Q0179	Zofran vial (inj) 2 mg	1	66.35
11/28/2006	35700	0750	0250	J3590	Percocet	14	63.00
11/28/2006	90850	0718	0270		Mini synder hemovac (JP)	1	31.00
11/28/2006	27907	0713	0300	80007	PA surgical profile	1	104.75
11/28/2006	27969	0713	0300	80058	PA liver profile	1	97.75
11/28/2006	59920	0780	0314	88304	P-gross & micro, diag sm	1	40.75
11/27/2006	2067	0770	0330	76000	XR fluro C-arm initial	2	464.00
11/27/2006	60006	0719	0360		OR time group VI	75	2514.00
11/27/2006	47070	0721	0370		Anesthesia	1	200.00
11/27/2006	85625	0720	0710		R-time recovery rm	60	346.80

Figure 5-20 Sample detailed itemized statement highlighting four sections of information generally reported on the statement.

them together for the purpose of obtaining accurate reimbursement and maintaining compliance with all billing and coding guidelines. Now that we have an understanding of the elements of the process, we will review the entire process from the time the patient is admitted to collection of accounts receivable.

BOX 5-13 ■ KEY POINTS

Claim Submission Methods

Manual

Paper claim sent by mail

Electronic Media Claim (EMC)

Claim sent by electronic data interchange (EDI)

HOSPITAL BILLING PROCESS

The hospital billing process begins with patient registration at admission, and it ends when payment is received for hospital services. The next section will review the billing process in order to provide a complete "big picture" understanding of how all the elements are related and how this relationship is critical to obtaining proper reimbursement and ensuring compliance. Figure 5-21 illustrates the billing process and indicates the departments involved in the process. The billing process consists of all functions required for claim submission and obtaining reimbursement. It includes patient admission/registration, patient care/ order entry, charge capture, chart review and coding, charge submission, reimbursement, and accounts receivable management.

Patient Admission and Registration

Patients are received at the hospital on an inpatient or outpatient basis. Non-patient services may be provided when a specimen is received for processing and the patient is not present. The process followed by the Admitting Department for each type of admission includes collection of demographic and insurance information. Patient registration involves entering all information into the hospital system. This information is utilized throughout the patient stay for the purpose of providing patient care services and posting charges for those services. The admission process is critical to ensure that accurate information is obtained that will be used for charge submission.

Patient Care Order Entry

Patient care services are rendered in accordance with the physician's orders. The physician's orders are entered into the hospital's information system and distributed to the appropriate departments. During the patient stay, hospital personnel from various clinical and ancillary departments are involved in providing care to the patient. Diagnostic and therapeutic services are provided by departments such as Radiology, Pathology/ Laboratory, and Rehabilitation. All patient care activities are recorded in the patient's medical record.

Charge Capture

All services and items provided during the patient stay are documented in the patient's record. Departments involved in providing patient care and HIM are responsible for posting charges to the patient's account through the chargemaster. Other departments such as Pharmacy and Sterile Supplies also post charges to the patient's account for items utilized for patient care, such as medications and supplies. As discussed previously, the chargemaster lists all services, procedures, items, and drugs that the hospital may provide. The items listed in the chargemaster are organized by department. Each item in the chargemaster is associated with the appropriate revenue code, procedure or item code, description, quantity, and charge.

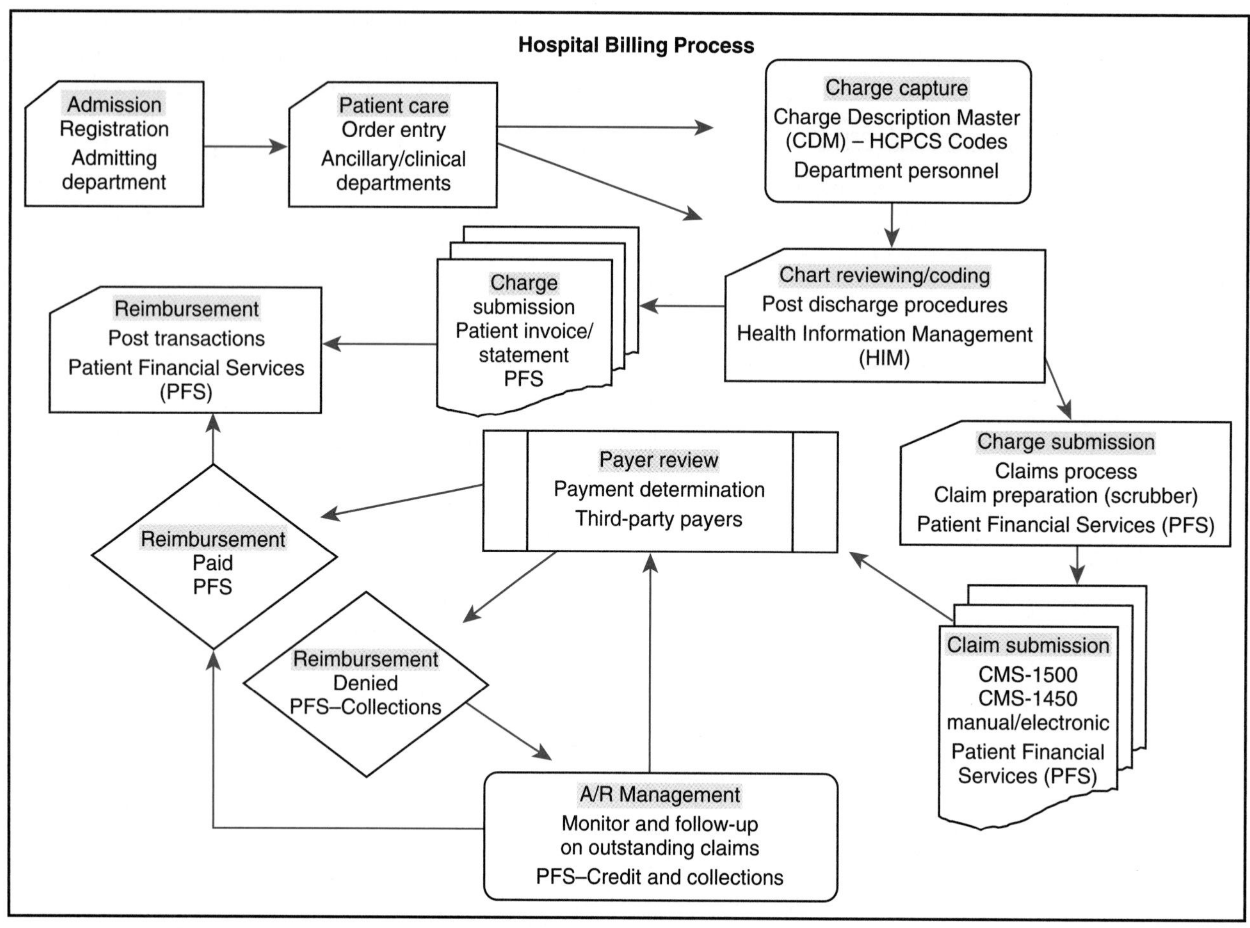

Figure 5-21 The hospital billing process: key functions and the primary departments involved in performing those functions. *(Revisions of illustration courtesy Sandra Giangreco.)*

Chart Review and Coding

The patient is released from the hospital when the attending physician provides written discharge orders and instructions. Once the patient is discharged, the completed medical record is forwarded to the HIM. HIM coding professionals review the patient's medical record for purposes of identifying and verifying charges. The coder then analyzes the medical record to abstract the patient's diagnosis(es) and significant procedure(s) from the record for the purpose of assigning procedure and diagnosis codes. A computer program called an **encoder** may be utilized to assist with code assignment. A program called the **grouper** is utilized for the assignment of a MS-DRG or APC based on the information entered such as diagnosis, procedure, and other patient information such as age, sex, and length of stay.

Charge Submission

The Patient Financial Services (PFS) Department utilizes information gathered during the patient stay to prepare appropriate documents required for charge submission. The patient invoice or statement is utilized to submit charges to the patient. Claim forms are utilized to submit charges to third-party payers.

Patient Invoice and Patient Statement

An invoice or statement is prepared and sent to advise the patient of an outstanding balance. A **patient invoice** is a document prepared by the hospital to advise the patient of an outstanding balance that includes details regarding current services, and it is generally sent out the first time a balance is billed to the patient, as illustrated in Figure 5-22. A **patient statement** is a document prepared by the hospital that provides details regarding account activity, including the previous balance, recent charges, payments, and the current balance. Hospitals generally send a patient statement monthly to notify the patient of a balance due.

A summary statement may also be sent to advise the patient of charges submitted to his or her insurance company or government program. The summary statement is a listing of charges posted during the patient stay, organized by revenue code category. Summary statements include the hospital name and address, patient name and account number, admission and dis-

TEST YOUR *Knowledge* BOX 5-4

UNIVERSALLY ACCEPTED CLAIM FORMS

1. Explain the purpose of a claim form.
2. List four areas of information required by payers on the CMS-1500.
3. Provide an explanation of the difference in format between the CMS-1500 and CMS-1450 (UB-04).
4. Outline the types of charges reported on the UB-04 versus those reported on the CMS-1500 claim form.
5. Discuss four sections of the UB-04.
6. Identify the section where procedure and diagnosis codes are listed on the UB-04 and list the form locators.
7. What section of the UB-04 is used to provide information about the charges to be submitted?
8. State the difference between a manual claim and electronic claim submission.
9. Explain what information is included on the detailed itemized statement and where the information on the statement comes from.
10. What is the term that describes the process of sending information from one party to another via computer?

charge dates, a summary of charges, payments, and adjustments, and the unpaid balance, as illustrated in Figure 5-23.

Patient invoices or statements are run in batches and sent to patients. A batch is a specified group of invoices or statements processed at one time. For example, invoices and statements for patient last names beginning with A through M may be run in the first batch. Invoices and statements for patient last names ning with N through Z may be run in another batch.

Claim Forms

Claim forms are utilized to submit charges to third-party payers, as outlined previously. The UB-04 is generally used to submit most hospital facility charges. The CMS-1500 is used to submit charges for professional services and other specified outpatient services. Claim forms are also prepared in batches, usually by payer type. Claim forms can be printed manually and sent to the payer by mail or fax or they can be submitted electronically. Most payers do not allow faxed claims unless they are resubmissions. Most hospital computer billing systems have computerized checks referred to as edits that are performed prior to submission of a claim. These edits are designed to detect potential claim problems. The computer system checks specific data against other data on the claim. Computer edits will vary by hospital.

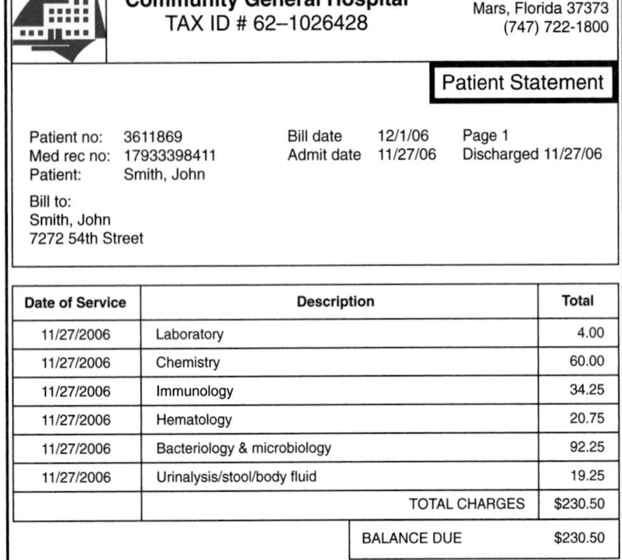

Community General Hospital
TAX ID # 62–1026428

8192 South Street
Mars, Florida 37373
(747) 722-1800

Patient Statement

Patient no: 3611869
Med rec no: 17933398411
Patient: Smith, John

Bill date 12/1/06
Admit date 11/27/06

Page 1
Discharged 11/27/06

Bill to:
Smith, John
7272 54th Street

Date of Service	Description	Total
11/27/2006	Laboratory	4.00
11/27/2006	Chemistry	60.00
11/27/2006	Immunology	34.25
11/27/2006	Hematology	20.75
11/27/2006	Bacteriology & microbiology	92.25
11/27/2006	Urinalysis/stool/body fluid	19.25
	TOTAL CHARGES	$230.50
	BALANCE DUE	$230.50

Figure 5-22 Sample hospital patient statement.

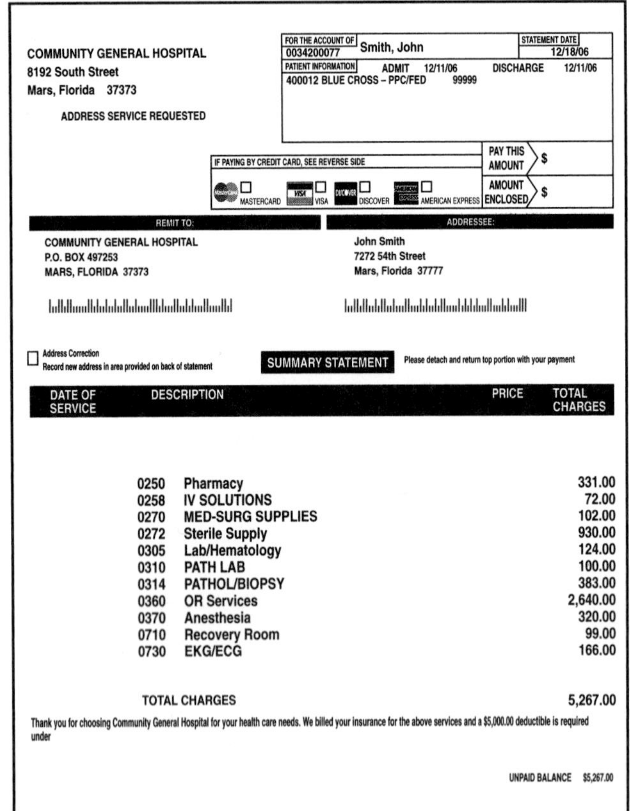

COMMUNITY GENERAL HOSPITAL
8192 South Street
Mars, Florida 37373

ADDRESS SERVICE REQUESTED

FOR THE ACCOUNT OF 0034200077 Smith, John
STATEMENT DATE 12/18/06
PATIENT INFORMATION ADMIT 12/11/06 DISCHARGE 12/11/06
400012 BLUE CROSS – PPC/FED 99999

IF PAYING BY CREDIT CARD, SEE REVERSE SIDE
☐ MASTERCARD ☐ VISA ☐ DISCOVER ☐ AMERICAN EXPRESS

PAY THIS AMOUNT $
AMOUNT ENCLOSED $

REMIT TO:
COMMUNITY GENERAL HOSPITAL
P.O. BOX 497253
MARS, FLORIDA 37373

ADDRESSEE:
John Smith
7272 54th Street
Mars, Florida 37777

☐ Address Correction
Record new address in area provided on back of statement

SUMMARY STATEMENT

Please detach and return top portion with your payment

DATE OF SERVICE	DESCRIPTION	PRICE	TOTAL CHARGES
0250	Pharmacy		331.00
0258	IV SOLUTIONS		72.00
0270	MED-SURG SUPPLIES		102.00
0272	Sterile Supply		930.00
0305	Lab/Hematology		124.00
0310	PATH LAB		100.00
0314	PATHOL/BIOPSY		383.00
0360	OR Services		2,640.00
0370	Anesthesia		320.00
0710	Recovery Room		99.00
0730	EKG/ECG		166.00
	TOTAL CHARGES		5,267.00

Thank you for choosing Community General Hospital for your health care needs. We billed your insurance for the above services and a $5,000.00 deductible is required under

UNPAID BALANCE $5,267.00

Figure 5-23 Sample hospital summary statement.

All computer edits are run for the purpose of identifying problems that can result in denial or inaccurate payment of a claim. The computer system will provide a report that outlines potential problems with the claim. Hospital billing and/or HIM staff will review the problem areas and make corrections prior to submission of the claim. The claim may be held while more information is requested.

BOX 5-14 ■ KEY POINTS

Computer Edits

Computer edits are designed to detect potential claim problems.

- Procedure versus patient's sex: to verify that the procedure is appropriate for the patient's sex
- Procedure versus patient's age: to ensure the procedure is age appropriate
- Procedure versus patient's diagnosis: to ensure the procedure is appropriate based on the patient's condition

Reimbursement

The purpose of the billing process is to submit hospital charges to patients and third-party payers for payment. As outlined in Chapter 4, payments are received and posted to the patient's account by the PFS Department. Patient payments are posted and balances owed are printed on a statement and sent to the patient until the balance is paid. Claims received by payers are processed after computer edits and manual review of the claim are performed. Payment determination is conducted by the payer after claim review edits are performed and can result in the following actions: the claim may be paid, the claim may be pended, or the claim may be denied.

Claim Paid

Payments received from a payer are accompanied by a document that explains the charges submitted, deductible, co-insurance, co-payment, allowed charges, and amount paid on the claim. The term for the document sent with payment is remittance advice. The remittance advice (RA) provides an explanation of the charges submitted and details regarding the payer's payment determination (Figure 5-24). Payers may use a variety of other names for this document, such as explanation of benefits, explanation of Medicare benefits, or Medicare summary notice. Payments are processed by the hospital as follows:

- Payment is posted to the patient's account
- Contractual adjustment is applied where applicable
- The balance is billed to the patient or to a secondary or tertiary payer where applicable

The payment is reviewed to determine whether the correct amount was paid. Payer payments will vary based on the specific guidelines for the policy or plan under which the patient is covered. Payments will also vary based on the participating provider agreements between the hospital and the payer, as discussed pre-

MEDICARE PART A

P.O. BOX 167953 TEMPE AR 72207 TEL# 800 660 4235 VER# 4010–A1

PROV #69542A PROVIDER NAME: Dr Martin Samerston PART A PAID DATE: 06/26/2006 REMIT#: 7654 PAGE:1

PATIENT NAME HIC NUMBER FROM DT THRU DT CLMSTATUS	PATIENT CNTRL NUMBER ICN NUMBERNACHG HICHG TOB COST COVDY NCOVDY	RC REM DRG# RC REM OUTCD CAPCD RC REM PROF COMP RC REM DRG AMT	DRG OUT AMT NEW TECH MSP PAYMT DEDUCTIBLES	COINSURANCE COVDCHGS NCOVD CHGS DENIED CHGS	PAT REFUND ESRD NET ADJ INTEREST PRE PAY ADJ	CONTRACT ADJ PER DIEM RTE PROC CD AMT NET REIMB
Smith John	7 9 4076922738872 084327777A 00					
109876543210		149	6,895.72	1,463.72	.00	4556.00
06/01/2005 06/05/2006	3 111					
6		M 45	.00	.00	.00	.00
		M 138	.00	.00	.00	.00
SUBTOTAL FISCAL YEAR-$000		45.03	876.00	5,432.00	.00	4,556.00
			.00	.00	.00	.00
			.00	.00	.00	.00
SUBTOTAL PART A		.00	.00	.00	.00	.00
			876.00	5,432.00	.00	4556.00
TOTAL PART A						

Figure 5-24 Sample remittance advice (RA), a document used by payers to communicate the payment determination on a claim to the provider.

viously in this chapter. If the payment is not correct, the hospital billing professional will gather information regarding the incorrect payment and pursue payment of the correct amount from the payer. Contact is made with the payer, generally in writing, to outline the details of the incorrect payment and to request the payment be corrected.

Claim Pended

When payers identify a potential problem with medical necessity or coverage based on the claim review, they may request additional information and put the claim in a pending status. The claim is put on hold until the requested information is received. The request for additional information is communicated on the RA that is sent to the provider along with an indication that payment cannot be processed until the requested information is received. Many payers send a notification to the patient to inform the patient about the pended status and the reason for nonpayment of the claim.

Claim Denied

A claim submitted to a payer may be denied entirely, or a specific charge on the claim may be denied. Claim denials are communicated on the RA that is sent to the provider. An explanation of the reason for denial is provided through the use of codes referred to as reason codes. A claim may be denied for many reasons:

- The patient's identification number and name may not match any in the payer file
- Coverage for the patient may not be in effect
- The plan may not provide coverage for a particular service or item
- The service or item may not be considered medically necessary
- Service may be included in a package and therefore not separately billable
- Services may be considered duplicate
- The hospital may not be a network provider through the plan

BOX 5-15 ▪ KEY POINTS

Payer Payment Determination

Payment determination is conducted by the payer after the claim passes all computer edits and can result in one of the following actions:

- Payment is processed for the claim
- The claim is put in a pending status until information requested is received
- The claim may be denied

BOX 5-16 ▪ KEY POINTS

Common Reasons for Claim Denials

Patient's identification number and name are incorrect
Coverage terminated prior to date of service
Service not covered under the plan
Service not considered medically necessary
Service included in a package
Duplicate services
Non-network provider

BOX 5-17 ▪ KEY POINTS

Accounts Receivable (A/R) Management

Performs functions required to monitor and follow-up on outstanding accounts In order to ensure that reimbursement is received in a timely manner

Accounts Receivable (A/R) Management

It is critical for hospitals to have accounts receivable management functions in place to ensure that payment is received in a timely manner. **Accounts receivable (A/R) management** refers to functions required for the monitoring and follow-up of outstanding accounts. A division under the PFS Department, commonly called Credit and Collections, is responsible for A/R management functions. Accounts are monitored by payer type, aging categories, and amount due. Computer-generated reports such as an aging report or a financial class report are printed to identify outstanding accounts based on specified criteria such as payer type or age of the accounts. Credit and collection personnel utilize these reports to identify accounts that require follow-up for the purpose of pursing payment. A/R management is discussed further in Chapter 6.

TEST YOUR *Knowledge* BOX 5-5

HOSPITAL BILLING PROCESS

1. Explain when the billing process begins and ends.
2. List five functions in the hospital billing process required to submit charges to third-party payers for reimbursement. Indicate what department is responsible for those functions.
3. Name the phase in the billing process that involves obtaining information required to submit claims to payers and bill patients.
4. Explain the role of the chargemaster in charge capture.
5. Name functions performed by the HIM Department relative to the billing process.
6. State the purpose of encoder and grouper programs.
7. Provide an explanation of the difference between billing patients and third-party payers.
8. What purpose does the patient summary statement serve?
9. Explain what it means to run invoices and claim forms in batches.
10. Describe the document prepared by payers that is sent with payment.

CHAPTER SUMMARY

The hospital billing process involves all functions performed to prepare and submit charges for services rendered. Services and items rendered are posted to the patient's account through the chargemaster. Charges are submitted to patients utilizing invoices and statements. Claim forms are utilized to submit charges to third-party payers such as insurance carriers or government programs. Claims may be submitted via mail, fax, or electronic data interchange (EDI). Coding systems are utilized to translate written descriptions of services and items into codes. Procedure and diagnosis codes are reported on the claim form to describe what services were performed and why they were performed. Third-party claims are reviewed and payment is determined based on the patient's coverage and the outcome of the claim form edits, or the claim can be denied or pended. Payers utilize various reimbursement methods to pay for services rendered. Outstanding accounts are monitored and hospital collection representatives pursue outstanding balances based on the account's age.

The purpose of the process is to obtain the appropriate reimbursement for services and items rendered. Hospital billing and coding professionals are required to have an understanding of the hospital's billing process, billing guidelines, payer specifications, and coding principles and guidelines. The insurance billing and coding industry is in constant motion, with changes in policies, procedures and guidelines occurring on a daily basis. As a result of the constant change, billing and coding professionals need to maintain a current knowledge base on payer guidelines and specifications.

CHAPTER REVIEW 5-1

True/False

1. The purpose of the hospital billing process is to obtain appropriate reimbursement for services rendered. T F
2. Accurate completion of the claim helps to ensure accurate reimbursement. T F
3. Patients are considered third-party payers. T F
4. The detailed itemized statement is an outline of all services and items posted to the patient's account during the patient stay. T F
5. The Charge Description Master does not include procedure codes. T F

Fill in the Blank

6. A claim that does not need to be investigated by the payer, passes all internal billing edits and payer-specific edits, and is paid without need of additional intervention is a ____________________.
7. The portion of a claim that the patient must pay is referred to as ____________________.
8. Two claim forms used to submit claims to third-party payers are ____________________ and ____________________.
9. The process of counting the number of days a claim is outstanding is known as ____________________.
10. Coding systems used to describe diagnosis and procedures on the UB-04 are ____________________, ____________________ and ____________________.

Match the Following Definitions With the Terms at Right

11. Reimbursement to the facility at a set rate as agreed to by the facility and the payer.
12. Reimbursement method that provides payment based on an established fee schedule for each service.
13. A reimbursement method used by Medicare to determine payment for inpatient cases.
14. A reimbursement method used by Medicare to determine payment for ambulatory surgery cases.
15. A reimbursement method in which a percentage of the total accrued charges are paid to the facility.

A. MS-DRG
B. Fee for service
C. Percentage of accrued charges
D. Contract rate
E. APC

Research Project

Utilize the participating provider agreement in Figures 5-3 and 5-4 and the hospital billing process information in this chapter. Perform a side-by-side comparison of the agreement with the billing process, and discuss how the hospital billing process is designed to meet provisions in the participating provider agreement. Conduct research as required through the Internet or through contact with a local hospital.

GLOSSARY

Accounts receivable (A/R) management Refers to functions required for the monitoring and follow-up on outstanding accounts to ensure that reimbursement is received in a timely manner.

Ambulatory Payment Classification (APC) The OPPS utilized by Medicare and other government programs to provide reimbursement for hospital outpatient services. Under the APC system, the hospital is paid a fixed fee based on the procedure(s) performed.

Ambulatory surgery Surgery is performed in a free-standing or hospital-based ambulatory surgery setting. Surgery is performed and the patient is discharged the same day.

Batch A specified group of invoices or statements processed at one time.

Billing process Involves all the functions required to prepare charges for submission to patients and third-party payers to obtain reimbursement.

Capitation A reimbursement method utilized that provides payment of a fixed amount, paid per member per month.

Case mix A term used to describe type of patient cases treated by the hospital.

Case rate A reimbursement method utilized that provides a set payment rate to the hospital for a case. The payment rate is based on the type of case and resources utilized to treat the patient.

Charge Description Master (CDM) Computerized system used by the hospital to inventory and record services and items provided by the hospital. The CDM is commonly referred to as the chargemaster.

Claims process The portion of billing that involves preparing claims for submission to payers.

Clean claim A claim that does not need to be investigated by the payer. A clean claim passes all internal billing edits and payer specific edits and is paid without need for additional intervention.

Clearinghouse A company that receives claim information from hospitals and other providers in various formats for conversion to a required format for submission to various payers.

Collections Involves monitoring accounts that are outstanding and pursuing payment from patients and third party payers. Collections is also referred to as accounts receivable (A/R) management.

Contract rate A reimbursement method utilized that provides a set payment rate to the hospital as agreed to by the hospital and payer.

Detailed itemized statement A listing of all charges incurred during the patient visit.

Electronic data interchange (EDI) Term used to describe the process of sending information from one place to another via computer.

Electronic media claim (EMC) Term used to describe the claim form that is sent via EDI.

Encoder A computer program utilized to assist with code assignment.

Facility charges Charges that represent cost and overhead for providing patient care services, including space, equipment, supplies, drugs and biologicals, and technical staff. Facility charges represent the technical component of the services.

Fee-for-service A reimbursement method that provides payment for hospital services based on an established fee schedule for each service.

Fee schedule A listing of established allowed amounts for specific medical services and procedures.

Flat rate A reimbursement method whereby the hospital is paid a set rate for a hospital admission regardless of charges accrued.

Form locator (FL) The name used to refer to each of the 81 fields (form locator(s) 1 through 81) on the UB-04.

Grouper A computer program utilized for the assignment of an MS-DRG or APC based on the information entered such as diagnosis, procedure, and other patient information like age, sex, and length of stay.

Health Care Common Procedure Coding System (HCPCS) The standard coding system used to report services and items to various payers. HCPCS consists of two levels: Level I, CPT codes, and Level II, Medicare National Codes.

Inpatient Prospective Payment System (IPPS) A Prospective Payment System established as mandated by the Tax Equity and Fiscal Responsibility Act (TEFRA) in 1983 to provide reimbursement for acute hospital inpatient services. The system implemented under IPPS is known as Medicare Severity Diagnosis Related Group (MS-DRG).

Medicare Severity Diagnosis Related Groups (MS-DRG) An Inpatient Prospective Payment System (IPPS) that is utilized by Medicare and other government programs to provide reimbursement for hospital inpatient services. The hospital is paid a fixed fee based on the severity of the patient's condition and relative treatment.

Outpatient Prospective Payment System (OPPS) Prospective Payment System implemented (effective August 2000) by CMS that provides reimbursement for hospital outpatient services. The system implemented under OPPS is known as ambulatory payment classification (APC).

Participating provider agreement A written agreement between the hospital and a payer that outlines the terms and specifications of participation for the hospital and the payer.

Patient invoice A document prepared by the hospital to advise the patient of an outstanding balance that includes details regarding current services. It is generally sent out the first time a balance is billed to the patient.

Patient statement A document prepared by the hospital that provides details regarding account activity, including the previous balance, recent charges, payments, and the current balance. The patient statement is generally sent monthly to notify the patient of a balance due.

Per diem A reimbursement method that provides payment of a set rate, per day to the hospital, rather than payment based on total charges.

Percentage of accrued charges A reimbursement method that calculates payment for charges accrued during a hospital stay. Payment is based on a percentage of approved charges.

Professional charges Charges that represent the professional component of patient care services performed by physicians and other non-physician clinical providers.

Prospective Payment System (PPS) A method of determining reimbursement to health care providers based on predetermined factors, not on individual services.

Reimbursement Term used to describe amount paid to the hospital by patients or third-party payers for services rendered.

Relative value scale (RVS) A reimbursement method that assigns a relative value to each procedure. It represents work, practice expense, and cost of malpractice insurance and is assigned to professional services.

Resource-based relative value scale (RBRVS) A payment method utilized by Medicare and other government programs to provide reimbursement for physician and some outpatient services. The RBRVS system consists of a fee schedule of approved amounts calculated based on relative values assigned to each procedure.

Revenue code A four-digit number assigned to each service or item provided by the hospital that designates the type of service or where the service was performed.

Third-party payer An organization or other entity that provides coverage for medical services, such as insurance companies, managed care plans, Medicare, and other government programs.

Usual, customary, and reasonable A reimbursement method whereby payment is determined by reviewing three fees: (1) the usual fee—the fee usually submitted by the provider of a service or item; (2) the customary fee—the fee that providers of the same specialty in the same geographic area charge for a service or item; and (3) the reasonable fee—the fee that is considered reasonable.

Chapter 6

Accounts Receivable (A/R) Management

The objective of this chapter is to provide an overview of patient account transactions and accounts receivable management. Hospitals provide services to patients for treatment of conditions utilizing highly specialized equipment and personnel. It is critical for hospitals to maintain an efficient cash flow by obtaining timely compensation for resources utilized in order to provide services in the hospital environment. Claim forms and patient statements are prepared to bill for services rendered on an outpatient and inpatient basis. Once the claim is submitted or patient statement is sent, the hospital must monitor outstanding accounts to ensure that payment is received within an appropriate time frame. This function is critical to maintaining a positive cash flow for the hospital. This chapter provides a brief overview of the life cycle of a hospital claim. A discussion of the payer's review of a claim and the remittance advice will provide an understanding of communications from the payer regarding a claim. Payer determinations are reviewed to provide an overview of issues handled by the Patient Financial Services and the Credit and Collection Departments. The chapter will close with a discussion of accounts receivable follow-up and the appeals process to provide a greater understanding of aspects involved in managing accounts receivable.

Chapter Objectives

- Define terms, phrases, abbreviations, and acronyms related to patient account transactions and accounts receivable follow-up.
- Demonstrate an understanding of the life cycle of a hospital claim.
- Discuss elements related to patient transactions.
- Provide an overview of key information found on an Explanation of Benefits or remittance advice.
- List common reasons for claim denials and delays.
- Demonstrate an understanding of A/R management.
- Provide an overview of the purpose and function of an accounts receivable report.
- Describe the process of monitoring and follow-up of outstanding accounts.
- Demonstrate an understanding of the appeals process.

Outline

Key Terms

Accounts receivable (A/R)
Accounts receivable (A/R) aging report
Accounts receivable ratio (A/R ratio)
Adjustment
Advance Beneficiary Notice (ABN)
Aging
Appeal
Balance billing
Clean claim
Contractual adjustment
CMS-1450 (UB-04)
CMS-1500
Days in accounts receivable (A/R)
Denied claim
Dun message
Electronic remittance advice (ERA)
Explanation of Benefits (EOB)
Fair Credit Billing Act
Fair Debt Collection Practices Act
Financial class
Hospital Issued Notice of Noncoverage (HINN)
Insurance claim tracer
Medicare Severity Diagnosis Related Groups (MS-DRG)
National Correct Coding Initiative (CCI)
Outstanding accounts
Payer data files
Pended claim
Prompt pay statutes
Rejected claim
Remittance advice (RA)
Statute of Limitations
Unbundling
Write-off

Acronyms and Abbreviations

ABN—Advance Beneficiary Notice
APC—Ambulatory Payment Classifications
A/R—Accounts receivable
CCI—National Correct Coding Initiative
CMS—Centers for Medicare and Medicaid Services
COB—Coordination of Benefits
EOB—Explanation of Benefits
EOMB—Explanation of Medicare Benefits
EMC—electronic media claim
ERA—electronic remittance advice
HIM—Health Information Management
HINN—Hospital Issued Notice of Noncoverage
MCE—Medicare Code Editor
MS-DRG—Medicare Severity Diagnosis Related Groups
OCE—Outpatient Code Editor
PFS—Patient Financial Services
RA—Remittance advice
TPP—third-party payer
UB-04—CMS-1450 Universal Bill implemented in 2007.

LIFE CYCLE OF A HOSPITAL CLAIM

The life cycle of a hospital claim begins when the patient arrives at the hospital for diagnosis and treatment of a condition(s) and ends when the claim is paid, as illustrated in Figure 6-1. As discussed in previous chapters, the Admissions Department is responsible for obtaining required demographic, financial, and insurance information from the patient. Another function that is equally important is obtaining appropriate referrals and authorizations. Information obtained by the Admissions Department is entered into the computer on the patient's account. Patient care services are rendered and documented by various departments within the hospital, and charges are generated. Most charges are posted at the department level through the chargemaster during the patient stay (Figure 6-2). Charges posted through the chargemaster are automatically dropped to the claim and submitted after the patient is discharged. Generally the hospital does not submit a claim or send a patient statement for inpatient services until after the patient is discharged. On discharge, the Health Information Management (HIM) Department receives the patient's chart for review and coding. The

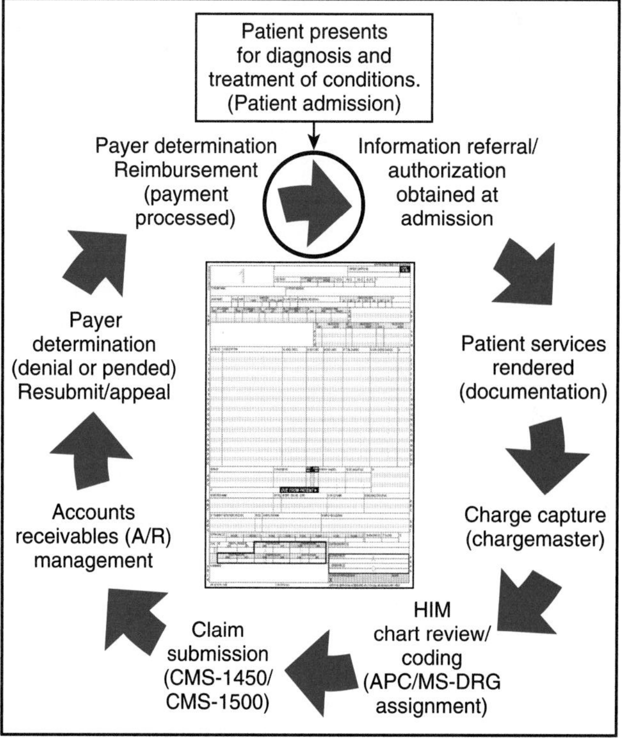

Figure 6-1 Life cycle of a hospital claim.

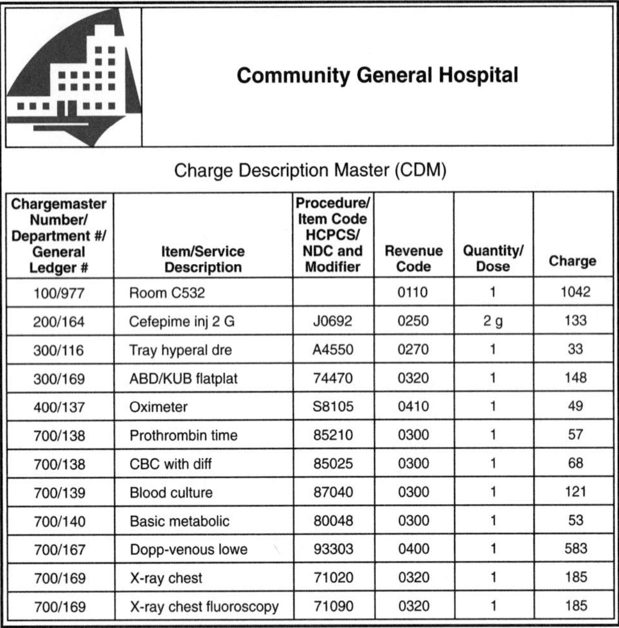

Community General Hospital

Charge Description Master (CDM)

Chargemaster Number/ Department #/ General Ledger #	Item/Service Description	Procedure/ Item Code HCPCS/ NDC and Modifier	Revenue Code	Quantity/ Dose	Charge
100/977	Room C532		0110	1	1042
200/164	Cefepime inj 2 G	J0692	0250	2 g	133
300/116	Tray hyperal dre	A4550	0270	1	33
300/169	ABD/KUB flatplat	74470	0320	1	148
400/137	Oximeter	S8105	0410	1	49
700/138	Prothrombin time	85210	0300	1	57
700/138	CBC with diff	85025	0300	1	68
700/139	Blood culture	87040	0300	1	121
700/140	Basic metabolic	80048	0300	1	53
700/167	Dopp-venous lowe	93303	0400	1	583
700/169	X-ray chest	71020	0320	1	185
700/169	X-ray chest fluoroscopy	71090	0320	1	185

Figure 6-2 Charge Description Master (CDM), commonly referred to as the chargemaster.

HIM Department codes services, procedures, and items that were not posted through the chargemaster, such as surgeries. The patient's diagnoses are also coded by the HIM Department. Coding is generally performed through an encoder program, which utilizes information entered by the HIM coder to assign procedure and diagnosis codes. The codes and other information entered are also used to assign Medicare Severity Diagnosis Related Group (MS-DRG) or Ambulatory Payment Classification (APC) to the hospital case.

BOX 6-1 ■ KEY POINTS

Hospital Encoder and Grouper Programs

An encoder program is computer software that allows the HIM professional to enter specified information regarding patient care services and the patient's condition. The program utilizes data entered to identify potential codes.

A Grouper program is software that allows the HIM professional to enter specified information regarding the patient's care including condition(s) and procedure(s). The program utilizes the information to assign MS-DRG or APC.

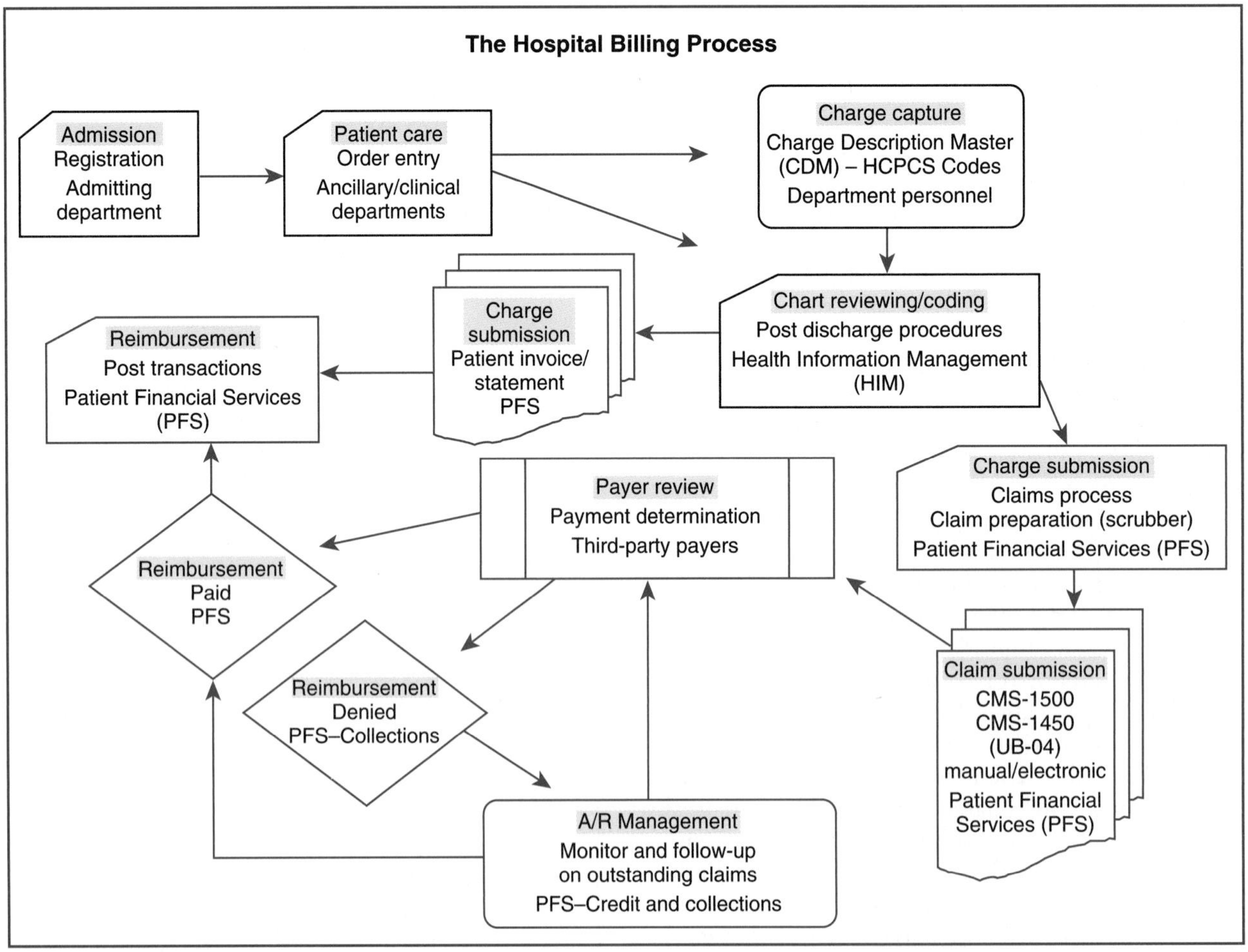

The Hospital Billing Process

Admission
Registration
Admitting department

Patient care
Order entry
Ancillary/clinical departments

Charge capture
Charge Description Master (CDM) – HCPCS Codes
Department personnel

Chart reviewing/coding
Post discharge procedures
Health Information Management (HIM)

Charge submission
Patient invoice/ statement
PFS

Reimbursement
Post transactions
Patient Financial Services (PFS)

Charge submission
Claims process
Claim preparation (scrubber)
Patient Financial Services (PFS)

Payer review
Payment determination
Third-party payers

Reimbursement
Paid
PFS

Reimbursement
Denied
PFS–Collections

Claim submission
CMS-1500
CMS-1450 (UB-04)
manual/electronic
Patient Financial Services (PFS)

A/R Management
Monitor and follow-up on outstanding claims
PFS–Credit and collections

Figure 6-3 Hospital billing process highlighting charge submission, payer review, A/R management, and reimbursement functions. *(Revision of illustration courtesy Sandra Giangreco.)*

HOSPITAL BILLING PROCESS

As discussed in previous chapters, the hospital billing process involves a series of functions required to submit charges for services rendered. The process involves collection of all financial, insurance, and medical information during the patient visit. Information obtained during the patient visit is utilized to submit charges to payers and patients. A critical part of the billing process is charge submission, which involves preparation of insurance claims and patient statements (Figure 6-3).

Insurance Claims and Patient Statements

Patient Financial Services (PFS) may also be referred to as the Business Office or the Patient Accounts Department. PFS is responsible for managing the hospital's patient financial transactions, which include charge submission, patient transactions, and accounts receivable (A/R) management. Charge submission involves preparation of insurance claims and patient statements (Figure 6-4).

BOX 6-2 ■ KEY POINTS

Hospital Billing Process

Patient admission
Patient care
Charge capture
Chart review/coding
Charge submission
A/R management
Payer processing and payment determination

BOX 6-3 ■ KEY POINTS

Patient Financial Services (PFS) Responsibilities

Charge Submission

- Insurance claim forms
- Patient statements

Patient Transactions

- Payments, adjustments, and write-offs

Accounts Receivable (A/R) Management

- Monitoring of and follow-up on outstanding accounts

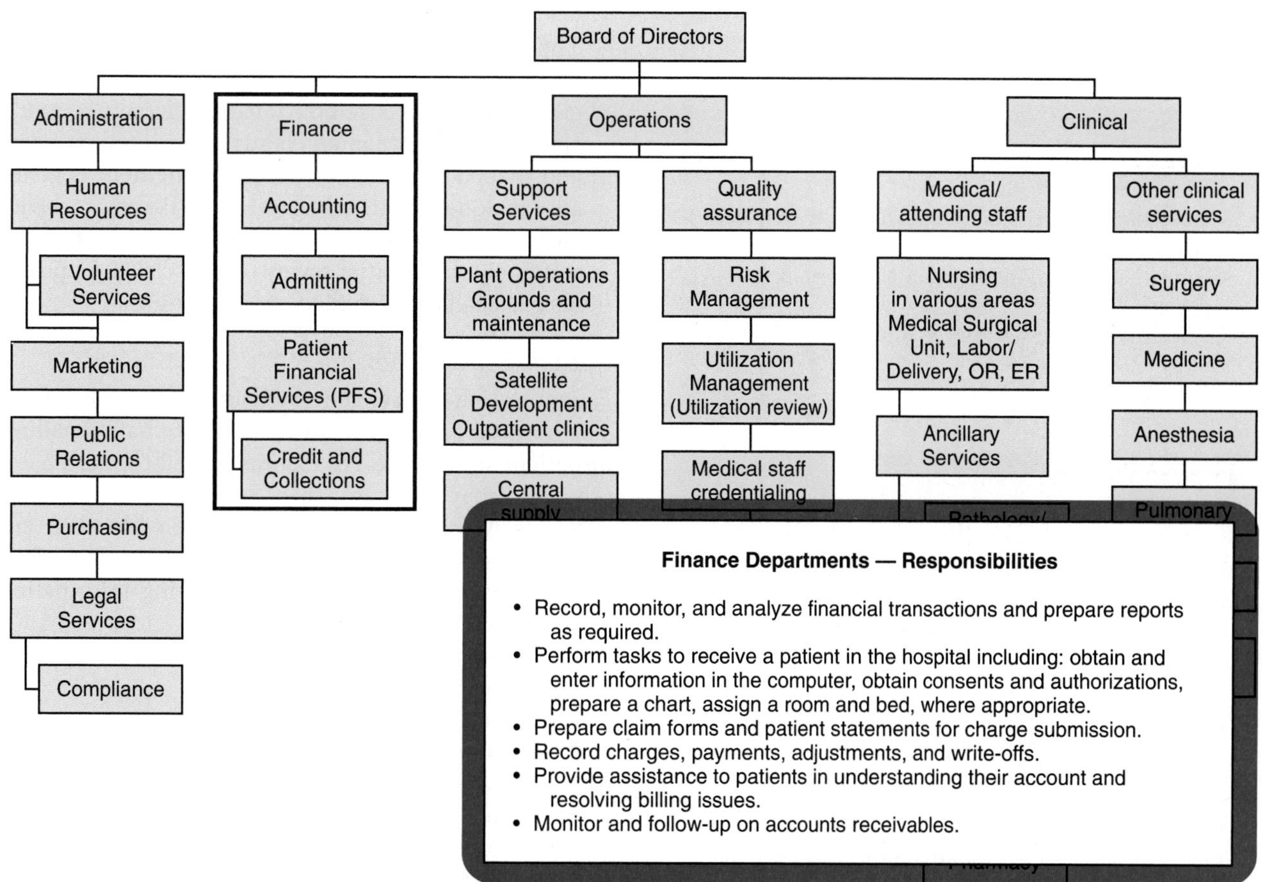

Figure 6-4 Hospital organizational chart illustrating the responsibilities of finance departments.

Insurance Claim Forms

A claim form is prepared for submission of charges to a third-party payer. The goal is to submit a clean claim the first time. A **clean claim** is defined as one that does not need to be investigated by the payer. The claim passes all internal billing edits and payer-specific edits and is paid without need for additional intervention. Claims that do not meet clean claim status may be denied, rejected, or pended. Preparation of insurance claim forms involves the following steps:

- A detailed itemized statement that outlines each item and service charged is prepared (Figure 6-5).
- The appropriate claim form is prepared. As discussed previously, claim form requirements vary by payer.
- The universally accepted claim form for submission of charges for physician and outpatient services is the **CMS-1500** (Figure 6-6).The **CMS-1450 (UB-04)** is the universally accepted claim used to submit facility charges for hospital outpatient and inpatient services (Figure 6-7).

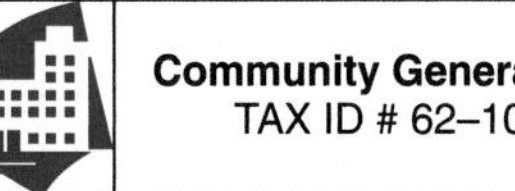

Community General Hospital
TAX ID # 62–1026428

8192 South Street
Mars, Florida 37373
(747) 722-1800

Detailed Itemized Statement

Patient no: 3611869
Med rec no: 17933398411
Patient: Smith, John

Bill date 12/1/06 Page 1
Admit date 11/27/06 Discharged 11/28/06
Bill type: Admit through discharge

Bill to:
Smith, John
7272 54th Street

Insurance: BC/BS P.O. Box 7272, Tampa, FL 34677

Date of Service	Charge-master #	Dept #	Revenue Code	HCPCS	Description	Qty/ Dose	Total Charges
11/27/2006	35466	0750	0250	33880551	Vistaril 25-100 mg inj	6	109.50
11/27/2006	35150	0750	0250	33820891	Docusate sodium	3	8.25
11/27/2006	32558	0750	0250	J3590	Cepacol loz	2	4.50
11/27/2006	35126	0750	0250	J1110	Diphenhydramine HCL	1	2.35
11/27/2006	34439	0750	0250	J2715	Demerol	2	21.70
11/27/2006	32444	0750	0250	J2250	Versed 1 mg/ml	1	19.50
11/28/2006	35422	0750	0250	Q0179	Zofran vial (inj) 2 mg	1	66.35
11/28/2006	35700	0750	0250	J3590	Percocet	14	63.00
11/28/2006	90850	0718	0270		Mini synder hemovac (JP)	1	31.00
11/28/2006	27907	0713	0300	80007	PA surgical profile	1	104.75
11/28/2006	27969	0713	0300	80058	PA liver profile	1	97.75
11/28/2006	59920	0780	0314	88304	P-gross & micro, diag sm	1	40.75
11/27/2006	2067	0770	0330	76000	XR fluro C-arm initial	2	464.00
11/27/2006	60006	0719	0360		OR time group VI	75	2514.00
11/27/2006	47070	0721	0370		Anesthesia	1	200.00
11/27/2006	85625	0720	0710		R-time recovery rm	60	346.80

Figure 6-5 Detailed itemized statement.

BOX 6-4 ■ KEY POINTS

Clean Claim

A claim that does not require further investigation by the payer. The claim passes all of the edits and is processed accordingly without any additional intervention.

Clean Claim Status

Examples of claims that do not meet clean claim status.

- Claims that require additional information
- Claims that require Medicare secondary payer (MSP) screening information
- Claims that require information to determine coverage
- Claims that do not pass payer edits

BOX 6-5 ■ KEY POINTS

Universally Accepted Claim Forms and Means of Submission

Claim Form

- CMS-1500 is the form utilized to submit physician and outpatient services
- CMS-1450 (UB-04) is the form utilized to submit facility charges for hospitals and other institutions

Methods for Submission

- Manual submission involves printing a paper claim that is sent by mail
- Electronic claims are submitted utilizing electronic data interchange (EDI)

- The claim forms are submitted to respective payers electronically or manually. Claim forms submitted electronically are referred to as electronic media claims (EMCs). Manual claims are printed on paper and mailed. A detailed itemized statement is generally included with paper claims. Payers receiving electronic claims may request a detailed itemized statement after initial review of the claim. Copies of insurance claims are filed for follow-up.

Patient Statements

Patient statements are generated and sent to the patient. The hospital generally has a schedule for batch mailings of patient statements. For example, the hospital's batch schedule may indicate that statements for patient accounts A to M should be mailed on Mondays and Wednesdays and N to Z on Tuesdays and Thursdays. Patient statements include the following information, as illustrated in Figure 6-8.

- Patient name, address, account number, and medical record number
- Admission and discharge date
- Description of services, including a procedure code and charge for each
- Payments and adjustments made on the account, listed along with the balance owed
- Message regarding outstanding balance or claim submission

1500
HEALTH INSURANCE CLAIM FORM
APPROVED BY NATIONAL UNIFORM CLAIM COMMITTEE 08/05

PICA | PICA | CARRIER

1. MEDICARE (Medicare #) | MEDICAID (Medicaid #) | TRICARE CHAMPUS (Sponsor's SSN) | CHAMPVA (Member ID#) | GROUP HEALTH PLAN (SSN or ID) | FECA BLK LUNG (SSN) | OTHER (ID)
1a. INSURED'S I.D. NUMBER (For Program in Item 1)
2. PATIENT'S NAME (Last Name, First Name, Middle Initial)
3. PATIENT'S BIRTH DATE MM DD YY SEX M F
4. INSURED'S NAME (Last Name, First Name, Middle Initial)
5. PATIENT'S ADDRESS (No., Street)
6. PATIENT RELATIONSHIP TO INSURED Self Spouse Child Other
7. INSURED'S ADDRESS (No., Street)
CITY STATE
8. PATIENT STATUS Single Married Other
CITY STATE
ZIP CODE TELEPHONE (Include Area Code) ( )
Employed Full-Time Student Part-Time Student
ZIP CODE TELEPHONE (Include Area Code) ( )
9. OTHER INSURED'S NAME (Last Name, First Name, Middle Initial)
10. IS PATIENT'S CONDITION RELATED TO:
11. INSURED'S POLICY GROUP OR FECA NUMBER
a. OTHER INSURED'S POLICY OR GROUP NUMBER
a. EMPLOYMENT? (Current or Previous) YES NO
a. INSURED'S DATE OF BIRTH MM DD YY SEX M F
b. OTHER INSURED'S DATE OF BIRTH MM DD YY SEX M F
b. AUTO ACCIDENT? YES NO PLACE (State)
b. EMPLOYER'S NAME OR SCHOOL NAME
c. EMPLOYER'S NAME OR SCHOOL NAME
c. OTHER ACCIDENT? YES NO
c. INSURANCE PLAN NAME OR PROGRAM NAME
d. INSURANCE PLAN NAME OR PROGRAM NAME
10d. RESERVED FOR LOCAL USE
d. IS THERE ANOTHER HEALTH BENEFIT PLAN? YES NO *If yes*, return to and complete item 9 a-d.

READ BACK OF FORM BEFORE COMPLETING & SIGNING THIS FORM.
12. PATIENT'S OR AUTHORIZED PERSON'S SIGNATURE I authorize the release of any medical or other information necessary to process this claim. I also request payment of government benefits either to myself or to the party who accepts assignment below.
SIGNED DATE
13. INSURED'S OR AUTHORIZED PERSON'S SIGNATURE I authorize payment of medical benefits to the undersigned physician or supplier for services described below.
SIGNED

PATIENT AND INSURED INFORMATION

14. DATE OF CURRENT: MM DD YY ILLNESS (First symptom) OR INJURY (Accident) OR PREGNANCY(LMP)
15. IF PATIENT HAS HAD SAME OR SIMILAR ILLNESS. GIVE FIRST DATE MM DD YY
16. DATES PATIENT UNABLE TO WORK IN CURRENT OCCUPATION FROM MM DD YY TO MM DD YY
17. NAME OF REFERRING PROVIDER OR OTHER SOURCE 17a. 17b. NPI
18. HOSPITALIZATION DATES RELATED TO CURRENT SERVICES FROM MM DD YY TO MM DD YY
19. RESERVED FOR LOCAL USE
20. OUTSIDE LAB? YES NO $ CHARGES
21. DIAGNOSIS OR NATURE OF ILLNESS OR INJURY (Relate Items 1, 2, 3 or 4 to Item 24E by Line)
1. 2. 3. 4.
22. MEDICAID RESUBMISSION CODE ORIGINAL REF. NO.
23. PRIOR AUTHORIZATION NUMBER

24. A. DATE(S) OF SERVICE From MM DD YY To MM DD YY	B. PLACE OF SERVICE	C. EMG	D. PROCEDURES, SERVICES, OR SUPPLIES (Explain Unusual Circumstances) CPT/HCPCS MODIFIER	E. DIAGNOSIS POINTER	F. $ CHARGES	G. DAYS OR UNITS	H. EPSDT Family Plan	I. ID. QUAL.	J. RENDERING PROVIDER ID. #
1								NPI	
2								NPI	
3								NPI	
4								NPI	
5								NPI	
6								NPI	

PHYSICIAN OR SUPPLIER INFORMATION

25. FEDERAL TAX I.D. NUMBER SSN EIN
26. PATIENT'S ACCOUNT NO.
27. ACCEPT ASSIGNMENT? (For govt. claims, see back) YES NO
28. TOTAL CHARGE $
29. AMOUNT PAID $
30. BALANCE DUE $
31. SIGNATURE OF PHYSICIAN OR SUPPLIER INCLUDING DEGREES OR CREDENTIALS (I certify that the statements on the reverse apply to this bill and are made a part thereof.)
SIGNED DATE
32. SERVICE FACILITY LOCATION INFORMATION a. NPI b.
33. BILLING PROVIDER INFO & PH # ( ) a. NPI b.

NUCC Instruction Manual available at: www.nucc.org
APPROVED OMB-0938-0999 FORM CMS-1500 (08-05)

Figure 6-6 CMS-1500 claim form utilized to submit charges for physician and outpatient services.

Third-Party Payer (TPP) Claim Processing

Third-party payer claim processing involves entering claim data into the payer's system, review of the payer's data file, performance of payer edits, and payment determination (Figure 6-9). Insurance claims can be transmitted electronically or sent by mail. Electronic claims are transmitted directly to the payer's computer system. Paper claims are scanned or entered manually into the payer's computer system. The payer's computer system performs a detailed review and electronic edits on each claim. The computerized review and edits are performed to check information on the claim for the purpose of identifying potential problems with the claim. First, the computer checks information on the claim against the payer's data files to verify patient coverage and eligibility. Then the payer's system performs computerized edits.

BOX 6-6 ■ KEY POINTS

Third-Party Payer Claim Processing

Claim data entered into payer system
Review of claim information
Payer edits
Payment determination

Payer's Data File

The computerized **payer data files** contain information regarding covered individuals, including a history of past claims submitted for the patient. Information submitted on the claim regarding the patient, the

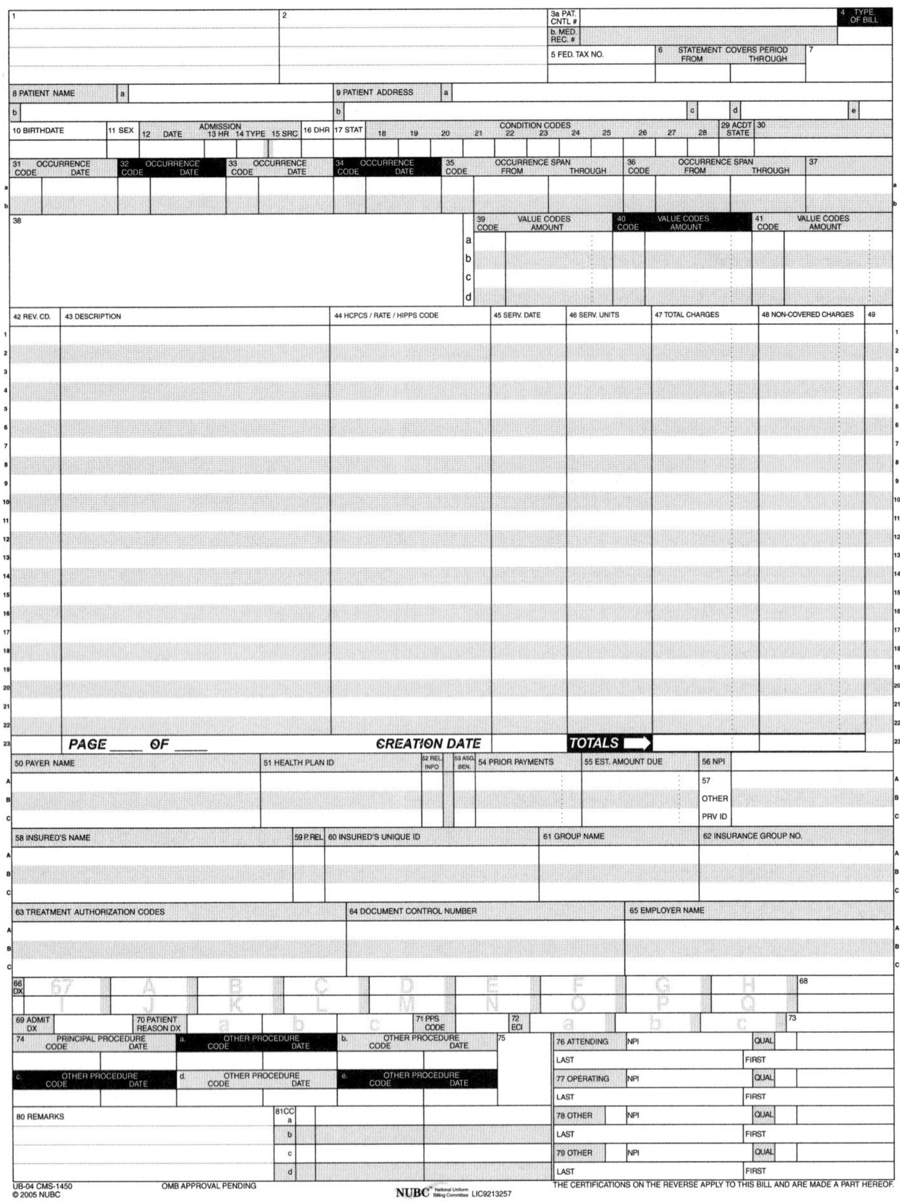

1 | 2 | 3a PAT. CNTL # | b. MED. REC. # | 4 TYPE OF BILL | 5 FED. TAX NO. | 6 STATEMENT COVERS PERIOD FROM THROUGH | 7

8 PATIENT NAME a b | 9 PATIENT ADDRESS a b c d e

10 BIRTHDATE | 11 SEX | ADMISSION 12 DATE 13 HR 14 TYPE 15 SRC | 16 DHR | 17 STAT | CONDITION CODES 18 19 20 21 22 23 24 25 26 27 28 | 29 ACDT STATE | 30

31 OCCURRENCE CODE DATE | 32 OCCURRENCE CODE DATE | 33 OCCURRENCE CODE DATE | 34 OCCURRENCE CODE DATE | 35 CODE OCCURRENCE SPAN FROM THROUGH | 36 CODE OCCURRENCE SPAN FROM THROUGH | 37

38 | 39 CODE VALUE CODES AMOUNT | 40 CODE VALUE CODES AMOUNT | 41 CODE VALUE CODES AMOUNT | a b c d

42 REV. CD. | 43 DESCRIPTION | 44 HCPCS / RATE / HIPPS CODE | 45 SERV. DATE | 46 SERV. UNITS | 47 TOTAL CHARGES | 48 NON-COVERED CHARGES | 49

1 2 3 4 5 6 7 8 9 10 11 12 13 14 15 16 17 18 19 20 21 22 23

PAGE ____ OF ____ CREATION DATE TOTALS

50 PAYER NAME | 51 HEALTH PLAN ID | 52 REL. INFO | 53 ASG. BEN. | 54 PRIOR PAYMENTS | 55 EST. AMOUNT DUE | 56 NPI | 57 OTHER PRV ID | A B C

58 INSURED'S NAME | 59 P.REL | 60 INSURED'S UNIQUE ID | 61 GROUP NAME | 62 INSURANCE GROUP NO. | A B C

63 TREATMENT AUTHORIZATION CODES | 64 DOCUMENT CONTROL NUMBER | 65 EMPLOYER NAME | A B C

66 DX | 67 A B C D E F G H I J K L M N O P Q | 68

69 ADMIT DX | 70 PATIENT REASON DX a b c | 71 PPS CODE | 72 ECI a b c | 73

74 PRINCIPAL PROCEDURE CODE DATE | a. OTHER PROCEDURE CODE DATE | b. OTHER PROCEDURE CODE DATE | 75 | 76 ATTENDING NPI QUAL LAST FIRST

c. OTHER PROCEDURE CODE DATE | d. OTHER PROCEDURE CODE DATE | e. OTHER PROCEDURE CODE DATE | 77 OPERATING NPI QUAL LAST FIRST

80 REMARKS | 81CC a b c d | 78 OTHER NPI QUAL LAST FIRST | 79 OTHER NPI QUAL LAST FIRST

UB-04 CMS-1450 © 2005 NUBC | OMB APPROVAL PENDING | NUBC National Uniform Billing Committee LIC9213257 | THE CERTIFICATIONS ON THE REVERSE APPLY TO THIS BILL AND ARE MADE A PART HEREOF.

Figure 6-7 CMS-1450 (UB-04) claim form utilized to submit facility charges for hospital services.

insurance, and the services billed is compared with information in the payer's data files to verify that the patient is covered under the plan, is eligible to receive benefits, and that all plan requirements are met. The following data are checked against the payer's data file:

- Patient name and identification number are checked to confirm that the patient is covered under the policy
- The date of service is checked to ensure that the services were provided within the benefit period and that the patient is eligible to receive benefits
- Preauthorization information is reviewed to ensure that plan requirements are met
- Dates of admission and discharge are checked against the plan coverage details to ensure that the length of stay is appropriate
- Procedure code data are reviewed to identify covered and noncovered items
- Services on the claim are also checked against the common data file to identify duplicate services

BOX 6-7 ■ KEY POINTS

Payer Data Files

Patient coverage is active.
Services were provided within coverage period and the patient is eligible to receive benefits.
Preauthorization requirements are met.
Length of stay is within plan criteria.
Services provided are covered and not duplicated.

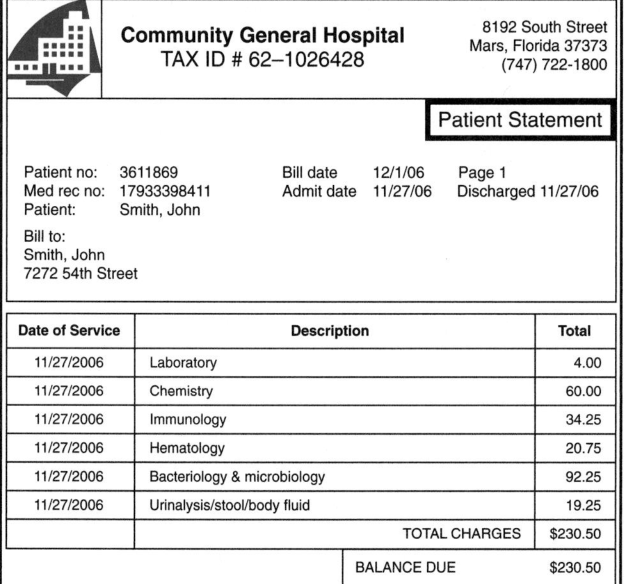

Community General Hospital
TAX ID # 62–1026428

8192 South Street
Mars, Florida 37373
(747) 722-1800

Patient Statement

Patient no: 3611869
Med rec no: 17933398411
Patient: Smith, John

Bill date 12/1/06
Admit date 11/27/06

Page 1
Discharged 11/27/06

Bill to:
Smith, John
7272 54th Street

Date of Service	Description	Total
11/27/2006	Laboratory	4.00
11/27/2006	Chemistry	60.00
11/27/2006	Immunology	34.25
11/27/2006	Hematology	20.75
11/27/2006	Bacteriology & microbiology	92.25
11/27/2006	Urinalysis/stool/body fluid	19.25
	TOTAL CHARGES	$230.50
	BALANCE DUE	$230.50

Figure 6-8 Sample patient statement.

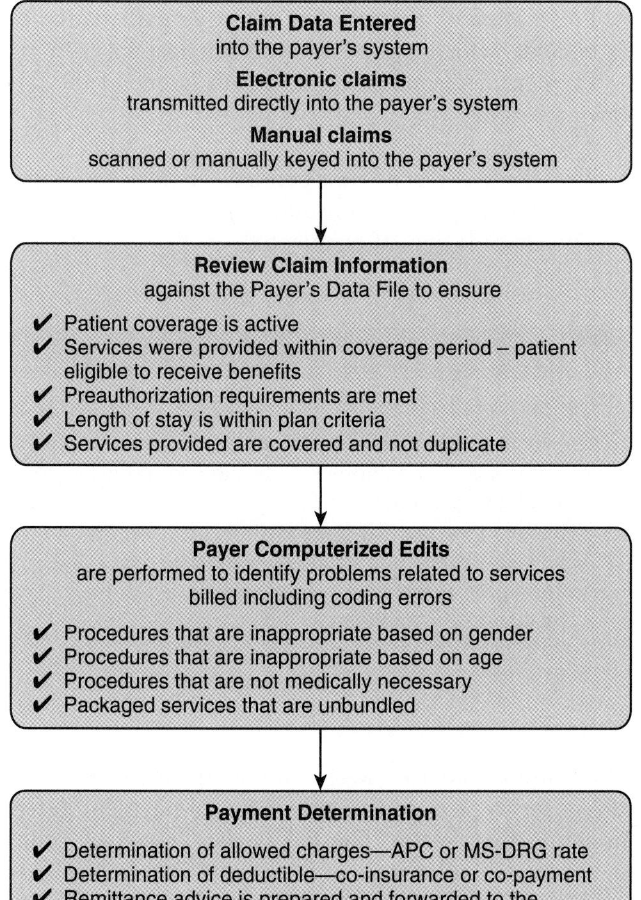

Figure 6-9 Phases of third-party payer claims processing include entering data, review of claim information, computerized edits, and payment determination.

Computer Edits

The payer's system performs computerized edits on the claim for the purpose of identifying problems relating to services billed such as coding errors or issues involving medical necessity. Payer computer edits vary according to the payer's criteria and system setup. For example, Medicare's system contains an Outpatient Code Editor (OCE) and a Medicare Code Editor (MCE). The OCE and MCE are used to identify data inconsistencies on hospital outpatient and inpatient claims. The OCE contains edits for hospital outpatient claims. The MCE contains edits for hospital inpatient claims (Figure 6-10). The following are examples of computer edits:

- Procedure conflicts with patient's sex. The procedure code is checked against the patient's sex to determine whether the procedure is appropriate. For example, a hysterectomy would not be performed on a male.
- Procedure conflict with patient's age. The procedure code is checked against the patient's age to verify that the procedure is age appropriate. For example, a hysterectomy would not normally be performed on a 10-year-old.

Medicare Outpatient Code Editor (OCE)	Medicare Code Editor (MCE)
Coding Edits ✔ Inpatient only procedure ✔ Invalid diagnosis or procedure code ✔ Age conflict ✔ Sex conflict ✔ Correct coding initiative edits **Coverage Edits** ✔ Non-covered procedures ✔ Questionable covered procedure **Clinical Edits** ✔ Invalid age ✔ Invalid sex **Claim Edits** ✔ Invalid date ✔ Date out of range ✔ Units of service edits ✔ Observation edits	**Inpatient Coding Edits** ✔ Invalid diagnosis or procedure code ✔ Invalid fourth or fifth digit for diagnosis codes ✔ E code used as a principal diagnosis ✔ Duplicate of the principal diagnosis ✔ Age conflict ✔ Sex conflict ✔ Manifestation code as principal diagnosis ✔ Nonspecific principal diagnosis ✔ Questionable admission ✔ Unacceptable principal diagnosis **Coverage Edits** ✔ Non-covered procedures ✔ Limited coverage ✔ Open biopsy ✔ Medicare secondary payer (MSP) alert **Inpatient Clinical Edits** ✔ Bilateral procedure ✔ Invalid age ✔ Invalid sex ✔ Invalid discharge status

Figure 6-10 Medicare Outpatient Code Editor (OCE) and Medicare Code Editor (MCE) computer edits are incorporated into Medicare's system. OCE is for outpatient claims, and MCE is for inpatient claims.

- Medical necessity. All services and items provided must be considered medically necessary to obtain third-party reimbursement. Diagnosis codes are checked against procedure codes to identify problems involving medical necessity.
- Bundled (packaged) services. Services and items billed are reviewed to identify cases of unbundling. **Unbundling** is the process of coding multiple codes to describe services that should be described with one code.

BOX 6-8 ■ KEY POINTS

Unbundling

The process of coding multiple codes to describe services that are described with one code. For example, reporting the following laboratory codes for three tests that were performed on one specimen at the same time.

- 82465, Cholesterol
- 83718, Lipoprotein
- 84478, Triglycerides

These tests should be reported as a Lipid Panel using CPT code 80061.

Many payers incorporate the National Correct Coding Initiatives edits into their system. The **National Correct Coding Initiative (CCI)** was developed by CMS for the purpose of promoting national coding guidelines and preventing improper coding. CCI outlines code combinations that are inappropriate (Figure 6-11).

National Correct Coding Intiative (CCI)

Symbol ■ Comprehensive versus component code
Misuse of column 2 with column 1

Column 1	Column 2
20605	J2001

Symbol ▼ Most extensive procedure

43632	43605

Symbol ✓ Mutually exclusive procedures

76856	76801

Symbol ✚ CPT/HCPCS coding manual guideline

87177	87015

Symbol ○ CPT separate procedure definition

91032	91000

Symbol ◆ CPT/HCPCS procedure code definitions

99218	99217

Symbol ❄ Standards of medical/surgical practice

G0101	99201

Figure 6-11 Examples of edits from the National Correct Coding Initiative (CCI).

BOX 6-9 ■ KEY POINTS

National Correct Coding Initiative (CCI)

Developed by CMS for the purpose of promoting national coding guidelines and preventing improper coding.

CCI outlines code combinations that are inappropriate, including services that are:

- Integral to a more comprehensive procedure
- Mutually exclusive
- Included in the surgical procedure
- Sequential procedures
- Bundled

Payment Determination

Determination of payment is conducted after the computer edits are performed. It includes the following steps:

- Determination of allowed charges, APC, MS-DRG rate
- Determination of deductible, co-insurance, or co-payment
- Preparation of a remittance advice or explanation of benefits, which is forwarded to the hospital

Payment determination may result in one of the following actions:

- The claim is paid
- The claim is placed in a pending or suspense status (pending requested information)
- The claim is denied or rejected

BOX 6-10 ■ KEY POINTS

Payer Payment Determination

Payment determination is conducted by the payer after the claim passes all computer edits and can result in one of the following actions.

- The claim payment is processed
- The claim is put in a pending status until requested information is received
- The claim is denied or rejected

Remittance Advice (RA)

A **remittance advice (RA)** is a document prepared by the payer to provide an explanation of payment determination for a claim. The RA is also known by other payers as an **Explanation of Benefits (EOB)** or Explanation of Medicare Benefits (EOMB). The RA includes detailed information about the charges submitted and an explanation of how the claim was processed. An RA can include information regarding several claims. It can be forwarded to the hospital electronically or it can be

TEST YOUR *Knowledge* BOX 6-1

LIFE CYCLE OF A HOSPITAL CLAIM; THIRD-PARTY PAYER CLAIM PROCESSING

1. Explain when the life cycle of a hospital claim begins.
2. Discuss the relationship between information obtained by the Admissions Department and the preparation of a claim form.
3. List the steps involved in processing a hospital claim form.
4. State what claim form(s) is used to submit facility charges for hospital outpatient and inpatient services.
5. Provide a brief overview of data found on a patient statement.
6. Discuss the purpose of checking claim information against the payer's common data file.
7. Explain the two types of review performed on a claim by the payer's computer system.
8. Explain the differences among the Medicare Code Editor (MCE), the Outpatient Code Editor (OCE), and the National Correct Coding Initiative (CCI).
9. State what items on the claim are checked to determine medical necessity.
10. List and discuss three steps in payment determination.

printed and sent to the hospital by mail. An **electronic remittance advice (ERA)** is a document that is electronically transmitted to the hospital to provide an explanation of payment determination for a claim.

BOX 6-11 ▪ KEY POINTS

Electronic Remittance Advice (ERA)

A document prepared by the payer to provide an explanation of payment determination for a claim. Also referred to as the following:
- Explanation of Benefits (EOB)
- Explanation of Medicare Benefits (EOMB)

Remittance Advice Data Elements

The design and content of an RA will vary by payer. Most include basic data regarding the patient, service provided, charges submitted, and explanation of the payment determination. Figure 6-12 illustrates the following data elements listed on a sample Medicare remittance advice:
- Date of the remittance advice and check number
- Patient's name and identification number
- Name of provider performing services, if not the same as the hospital
- Claim control number—a number given to the payer as a reference to the claim when the hospital inquires about a claim

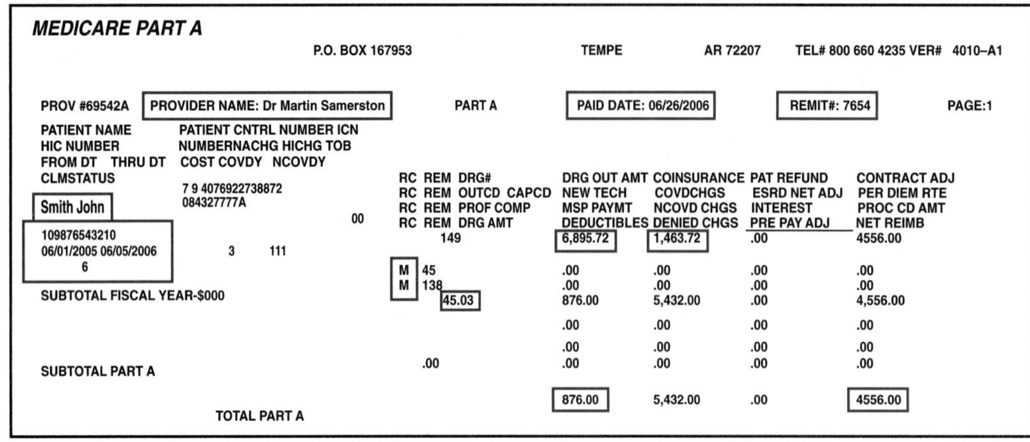
MEDICARE PART A
P.O. BOX 167953 TEMPE AR 72207 TEL# 800 660 4235 VER# 4010–A1

PROV #69542A PROVIDER NAME: Dr Martin Samerston PART A PAID DATE: 06/26/2006 REMIT#: 7654 PAGE:1

PATIENT NAME PATIENT CNTRL NUMBER ICN
HIC NUMBER NUMBERNACHG HICHG TOB
FROM DT THRU DT COST COVDY NCOVDY
CLMSTATUS

			RC REM DRG#	DRG OUT AMT	COINSURANCE	PAT REFUND	CONTRACT ADJ
	7 9 4076922738872		RC REM OUTCD CAPCD	NEW TECH	COVDCHGS	ESRD NET ADJ	PER DIEM RTE
Smith John	084327777A		RC REM PROF COMP	MSP PAYMT	NCOVD CHGS	INTEREST	PROC CD AMT
		00	RC REM DRG AMT	DEDUCTIBLES	DENIED CHGS	PRE PAY ADJ	NET REIMB
109876543210 06/01/2005 06/05/2006 6	3 111		149	6,895.72	1,463.72	.00	4556.00
			M 45	.00	.00	.00	.00
			M 138	.00	.00	.00	.00
SUBTOTAL FISCAL YEAR-$000			45.03	876.00	5,432.00	.00	4,556.00
				.00	.00	.00	.00
				.00	.00	.00	.00
SUBTOTAL PART A			.00	.00	.00	.00	.00
TOTAL PART A				876.00	5,432.00	.00	4556.00

Figure 6-12 Sample Medicare remittance advice (RA) illustrating data elements (page 1).

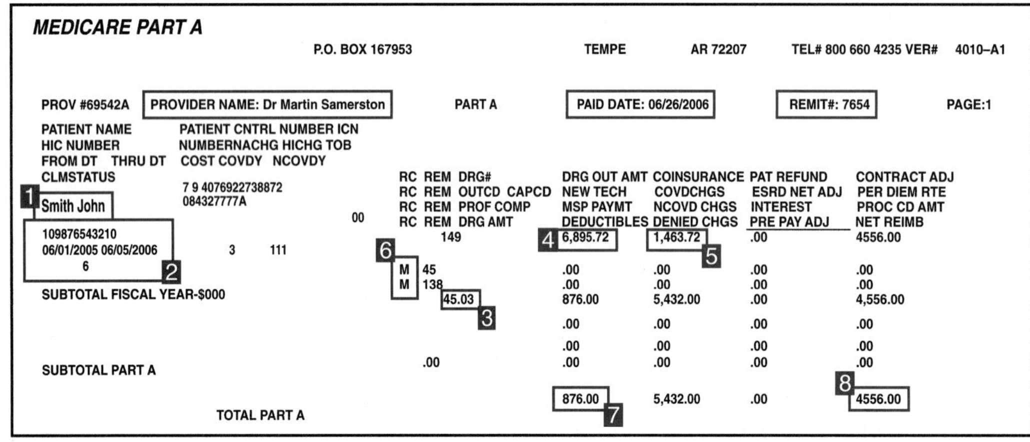
MEDICARE PART A
P.O. BOX 167953 TEMPE AR 72207 TEL# 800 660 4235 VER# 4010–A1

PROV #69542A PROVIDER NAME: Dr Martin Samerston PART A PAID DATE: 06/26/2006 REMIT#: 7654 PAGE:1

PATIENT NAME PATIENT CNTRL NUMBER ICN
HIC NUMBER NUMBERNACHG HICHG TOB
FROM DT THRU DT COST COVDY NCOVDY
CLMSTATUS

			RC REM DRG#	DRG OUT AMT	COINSURANCE	PAT REFUND	CONTRACT ADJ
	7 9 4076922738872		RC REM OUTCD CAPCD	NEW TECH	COVDCHGS	ESRD NET ADJ	PER DIEM RTE
1 Smith John	084327777A		RC REM PROF COMP	MSP PAYMT	NCOVD CHGS	INTEREST	PROC CD AMT
		00	RC REM DRG AMT	DEDUCTIBLES	DENIED CHGS	PRE PAY ADJ	NET REIMB
109876543210 06/01/2005 06/05/2006 6 2	3 111		6 149	4 6,895.72	1,463.72 5	.00	4556.00
			M 45	.00	.00	.00	.00
			M 138	.00	.00	.00	.00
SUBTOTAL FISCAL YEAR-$000			45.03 3	876.00	5,432.00	.00	4,556.00
				.00	.00	.00	.00
				.00	.00	.00	.00
SUBTOTAL PART A			.00	.00	.00	.00	.00
TOTAL PART A				876.00 7	5,432.00	.00	8 4556.00

Figure 6-13 Sample Medicare remittance advice (RA) (page 1) illustrating the steps (*1 through 8*) in analyzing a remittance advice.

- ICD-9-CM procedure or HCPCS codes and modifiers describing the billed services or items
- Explanation code or reason code that explains the claim processing, such as whether the claim is denied or reduced
- The amount of deductible the patient is responsible to meet
- The co-insurance amount the patient is responsible to pay
- The payment amount, which is the total amount paid for all claims outlined on the remittance advice

Analyzing a Remittance Advice

It is important for hospital billing professionals to understand the elements of an RA. Information on the RA is carefully analyzed to ensure that the claim was processed appropriately. This task is complicated by the fact that each payer may adopt a different type of form. Information on the RA is used to post payments to the patient's account. An RA may be several pages long, and it may contain information regarding several patients and several claims (Figures 6-13 and 6-14). Following is an overview of how to analyze the RA.

1. Identify the patient's name and number for the purpose of opening the correct patient account on the computer system.
2. Match the date of service on the RA to the date of service on the patient's account.
3. Compare the procedure code indicated on the RA with that listed on the patient's account to ensure that the claim was paid based on the correct service.
4. Review the charge billed on the RA against the charge listed on the patient's account.
5. Analyze the approved amount and noncovered charges. These amounts indicate what the payer is approving for the service. The payment is determined based on the approved amount.
6. An explanation of the approved amount is indicated using some type of coding system commonly referred to as explanation or reason codes. Definitions of the reason codes are listed on the bottom or the back of the RA, as illustrated in Figure 6-15. The reason X2 on the ABC Insurance RA tells the hospital that the allowed amount was determined based on the contract.

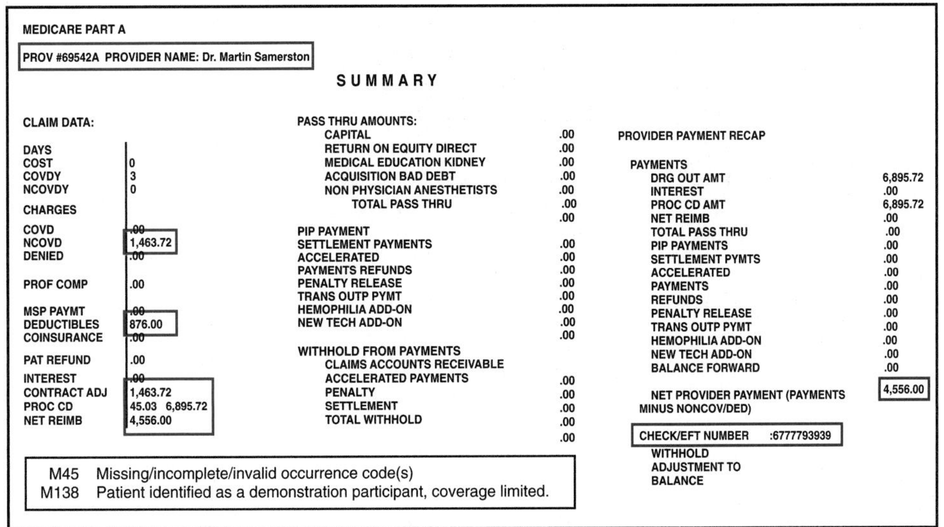

MEDICARE PART A

PROV #69542A PROVIDER NAME: Dr. Martin Samerston

SUMMARY

CLAIM DATA:	
DAYS	
COST	0
COVDY	3
NCOVDY	0
CHARGES	
COVD	.00
NCOVD	1,463.72
DENIED	.00
PROF COMP	.00
MSP PAYMT	.00
DEDUCTIBLES	876.00
COINSURANCE	.00
PAT REFUND	.00
INTEREST	.00
CONTRACT ADJ	1,463.72
PROC CD	45.03 6,895.72
NET REIMB	4,556.00

PASS THRU AMOUNTS:	
CAPITAL	.00
RETURN ON EQUITY DIRECT	.00
MEDICAL EDUCATION KIDNEY	.00
ACQUISITION BAD DEBT	.00
NON PHYSICIAN ANESTHETISTS	.00
TOTAL PASS THRU	.00
	.00
PIP PAYMENT	
SETTLEMENT PAYMENTS	.00
ACCELERATED	.00
PAYMENTS REFUNDS	.00
PENALTY RELEASE	.00
TRANS OUTP PYMT	.00
HEMOPHILIA ADD-ON	.00
NEW TECH ADD-ON	.00
	.00
WITHHOLD FROM PAYMENTS	
CLAIMS ACCOUNTS RECEIVABLE	
ACCELERATED PAYMENTS	.00
PENALTY	.00
SETTLEMENT	.00
TOTAL WITHHOLD	.00
	.00

PROVIDER PAYMENT RECAP	
PAYMENTS	
DRG OUT AMT	6,895.72
INTEREST	.00
PROC CD AMT	6,895.72
NET REIMB	.00
TOTAL PASS THRU	.00
PIP PAYMENTS	.00
SETTLEMENT PYMTS	.00
ACCELERATED	.00
PAYMENTS	.00
REFUNDS	.00
PENALTY RELEASE	.00
TRANS OUTP PYMT	.00
HEMOPHILIA ADD-ON	.00
NEW TECH ADD-ON	.00
BALANCE FORWARD	.00
NET PROVIDER PAYMENT (PAYMENTS MINUS NONCOV/DED)	4,556.00

CHECK/EFT NUMBER :6777793939

WITHHOLD
ADJUSTMENT TO
BALANCE

M45 Missing/incomplete/invalid occurrence code(s)
M138 Patient identified as a demonstration participant, coverage limited.

Figure 6-14 Sample Medicare remittance advice (RA) (page 2) illustrating claim data related to payment.

ABC Insurance

Claim #	Patient Name (ID Number)	Service Date	Procedure	Amount Billed	Amount Approved	Reason	Deductible	Coinsurance	Payment Amount
1	S. DAVIS 422-07-7904A	12 19 20XX	11020	$61.00	$43.30	X2	$0.00	$8.66	$34.64
2	X. PALATE 662-07-1234A	08 19 20XX	90050	$28.00	$25.00	X2 A1	$25.00	$0.00	$0.00
3	K. TELLAR 662-07-1234A	11 19 20XX	99205	$235.00	$152.00	Z90	$0.00	$30.40	$121.60
4	F. SIMPSON 662-07-1234A	10 19 20XX	99213	$125.00	$0.00	Z81	$0.00	$0.00	$0.00
			69210	$1,762.00	$1,533.00	X2	$500.00	$206.60	$826.40
5	H. DEAN 662-07-1234A	8 31 19 20XX	80053	$275.00	$175.00	X2	$0.00	$35.00	$140.00
			82247	$56.00	$0.00	X10	$0.00	$0.00	$0.00
			82310	$75.00	$0.00	X10	$0.00	$0.00	$0.00

Reason Codes
A1 - amount applied to deductible
X2 - allowed amount determined based on contract
X10 - payment reduced-test considered part of panel
Z81 - service bundled
Z90 - reduced payment-level of service not medically necessary

Figure 6-15 ABC Insurance remittance advice (RA) illustrating reason codes and their explanations.

7. Information on the RA regarding the deductible and co-insurance explains amounts that are billable to the patient.
8. The payment amount on the bottom of the page is the total payment for all claims listed on the RA.

BOX 6-12 ■ KEY POINTS

Patient Transactions

The Patient Financial Services (PFS) Department is responsible for posting transactions to the patient's account. Patient transactions include the following.

- Patient payments
- Third-party payer payments

The account balance will be billed to the patient (balance billing) when appropriate or to a secondary or tertiary insurance (secondary billing).

PATIENT TRANSACTIONS

The PFS Department is responsible for processing transactions including payments, adjustments, and other transactions to the patient's account. Patient payments and third-party payments are posted to the patient's account by PFS. The process followed is outlined below:

- Payment is posted to the patient's account
- A contractual adjustment is applied where applicable
- The balance is billed to the patient or sent to a secondary or tertiary payer when applicable
- Denials and information requests are researched and processed as appropriate
- If the claim is denied appropriately, the claim may need to be submitted to a secondary insurance

Patient Payments

Patient payments are posted to the patient's account when payment is received. The patient may pay the entire amount or part of the balance owed. When the entire amount is not paid, a statement reflecting the balance will be sent to the patient in the next billing period. Adjustments may be posted to the patient's account to reflect discounts or amounts that are uncollectible, as discussed later in this section.

Third-Party Payer Payments

Payments from third-party payers are posted to the patient's account when an RA and check are received from the payer. Payment on a claim is processed in accordance with the payer's determination. The payer may process payment for the claim as appropriate or the payment amount may be lower than expected by the hospital. This may occur when services are billed separately that are bundled or when medical necessity criteria are not met for a higher level of service. If the correct amount is not paid by the payer, a hospital representative will pursue correction of the claim.

Incorrect Payment Level

When the payer processes a claim at a reduced level or payment is not made for a service reported on the claim, a hospital representative must investigate the reason for the reduced payment or nonpayment. Common situations when a claim may be paid at a reduced level are outlined as follows:

- The diagnosis code(s) submitted does not meet medical necessity criteria for the service level billed
- Services are billed with more than one code when they should be described with a single code
- A service that is considered part of a more comprehensive service is billed separately

The ABC Insurance RA #1 illustrated in Figure 6-16 highlights a reduced payment situation. The RA reason, code Z81, indicates that the payer did not pay on procedure 99213, "Evaluation and Management" (E/M) service. The reason for nonpayment is that the payer considered the E/M to be part of the surgical package. The surgical package outlines services that are bundled into the surgery code.

The hospital cannot balance bill the patient for this amount if it participates with the insurance company. Upon investigation, it may be determined that the service should not have been considered part of the surgical package, and payment should have been made. If the E/M service was not related to the surgery or if the decision for surgery was made during the E/M service, the hospital may request that the claim be reprocessed with a modifier attached to the E/M code, or the hospital may appeal the claim.

BOX 6-13 ■ KEY POINTS

Common Reasons for Reduced Claim Payments

Level of service is not supported by the patient's condition

Service may be bundled, such as services included in the surgical package

Service may be considered an integral part of a larger procedure

ABC Insurance

Claim #	Patient Name (ID Number)	Service Date	Procedure	Amount Billed	Amount Approved	Note	Deductible	Coinsurance	Payment Amount
1	S. DAVIS 422-07-7904A	12 19 20XX	11020	$61.00	$43.30	X2	$0.00	$8.66	$34.64
2	X. PALATE 662-07-1234A	08 19 20XX	90050	$28.00	$25.00	X2 A1	$25.00	$0.00	$0.00
3	K. TELLAR 662-07-1234A	11 19 20XX	99205	$235.00	$152.00	Z90	$0.00	$30.40	$121.60
								Service bundled	
4	F. SIMPSON 662-07-1234A	10 19 20XX	99213	$125.00	$0.00	Z81	$0.00	$0.00	$0.00
			69210	$1,762.00	$1,533.00	X2	$500.00	$206.60	$826.40
5	H. DEAN 662-07-1234A	8 31 19 20XX	80053	$275.00	$175.00	X2	$0.00	$35.00	$140.00
			82247	$56.00	$0.00	X10	$0.00	$0.00	$0.00
			82310	$75.00	$0.00	X10	$0.00	$0.00	$0.00

Reason Codes

A1 - amount applied to deductible
X2 - allowed amount determined based on contract
X10 - payment reduced-test considered part of panel
Z81 - service bundled
Z90 - reduced payment-level of service not medically necessary

Figure 6-16 ABC Insurance remittance advice (RA) #1 highlighting a service the payer bundled into another service. The hospital cannot balance bill the patient for this amount if it participates with insurance.

Adjustments

An **adjustment** is the process of reducing the original amount charged by a specified amount. There are several types of adjustments that may be posted to a patient's account, such as discount, contractual adjustment, or write-off.

> **BOX 6-14 ■ KEY POINTS**
>
> **Adjustments**
>
> The original amount charged is reduced by a specified amount. Types of adjustments are as follows.
> - Discount
> - Contractual adjustment
> - Write-off

Discount

The original charge may be discounted by a specific amount as an agreement between the patient and the hospital. For example, a hospital may offer a discount to self-pay patients who are responsible for the entire hospital bill. The hospital may offer a 20% discount to the patient for payment of the entire balance. When the payment is received, the adjustment is made to the patient's account to reduce the original charge by the discounted amount.

Contractual Adjustment

A **contractual adjustment** is a reduction made to the original charge in accordance with the hospital's contract with a payer. Payer contracts include provisions regarding the amount the hospital is required to accept as payment in full, commonly referred to as the approved amount. The approved amount may represent a case rate, contract rate, MS-DRG or APC rate, or fee schedule amount. In accordance with the contract, the hospital agrees to follow those provisions and therefore may not bill patients for amounts over the approved amount. The difference between the approved amount and the hospital's original charge must be adjusted off the patient's account. The hospital posts a contractual adjustment to the patient's account to reduce the original charge. Most hospitals program the computer billing system to calculate and deduct the contractual amount as required by agreement with the payer.

The ABC Insurance RA #2 illustrated in Figure 6-17 highlights a contractual adjustment situation. The difference between the billed amount of $61.00 and the approved amount of $43.30 on claim number 1 is $17.70. A contractual adjustment in the amount of $17.70 must be posted to the patient account if the hospital is participating with the insurance company. The reduction of the claim by $17.70 is a contractual adjustment that is made in accordance with the hospital's contract with the payer.

Write-Off

A **write-off** is the process of reducing a patient's balance to zero. Write-offs are made when the balance is deemed uncollectible. In accordance with most contracts, the hospital is not allowed to forgive or write-off a patient deductible, co-insurance, and co-payment amount.

Contractual adjustment – $17.70
Difference between amount charged and approved amount

ABC Insurance

Claim #	Patient Name (ID Number)	Service Date	Procedure	Amount Billed	Amount Approved	Reason	Deductible	Coinsurance	Payment Amount
1	S. DAVIS 422-07-7904A	12 19 20XX	11020	$61.00	$43.30	X2	$0.00	$8.66	$34.64
2	X. PALATE 662-07-1234A	08 19 20XX	90050	$28.00	$25.00	X2 A1	$25.00	$0.00	$0.00
3	K. TELLAR 662-07-1234A	11 19 20XX	99205	$235.00	$152.00	Z90	$0.00	$30.40	$121.60
4	F. SIMPSON 662-07-1234A	10 19 20XX	99213 69210	$125.00 $1,762.00	$0.00 $1,533.00	Z81 X2	$0.00 $500.00	$0.00 $206.60	$0.00 $826.40
5	H. DEAN 662-07-1234A	8 31 19 20XX	80053 82247 82310	$275.00 $56.00 $75.00	$175.00 $0.00 $0.00	X2 X10 X10	$0.00 $0.00 $0.00	$35.00 $0.00 $0.00	$140.00 $0.00 $0.00

Reason Codes
- A1 - amount applied to deductible
- X2 - allowed amount determined based on contract
- X10 - payment reduced-test considered part of panel
- Z81 - service bundled
- Z90 - reduced payment-level of service not medically necessary

Figure 6-17 ABC Insurance RA #2 illustrating a contractual adjustment in the amount of $17.70 (the difference between the amount billed and the amount approved).

The hospital is required to follow the necessary steps required to make every attempt to collect the amount for which the patient is responsible. When all efforts are exhausted to collect the patient's responsibility, the hospital may then write-off the balance. These write-offs are considered a bad debt. Hospitals establish policies and procedures regarding write-offs that detail the necessary steps required to collect the patient balance and the criteria for write-offs.

Balance Billing

Balance billing refers to billing the patient for a balance in excess of the payer's approved amount in accordance with the payer contract. When the hospital is participating with the payer, the contractual agreement prohibits balance billing a patient for the following amounts:

- The difference between the original charge and the approved amount
- The amount of hospital charges that are greater than an MS-DRG payment rate
- The amount of hospital charges that are greater than an APC payment rate

The hospital is required to bill a patient for amounts related to co-payments, co-insurance, and deductible amounts. In some cases, charges for services that are not covered may also be billed. Medicare requires that beneficiaries be given an Advance notice of services that Medicare may not cover due to medical necessity. The notice required by Medicare is the Advance Beneficiary Notice (ABN) or Hospital Issued Notice of Noncoverage (HINN).

BOX 6-15 ■ KEY POINTS

Balance Billing

Law prohibits balance billing Medicare patients for the following amounts:

- The difference between the original charge and the approved amount
- The amount of hospital charges that are greater than a MS-DRG payment
- The amount of hospital charges that are greater than an APC payment

Advance Beneficiary Notice (ABN)

An **Advance Beneficiary Notice** is a written notice that is presented to a Medicare beneficiary before Medicare Part B services are furnished, to inform the beneficiary that the provider believes Medicare will not pay for some or all of the services to be rendered because they are not reasonable and necessary. Figure 6-18 illustrates Medicare's ABN. Hospitals are required to present this form for signature to the beneficiary before services are rendered. The hospital cannot bill the patient for these services if the ABN is not completed and on file.

Hospital Issued Notice of Noncoverage (HINN)

The **Hospital Issued Notice of Noncoverage (HINN)** is a written notice that is presented to a Medicare beneficiary before Medicare Part A services are furnished to inform the beneficiary that the provider believes that Medicare will not pay for some or all of the services to be rendered because they are not reasonable and necessary. The HINN is required by Medicare for hospital Part A services that may not be covered due to medical necessity. The HINN is written in letter form, and it must be presented and signed by the beneficiary before services are rendered. The content of an HINN varies based on the type of services that may not be covered; for example, an admission. Figure 6-19 illustrates a sample HINN.

Secondary Billing

Secondary billing may occur when the patient has a supplemental insurance that is designed to cover expenses not covered by the primary insurance. When payment is processed from the primary payer, the hospital representative may initiate billing to a secondary or tertiary payer. Coordination of Benefits (COB) provisions for the plan must be followed. Coordination of Benefits is a clause written into an insurance policy or government program that defines how benefits will be paid when the member or beneficiary is covered under multiple plans. Medicare secondary payer guidelines must also be followed. Coordination of benefits and Medicare secondary payer guidelines will be discussed later in this text in the payer chapters.

BOX 6-16 ■ KEY POINTS

Advance Beneficiary Notice (ABN) and Hospital Issued Notice of Noncoverage (HINN)

ABN

A written notice presented to a Medicare beneficiary before Part B services are furnished to inform the beneficiary that Medicare may not pay for some or all of the services to be rendered because they are not reasonable and necessary.

HINN

A written notice presented to a Medicare beneficiary before Part A services are furnished to inform the beneficiary that Medicare will not pay for some or all of the services to be rendered because they are not reasonable and necessary.

(A) **Notifier(s):**
(B) **Patient Name:** *(C)* **Identification Number:**

ADVANCE BENEFICIARY NOTICE OF NONCOVERAGE (ABN)

NOTE: If Medicare doesn't pay for ***(D)***_____________ below, you may have to pay.

Medicare does not pay for everything, even some care that you or your health care provider have good reason to think you need. We expect Medicare may not pay for the ***(D)***____________ below.

*(D)*_______________	***(E)* Reason Medicare May Not Pay:**	***(F)* Estimated Cost:**

WHAT YOU NEED TO DO NOW:

- Read this notice, so you can make an informed decision about your care.
- Ask us any questions that you may have after you finish reading.
- Choose an option below about whether to receive the ***(D)***_____________listed above.

  Note: If you choose Option 1 or 2, we may help you to use any other insurance that you might have, but Medicare cannot require us to do this.

***(G)* OPTIONS:** **Check only one box. We cannot choose a box for you.**
☐ **OPTION 1.** I want the ***(D)***__________ listed above. You may ask to be paid now, but I also want Medicare billed for an official decision on payment, which is sent to me on a Medicare Summary Notice (MSN). I understand that if Medicare doesn't pay, I am responsible for payment, but **I can appeal to Medicare** by following the directions on the MSN. If Medicare does pay, you will refund any payments I made to you, less co-pays or deductibles.
☐ **OPTION 2.** I want the ***(D)***__________ listed above, but do not bill Medicare. You may ask to be paid now as I am responsible for payment. **I cannot appeal if Medicare is not billed.**
☐ **OPTION 3.** I don't want the ***(D)***_________ listed above. I understand with this choice I am **not** responsible for payment, and **I cannot appeal to see if Medicare would pay.**

***(H)* Additional Information:**

This notice gives our opinion, not an official Medicare decision. If you have other questions on this notice or Medicare billing, call **1-800-MEDICARE** (1-800-633-4227/**TTY**: 1-877-486-2048).

Signing below means that you have received and understand this notice. You also receive a copy.

***(I)* Signature:**	***(J)* Date:**

According to the Paperwork Reduction Act of 1995, no persons are required to respond to a collection of information unless it displays a valid OMB control number. The valid OMB control number for this information collection is 0938-0566. The time required to complete this information collection is estimated to average 7 minutes per response, including the time to review instructions, search existing data resources, gather the data needed, and complete and review the information collection. If you have comments concerning the accuracy of the time estimate or suggestions for improving this form, please write to: CMS, 7500 Security Boulevard, Attn: PRA Reports Clearance Officer, Baltimore, Maryland 21244-1850.

Form CMS-R-131 (03/08) Form Approved OMB No. 0938-0566

Figure 6-18 Advance Beneficiary Notice (ABN), required for Medicare Part B services. *(From www.cms.hhs.gov.)*

ACCOUNTS RECEIVABLE (A/R) MANAGEMENT

Accounts receivable is a term used to describe revenue owed to the hospital by patients and third-party payers. Accounts receivable is commonly referred to as A/R. A/R management is a vital function required to monitor and follow-up on outstanding accounts. The financial stability of a hospital is highly dependent on maintaining a positive cash flow. The hospital must maintain a steady flow of revenue (income) to cover expenses required to provide patient care services. To accomplish this, the hospital monitors the revenue cycle. As illustrated in Figure 6-20, the hospital revenue cycle begins when the patient arrives at the hospital for patient care services and ends when payment is received. The primary objective of A/R management is to minimize the amount of time that accounts are outstanding. **Outstanding accounts** are accounts that have been billed to the patient or third-party payer but no payment has been recceived. A/R management involves tracking accounts that have not been paid, assessing action required to secure payment, and implementing procedures to secure payment.

Accounts Receivable (A/R) Reports

Hospitals utilize various computerized reports to monitor accounts that have not been paid, such as an unbilled accounts report, financial class report, denials management report, and accounts receivable aging reports.

COMMUNITY HOSPITAL
8192 South Street
Mars, Florida 37373
(747) 722-1800

HOSPITAL ISSUED NOTICE OF NONCOVERAGE (HINN)

December 15, 2005

Patient name: Zalma Jerzon
Address: 4949 South Street
Philadelphia, PA 72929

Admission Date: December 15, 2005 Health Insurance Claim (HIC) Number: 67945221
Attending Physician: Dr. Jason James

YOUR IMMEDIATE ATTENTION IS REQUIRED

Dear Ms. Jerson:

The purpose of this notice is to inform you that we find that your admission for (a total knee replacement) is not covered under Medicare for the following reason(s) MEDICAL NECESSITY. This determination was based upon our understanding and interpretation of available Medicare coverage policies and guidelines. You should discuss with your attending physician other arrangements for any further health care you may require. If you decide to (be admitted to/remain in) the hospital, you will be financially responsible for all customary charges for services furnished during the stay, except for those services for which you are eligible under Part B.

This notice, however, is not an official Medicare determination. The QIO Organization is the quality improvement organization (QIO) authorized by the Medicare program to review inpatient hospital services provided to Medicare patients in the State of (Pennsylvania), and to make that determination.

If you disagree with our conclusion: (Select as appropriate)
Preadmission:
- ☐ Request immediately, but no later than 3 calendar days after receipt of this notice, or, if admitted, at any point in the stay, an immediate review of the facts in your case. You may make this request through us or directly to the QIO by telephone or in writing to the address listed below.
- ☐ Admission:
- ☐ Request immediately, or at any point during your stay, an immediate review of the facts in your case. You may make this request through us or directly to the QIO by telephone or in writing to the address listed below.

If you do not wish an immediate review:
- ☐ You may still request a review within 30 calendar days from the date of receipt of this notice by telephoning or writing to the address specified below.

Results of the QIO Review:
- ☐ The QIO will send you a formal determination of the medical necessity and appropriateness of your hospitalization, and will inform you of your reconsideration and appeal rights.
- ☐ IF THE QIO DISAGREES WITH THE HOSPITAL (i.e., the QIO determines that your care is covered), you will be refunded any amount collected except for any applicable amounts for deductible, coinsurance, and convenience services or items normally not covered by Medicare.
- ☐ IF THE QIO AGREES WITH THE HOSPITAL, you are responsible for payment for all services beginning on December 15, 2005.

ACKNOWLEDGMENT OF RECEIPT OF NOTICE
This is to acknowledge that I received this notice of non-coverage of services from the Community Hospital on 12/15/04 at 8:35 a.m. I understand that my signature below does not indicate that I agree with the notice, only that I have received a copy of the notice.

(Signature of beneficiary or Representative) Date Time

cc: QIO and Attending Physician

Figure 6-19 Hospital Issued Notice of Noncoverage (HINN), CMS Hospital Manual required for Medicare Part A services. *(Modified from Centers for Medicare & Medicaid Services:* Hospital-issued notice of noncoverage, *www.cms.hhs.gov.)*

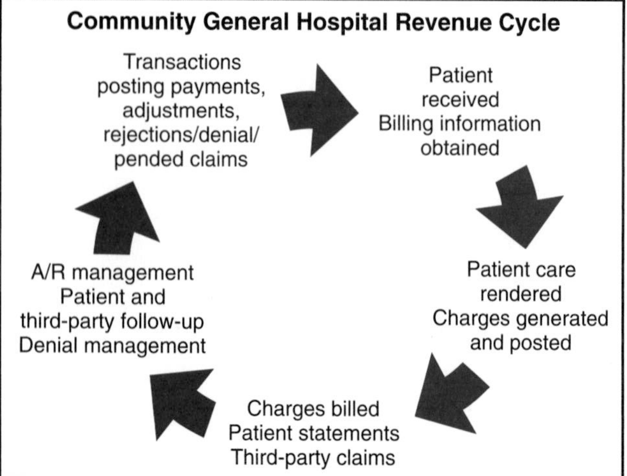

Figure 6-20 Hospital revenue cycle.

BOX 6-17 ■ KEY POINTS

Accounts Receivable (A/R) Management

Functions required to monitor and follow-up on outstanding accounts to ensure that reimbursement is received in a timely manner.

Accounts Receivable (A/R) Reports

UNBILLED ACCOUNTS
Listing of patient accounts that have not been billed

FINANCIAL CLASS
Outlines claim information such as charges, payments, and outstanding balances, grouped according to type of payer

DENIALS MANAGEMENT
Listing of claims that have been denied

ACCOUNTS RECEIVABLE (A/R) AGING
Outstanding accounts are categorized based on the number of days the balance is outstanding

Accounts Receivable (A/R) Aging Report

Computer-generated A/R aging reports are utilized to identify and analyze outstanding accounts. The **A/R aging report** is a listing of outstanding accounts based on the age of the account. The term **aging** refers to the number of days the account has been outstanding. The computer system counts the number of days the account is outstanding from the date the claim or statement is sent. A/R reports can be run for specified patient accounts or by payer type. The report categorizes accounts based on aging categories in increments of 30 days, as outlined below:

- 0 to 30 days
- 31 to 60 days
- 61 to 90 days
- 91 to 120 days
- 121 to 150 days
- 151 to 180 days

Table 6-1 illustrates an A/R aging report based on patient billed date. The report outlines outstanding accounts by patient and includes the account number, patient name, and phone number. Outstanding amounts owed on the patient account are reported in the column that reflects the aging category of the amount owed. Table 6-2 illustrates an A/R report based on payer type. Payer-based A/R reports outline outstanding accounts by payer and include the payer name, payer code, and phone number. Outstanding amounts are reported in the appropriate aging category. A/R reports provide a percentage of aging in each of the aging categories.

Hospital policies and procedures outline priorities for follow-up on outstanding accounts. Priorities are set based on two factors—the age and dollar amount of outstanding accounts. For example, the initial focus is

TABLE 6-1 Community General Hospital Patient A/R Report, December 30, 2005

				DAYS OUTSTANDING						
Account Number	**Name**	**Phone**	**Current**	**31-60**	**61-90**	**91-120**	**121-150**	**151-180**	**180+**	**Total Balance**
05962	Applebee, Carla	(813) 797-4545							724.45	724.45
23456	Borden, Andrew	(813) 423-9678		200.00			47.52			247.52
16955	Cox, Anthony	(813) 233-7794	175.00		695.00		199.53			1069.53
14355	Freeman, Tina	(727) 665-7878					592.14			592.14
00876	Holtsaver, Marshall	(727) 874-2945	485.72		400.00				1583.66	2469.38
00023	James, John	(813) 201-2054			350.00		963.68			1313.68
10245	Marcus, Xavier	(727) 779-3325		2745.21						2745.21
19457	Peters, Samantha	(413) 544-2243			1545.23		1022.69			2567.92
99645	Snowton, Michael	(941) 333-4325			1314.00	3254.00				4568.00
	Report Totals		660.72	2945.21	4304.23	3254	2825.56	0	2308.11	16297.83
	% Aged		4.05%	18.07%	26.41%	19.97%	17.34%	0.00%	14.16%	

typically directed toward accounts that fall within the 61- to 90-day aging category, then the 91- to 120-day category, and then 120+ days. Accounts with large balances are generally considered a priority. Hospitals utilize the A/R ratio and the days in A/R formula to assess the efficiency of A/R management activity, as illustrated in Figure 6-21.

Denials Management Report

Denials management reports are utilized to identify claims that have been denied, rejected, or pended. Claims identified with this report are investigated to determine why the claim was denied, rejected, or pended (Table 6-3).

Financial Class Reports

Hospitals utilize financial class reports to identify outstanding accounts based on the type of payer, or financial class. A **financial class** is a classification system used to categorize accounts by payer types. A financial class is assigned to all hospital accounts to identify the type of payer. For example, a patient who has a commercial insurance plan would be assigned to the financial class "Commercial." Financial classes may also be referred to as financial buckets. Common financial classes are Commercial, Blue Cross/Blue Shield, Medicaid, Medicare, TRICARE, Auto, and Worker's Compensation. Managed care plans may also be assigned a separate financial class of "Managed Care." Designation of a financial class allows detailed tracking and reporting of charges, payments, and outstanding balances per payer type, as illustrated in Table 6-4. Financial class reports help to identify payer-specific problems with outstanding claims for each financial class.

Unbilled Accounts Report

Unbilled accounts reports are utilized to track accounts that have not been billed since the patient was discharged. This report is utilized to identify reasons why accounts are not billed (Table 6-5). Some common reasons an account may be in an unbilled status are as follows:

- The claim is on hold. The claim may be on hold pending insurance verification or authorization. Insurance companies will not pay if the patient is not covered or if the appropriate authorizations have not been obtained. Managers will identify problems that cause delays in obtaining verifications or authorization and implement systems to correct the problems.

TEST YOUR *Knowledge* BOX 6-2

REMITTANCE ADVICE (RA); PATIENT TRANSACTIONS

1. Define an electronic remittance advice.
2. List various names used to describe the document provided by the payer that explains how a claim was processed.
3. Explain the process of posting patient and third-party payments to the patient's account by the PFS.
4. Explain why it is important to compare the procedures listed in a remittance advice with those listed on the patient's account.
5. Describe the purpose of reason codes.
6. List common reasons why a payer may process payment at an incorrect level.
7. Discuss why it is important for a hospital representative to analyze payment made by an insurance company.
8. Outline the actions required when payment is received at the incorrect level.
9. Provide an explanation of an adjustment.
10. List three types of adjustments a hospital may make to a patient's account.
11. Describe contractual adjustment and explain when this type of adjustment is made to a patient account.
12. State when a hospital may write off a balance.
13. Provide a brief explanation of balance billing.
14. Explain the purpose of an ABN.
15. Discuss the difference between an ABN and an HINN.

TABLE 6-2 **Community General Hospital Third-Party Payer A/R Report, December 30, 2005**

				DAYS OUTSTANDING						
Payer	**Payer Code**	**Phone**	**Current**	**31-60**	**61-90**	**91-120**	**121-150**	**151-180**	**180+**	**Balance**
Aetna	AETNA	(800) 797-4545							724.45	724.45
BlueCross/ Blue Shield	BCBS	(800) 423-9678		24224.34	29666.59	45987.65	32456.78	15765.12	27459.44	175559.92
Champus	CHMPV	(800) 233-7794	6759.25		695.00		199.53			7653.78
Fed Emp Trust	FET	(800) 665-7878					592.14			592.14
Medicaid	MDCD	(800) 874-2945	2459.32	1456.00	14245.00	11727.00	1600.00	792.80	1435.00	33715.12
Medicare	MDCR	(800) 201-2054	34567.00	52000.00	37456.32	64456.00	60797.00	45511.00	27564.88	322352.2
Metropolitan	MET	(800) 779-3325		16453.22	274.00	6400.00	7329.00	14676.11	22453.29	67585.62
Nationwide	NAT	(800) 544-2243			1545.23		1022.69			2567.92
Workers Comp	WCMP	(800) 333-4325	6600.00	47243.00	82899.00	3254.00	64222.00	24214.55	17243.56	245676.11
	Report Totals		50385.57	141376.56	166781.14	131824.65	168219.14	100959.58	6880.62	856427.26
	% Aged		5.88%	16.51%	19.47%	15.39%	19.64%	0.00%	14.16%	

A/R Ratio

The A/R ratio is a formula that calculates the percentage of accounts receivables in comparison with total charges.

Total charges − net collections = A/R
A/R ÷ average monthly charges = A/R ratio

Days in A/R

Days in A/R is another formula used to determine the number of days it takes to collect outstanding accounts.

Average monthly charges ÷ by 30 = average daily charges
Total A/R ÷ by average daily charges = days in A/R

Figure 6-21 Formulas used to assess accounts receivable mangement activity. A/R ratio and days in A/R.

- Chargemaster data are inaccurate. Hospitals continually monitor chargemaster data to ensure that the correct information is listed in the chargemaster. For example, Medicare requires HCPCS level II codes for specific services. The chargemaster may not have all the current codes listed.
- Coding from the medical record may be delayed due to incomplete documentation. Claims cannot be submitted without diagnosis and procedure codes. The HIM Department may have to seek clarification of information in the medical record to code the case accurately.
- Errors may have been made in entering data. Incorrect data such as the wrong patient identification number or codes can delay claim submission.

BOX 6-18 ■ KEY POINTS

Unbilled Accounts

Common reasons that accounts are unbilled:
- Pending insurance verification
- Incorrect chargemaster data
- Delayed coding
- Data entry errors

Accounts Receivable (A/R) Procedures

Hospitals establish policies and procedures for A/R follow-up to ensure that payment is received within an appropriate time frame. Basic procedures for monitoring and follow-up include identifying accounts that are outstanding. Hospital procedures outline specific guidelines on actions required to pursue payment on accounts that are outstanding, including lost, denied, rejected, and pended claims. The next section outlines procedures to follow to secure payments in these situations.

BOX 6-19 ■ KEY POINTS

A/R Procedures

Hospitals establish policies and procedures for accounts receivable follow-up activities involving the types of following claims:
- Lost
- Rejected
- Denied
- Pended

TABLE 6-3 Community General Hospital
Denial Management Report, 01/01/06 to 06/30/06

Denial Code	Patient Name	Service Date	Total Charges	Payment	Action Code 1	Status Code
19 WK IN	Harold, A	02/02/2006	$1,356.50	$0.00	CO INQ	PEND
19 WK IN	Sanders, P	03/17/2006	$27,865.00	$0.00	CO INQ	PEND
19 WK IN	Thomas, J	06/22/2006	$42,677.97	$0.00	CO INQ	PEND
19 WK IN	Peters, X	02/25/2006	$18,433.56	$0.00	CO INQ	RESUB
19 WK IN	Hanson, T	05/31/2006	$879.97	$0.00	CO INQ	APPEAL
31 PTNCOV	Martel, B	06/22/2006	$42,677.97	$0.00	LTR	PEND INS
31 PTNCOV	Morris, B	03/17/2006	$27,865.00	$0.00	LTR	PEND INS
31 PTNCOV	Hanna, J	02/25/2006	$18,433.56	$0.00	LTR	PEND INS
31 PTNCOV	Halbert, A	02/02/2006	$1,356.50	$0.00	LTR	PEND INS
31 PTNCOV	Yandic, M	05/31/2006	$879.97	$0.00	LTR	PEND INS
39 AUTH RQ	Steff, H	02/02/2006	$572.00	$0.00	OB AU	REQ AUTH
39 AUTH RQ	Albert, A	03/17/2006	$877.97	$0.00	OB AU	REQ AUTH
39 AUTH RQ	Baxter, M	06/22/2006	$256.34	$0.00	OB AU	REQ AUTH
39 AUTH RQ	Parcon, M	02/25/2006	$72.82	$0.00	OB AU	NO AUTH
39 AUTH RQ	Smith, J	05/31/2006	$10,423.00	$0.00	OB AU	RESUB WA

TABLE 6-4 Community General Hospital
Payer Financial Class Report, 01/01/06 to 06/30/06

Financial Class	Patient Name	Service Date	Total Charges	Payment	Contractual Adjustment	Balance
01 BC/BS	Adams, Harold	02/02/2006	$1,356.50	$868.16	$271.30	$217.04
	Boyter, Susan	03/17/2006	$27,865.00	$17,833.60	$5,573.00	$4,458.40
	Johns, Tina	06/22/2006	$42,677.97	$27,313.90	$8,535.59	$6,828.48
	Xavier, George	02/25/2006	$18,433.56	$11,797.48	$3,686.71	$2,949.37
	Yohanson, Phil	05/31/2006	$879.97	$563.18	$175.99	$140.80
02 Commercial	Beard, Bobby	06/22/2006	$42,677.97	$27,313.90	$8,535.59	$6,828.48
	Baxter, Morris	03/17/2006	$27,865.00	$17,833.60	$5,573.00	$4,458.40
	James, John	02/25/2006	$18,433.56	$11,797.48	$3,686.71	$2,949.37
	Hatley, Hanna	02/02/2006	$1,356.50	$868.16	$271.30	$217.04
	Mannie, Minnie	05/31/2006	$879.97	$563.18	$175.99	$140.80
03 Medicaid	Harold, Adam	02/02/2006	$572.00	$171.60	$400.40	$0.00
	Harpo, Harold	03/17/2006	$877.97	$0.00	$614.58	$263.39
	Morris, Baxter	06/22/2006	$256.34	$76.90	$179.44	$0.00
	Polo, Marco	02/25/2006	$72.82	$0.00	$50.97	$21.85
	Smith, Ima	05/31/2006	$10,423.00	$0.00	$7,296.10	$3,126.90
04 Medicare	Anson, Annie	02/02/2006	$1,356.50	$868.16	$271.30	$217.04
	Chan, William	02/25/2006	$18,433.56	$11,797.48	$3,686.71	$2,949.37
	Cater, Cody	03/17/2006	$27,865.00	$17,833.60	$5,573.00	$4,458.40
	Janson, Jonnie	05/31/2006	$879.97	$563.18	$175.99	$140.80
	Williams, Meta	06/22/2006	$42,677.97	$27,313.90	$8,535.59	$6,828.48

TABLE 6-5 **Community General Hospital Unbilled Accounts Report, 07/01/06 to 07/31/06**

Account Number	Patient Name	Service Date	Total Charges	Service Code	Account Balance	Status
825473	Adams, Harold	02/02/2006	$1,356.50	OUTSUR	$271.30	SECINS
649782	Boyter, Susan	03/17/2006	$27,865.00	INPT	$5,573.00	MR INFO
215673	Johns, Tina	06/22/2006	$42,677.97	INPT	$8,535.59	SECINS
692777	Xavier, George	02/25/2006	$18,433.56	INPT	$3,686.71	APPEAL
625713	Yohanson, Phil	05/31/2006	$879.97	ANC	$175.99	ADD
228792	Beard, Bobby	06/22/2006	$42,677.97	INPT	$42,677.97	MR COMP
664392	Baxter, Morris	03/17/2006	$27,865.00	INPT	$27,865.00	MR COMP
865312	James, John	02/25/2006	$18,433.56	INPT	$18,433.56	PHY
296454	Hatley, Hanna	02/02/2006	$1,356.50	ER	$1,356.50	AUTH
572658	Mannie, Minnie	05/31/2006	$879.97	ANC	$879.97	AUTH

Community General Hospital Procedures – Accounts Receivable

Lost Claim

Payer has no receipt of claim on file

Submit copy of the original claim

Rejected Claim

Payer rejected the claim due to technical error or other reason it could not be processed

Investigate reason for rejection of correct claim and resubmit

Denied Claim

Payer denied the entire claim or specified charges on the claim

Investigate reason for denial and submit an appeal where appropriate

Pended Claim

Payer placed claim in a "suspended" hold status pending additional information

Obtain copies of information from the patient record and submit to the payer

Figure 6-22 Hospital accounts receivable (A/R) procedures for lost, denied, rejected, and pended claims.

LOST, REJECTED, DENIED, AND PENDED CLAIMS

Payment determination for a claim may result in the claim being rejected or denied. The payer may also place the claim in a pending status and request more information for the claim. These situations are handled in accordance with hospital policy, as outlined below (Figure 6-22).

Lost Claim

The follow-up on a claim may result in the payer indicating that the claim is not on file. This happens when the claim was not received by the payer or when the claim was not entered as a result of a backlog in processing claims. If the claim is not on file and there is no backlog, the hospital representative should submit a copy of the original claim to the payer. Many payers require a note indicating the claim is a copy of an original claim and the date the claim was originally submitted. It is important to remember that payers require claims to be submitted within specified time periods known as the timely filing period. For this reason, it is critical to ensure that lost claim issues are resolved and receipt of the claim is acknowledged by the payer within the timely filing period.

Rejected Claim

A **rejected claim** is a claim that is returned to the hospital by the payer because the claim contained a technical error or could not be processed because it was not completed in accordance with payer guidelines. Outlined below are circumstances when claims are rejected.

- The patient identification number on the claim does not match a patient listed in the payer's data file.
- Diagnosis or procedure codes do not match the payer's data file.
- The place of service, date of service, or provider number are not valid or do not match the payer's data files.

The PFS and Credit and Collection Departments are responsible for investigating reasons for claim rejections to determine whether the claim was rejected appropriately (see Figure 6-22). If it is found during the investigation that the reason for rejection is inaccurate, the claim may be corrected and resubmitted. For example, a claim may be rejected with an indication that no patient with the identification number 6597732 is covered by the plan. On investigation, it is determined that the correct identification number for the patient is 6997732. The correction is made in the system, and the claim can be resubmitted.

BOX 6-20 ■ KEY POINTS

Claim Rejections

Common reasons for claim rejections:
- Incorrect or missing patient identification number
- Incorrect or missing diagnosis or procedure codes
- The place of services is invalid or not indicated
- Incorrect format for the date of service
- Incorrect or missing provider number

Denied Claim

A **denied claim** is a claim processed by the payer resulting in a determination that no payment will be made on the claim. A claim submitted to a payer may be denied entirely or a specific charge on the claim may be denied. Claim denials are communicated on the RA that is forwarded to the hospital. A claim may be denied for various reasons. Some common circumstances where a claim can be denied are outlined below:
- The diagnosis code submitted does not meet medical necessity criteria
- Services submitted were unbundled
- Required authorization was not obtained

Claim denials must also be investigated to determine whether the denial is appropriate. Upon investigation, the hospital representative may find that the reason for denial is not valid. For example, a claim may be denied stating that the required authorizations were not obtained. Review of the patient record indicates that an authorization was obtained for the service and an authorization number was provided by the payer's representative. The claim may be resubmitted or appealed with the authorization number recorded in the patient's file.

BOX 6-21 ■ KEY POINTS

Claim Denials

Common reasons for claim denials:
- Medical necessity criteria not met
- Procedure is bundled in a more comprehensive procedure
- Service was not authorized

Pended Claim

A **pended claim** is a claim that is placed on hold by the payer, pending receipt of additional information. When payers identify a potential problem with medical necessity or coverage, based on the claim review, they may request additional information and put the claim in a pending status or what is commonly referred to as a "suspended claim." The claim is put on hold until the information requested is received. The request for additional information is usually communicated on the RA that is sent to the hospital along with an indication that payment cannot be processed until the requested information is received. The requested information should be copied from the patient's medical record and forwarded to the payer.

COLLECTION ACTIVITIES

Collection activities are vital functions performed by the hospital Credit and Collections Department to ensure that timely payments are received from patients and third-party payers. Hospital policies and procedures for collections vary by hospital; however, they generally include the following, as outlined in Figure 6-23:
- Collection activity priorities
- Patient and third-party payer follow-up procedures
- Procedures for uncollected accounts
- Insurance commissioner inquiries

Community General Hospital Policies and Procedures
Collection Activities

Section I
Collection Activity Priorities
- Age status
- Account balance

Section II
Patient Follow-up Procedures
- Written follow-up
- Phone contact
- Problem resolution

Third-party Payer Follow-up Procedures
- Written follow-up
- Phone contact
- Problem resolution
- Appeals

Section III
Procedures for Handling Uncollectible Patient Accounts
- When the account may be turned over to a collection agency
- Process to follow to assign an account to the collection agency

Section IV
Insurance Commissioner Inquiries
- Criteria for submission of inquiry
- Procedures for submission of inquiry

Figure 6-23 Hospital policies and procedures covering collection activities.

TEST YOUR *Knowledge* BOX 6-3

ACCOUNTS RECEIVABLE MANAGEMENT; LOST, REJECTED, DENIED, AND PENDED CLAIMS

1. Define accounts receivable.
2. Explain the primary objective of A/R management.
3. What is an A/R report?
4. Discuss accounts receivable and why it is important to monitor it.
5. Explain the relationship between an aging report and follow-up on outstanding claims.
6. Discuss how accounts are aged.
7. Provide an explanation of the aging categories found on the accounts receivable report.
8. List and provide an explanation of information found on a third-party payer accounts receivable report.
9. Discuss two factors that are considered in determining what accounts require follow-up.
10. Name two formulas used to assess the efficiency of A/R management activity.
11. What is a denials management report?
12. What are the four common reasons an account may be in an unbilled status?
13. List common reasons for rejected claims.
14. Discuss what actions hospital personnel should take when a claim is denied.
15. Describe a pended claim and explain why a payer may put a claim in pending status.

Prioritizing Collection Activities

Timely follow-up on outstanding accounts is essential to obtaining payment in a reasonable time frame. The collection process begins with identifying accounts that require follow-up. Hospital policies and procedures outline criteria for prioritizing collection activities based on the age and the amount outstanding on the account. The department utilizes A/R aging reports to identify accounts that require follow-up. As discussed earlier, the criteria will vary by hospital. Generally accounts in the aging category of 61 to 90 days with a higher dollar value are pursued first.

BOX 6-22 ■ KEY POINTS

Collection Activities

Hospital policies and procedures for collections include guidelines that outline the following:

- Criteria for prioritizing collection activities
- Establishment of patient and third-party follow-up procedures
- Procedures for handling uncollectible patient accounts
- Insurance Commissioner inquiries procedures

The Credit and Collection Department performs various collection functions to ensure that timely payment is received.

Patient and Third-Party Follow-up Procedures

Procedures are defined by the hospital regarding the follow-up on outstanding patient accounts and third-party claims. Hospital procedures outline methods for follow-up that generally include:

- Written follow-up
- Phone contact
- Problem resolution

Hospital follow-up procedures are developed in accordance with credit and collection laws. Procedures followed for outstanding patient accounts vary from those for claims involving third-party responsibility. Follow-up procedures and credit and collection laws will be discussed in detail later in this chapter.

BOX 6-23 ■ KEY POINTS

Patient and Third-Party Payer Follow-up Procedures

Hospital policies and procedures outline guidelines and methods for follow-up on outstanding accounts, including the following methods:

- Written follow-up
- Phone contact
- Problem resolution
- Appeals

Uncollectible Patient Accounts

Patient account balances may be deemed uncollectible after all efforts to pursue payment on the account are exhausted. Hospital policies define when an account is to be written off as a bad debt and when an account should be forwarded to a collection agency. Hospitals may contract with an outside collection agency to pursue patient accounts as a last resort, prior to initiating a write-off. Hospital procedures for submission of outstanding accounts to a collection agency may include:

- When the account may be turned over
- The process to follow to assign an account to the collection agency

Hospital policies dictate circumstances under which an account should not be sent to collection. For example, if a patient submits documentation showing financial hardship, the hospital may elect to write the balance off. If the case does not involve financial hardship, the account may be turned over to collection. The hospital will outline the time frame and procedures that must be followed before an account can be assigned to a collection agency. The process will include documentation required and necessary authorization from management to assign an account to a collection agency.

Insurance Commissioner Inquiries

Insurance companies are regulated by the Department of Insurance within each state (Figure 6-24). The Department of Insurance is also known as the Insurance Commissioner. The Insurance Commissioner is a state department that monitors activities of insurance companies to make sure the interests of the policy-holders are protected. Hospital collection personnel may need to pursue resolution to an outstanding claim through the Insurance Commissioner. Two of the most common circumstances that require hospital personnel to submit an inquiry to the Insurance Commissioner are:

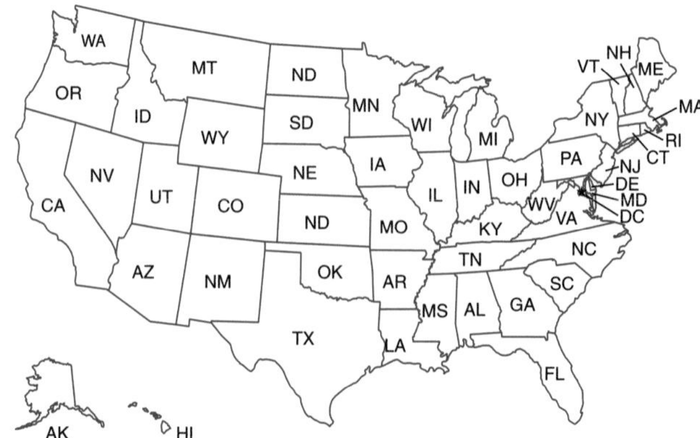

Figure 6-24 Each state has its own insurance commissioner. The website www.naic.org has a link to each state's department of insurance.

1. Delay in settlement of a claim, after proper appeal has been made
2. Improper denial of a claim or settlement for an amount less than indicated by the policy, after proper appeal has been made

Hospital collection personnel may submit an inquiry or complaint to the Insurance Commissioner regarding a claim(s) after all efforts to rectify the situation have been exhausted. Complaints must be submitted in writing and they must include the following information:

- Patient or policyholder's name, address, and telephone number
- Insured's name, address, and telephone number
- Name of the insurance company and representative involved with the claim, as well as the address and phone number of the insurance company
- Details regarding the complaint with appropriate documentation such as a claim form, explanation of benefits, and copies of the medical bill and/or insurance policy
- Claim number and policy number
- Date of service
- Patient's signature and date

BOX 6-24 ■ KEY POINTS

Insurance Commissioner Inquiries

Delay in settlement of a claim, after prompt appeal has been made

Improper denial of a claim or settlement for an amount less than indicated by the policy, after proper appeal has been made

CREDIT AND COLLECTION LAWS

Hospital collection personnel must be aware of legal and regulatory issues that apply to collection procedures. Hospital collection activities are generally divided into two categories:

- Outstanding patient accounts
- Outstanding third-party claims

Legal and regulatory issues vary for outstanding patient accounts and outstanding third-party claims. Collection activities involving patient accounts are governed by many state and federal laws, including Statute of Limitations, the Fair Credit Billing Act, and the Fair Debt Collection Practices Act.

BOX 6-25 ■ KEY POINTS

Credit and Collections Laws

Statute of Limitations
Fair Credit Billing Act
Fair Debt Collection Practices Act

Statute of Limitations

Statute of Limitations legislation is passed at the state level establishing the time period in which legal collection procedures may be filed against a patient (Figure 6-25). The time period (number of years) varies in accordance with state law. For example, the statute of limitations in Florida is 5 years. This means that legal collection procedures cannot be filed against a patient if the 5-year period has passed.

Fair Credit Billing Act

The **Fair Credit Billing Act** is federal legislation that outlines the patient's rights regarding errors on a bill. The Act states that the patient has 60 days from receipt of a statement to submit notification of an error. The notification must be in writing. The hospital is required to acknowledge the notification of error within 30 days of receipt. The hospital must contact the patient and explain why the bill is correct. If the bill is not correct, the hospital is required to correct the error within two billing cycles. The maximum number of days to correct an error is 90.

Fair Debt Collection Practices Act

The **Fair Debt Collection Practices Act** is federal legislation that was passed to protect consumers from inappropriate collection activities such as harassment or deception. As shown in Figure 6-26, the Act provides guidelines for appropriate collection practices as outlined below:

- Patient (debtor) may be contacted only once per day.
- Calls should be made after 8:00 AM and before 9:00 PM.
- Patient (debtor) may not be contacted on Sundays or holidays.
- Hospital personnel are required to identify themselves and the hospital they represent.
- Contact of a patient (debtor) at work is only appropriate when the patient cannot be contacted elsewhere or if the patient requests that he or she be contacted at work.
- If the patient (debtor) is represented by an attorney, the attorney should be contacted.
- Hospital personnel should not use a threatening tone or inappropriate language.
- Correspondence regarding debt must be kept private; therefore, postcards are not acceptable forms of correspondence.
- Collect calls to a patient are not appropriate.
- Never leave messages with details regarding outstanding debt with individuals other than the patient, on an answering machine, or at an individual's workplace. Messages should include a name, a phone

Fair Debt Collection

Statute of Limitations (SoL) listed by state and type of debt including Virgin Islands and Ontario with state civil code references.

Statute of Limitations apply to open ended contracts such as credit cards and store credit accounts and contracts for sale under the Uniform Commercial Code (UCC). Also covered under most State's statutes of limitation are oral agreements, promissory notes, written contracts, loans, mortgages and car payments as we... circumstances the statue of limitations can be renewed for just abo...

Clicking on your State link to see the statute of limitations.

Alabama	Hawaii	Michigan
Alaska	Iowa	Minnesota
Arizona	Idaho	Mississippi
Arkansas	Illinois	Missouri
California	Indiana	Montana
Colorado	Kansas	Nebraska
Connecticut	Kentucky	Nevada
Delaware	Louisiana	New Hampshire
D.C.	Maine	New Jersey
Florida	Maryland	New Mexico
Georgia	Massachusetts	New York

In-depth explanation each section of the **The fair debt collection practi...**

STATE STATUTE OF LIMITATONS

State	Open	Written	State	Open	Written
Alabama	3 years	6 years	Montana	5 years	8 years
Alaska	6 years	6 years	Nebraska	4 years	5 years
Arizona	3 years	6 years	Nevada	4 years	6 years
Arkansas	3 years	5 years	New Hampshire	6 years	6 years
California	4 years	4 years	New Jersey	6 years	6 years
Colorado	6 years	6 years	New Mexico	4 years	6 years
Connecticut	6 years	6 years	New York	6 years	6 years
Delaware	3 years	6 years	North Carolina	3 years	3 years
District of Columbia	3 years	3 years	North Dakota	6 years	6 years
			Ohio	6 years	15 years
Florida	4 years	5 years	Oklahoma	3 years	5 years
Georgia	4 years	6 years	Oregon	6 years	6 years
Hawaii	6 years	6 years	Pennsylvania	6 years	6 years
Idaho	4 years	5 years	Rhode Island	6 years	6 years
Illinois	5 years	10 years	South Carolina	6 years	6 years
Indiana	6 years	10 years	South Dakota	6 years	6 years
Iowa	5 years	10 years	Tennessee	6 years	6 years
Kansas	3 years	5 years	Texas	4 years	4 years
Kentucky	5 years	15 years	Utah	4 years	6 years
Louisana	6 years	6 years	Vermont	6 years	6 years
Maine	6 years	6 years	Virginia	3 years	5 years
Maryland	3 years	3 years	Washington	3 years	6 years
Massachusetts	6 years	6 years	West Virginia	5 years	10 years
Michigan	6 years	6 years	Wisconsin	6 years	6 years
Minnesota	6 years	6 years	Wyoming	8 years	10 years
Mississippi	3 years	6 years			
Missouri	5 years	10 years			

Figure 6-25 State statute of Limitations. *(From Fair Debt Collection:* Statue of Limitations by State, *http://www.fair-debt-collection.com/SOL-by-State.html, 2005 and Adams WL*: Adams' coding and reimbursement, a simplified approach, *ed 2, St Louis, 2005, Elsevier.)*

Fair Debt Collection Practices Act

1. Contact debtors only once a day; in some states, repeated calls on the same day or the same week could be considered harassment.
2. Place calls after 8 AM and before 9 PM.
3. Do not contact debtors on Sunday or any other day that the debtor recognizes as a Sabbath.
4. Identify yourself and the medical practice represented; do not mislead the patient.
5. Contact the debtor at work only if unable to contact the debtor elsewhere; no contact should be made if the employer or debtor disapproves.
6. Contact the attorney if an attorney represents the debtor; contact the debtor only if the attorney does not respond.
7. Do not threaten or use obscene language.
8. Do not send postcards for collection purposes; keep all correspondence strictly private.
9. Do not call collect or cause additional expense to the patient.
10. Do not leave a message on an answering machine indicating that you are calling about a bill.
11. Do not contact a third party more than once unless requested to do so by the party or the response was erroneous or incomplete.
12. Do not convey to a third party that the call is about a debt.
13. Do not contact the debtor when notified in writing that a debtor refuses to pay and would like contact to stop, except to notify the debtor that there will be no further contact or that there will be legal action.
14. Stick to the facts; do not use false statements.
15. Do not prepare a list of "bad debtors" or "credit risks" to share with other health care providers.
16. Take action immediately when stating that a certain action will be taken (e.g., filing a claim in small claims court or sending the patient to a collection agency).
17. Send the patient written verification of the name of the creditor and the amount of debt within 5 days of the initial contact.

Figure 6-26 Guidelines for collection procedures outlined under the Fair Debt Collection Practices Act. *(From Fordney M: Insurance handbook for the medical office, ed 8, St Louis, 2003, Elsevier.)*

number, and a brief statement that you are calling about a bill.

- Contact of third parties should be recorded in the patient's record and should only be made once. No details regarding the debt may be provided to the third party.
- The patient (debtor) may notify the hospital, in writing, that he or she has no intent to pay and may request that all contact be stopped. The hospital may not contact the patient after this notification is received.
- Never use false statements. Only facts should be used in communicating with a patient regarding the debt.
- Written notification may be sent to the patient to advise that action will be taken if the debt is not paid within a specified time frame.

Collection activities involving insurance claims are considered business collections since they involve provisions outlined in the contract between the hospital and a payer. The contract legally binds both parties to the provisions in the contract. As discussed in previous chapters, the payer contract outlines provisions that a provider must follow; for example, timely submission requirements, collection of deductibles, co-insurance, and co-payments, and accepting the approved amount as payment in full. The payer contract also outlines provisions that must be followed by the payer, such as statute and prompt pay provisions. Statute provisions outline when the payer is responsible for secondary claims and how the benefits will be processed and paid. Prompt pay provisions indicate the maximum amount of time the payer has to submit payment on a claim.

OUTSTANDING PATIENT ACCOUNTS

Hospital policies established for collecting outstanding patient accounts vary by hospital. Policies define procedures to be followed to pursue collection of outstanding patient balances. Basic policies include guidelines for

TEST YOUR *Knowledge* BOX 6-4

COLLECTION ACTIVITIES; CREDIT AND COLLECTION LAWS

1. What hospital department is responsible for monitoring and follow-up on outstanding accounts?
2. Explain how a hospital may use a collection agency.
3. Briefly discuss what an uncollectible account is.
4. Provide an explanation of the relationship between the Insurance Commissioner and outstanding claims.
5. State two situations that would require intervention by the Insurance Commissioner.
6. List and discuss two categories of collection activities.
7. Outline three credit and collection laws.
8. Give the law that defines the maximum period of time that legal collection actions can be filed against a patient.
9. Name the law that outlines the period of time a patient has to notify the hospital of an error on his or her statement.
10. State what law was designed to protect consumers from unfair collection activities.

collection: sending patient statements, phone contact, and collection letters (Figure 6-27).

Patient Statements

As discussed previously, patient statements are utilized to bill patients for amounts the patient is responsible to pay. Patient statements are sent after the patient is discharged when the patient has no third-party coverage. When a third-party payer is involved, the patient statement is sent after payment determination is received from the payer, when appropriate. If the patient balance is not paid within 30 days after a statement is sent, the hospital will send another statement at 60 days and at 90 days. Second and third statements generally include dun messages.

Dun Messages

A **dun message** is a message recorded on a patient statement regarding the status of an outstanding account and action required. Examples of dun messages are:

- Your account balance is due and payable within 10 days
- Your account is 60 days past due; please contact us regarding payment
- Your account is now 90 days past due; please remit payment within 10 days

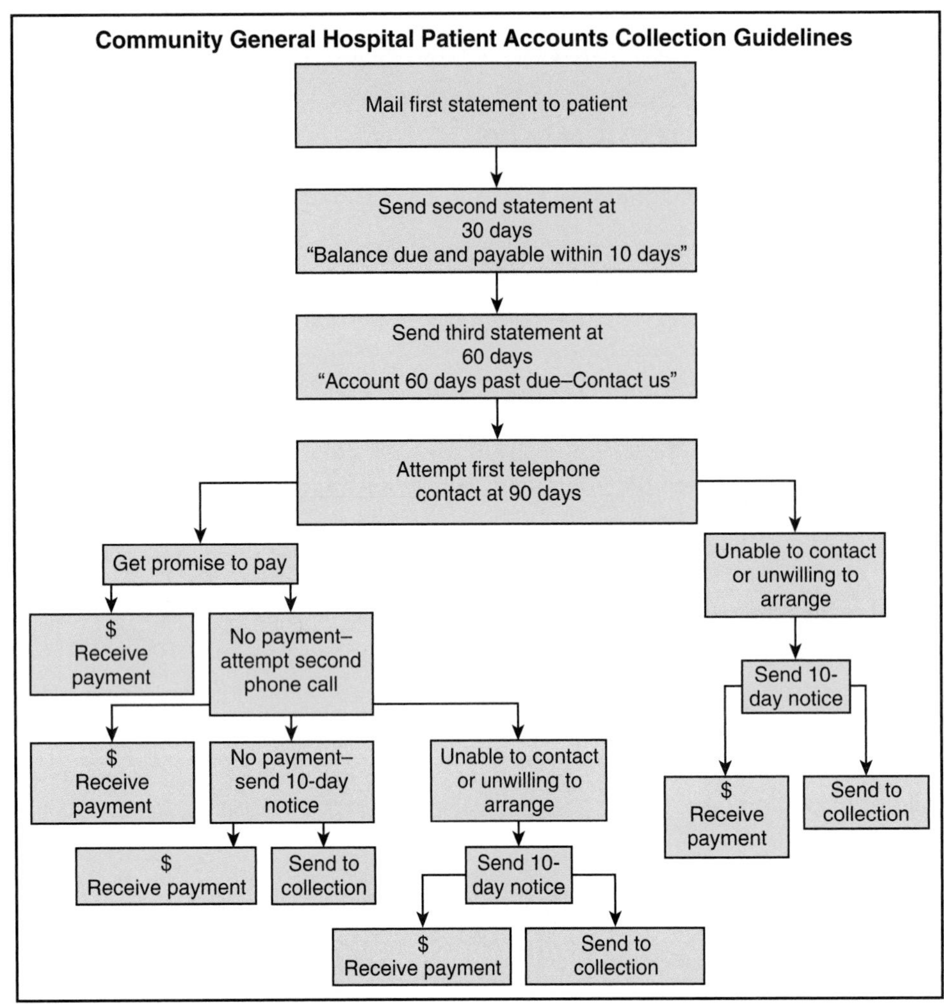

Figure 6-27 Sample hospital guidelines for patient accounts collection activities. *(Modified from Fordney M:* Insurance handbook for the medical office, *ed 11, St Louis, 2010, Elsevier.)*

Payment Options

Hospitals very often include information on the patient statement regarding payment options. For example, the statement may read: "For your convenience we accept MasterCard, Visa, and Discover."

Patient Phone Contact

When payment is not received on a patient account and the patient does not respond to statements, phone contact may be required. It is important to have a friendly and helpful tone. The purpose of the phone contact is to remind the patient of the outstanding balance and determine when and how much the patient will pay. Hospital policies provide guidelines for making patient phone contact. Figure 6-28 illustrates a sample page from a hospital training manual detailing the following regarding patient phone contact:

- Required preparation before contact is made
- Information to be provided to the patient when contact is made
- Patient's response statement and appropriate reply from the hospital representative

It is important for hospital representatives to have a friendly and helpful disposition toward the patient. Patient phone contacts are made in accordance with credit and collection laws, as discussed previously. When the patient cannot be contacted by phone or if the patient does not send payment, a collection letter is sent.

Collection Letters

Hospital collection procedures include the use of collection letters. A series of letters are developed that are designed to advise the patient of an outstanding balance and encourage the patient to make payment within a specified time frame. Hospitals may develop several letters or they may have a form letter that includes a series of statements. The content of a collection letter may range from a simple reminder to a statement indicating the consequence of failure to pay. Figure 6-29 illustrates a sample collection letter.

Community General Hospital Training Manual
Patient Phone Contact

Section I

Required Preparation

- Have details regarding the charges available
- Note whether insurance has paid and be prepared to explain the balance
- Remember the purpose of the call is to collect full payment or set a schedule for payments to be made

Section II

Information to be Provided to the Patient when Contact Is Made

- Identify yourself and the hospital you represent
- Confirm that the individual on the phone is the patient
- Advise the patient you are calling about an outstanding balance and give the patient the date of service and the amount outstanding
- Ask the patient when payment can be expected

Patient's Response and Reply

- Payment was sent
  When the patient indicates the payment was sent, inquire as to the date payment was sent and the amount. Thank the patient for his/her time and note the information in the patient's account.
- Patient does not understand charges or has questions regarding charges
  It may be necessary to explain the charges or answer specific questions regarding the charges. Once all answers are provided to the patient, inquire as to when payment will be sent.
- Patient is unable to pay the entire balance
  When the patient indicates he/she is unable to pay the entire balance, recommend a payment plan or budget in accordance with hospital policies. Advise the patient of the minimum payment that can be made and the time interval for which payments should be made.
- Patient has no intent to pay
  If the patient indicates he/she has no intention of paying, try to find out why. These situations will be handled according to hospital policy based on the reason the patient is not going to pay.

Figure 6-28 Sample hospital training manual outlining guidelines for contacting patients by phone for collection purposes.

Community General Hospital
7979 First Place
Tampa, Florida 33697

November 21, 2005

Sam Jones
22 Harold Place
Tampa, FL 33429

Dear Mr. Jones:

I am writing regarding your account, which is currently past due. We have made several attempts to contact you with no success. We realize this may be an oversight. If you have questions regarding the balance on your account please do not hesitate to contact us at (747) 721-1800.

If this is an oversight, please remit payment within 10 days.

Thank you for your cooperation.

Sincerely,

Pam James
Patient Account Representative

Alternative Statements

Your account is now 90 days past due. Please remit payment within 10 days.

Your account is seriously past due. Please remit payment within 10 days to avoid legal action.

Your account requires immediate attention. Please remit full payment within 10 days. Delinquent accounts are turned over to our legal department 30 days after this notice is sent.

Figure 6-29 Sample collection letter illustrating alternative statements regarding action required.

OUTSTANDING THIRD-PARTY CLAIMS

Timely follow-up on outstanding claims is critical to obtaining payment within an appropriate time frame and also to prevent further delay of a claim. Third-party payers are required to process timely payment in accordance with prompt pay statutes.

Prompt Pay Statutes

Prompt pay statutes outline the required language in contracts regarding timely payment on claims. Prompt pay statutes vary by state. As outlined in Figure 6-30, statutes generally include provisions for the following:

- Maximum number of days, after receipt of the claim, a payer has to process payment
- Maximum number of days, after receipt of additional information requested, to process payment
- Number of days a payer has to pay or deny a claim
- Interest rate on overpayments
- Terms for which the payer will investigate claims of improper billing

In accordance with prompt pay statutes, payment on claims should be made within an appropriate time frame. Electronic claims are generally processed within 2 to 3 weeks. Paper claims may take 4 to 6 weeks for processing. Follow-up on outstanding claims may be made by phone or computer or through submission of an insurance claim tracer. The status may be determined utilizing one of these methods.

Insurance Telephone Claim Inquiry

Some payers allow follow-up on outstanding claims to be performed by phone contact. Payers may allow follow-up on several claims during a phone conversation. It is necessary to have the following information available for each claim:

Florida Prompt Pay Statutes

Title XXXVII INSURANCE

Chapter 627 INSURANCE RATES AND CONTRACTS

627.613 Time of payment of claims.

(1) The contract shall include the following provision:

"Time of Payment of Claims: After receiving written proof of loss, the insurer will pay monthly all benefits then due for (type of benefit). Benefits for any other loss covered by this policy will be paid as soon as the insurer receives proper written proof."

(2) Health insurers shall reimburse all claims or any portion of any claim from an insured or an insured's assignees, for payment under a health insurance policy, within 45 days after receipt of the claim by the health insurer. If a claim or a portion of a claim is contested by the health insurer, the insured or the insured's assignees shall be notified, in writing, that the claim is contested or denied, within 45 days after receipt of the claim by the health insurer. The notice that a claim is contested shall identify the contested portion of the claim and the reasons for contesting the claim.

(3) A health insurer, upon receipt of the additional information requested from the insured or the insured's assignees shall pay or deny the contested claim or portion of the contested claim, within 60 days.

(4) An insurer shall pay or deny any claim no later than 120 days after receiving the claim.

(5) Payment shall be treated as being made on the date a draft or other valid instrument which is equivalent to payment was placed in the United States mail in a properly addressed, postpaid envelope or, if not so posted, on the date of delivery.

(6) All overdue payments shall bear simple interest at the rate of 10 percent per year.

(7) Upon written notification by an insured, an insurer shall investigate any claim of improper billing by a physician, hospital, or other health care provider. The insurer shall determine if the insured was properly billed for only those procedures and services that the insured actually received. If the insurer determines that the insured has been improperly billed, the insurer shall notify the insured and the provider of its findings and shall reduce the amount of payment to the provider by the amount determined to be improperly billed. If a reduction is made due to such notification by the insured, the insurer shall pay to the insured 20 percent of the amount of the reduction up to $500.

History.--s. 556, ch. 59-205; s. 3, ch. 76-168; s. 1, ch. 77-457; ss. 2, 3, ch. 81-318; ss. 462, 497, 809(2nd), ch. 82-243; s. 79, ch. 82-386; s. 2, ch. 90-85; s. 5, ch. 91-296; s. 114, ch. 92-318.

Figure 6-30 Sample prompt pay statutes for the state of Florida. *(From The Florida State Senate, Florida Prompt Pay Statues, www.flsenate.gov/statutes.)*

- Hospital's provider identification number
- Patient's name and date of birth
- Insurance identification number and group or contract name and number
- Date of service on each claim
- Dollar amount of each claim
- Claim information such as procedures and diagnosis codes

Insurance Computer Claim Inquiry

Many payers have Internet Web sites on which claim status can be researched. The payer provides the Web address and procedures to sign on and obtain claim status information. All information regarding the patient and claim are required as outlined above.

Insurance Claim Tracer

A form utilized to submit a claim inquiry to a payer, referred to as an **insurance claim tracer,** may be required by payers for claim inquiries. Figure 6-31 illustrates a sample insurance claim tracer. The insurance claim tracer requires information regarding the patient and claim. The form generally includes a list of options regarding the reason for the inquiry.

When the claim status is known, the hospital representative can pursue resolution of the claim as discussed previously. Claim status may include the following:

- Payment was processed and sent
- Claim is not on file
- Claim was denied or rejected
- Claim is in a pending status and more information is required

The purpose of claims inquiry is to determine whether payment was processed. If payment was not processed, the hospital representative will request information about the delay in processing the claim. After contact is made with the payer about the status of an outstanding claim, the hospital representative will record information about the contact on the patient's account and will work to resolve the delay.

APPEALS PROCESS

An **appeal** is a request submitted to the payer by the hospital for reconsideration of a claim denial or rejection or an incorrect payment. Payers provide hospitals with procedures required to file an appeal (Figure 6-32). The procedures generally include provisions regarding the type of claim that can be appealed, who can file an appeal, the time frame for submission of appeals, and the levels of appeals.

BOX 6-26 ■ KEY POINTS

Appeals

Claim determinations that can be appealed:

- Denied claims, reason unclear
- Incorrect payment
- Denial based on preexisting conditions
- Denial based on authorization or precertification requirements

Claim Determinations That Can Be Appealed

Payers include provisions in their contract outlining the type of claim determinations that can be appealed. Common types of claim determinations that can be appealed are as follows:

- Payment is denied for reasons that are not clear to the hospital or the hospital has more information to prove that the denial is in error
- Payment was processed at an incorrect level
- Services are denied based on the payer's preexisting condition provisions
- Claim is denied for reasons relating to authorization or precertification requirements

COMMUNITY GENERAL HOSPITAL
8192 South Street
Mars, Florida 37373

Telephone (555) 486-9002 **Fax (555) 487-8976**

INSURANCE CLAIM TRACER

INSURANCE COMPANY NAME American Insurance DATE 09/14/XX
ADDRESS P.O. Box 5300, New York, New York 12345

Patient: Marcella Austin
Insured: Marcella Austin
Employer: T C Corporation
Policy/certificate no. 9635 402-A
Group name/no. B0105
Date of initial claim submission: 08/02/XX
Amount of claim: $536.24

An inordinate amount of time has passed since the submission of our original claim. We have not received a request for additional information and still await payment of this assigned claim. Please review the attached duplicate and process for payment within 7 days.

If there is any difficulty with this claim, please check the reason below and return this letter to our office. Thank you.

- ☐ No record of claim.
- ☐ Claim received and payment is in process.
- ☐ Claim is in suspense (comment please).
- ☐ Claim is in review (comment please).
- ☐ Additional information needed (comment please)
- ☐ Claim paid. Date:______ Amount:$______ To whom:______
- ☐ Claim denied (comment please).

Comments:______

Thank you for your assistance in this important matter. Please contact the insurance specialist named below if you have any questions regarding this claim.

Katelyn Chang — Insurance Specialist (555) 486-9002 Ext. 236
Gene Ullibarri, MD — Treating Physician

Figure 6-31 Sample insurance claim tracer. *(Modified from Fordney MT:* Insurance Handbook for the Medical Office, *ed 9, St Louis, 2005, Elsevier.)*

Medicare Levels of Appeal

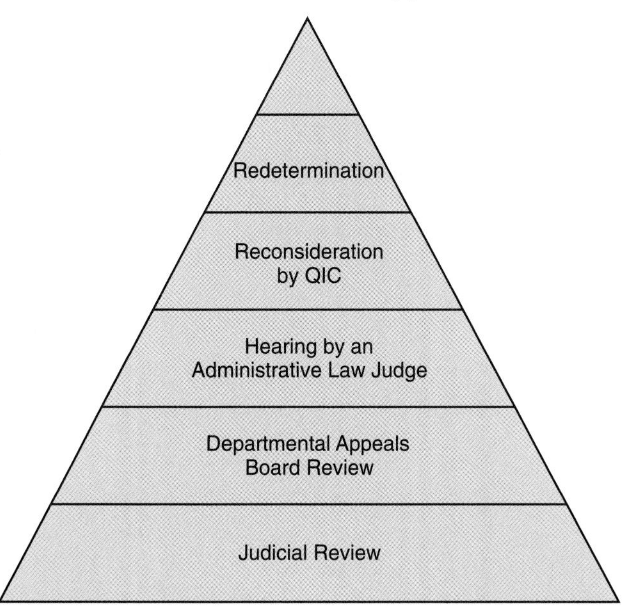

Figure 6-32 Appeal levels and procedures vary by payer. Medicare appeal procedures outline five levels of appeal.

Who Can Request an Appeal

Payers determine the appropriate party to appeal a claim based on whether the claim is assigned or nonassigned, as outlined below:

- Assigned claims can be appealed by the hospital or by the patient
- Nonassigned claims can be appealed by the patient or by the hospital when the patient has given consent for the appeal and when the provider is liable for the amount not paid

Time Requirement for Appeal Submission

Payers require submission of appeals within a specified time period after the claim was processed. Time requirements vary by payer, and they may also vary based on the level of appeal. For example, Medicare requires that a request for redetermination be submitted within 120 days of the date of the original claim determination.

Levels of Appeals

Payers may have various levels of appeals. Time requirements and procedures are specified for each level. For example, Medicare has five levels of appeals:

1. Redetermination by Medicare Administrative Contractor (MAC)
2. Reconsideration by a Qualified Independent Contractor (QIC)
3. Administrative law judge hearing
4. Departmental Appeals Board review
5. Judicial review in U.S. District Court

Appeal Submission Procedures

The appeal submission procedures vary by payer and by type of review requested. The hospital representative should contact the payer to determine the procedure for filing an appeal. For example Medicare requires form CMS-20027 for a Redetermination and form CMS-20033 for a Reconsideration. Basic steps to filing an appeal are outlined below:

- Prepare letter or form required by payer that outlines the reason for the appeal
- Prepare all supporting documentation such as the RA, copy of the policy, publications, and resources regarding billing and coding guidelines
- If similar claim denials were successfully appealed by the insurance company, send information regarding those cases
- Contact the insurance company to identify the appropriate person and department the appeal should be sent to.
- Keep copies of the appeal and all information submitted

It is necessary to monitor the status of an appeal until a decision is made. If the appeal is not successful at the level submitted, the hospital may elect to submit an appeal at the next level.

CHAPTER SUMMARY

A/R management is a vital function of a hospital to ensure that payment is received in an appropriate time frame. The life cycle of a claim starts when the patient arrives and ends when payment is received for services rendered. Once charges are billed to a patient or third-party payer, accounts must be monitored carefully to prevent an unreasonable period of time from passing before payment is received. Delayed payment on accounts will have a negative effect on the hospital's revenue cycle. To maintain financial stability, the hospital must have an efficient flow of revenue.

The PFS Department is responsible for managing the hospital's patient financial transactions, which include charge submission and A/R management. Hospital policies and procedures are established for patient transactions. Payments received from the patient and third-party payers are posted to the patient's account and balances are billed to the patient or other payers. Adjustments may be required to reduce the original charge by a specified amount based on payer contracts, the patient's ability to pay, or inability to collect patient balances. The Credit and Collections Department is responsible for monitoring and follow-up on outstanding accounts.

Hospital policies are also established regarding monitoring outstanding accounts and collection activities that are hospital specific and they are developed within the parameters defined by payers and various legal and regulatory agencies. Hospitals utilize various A/R reports to monitor outstanding accounts such as the unbilled accounts, denials management, and A/R aging reports.

Hospital personnel must have knowledge of all aspects of the life cycle of a claim, including posting transactions and collections procedures. Hospital personnel must also have knowledge of federal and state laws that govern collection activities in order to ensure that proper collection procedures are followed. This chapter provides a basic overview of various aspects of patient transactions, A/R management, and collection activities.

TEST YOUR *Knowledge* BOX 6-5

OUTSTANDING THIRD-PARTY CLAIMS; APPEALS PROCESS

1. Discuss the function of patient statements in pursuing outstanding patient accounts.
2. Define and discuss the purpose of dun messages.
3. Patient phone contact must be made in accordance with what laws?
4. Briefly discuss prompt pay statutes.
5. List three methods utilized for claim inquiries.
6. Discuss the purpose of an appeal.
7. List four claim determinations that can be appealed.
8. Who can request an appeal?
9. List five levels of Medicare appeals.
10. Briefly explain procedures required for submission of an appeal.

CHAPTER REVIEW 6-1

True/False

1. Patient statements are generated in batches and sent periodically. T F
2. A remittance advice is also known as a payment document. T F
3. Adjustments are when the original charge is reduced by a specified amount. T F
4. Unbilled accounts may be the result of delays in coding. T F
5. Old accounts with a high dollar amount receive priority collection status. T F

Fill in the Blank

6. A ____________________. adjustment is required when a participating hospital's original charge is greater than the approved amount.
7. Payment determination that indicates no payment will be made is referred to as a ____________________. claim.
8. Claims may be in a ____________________. status until requested information is sent to the payer.
9. A process that can be followed to request that a payer reconsider determination on a claim is referred to as a ____________________. process.
10. Filing requirements for appeals vary by payer. Medicare requires that redetermination requests be submitted within ____________________. days.

Match the Following Definitions With the Terms at Right

11. ___ The law that indicates a patient may submit notification of an error on a statement within 60 days and that the hospital must acknowledge receipt within 30 days.
12. ___ The law that indicates language that must be in a payer's contract regarding timely payment.
13. ___ Complaints regarding claims may be forwarded to this agency after appeals have been exhausted
14. ___ Law passed to protect consumers from unfair collection activities.
15. ___ Outlines the time frame in which a legal action can be filed against a patient.

A. Statute of Limitations
B. Prompt pay statutes
C. Fair Credit Billing Act
D. Fair Debt Collection Practices Act
E. Insurance Commissioner

Research Project

Refer to the CMS Web site at: http://www.cms/gov/medlearn. Search for information on appeals. Discuss five appeal levels for Medicare claims, including: who can appeal, when the appeal must be filed, and how it should be filed.

GLOSSARY

Accounts receivable (A/R) A term used to describe revenue owed to the hospital by patients and third-party payers.

Accounts receivable (A/R) aging report A listing of outstanding accounts based on the age of the account.

Accounts receivable ratio (A/R ratio) A formula that calculates the percentage of accounts receivable in comparison with total charges.

Adjustment The process of reducing the original amount charged by a specified amount.

Advance Beneficiary Notice (ABN) Written notice that is presented to a Medicare beneficiary before Medicare Part B services are furnished, to inform the beneficiary that the provider believes that Medicare will not pay for some or all of the services to be rendered because they are not reasonable and necessary.

Aging Term used to describe the number of days the account is outstanding from the date the claim or statement is sent.

Appeal A request submitted to the payer by the hospital for reconsideration of a claim denial, rejection, or incorrect payment.

Balance billing Refers to billing the patient for a balance in excess of the payer's approved amount in accordance with the payer contract.

Clean claim A claim that does not need to be investigated by the payer. The claim passes all internal billing edits and payer-specific edits and is paid without need for additional intervention.

CMS-1450 (UB-04) The universally accepted claim form utilized to submit facility charges for hospital outpatient and inpatient services.

CMS-1500 The universally accepted claim form utilized to submit charges for physician and outpatient services.

Contractual adjustment A reduction made to the original charge in accordance with the hospital's contract with a payer.

Days in accounts receivable (A/R) A formula used to determine the number days it takes to collect outstanding accounts.

Denials management report Report utilized to identify claims that have been denied, rejected, or pended. Claims on the report are investigated to determine the reason for nonpayment.

Denied claim A claim processed by the payer resulting in a determination that no payment will be made on the claim.

Dun message A message recorded on a patient statement regarding the status of an outstanding account.

Electronic remittance advice (ERA) A document electronically transmitted to the hospital to provide an explanation of payment determination for a claim.

Explanation of Benefits (EOB) A document prepared by the payer to provide an explanation of payment determination for a claim. An EOB is also referred to as a remittance advice (RA).

Fair Credit Billing Act Federal legislation that outlines the patient's rights regarding errors on a bill.

Fair Debt Collection Practices Act Federal legislation that was passed to protect consumers from inappropriate collection activities such as harassment or deception.

Financial class A classification system used to categorize accounts by payer types. Financial classes may also be referred to as financial buckets.

Hospital Issued Notice of Noncoverage (HINN) A written notice that is presented to a Medicare beneficiary before Part A services are furnished, to inform the beneficiary that the provider believes that Medicare will not pay for some or all of the services to be rendered because they are not reasonable and necessary.

Insurance claim tracer A form utilized to submit a claim inquiry to a payer.

National Correct Coding Initiative (CCI) Developed by CMS for the purpose of promoting national coding guidelines and preventing improper coding. CCI outlines code combinations that are inappropriate.

Outstanding accounts Accounts that have been billed to the patient or third-party payer and no payment is received.

Payer data files Payer files that contain information regarding covered individuals including a history of past claims submitted for the patient.

Pended claim A claim that is placed on hold by the payer, pending receipt of additional information.

Prompt pay statutes State statutes that outline required language in contracts regarding timely payment on claims. Prompt pay statutes vary by state.

Rejected claim A claim that is returned to the hospital by the payer because the claim contained a technical error or could not be processed because it was not completed in accordance with payer guidelines.

Remittance advice (RA) A document prepared by the payer to provide an explanation of payment determination for a claim. The payer forwards this document to the hospital. RA is also referred to as an explanation of benefits (EOB).

Statute of Limitations State legislation that establishes the time period in which legal collection procedures may be filed against a patient.

Unbilled accounts report A report utilized to track accounts that have not been billed since the patient was discharged.

Unbundling The process of coding multiple codes to describe multiple services using one code.

Write-off The process of reducing a patient's balance to zero.

SECTION THREE

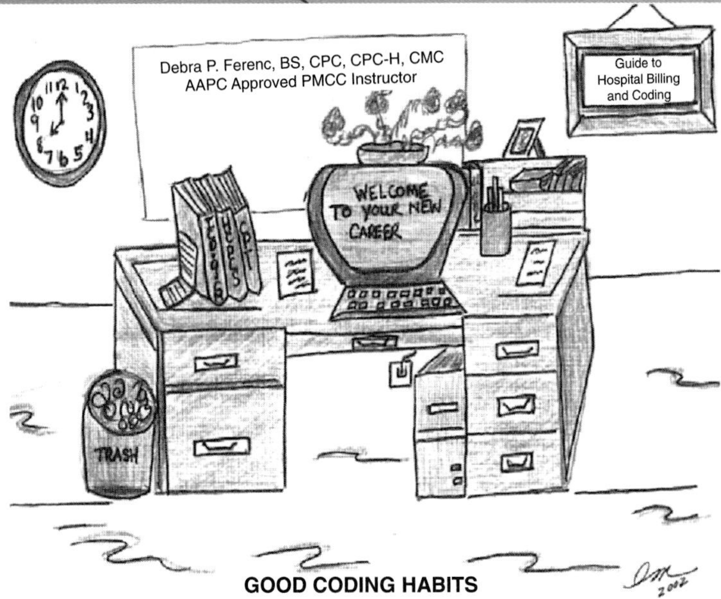

- ✔ DO NOT ASSUME
- ✔ Identify all possible codes in the index (Volume II)
- ✔ NEVER EVER code only from the index (Volume II)
- ✔ Review each code in the tabular list (Volume II)
- ✔ Review all codes in the range
- ✔ WHEN IN DOUBT ASK
- ✔ Never use an E code as the first listed condition
- ✔ Consistency is critical

Coding

Coding Medical Conditions (Diagnosis Coding)

Coding Procedures, Services, and Items (Procedure Coding)

Coding Guidelines and Applications

Chapter 7

Coding Medical Conditions (Diagnosis Coding)

Diagnosis coding has been around for hundreds of years, and it has evolved to serve many purposes in the health care industry. Hospital coding and billing professionals are required to have an understanding of the ICD-9-CM coding system. The ability to understand and apply coding principles and guidelines is essential to ensure patients' conditions are described accurately and to make sure the hospital is in compliance with coding guidelines.

The objective of this chapter is to provide an overview of the history and purpose of coding medical conditions using ICD-9-CM. A review of how coding relates to documentation, medical necessity, claim form submission, and reimbursement will demonstrate the importance of coding conditions in the hospital. The content of the ICD-9-CM Volume I and II coding manual is outlined to review the coding system and how it is organized. A detailed discussion on ICD-9-CM coding conventions is important to understand how the conventions are used to communicate instructions to the coder. The basic steps to coding conditions using ICD-9-CM will be reviewed to provide an enhanced understanding of the coding process. The chapter will end with a brief discussion of ICD-10. The chapter's focus is on diagnosis coding utilizing ICD-9-CM Volume I and II. Coding of procedures will be discussed in Chapter 8, and ICD-9-CM Volume III procedure coding will be included in that discussion.

Outline

Chapter Objectives

- Define terms, phrases, abbreviations, and acronyms related to coding conditions for hospital services.
- Demonstrate an understanding of the history and purpose of diagnosis coding.
- Discuss how ICD-9-CM coding data are utilized for research, education, and administrative purposes.
- Provide an explanation of the relationship among documentation, medical necessity, claim forms, reimbursement, and coding.
- Outline the content of ICD-9-CM Volume I and II.
- Demonstrate an understanding of ICD-9-CM coding conventions.
- Demonstrate an understanding of ICD-9-CM coding principles.
- Demonstrate an understanding of coding utilizing the ICD-9-CM diagnosis coding system.

Key Terms

Admitting diagnosis
Adverse reaction
Benign hypertension
Benign neoplasm
Chief complaint (CC)
Coding
Co-morbidity
Complication
Convention
Diagnosis coding
Documentation
First-Listed Condition
Hypertension
International Classification of Diseases, 9th Revision, Clinical Modification (ICD-9-CM)
International Classification of Diseases (ICD)
International List of Causes of Death
London Bills of Mortality
Main term
Malignant hypertension
Malignant neoplasm
Medical necessity
Medicare Severity Diagnosis Related Groups (MS-DRG)
Morbidity
Mortality
Neoplasm
Poisoning
Principal diagnosis
Sequencing
World Health Organization (WHO)

Acronyms and Abbreviations

AHA—American Hospital Association
AHIMA—American Health Information Management
CC—complication and co-morbidity
CDC—Centers for Disease Control
CMS—Centers for Medicare and Medicaid Services
DHHS—Department of Health and Human Services
FL—form locator
ICD—International Classification of Diseases
ICD-9-CM—International Classification of Diseases, 9th Revision, Clinical Modification
ICD-10—International Classification of Diseases, 10th Revision (ICD-10)
MS-DRG—Medicare Severity Diagnosis Related Groups
MSP—Medicare secondary payer
NCHS—National Center for Health Statistics
PPS—Prospective Payment System
SNDO—Standard Nomenclature of Diseases and Operations
UB-04—CMS-1450 Universal Bill implemented in 2007.
WHO—World Health Organization

HISTORY AND PURPOSE OF DIAGNOSIS CODING

The evolution of classification systems for coding medical conditions dates back to the 17th century, when systems were originally developed to track the number of deaths in children. **Coding** is the assignment of numeric or alphanumeric codes to all health care data elements of inpatient and outpatient care. All coding systems are encompassed in this definition. Coded health care data were originally intended for use in research and study. Today the value of such data has expanded beyond just the classification of diseases. The primary key to reimbursement and statistical analysis by hospitals, insurance companies, health care facilities, and other relevant businesses is coded health care data. The resulting codes serve two major uses: (1) statistical, in which patient information is aggregated by code number; and (2) clinical, in which the codes assigned to patient information are used individually. Statistical uses of codes include the study of etiology (cause) and incidences of disease, health care planning, and quality control of health care. The clinical use of codes includes completion of claim forms for reimbursement and indexing individual patient records; both are significant applications in the United States. Quality coding is utilized as an accurate and reliable data base for budgeting, clinical research, credentialing, peer review, education, financial analysis, marketing, patient care, quality assurance and risk management statistics, strategic planning, utilization management, and other internal or external facility purposes.

Diagnosis coding is a vital function in the hospital billing process, as discussed previously. Accurate and timely coding ensures appropriate reimbursement for health care services. Hospital coding professionals are responsible for coding patient conditions for the purpose of describing the reason why services and items were provided. Hospital coding professionals strive to master an understanding of coding principals and the application of coding guidelines to ensure that an accurate description of the patient's condition is presented, to comply with coding guidelines, and to obtain proper reimbursement. Hospital billing professionals need to achieve a good understanding of coding classification systems in order to ensure that payer coding guidelines are satisfied when the claim is submitted and to communicate with payers regarding reimbursement issues.

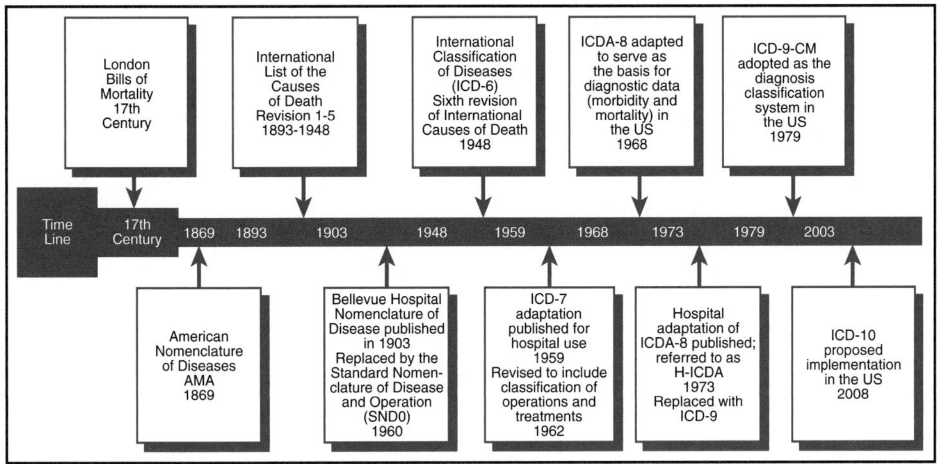

Figure 7-1 Evolution of diagnosis classifications systems. *(Modified from Fordney MT, French LL: Medical insurance billing and coding, ed 1, St Louis, 2003, Saunders.)*

BOX 7-1 ■ KEY POINTS

Diagnosis Coding and Hospital Coding and Billing Professionals

Hospital Coding Professionals

Must master coding principals and applications to describe patient conditions accurately, ensure compliance with coding guidelines, and obtain proper reimbursement

Hospital Billing Professionals

Must understand diagnosis coding to ensure compliance with billing guidelines and to obtain accurate reimbursement

Major Diagnosis Classifications

I. International List of Causes of Death
Revisions 1–5
1838–1958

II. International Classification of Diseases (ICD) published by the World Health Organization (WHO)
Revisions 6–9
1958–1978

III. International Classification of Diseases, 9th Revision, Clinical Modification
Developed in the United States and adopted for coding diagnosis
1979

Figure 7-2 Three major diagnosis classification systems.

History of Diagnosis Coding

The classification and coding of medical conditions (diseases) began in England in the 17th century with the work of John Graunt on the **London Bills of Mortality,** who developed them in an attempt to estimate the proportion of live-born children who died before reaching the age of 6 years. As centuries passed, the attempts to classify causes of death and diseases continued. Many systems were developed, such as the International List of the Causes of Death, American Nomenclature of Diseases, International Classification of Diseases (ICD), Standard Nomenclature of Diseases and Operations (SNDO), and International Classification of Diseases, 9th Revision, Clinical Modification (ICD-9-CM). This evolution, which continues into the 21st century is illustrated in Figure 7-1. The three major diagnosis classification systems that have been utilized over the centuries are the International List of the Causes of Death, the International Classification of Diseases, and the International Classification of Diseases, 9th Revision, Clinical Modification (Figure 7-2).

International List of the Causes of Death

The **International List of the Causes of Death** is a classification of causes of death that was based on the London Bills of Mortality. A committee chaired by Jacques Bertillion utilized the London Bills of Mortality to develop it. The International List of the Causes of Death was presented at the International Statistical Institute and was adopted in 1893. Several countries adopted the list during the 19th century. Six revisions were made to the International List of the Causes of Death through 1948, and the sixth revision included a name change to the International Classification of Diseases.

International Classification of Diseases (ICD)

The **International Classification of Disease (ICD)** is a classification system that was utilized to collect data regarding the causes of death for statistical purposes. It was a revised version of the International List of the Causes of Death. The ICD was published by the

World Health Organization (WHO). The Interim Commission of WHO was given the responsibility for the sixth revision and also for the establishment of a List of Causes of Morbidity for international use. In 1948, WHO published ICD-6, which was a combined classification of causes of death (mortality) and disease (morbidity). With this publication came internationally accepted rules for selecting the underlying cause of death. The National Committee on Vital and Health Statistics (NCHS) was established to serve as a liaison between national statistical institutions and WHO. From 1948 to today, there have been several revisions of the ICD. Information about WHO can be viewed on their Web site at http://www.who.int.

During the 1950s, hospitals began to describe diseases and procedures utilizing the ICD-7. A revision was made in 1962 that included the first "Classification of Operations and Treatments" for hospital use. In 1968, the United States Public Health Service published ICD-8, and later the Commission on Professional and Hospital Activities (CHA) published the Hospital Adaptation of the ICD-A based on both the original ICD-8 and ICDA-8. The ICD-A provided greater detail for coding of hospital and morbidity data. The hospital adaptation of the ICDA-8 was published in 1973, and it was referred to as the H-ICDA. The International Classification of Diseases (ICD-8) was the coding system used for coding diseases until the late 1970s. The ICD-9 was published by WHO. The United States modified ICD-9 and adopted it as the diagnosis classification system for the United States in 1979. The modified version is known as the International Classification of Diseases, 9th Revision, Clinical Modification (ICD-9-CM).

BOX 7-2 ■ KEY POINTS

Evolution of ICD-9-CM

International List of the Causes of Death (Revisions 1–6)

↓

International Classification of Diseases (Revisions 6–9)

↓

International Classification of Diseases, 9th Revision, Clinical Modification

International Classification of Diseases, 9th Revision, Clinical Modification (ICD-9-CM)

Diseases listed in the ICD-9 were primarily acute and related to conditions resulting from infectious diseases. The types of conditions seen in Europe were different from those in the United States. As discussed in Chapter 1, medical and technological advances led to new knowledge about diseases. A modification to the ICD-9 was required to include more detailed information regarding diseases and procedures that would be more reflective of the conditions seen in the United States. The ICD was "clinically" modified to enhance the classification and collection of morbidity data and for indexing medical records. The Department of Health and Human Services published the modified version of the ICD-9 called the International Classification of Diseases, 9th Revision, Clinical Modification (ICD-9-CM) in 1979, and it is the standard coding system currently utilized in the United States by hospitals and other providers to describe a patient's condition, injury, illness, disease or other reason the patient is receiving health care services.

The ICD-9-CM Coordination and Maintenance Committee

Maintenance and update of the ICD-9-CM is the result of a collaborative effort of members of the ICD-9-CM Coordination and Maintenance Committee. The committee consists of representatives from four organizations: the National Center for Health Statistics (NCHS), the Centers for Medicare and Medicaid Services (CMS), the American Hospital Association (AHA), and the American Health Information Management Association (AHIMA). The organizations are referred to as cooperating parties. Table 7-1 outlines the cooperating parties and responsibilities of each organization. Information regarding the ICD-9-CM Coordination and Maintenance Committee can be viewed on their Web site, at http://www.cdc.gov/nchs/icd/icd9cm_maintenance.htm.

International Classification of Diseases, 10th Revision (ICD-10)

In 1993 WHO published the newest version of the International Classification of Diseases, 10th Revision (ICD-10). The ICD-10 is being used in some European countries, and implementation in the United States is scheduled for 2013 as outlined on the CDC website: http://www.cdc.gov/nchs/icd/icd10cm.htm.

BOX 7-3 ■ KEY POINTS

ICD-9-CM Data Classifications

International Classification of Diseases, 9th Revision, Clinical Modification (ICD-9-CM) allows the collection of data regarding:

- Morbidity (patient illness or disease)
- Mortality (factors that contribute to death)
- Hospital procedures (significant procedures performed in the hospital such as surgery).

Purpose of Diagnosis Coding

Coding systems are designed to provide a standardized system for describing and classifying data. The use of coding classification systems provides an efficient

TABLE 7-1 The ICD-9-CM Coordination and Maintenance Committee ICD-9-CM Cooperating Parties

Organization	Responsibilities
National Center for Health Statistics (NCHS)	• Maintains the disease classification • Approves official coding guidelines
Centers for Medicare and Medicaid Services (CMS)	• Maintains the procedure classification • Approves official coding guidelines
American Hospital Association (AHA)	• Maintains Central Office on ICD-9-CM • Approves official coding guidelines • Publishes *Coding Clinic*
American Health Information Management Association (AHIMA)	• Offers coding certifications • Provides coding education • Sponsors Council on Coding and Classification and the Society for Clinical Coding • Approves official coding guidelines

Data from Abdelhak M, Grostick S, Hanken MA, Jacobs E, editors: Health information: management of a strategic resource, *ed 2, St Louis, 2001, Saunders.*

method to collect, track, research, and analyze specified data. Coding medical conditions (diagnosis) involves assigning codes to written descriptions of the patient's signs, symptoms, illness, injury, disease, condition, or other reason for patient care services. Diagnosis codes are used to describe patient conditions and to explain the medical necessity for services and items provided to third-party payers. The ICD-9-CM classification allows advanced applications using the data for research, education, and administration of all aspects of health care such as indexing of patient records based on diagnosis and monitoring of health care costs. The ICD-9-CM allows for the collection of data regarding morbidity, mortality, and hospital procedures.

Morbidity

The term **morbidity** refers to the patient's illness or disease. ICD-9-CM Volume I and II is a classification of patient conditions, including signs, symptoms, illness, injury, diseases, and other reasons patients seek health care services. Data collected through ICD-9-CM can be retrieved and utilized to track diseases for various reasons such as the identification of possible epidemics or linking certain conditions with environmental factors.

Mortality

The term **mortality** refers to death. ICD-9-CM Volume I and II also classifies patient conditions that may be the cause of death. Tracking of patient conditions using ICD-9-CM also helps to identify other factors that contribute to death or health risk factors.

Hospital Procedures

Significant procedures performed in the hospital during a hospital stay are coded utilizing ICD-9-CM Volume III procedure codes. Surgery is an example of a significant procedure. Data collected using Volume III can be utilized to conduct research or analysis of patient conditions and outcomes of treatments for those conditions.

Utilization of Diagnosis Code Data

Data collected through the use of the ICD-9-CM coding system are utilized in a number of ways, as outlined in Figure 7-3. Various organizations and other entities such as government agencies, research organizations, medical associations, and insurance companies use data collected for purposes such as research, education, and administration.

Research

Data from coding systems are used to research various patterns in diagnosis and treatment of conditions. Researchers can monitor various treatments provided for specific conditions to determine outcomes. Research data are also used to study conditions and develop new treatments and technology. By monitoring these data, researchers can identify various risk factors related to specific procedures, services, or items. Analysis of health care data is critical to predicting trends in the health care industry.

Education

Data from coding systems can be utilized to educate health care professionals such as medical students, nurses, and doctors. Education of health care professionals can be enhanced through knowledge gained by analyzing ICD-9-CM data related to conditions and treatments. New treatments, supplies, and medications can be monitored for assessment of outcomes, both positive and negative. These data can also be utilized to

TEST YOUR *Knowledge* BOX 7-1

HISTORY OF DIAGNOSIS CODING

1. Discuss the original intent of coded health care data and how that differs from its value today.

2. Explain three reasons why it is important for hospital coding and billing professionals to master an understanding and application of diagnosis coding principles.

3. Name the classification system that was the basis for the development of the International List of Causes of Death.

4. What classification system was utilized to collect data regarding the causes of death for statistical purposes during the 1900s?

5. What organization published the International Classification of Diseases (ICD)?

6. Explain what mortality and morbidity refers to in ICD-6.

7. When did hospitals begin using the ICD?

8. Provide an explanation of when procedures, "Operations and Treatments," were included in a classification system. Name the system.

9. Explain the difference between International Classification of Diseases (ICD) and International Classification of Diseases, 9th Revision, Clinical Modification (ICD-9-CM).

10. Who published the ICD-9-CM?

11. The ICD-9-CM Coordination and Maintenance Committee is responsible for ______________.

List the four organizations represented on the ICD-9-CM Coordination and Maintenance Committee.

12. ______________.

13. ______________.

14. ______________.

15. ______________.

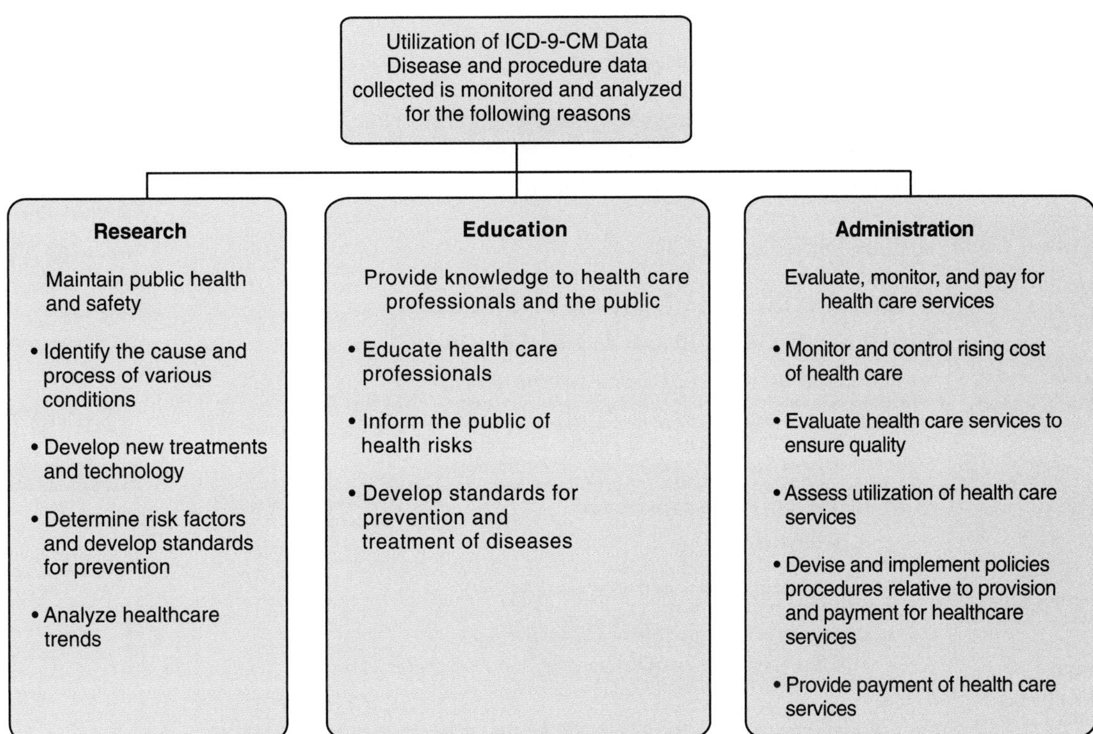

Utilization of ICD-9-CM Data
Disease and procedure data collected is monitored and analyzed for the following reasons
Research
Maintain public health and safety
• Identify the cause and process of various conditions
• Develop new treatments and technology
• Determine risk factors and develop standards for prevention
• Analyze healthcare trends
Education
Provide knowledge to health care professionals and the public
• Educate health care professionals
• Inform the public of health risks
• Develop standards for prevention and treatment of diseases
Administration
Evaluate, monitor, and pay for health care services
• Monitor and control rising cost of health care
• Evaluate health care services to ensure quality
• Assess utilization of health care services
• Devise and implement policies procedures relative to provision and payment for healthcare services
• Provide payment of health care services

Figure 7-3 Utilization of ICD-9-CM data for research, education and administrative purposes.

identify and target specific educational needs of the public such as risk factors related to heart disease or breast cancer. Standards for the prevention and treatment of disease are developed as a result of research utilizing data from various coding systems.

Administration

There are various administrative uses of data collected from coding systems. Data can be used to evaluate, monitor, and pay for health care services. Utilization of services is a major focus area of data analysis to ensure quality of care and to control health care costs. Data are used to measure and assess the quality of health care services. The development and implementation of policies and procedures related to the provision of patient care services and payment for those services are the result of analysis of ICD-9-CM data. Many payers utilize data collected through these systems to determine appropriate services provided for specific conditions and to make payment determinations.

BOX 7-4 ■ KEY POINTS

ICD-9-CM Data Utilization

Data collected through the use of the ICD-9-CM coding system are utilized for:

- Research
- Education
- Administration

Organizations Utilizing Diagnosis Code Data

The Centers for Disease Control and Prevention (CDC) and the Centers for Medicare and Medicaid Services (CMS) are examples of two organizations that depend on the data collected through the use of ICD-9-CM and other coding systems for purposes of research, education, and administration.

Centers for Disease Control and Prevention (CDC)

The CDC is an agency of the U.S. government that provides facilities and services for the investigation, identification, prevention, and control of disease. The CDC is primarily concerned with communicable diseases, environmental health, and foreign quarantine activities. The CDC also works with state and local agencies, and it provides consultation, education, and training on communicable disease issues. For example, the CDC has established recommendations (standards) called "Universal Precautions" that specify how to minimize the risk of contracting acquired immunodeficiency syndrome (AIDS). Data from the ICD-9-CM are utilized by the CDC for many reasons such as the identification of potential epidemics such as SARS or anthrax and to predict trends regarding disease. Information regarding the CDC can be obtained from the Web site, at http://www.cdc.gov/nchs/icd/icd9cm.htm, as illustrated in Figure 7-4.

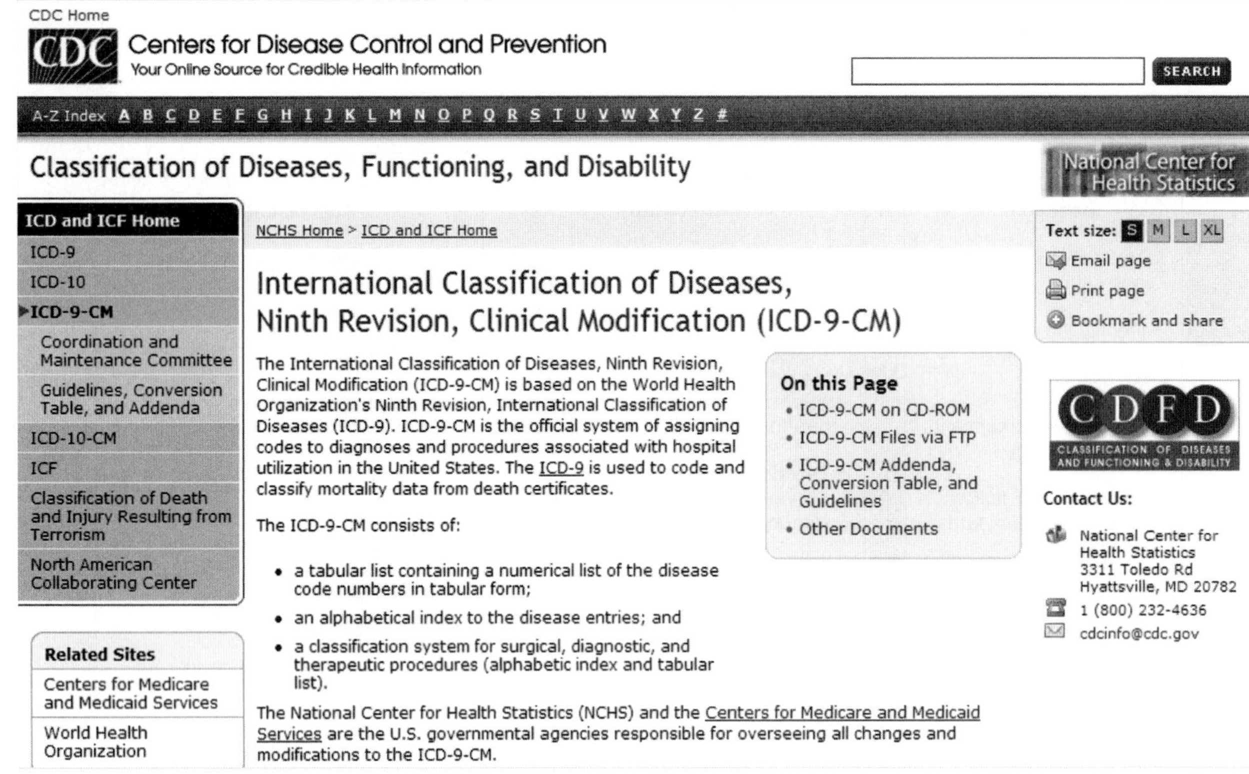

Figure 7-4 The Centers for Disease Control (CDC) Web site.

Centers for Medicare and Medicaid Services (CMS)

The U.S. Department of Health and Human Services created the Health Care Financing Administration (HCFA), now known as the CMS, for the purpose of administering the Medicare and Medicaid programs. Data from ICD-9-CM are used by the CMS for many purposes, such as utilization and monitoring of health care costs and reimbursement. The government is one of the largest payers for health care services, and CMS is responsible for ensuring appropriate utilization of health care services and controlling health care costs. ICD-9-CM codes provide explanations of why services were provided. They are utilized by providers to communicate with payers regarding the medical necessity of services provided. CMS must also monitor health care costs for the Medicare and Medicaid programs to ensure that federal budgets are in balance. Reimbursement methods implemented under the Prospective Payment System (PPS) were developed utilizing data from various coding systems. For example, Medicare Severity Diagnosis Related Groups (DRG) were developed through the classification of diseases, and payments are determined based on that classification. Information regarding CMS can be obtained from the Web site, at http://www.cms.gov, as illustrated in Figure 7-5.

BOX 7-5 ■ KEY POINTS

Organizations That Utilize ICD-9-CM Data

The Centers for Disease Control (CDC)
The Centers for Medicare and Medicaid Services (CMS)

Diagnosis Coding Defined

Coding medical conditions is referred to as diagnosis coding. **Diagnosis coding** is the process of translating written descriptions of signs, symptoms, illness, injury, disease, and other reasons for health care services from the patient's record into codes. The system utilized for diagnosis coding is the International Classification of Diseases, 9th Revision, Clinical Modification (ICD-9-CM).

Diagnosis coding is essential to describe why the patient is receiving health care services. The process begins when the patient arrives at the hospital with a health care issue(s) that requires attention or for a service involving health care status. **Chief complaint (CC)** is the term used to describe the main reason (medical condition or symptoms) why the patient is seeking health care services. A clinical interview is conducted with the patient for the purpose of obtaining information regarding the patient's chief complaint and

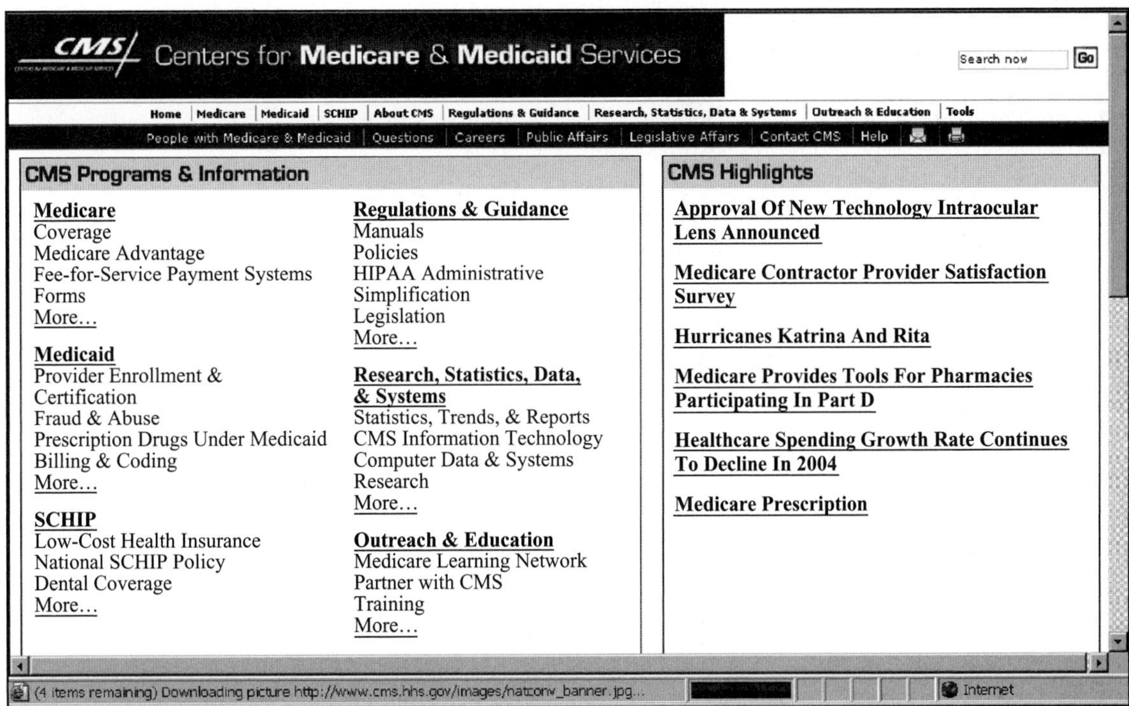

Figure 7-5 The Centers for Medicare and Medicaid Services (CMS) Web site. *(From Centers for Medicare and Medicaid Services: www.cms.hhs.gov.)*

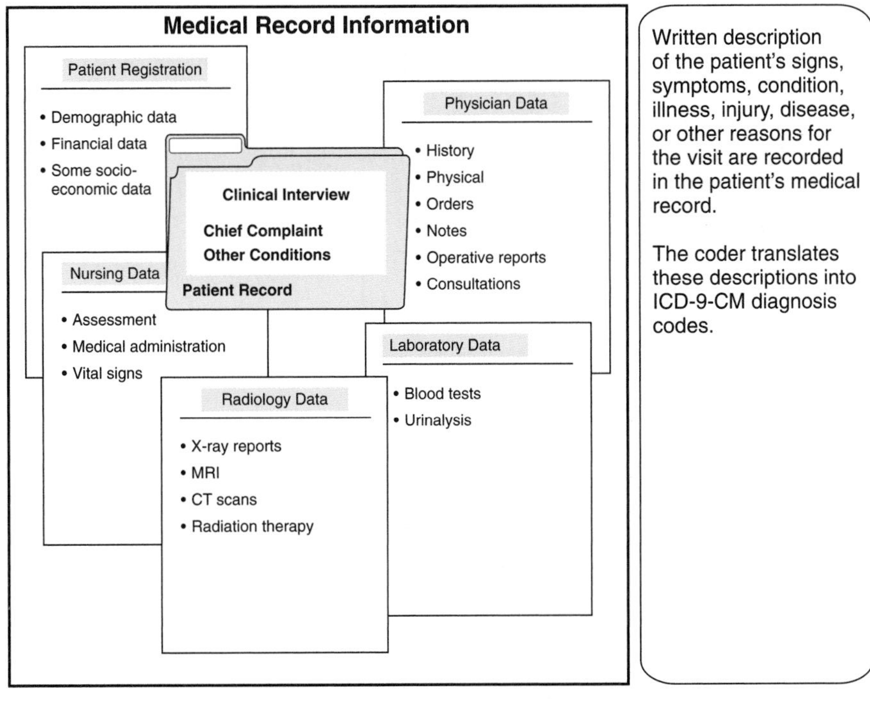

Figure 7-6 Information in the patient's medical record that is utilized for diagnosis coding. *(Modified from Davis N, LaCour M: Introduction to health information technology, ed 1, St Louis, 2002, Saunders.)*

the history of the illness. Details about the chief complaint can include when the condition occurred, how bad the condition is, and if it gets worse during certain activities or at particular times. Information regarding other conditions that may relate to the main condition is also obtained. The physician or other provider reviews the history, performs an examination, and prepares a plan of care. Other patient care services may be provided. Written descriptions of the patient's signs, symptoms, conditions, illness, injury, disease, or other reason for the visit, as well as procedures, services, and items, are recorded in the patient's medical record. The coder translates descriptions of medical conditions into diagnosis codes (Figure 7-6).

ICD-9-CM Volume I and II is the coding system utilized to identify codes that describe the patient's condition. ICD-9-CM codes are three- to five-digit codes that represent the patient's condition. Submission of claim forms for services rendered requires codes representing all conditions treated and those that affect treatment. A review of the ICD-9-CM coding system, contents, and guidelines will be presented in the next section of this chapter.

BOX 7-6 ■ KEY POINTS

Diagnosis Coding Defined

Coding is the assignment of numeric or alphanumeric codes to all health care data elements of outpatient and inpatient care.

The coding of medical conditions (diagnosis) involves assigning codes to written descriptions of the patient's sign, symptom, illness, injury, disease, condition, or other reason for patient care services.

DIAGNOSIS CODING RELATIONSHIPS

The ICD-9-CM is the standard coding system used by providers and facilities to describe a patient's condition, injury, illness, disease, or other reasons the patient is receiving health care services. The coding of signs, symptoms, illness, injury, conditions, diseases, or other reasons that patient seeks health care services requires knowledge of medical terminology, anatomy and physiology, pharmacology, and coding principles and guidelines. To code effectively, it is first important to have an understanding of the relationship of diagnosis coding to documentation, medical necessity, claim forms, and reimbursement (Figure 7-7).

Documentation

Documentation is the term used to describe information regarding the patient's condition, treatment, and response to treatment. This information is recorded in the patient's medical record. The patient's medical record is the foundation for coding. The Golden Rule in coding is **IF IT IS NOT DOCUMENTED, DO NOT CODE IT**. When coding patient conditions it is necessary to read the record to identify the condition(s) that is being treated and the condition(s) that can affect treatment. A code(s) is then selected from the ICD-9-CM that accurately describes the statement in the medical record. Examples of information recorded in the patient's medical record and the code assignments are illustrated in Figure 7-8.

- Example #1. This record is assigned code 458.0 to describe the diagnosis "Orthostatic hypotension." This code is selected as opposed to a code describing only "hypotension" because the statement in the record indicates that the patient's blood pressure drops excessively when assuming a standing position.
- Example #2. This record is assigned a code 796.2, "Elevated blood pressure reading without diagnosis of hypertension." This code assignment is appropriate rather than a diagnosis of hypertension because the record did not indicate a diagnosis of hypertension.

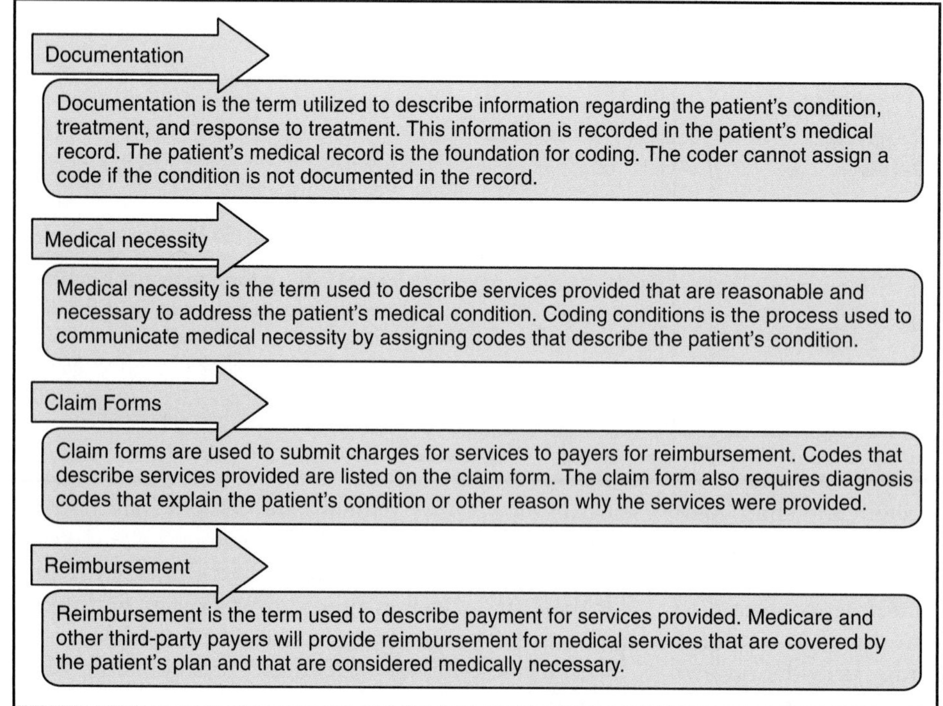

Documentation
Documentation is the term utilized to describe information regarding the patient's condition, treatment, and response to treatment. This information is recorded in the patient's medical record. The patient's medical record is the foundation for coding. The coder cannot assign a code if the condition is not documented in the record.
Medical necessity
Medical necessity is the term used to describe services provided that are reasonable and necessary to address the patient's medical condition. Coding conditions is the process used to communicate medical necessity by assigning codes that describe the patient's condition.
Claim Forms
Claim forms are used to submit charges for services to payers for reimbursement. Codes that describe services provided are listed on the claim form. The claim form also requires diagnosis codes that explain the patient's condition or other reason why the services were provided.
Reimbursement
Reimbursement is the term used to describe payment for services provided. Medicare and other third-party payers will provide reimbursement for medical services that are covered by the patient's plan and that are considered medically necessary.

Figure 7-7 The relationship of diagnosis coding to documentation, medical necessity, claim forms and reimbursement.

TEST YOUR *Knowledge* BOX 7-2

PURPOSE OF DIAGNOSIS CODING; DIAGNOSIS CODING DEFINED

1. Explain the purpose of diagnosis coding.
2. List three types of data that are classified in the ICD-9-CM coding system.
3. State the difference between mortality and morbidity.
4. Discuss three ways diagnosis code data are utilized.
5. Outline two organizations that utilize diagnosis code data, and provide an example.
6. Provide a brief explanation of how CMS utilizes diagnosis code data.
7. Provide a definition of diagnosis coding.
8. What coding system is utilized to code a diagnosis?
9. Explain what information found in a medical record is assigned a diagnosis code.
10. ICD-9-CM codes contain how many digits?

The challenge for coders is to be absolutely certain the code assignment represents what is in the record. It is important that the coder does not read into the scenario and code a condition that is not documented appropriately. If the record lacks specific information required to select a code, the coder should pursue more specific information from the physician or other provider. Coders should always follow good coding habits, such as **WHEN IN DOUBT, ASK.**

BOX 7-7 ■ KEY POINTS

Golden Rule in Coding

IF IT IS NOT DOCUMENTED, DO NOT CODE IT

Good Coding Habits

- DO NOT ASSUME.
- Identify all possible codes in the index (Volume II).
- NEVER EVER code from the index (Volume II).
- Review each code in the tabular list (Volume I).
- Review all codes in the range.
- WHEN IN DOUBT, ASK.
- Never use an E code as the first-listed condition.

Medical Necessity

Medical necessity is the term used to describe procedures or services performed that are reasonable and necessary to address the patient's medical condition. Medical necessity guidelines are generally determined based on standards of medical care. Payer guidelines regarding medical necessity will vary by payer. Coding conditions is the process used to communicate on the claim form the conditions for which the patient is seeking health care services. Codes selected should be specific in order to describe the patient's condition completely and to establish medical necessity.

Example #1

Medical Record of Jon Jamerstonig

Mr. Jamerstonig presents with abnormally low blood pressure. The patient's blood pressure drops excessively when the patient stands. Tests were ordered to assess the cause of the abnormally low blood pressure. Diagnosis: orthostatic hypotension.

Johnathan Sampson, M.D.

Code assignment: 458.0
"Orthostatic hypotension"

Example #2

Medical Record of Sara Sopterson

Ms. Sopterson presents today for a blood pressure check. Her blood pressure was elevated last visit. Her blood pressure today is still high, but not as high as last week. She may have hypertension. Ms. Sopterson will be scheduled for a blood pressure check next week. Diagnosis: elevated blood pressure.

Tamara Johnson-Meeks, M.D.

Code assignment: 796.2
"Elevated Blood Pressure"

Figure 7-8 Examples of coding conditions from the medical record.

BOX 7-8 ■ KEY POINTS

Medical Necessity

Medically necessary services are those that are reasonable and medically necessary to address the patient's medical condition.

Medical necessity is determined based on standards of medical practice.

Diagnosis codes explain the medical necessity for services or items provided.

Claim Forms

A CMS-1500 or CMS-1450 (UB-04) is used to submit charges for services rendered to payers for reimbursement. Codes that describe services provided are listed on the claim form. Diagnosis codes that explain the patient's condition or other reason why the services were provided are also required on the claim form, as illustrated in Figures 7-9 and 7-10. Diagnosis codes reported on the claim form may represent the primary, admitting, or principal diagnosis and other secondary diagnoses.

BOX 7-9 ■ KEY POINTS

Claim Forms

CMS-1500

Used for submission of physician and outpatient services

CMS-1450 (UB-04)

Used for submission of facility charges for most hospital services

First-Listed Condition

The **first-listed condition** is the major most significant reason why the patient is seeking health care services. First-listed condition is a term generally associated with physician and outpatient services. For example, if a patient presents with chest pain and knee pain, chest pain is the primary diagnosis as it is the major most significant reason for the visit (Figure 7-11). Hospital inpatient coding involves an admitting diagnosis.

Admitting Diagnosis

The **admitting diagnosis** is the major most significant reason why the patient is being admitted. For example, if a patient is admitted because he or she is experiencing rapid heart beat and a fever, rapid heart beat would be the admitting diagnosis as it is the major most significant reason for the admission (Figure 7-12).

Principal Diagnosis

The **principal diagnosis** is the condition determined after study. Study refers to the examination and other diagnostic testing used to determine the patient diagnosis. For example, a patient is admitted to the hospital for chest pain. After diagnostic tests are performed, the physician records a diagnosis of arteriosclerosis. The principal diagnosis is the condition determined after study, which is arteriosclerosis (Figure 7-13).

Other Secondary Diagnoses

Additional diagnosis codes may be required to describe other conditions that are treated or those that affect treatment. Other diagnosis may describe a complication or co-morbidity.

Complication

A **complication** is a disease or condition that develops during the course of a hospital stay. Complications may prolong the patient's length of stay, usually by 1 day in 75 percent of cases. Complications generally have an affect on the DRG assignment. An example of a complication would be when the patient develops an infection of a surgical wound (postoperative infection; Figure 7-14).

BOX 7-10 ■ KEY POINTS

Diagnoses

First-Listed Condition

The major most significant reason for the visit

Admitting

The major most significant reason for the hospital admission

Principal

The condition determined after study

Other Secondary Diagnoses

Complications and coexisting conditions (co-morbidities)

1500
HEALTH INSURANCE CLAIM FORM
APPROVED BY NATIONAL UNIFORM CLAIM COMMITTEE 08/05

PICA PICA

CARRIER

1. MEDICARE (Medicare #) MEDICAID (Medicaid #) TRICARE CHAMPUS (Sponsor's SSN) CHAMPVA (Member ID#) GROUP HEALTH PLAN (SSN or ID) FECA BLK LUNG (SSN) OTHER (ID)
1a. INSURED'S I.D. NUMBER (For Program in Item 1)
2. PATIENT'S NAME (Last Name, First Name, Middle Initial)
3. PATIENT'S BIRTH DATE MM DD YY SEX M F
4. INSURED'S NAME (Last Name, First Name, Middle Initial)
5. PATIENT'S ADDRESS (No., Street)
6. PATIENT RELATIONSHIP TO INSURED Self Spouse Child Other
7. INSURED'S ADDRESS (No., Street)
CITY STATE
8. PATIENT STATUS Single Married Other
CITY STATE
ZIP CODE TELEPHONE (Include Area Code) ( )
Employed Full-Time Student Part-Time Student
ZIP CODE TELEPHONE (Include Area Code) ( )
9. OTHER INSURED'S NAME (Last Name, First Name, Middle Initial)
10. IS PATIENT'S CONDITION RELATED TO:
11. INSURED'S POLICY GROUP OR FECA NUMBER
a. OTHER INSURED'S POLICY OR GROUP NUMBER
a. EMPLOYMENT? (Current or Previous) YES NO
a. INSURED'S DATE OF BIRTH MM DD YY SEX M F
b. OTHER INSURED'S DATE OF BIRTH MM DD YY SEX M F
b. AUTO ACCIDENT? PLACE (State) YES NO
b. EMPLOYER'S NAME OR SCHOOL NAME
c. EMPLOYER'S NAME OR SCHOOL NAME
c. OTHER ACCIDENT? YES NO
c. INSURANCE PLAN NAME OR PROGRAM NAME
d. INSURANCE PLAN NAME OR PROGRAM NAME
10d. RESERVED FOR LOCAL USE
d. IS THERE ANOTHER HEALTH BENEFIT PLAN? YES NO *If yes, return to and complete item 9 a-d.*

PATIENT AND INSURED INFORMATION

READ BACK OF FORM BEFORE COMPLETING & SIGNING THIS FORM.
12. PATIENT'S OR AUTHORIZED PERSON'S SIGNATURE I authorize the release of any medical or other information necessary to process this claim. I also request payment of government benefits either to myself or to the party who accepts assignment below.
SIGNED DATE
13. INSURED'S OR AUTHORIZED PERSON'S SIGNATURE I authorize payment of medical benefits to the undersigned physician or supplier for services described below.
SIGNED

14. DATE OF CURRENT: MM DD YY ILLNESS (First symptom) OR INJURY (Accident) OR PREGNANCY(LMP)
15. IF PATIENT HAS HAD SAME OR SIMILAR ILLNESS. GIVE FIRST DATE MM DD YY
16. DATES PATIENT UNABLE TO WORK IN CURRENT OCCUPATION FROM MM DD YY TO MM DD YY
17. NAME OF REFERRING PROVIDER OR OTHER SOURCE 17a. 17b.
18. HOSPITALIZATION DATES RELATED TO CURRENT SERVICES FROM MM DD YY TO MM DD YY
21. DIAGNOSIS OR NATURE OF ILLNESS OR INJURY (RELATIVE ITEMS 1, 2, 3, OR 4 TO ITEM 24E BY LINE)
20. OUTSIDE LAB? YES NO $ CHARGES
21. DIAGNOSIS OR NATURE OF ILLNESS OR INJURY (Relate Items 1, 2, 3 or 4 to Item 24E by Line)
1. 3.
2. 4.
22. MEDICAID RESUBMISSION CODE ORIGINAL REF. NO.
23. PRIOR AUTHORIZATION NUMBER
24. A. DATE(S) OF SERVICE From MM DD YY To MM DD YY B. PLACE OF SERVICE C. EMG D. PROCEDURES, SERVICES, OR SUPPLIES (Explain Unusual Circumstances) CPT/HCPCS MODIFIER E. DIAGNOSIS POINTER F. $ CHARGES G. DAYS OR UNITS H. EPSDT Family Plan I. ID. QUAL. J. RENDERING PROVIDER ID. #
1 NPI
2 NPI
3 NPI
4 24. A-J PROCEDURES, SERVICES, OR SUPPLIES NPI
5 LINK EACH PROCEDURE CODE TO DIAGNOSIS POINTER IN 24E NPI
6 NPI

PHYSICIAN OR SUPPLIER INFORMATION

25. FEDERAL TAX I.D. NUMBER SSN EIN
26. PATIENT'S ACCOUNT NO.
27. ACCEPT ASSIGNMENT? (For govt. claims, see back) YES NO
28. TOTAL CHARGE $
29. AMOUNT PAID $
30. BALANCE DUE $
31. SIGNATURE OF PHYSICIAN OR SUPPLIER INCLUDING DEGREES OR CREDENTIALS (I certify that the statements on the reverse apply to this bill and are made a part thereof.)
SIGNED DATE
32. SERVICE FACILITY LOCATION INFORMATION a. NPI b.
33. BILLING PROVIDER INFO & PH # ( ) a. NPI b.
NUCC Instruction Manual available at: www.nucc.org
APPROVED OMB-0938-0999 FORM CMS-1500 (08-05)

Figure 7-9 CMS-1500 claim form illustrating Blocks 21, 24, and 24E used to record and link services to diagnosis.

Co-Morbidity

Co-morbidity is a secondary condition that coexists with the condition for which the patient is seeking health care services. Co-morbidities may prolong the patient's length of stay, usually by 1 day in 75 percent of cases, which will affect the MS-DRG assignment. An example of co-morbidity is a patient presenting with atherosclerosis of an extremity who also has malignant hypertension. Malignant hypertension would be coded as the secondary diagnosis (Figure 7-14).

The first-listed condition, admitting, principal, and other secondary diagnoses are recorded on the appropriate claim form for the purpose of explaining to the payer why services were provided. As discussed in previous chapters, the claim form utilized varies based on the type of service or the type of provider. The diagnosis recorded on the form is determined by which form is used, the CMS-1500 or (UB-04). It is important for coders to understand what diagnosis is required for the claim form, where the diagnosis code is recorded, and what coding guidelines apply to the patient case, as illustrated in Table 7-2.

CMS-1500

The CMS-1500 is utilized to submit charges for physician and outpatient services. Completion of the CMS-1500 requires the patient diagnosis to be recorded in Block 21. The term first-listed condition is generally used in the physician and outpatient settings. Block 21

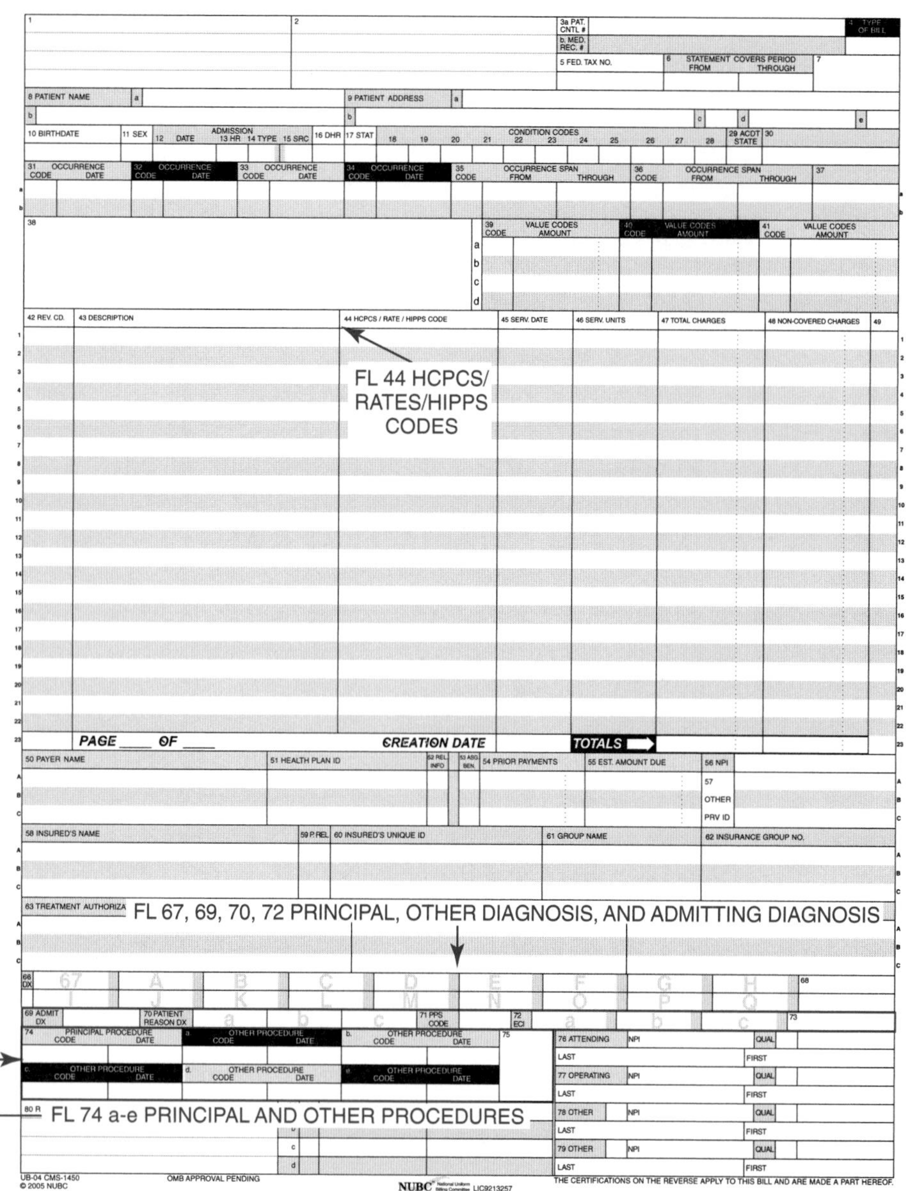

Figure 7-10 CMS-1450 (UB-04) claim form illustrating FL 67-72 used to record the admitting, principal, and other diagnosis. FL 44 is used to record HCPCS and FL 74a–e to record principal and other procedures.

> **Medical Record**
>
> Patient presents with chest pain and knee pain.
>
> First-listed condition: chest pain
>
> *Johnathan Sampson, M.D.*
>
> **First-Listed Condition Code assignment: 786.50 "Chest pain, unspecified"**
>
> Note: Code 719.46 "Pain, joint, knee" would also be assigned to explain the secondary condition.

Figure 7-11 Example of a first-listed condition code assignment.

> **Medical Record**
>
> Patient admitted to the hospital experiencing rapid heart beat and a fever.
>
> Admitting diagnosis: rapid heart beat
>
> *Johnathan Sampson, M.D.*
>
> **Admitting Diagnosis Code assignment: 785.0 "Tachycardia, unspecified"**

Figure 7-12 Example of an admitting diagnosis code assignment.

provides four areas to record the first-listed condition and other diagnosis (or diagnoses). These areas are marked with numbers referred to as reference line numbers 1, 2, 3, and 4. The first-listed condition diagnosis is listed in reference line number 1. Other secondary diagnoses are listed in order of severity in reference lines 2 to 4.

Procedure codes that describe services rendered are recorded in Block 24D. Diagnosis codes are linked to procedure codes in Block 24E. The reference line

Medical Record

Patient admitted to the hospital for chest pain. Examination and diagnostic studies reveal arteriosclerosis.

Principal diagnosis: arteriosclerosis.

Johnathan Sampson, M.D.

Principal Diagnosis Code assignment: 440.9 "Generalized and unspecified atherosclerosis"

Note: Code range 440 includes arteriosclerosis.

Figure 7-13 Example of a principal diagnosis code assignment.

Medical Record

Patient admitted to the hospital for atherosclerosis of extremity. Patient also has malignant hypertension. Medications for hypertension ordered. Bypass surgery performed. Patient developed postoperative wound infection.

Secondary condition (co-morbidity): malignant hypertension
Complication: postoperative wound infection

Johnathan Sampson, M.D.

Co-morbidity Diagnosis Code assignment: 401.0 "Hypertension, malignant"
Complication Diagnosis Code assignment: 998.59 "Postoperative infection"

Note: Principal diagnosis code assignment: 440.20 "Atherosclerosis of extremity, unspecified."

Figure 7-14 Example of other secondary diagnosis coding assignment involving a complication and co-morbidity.

TABLE 7-2 Claim Variations for ICD-9-CM Diagnosis Codes

ICD-9-CM diagnosis codes are used to report patient conditions or other reason for the visit for all (outpatient, inpatient, or nonpatient) services.

	CLAIM FORMS		
Diagnosis Coding	**CMS-1500 Diagnosis Code Block**	**CMS-1450 (UB-04) Diagnosis Code FL**	**ICD-9-CM Guidelines Applied**
First-Listed Condition			
The major most significant reason for the visit	Block 21 Reference line 1		General coding guidelines Coding guidelines for **outpatient** services
Admitting Diagnosis			
The major most significant reason for the visit		Form locator 69	General coding guidelines Coding guidelines for **inpatient**, short-term, acute care, and long-term care hospital records
Principal Diagnosis			
The condition determined after study		Form locator 67	General coding guidelines Coding guidelines for **inpatient**, short-term, acute care, and long-term care hospital records
Other Diagnosis			
Secondary diagnosis, co-existing conditions	Block 21 Reference lines 2–4		General coding guidelines Coding guidelines for **outpatient** services
Other diagnosis, complications and co-morbidities (co-existing conditions)		Form locators FL 67A–Q FL 70 FL 72	General coding guidelines Coding guidelines for **inpatient**, short-term, acute care, and long-term care hospital records

number from Block 21 is listed in 24E for the diagnosis that explains the reason the service was performed. Claim forms are carefully reviewed by the payer to identify potential reimbursement issues. Block 21 is compared against Block 24 to determine whether the service provided was medically necessary. Figure 7-15 illustrates Blocks 21, 24, and 24E on the CMS-1500. The ICD-9-CM general coding guidelines and the guidelines for outpatient services should be followed. Procedure coding will be discussed in the next chapter.

CMS-1500 (Physician and Outpatient Services)

21. DIAGNOSIS OR NATURE OF ILLNESS OR INJURY, (RELATE ITEMS 1, 2, 3 OR 4 TO ITEM 24E BY LINE) -------

1. 610 .0 3. ___ .

2. V16 .3 4. ___ .

24.	A	B	C	D		E	F	
	DATE(S) OF SERVICE From To MM DD YY MM DD	Place of Service	Type of Service	PROCEDURES, SERVICES, OR SUPPLIES (Explain Unusual Circumstances) CPT/HCPCS MODIFIER		DIAG-NOSIS CODE	$ CHARGE	
1	09 27 06 09 27 06	11	1	99212	25	1 2	120 00	1
2	09 27 06 09 27 06	11	1	19000		1 2	250 00	1
3								

Medical Record

An established patient presents with a lump in the left breast. She indicates she has a family history of breast cancer on her mother's side. Problem focus exam performed. A puncture aspiration of the solitary cyst was performed. Patient scheduled in one week for follow-up.

Diagnosis: Solitary cyst of the left breast.

Johnathan Sampson, M.D.

First Listed Condition Code assignment: Cyst 610.0
Secondary Diagnosis: Family History Malignant Neoplasm V16.3
E/M Problem Focused 99212
Puncture Aspiration left breast 19000
Patient Insurance Blue Cross/Blue Shield

Figure 7-15 Diagnosis codes are recorded on the CMS-1500 in Blocks 21 and 24E. The first-listed condition is recorded in Block 21, on reference line 1. The secondary diagnosis is recorded in Block 21, on reference line 2. The diagnosis code that explains why the service was performed is linked to the procedure in 24E.

CM5-1450 (UB-04)
(Facility Charges for Outpatient, Inpatient, and Non-Patient Services)

67 PRIN. DIAG. CD.	67 A-Q OTHER DIAG. CODES.				69 ADM. DIAG. CODE	72 E-CODE
440.20	401.0	998.59			440.20	

Medical Record

Patient admitted to the hospital for atherosclerosis of extremity. Patient also has malignant hypertension. Medications for hypertension ordered. Bypass surgery performed. Patient developed postoperative wound infection.

Johnathan Sampson, M.D.

Code assignment:
Principal diagnosis:
440.20 "Atherosclerosis of extremity, unspecified"
Other Secondary diagnosis:
401.0 "Malignant Hypertension"
998.59 "Postoperative infection "

Figure 7-16 Diagnosis codes are recorded on the CMS-1450 (UB-04) in FL 67, 69, 70, 72 as outlined below. Diagnosis codes must provide an explanation for the patient admission, services, and items provided during the admission.

BOX 7-11 ■ KEY POINTS

Complications and Co-morbidities

A complication is a disease or condition that develops during the course of a hospital stay.

A co-morbidity is a secondary condition that coexists with the condition for which the patient is seeking health care services.

CMS-1450 (UB-04)

The CMS-1450 (UB-04) is utilized to submit facility charges for outpatient, non-patient, and inpatient services provided by a hospital or other facility. The UB-04 contains 81 fields referred to as form locators (FL). Completion of the UB-04 requires that all patient diagnoses be recorded to explain the medical reason for the admission and services provided. Procedure codes are also recorded on the claim form to describe the services or items rendered. Procedure coding will be discussed in the next chapter. Figure 7-16 illustrates how diagnosis code(s) are recorded on the UB-04.

The patient's principal diagnosis is recorded in FL 67. The term *principal diagnosis* is generally used for facility claims. Inpatient claims also require a present on admission indicator (POA). FL 67A–Q are used to record other diagnosis codes representing complications, co-morbidities, or other reasons for the admission. The admitting diagnosis is recorded in FL 69. The patient reason diagnosis is recorded in FL 70 on outpatient claims. If there is an external cause of injury, the appropriate code to describe it is recorded in FL 72. Principal and other procedure codes listed in FL 74a-e are designed to explain the principal and other procedures. The payer will carefully review and compare these fields to determine whether the admission and services provided meet medical necessity requirements.

Reimbursement

Reimbursement is the term used to describe payment for services provided. Claim forms are submitted to third-party payers such as insurance companies, Medi-

Medical Record

A patient presents complaining of pain in the left breast. She indicates she has a family history of breast cancer on her mother's side. Problem focus exam performed that revealed a lump in the left breast. A puncture aspiration of the solitary cyst was performed. Patient scheduled in one week for follow-up.

Diagnosis: solitary cyst of the left breast.

Johnathan Sampson, M.D.

First-Listed Condition Code assignment: Cyst 610.0
Secondary Diagnosis: Family History Malignant Neoplasm V16.3
E/M Problem Focused 99212
Puncture Aspiration left breast 19000

Patient Insurance Blue Cross/Blue Shield

Figure 7-17 Example of medical record documentation illustrating medical necessity.

care, and other government payers to obtain reimbursement for services provided. Diagnosis codes are utilized on the claim form to explain why the services were provided. They are also used to explain the medical necessity of services provided. Payers provide reimbursement for services that are covered by the patient's plan and that are considered medically necessary based on standards of medical care. Therefore, it is critical to ensure that the codes submitted completely describe the patient's medical condition(s) to explain why the services were necessary. Figure 7-17 highlights an example of how the record contains information that explains why the service was required. The patient has a lump in her left breast and she has a family history of breast cancer. If the claim was submitted with a diagnosis of pain in left breast, the payer might not consider the puncture aspiration medically necessary. The submission of diagnosis codes describing the lump and family history of breast cancer provide a clear explanation of why the aspiration was required.

ICD-9-CM CONTENT

The International Classification of Diseases, 9th Revision, Clinical Modification (ICD-9-CM) consists of three sections referred to as volumes. Volumes I and II are used to code descriptions of the patient's signs, symptoms, injury, illness, disease, or other reason the patient is seeking health care services. Volume III is used to code descriptions of procedures performed during a hospital visit (Figure 7-18). Physician and outpatient providers utilize Volumes I and II. Hospitals and other facilities utilize Volumes I, II, and III of the ICD-9-CM to report procedures, items, and a description of the patient's condition that explains why the service or item was provided. The ICD-9-CM can be purchased with Volumes I and II only for physician and outpatient coding or with all three volumes for use by hospitals and facilities (Figure 7-19).

ICD-9-CM
International Classification of Diseases, 9th Revision, Clinical Modification

Volume I
Tabular List of Diseases

Volume II
Alphabetic Index to Diseases

Volume III
Alphabetic and Tabular List of Procedures

(for hospitals and other facilities)

Figure 7-18 ICD-9-CM manual.

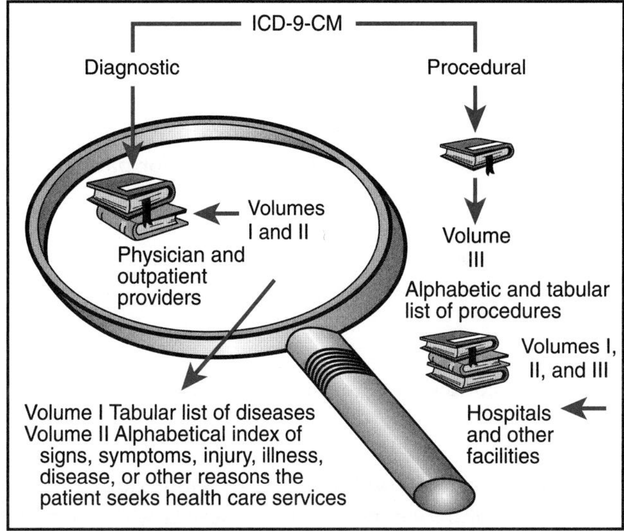

Figure 7-19 ICD-9-CM Content Volumes I, II, and III. *(Modified from Radcode Inc.: Content of ICD-9CM, www.radcodeinc.com/page2.html, 2005.)*

BOX 7-12 ■ KEY POINTS

ICD-9-CM Volumes I, II, and III

Volume I

Includes the tabular list of diseases, two supplemental classifications, and appendices.

Volume II

Contains an alphabetic index to diseases, three tables, and an alphabetic index to external causes of injury as outlined.

Volume III

Contains an alphabetical and tabular listing of procedures

ICD-9-CM Volume I Content

Volume I is the Tabular List of Diseases generally located in the middle of the ICD-9-CM coding book. It is listed in the middle of the book because the coder will reference Volume II, the alphabetical index, first to

TEST YOUR *Knowledge* BOX 7-3

DIAGNOSIS CODING RELATIONSHIPS

Provide a brief explanation of the relationship between diagnosis coding and the following:

1. Documentation
2. Medical necessity
3. Claim forms
4. Reimbursement.

Fill in the blank: provide a term for the following definitions:

5. The major most significant reason for patient care services rendered in a physician's office is the ____________ diagnosis.
6. The major most significant reason for a hospital admission is the ____________ diagnosis.
7. The condition determined after study is the ____________ diagnosis.
8. A disease or condition that develops during the course of a hospital stay is ____________.
   A secondary condition that coexists with the first-listed or principal condition is ____________.
9. Explain how diagnosis codes are linked to procedures on the CMS-1500.
10. Describe where diagnosis codes are recorded in the following claim forms:
    CMS-1500
    CMS-1450 (UB-04).

identify possible codes. Volume I is used to review codes identified in the index (Volume II) for selection of the code that most accurately describes the diagnostic statement in the record. Volume I contents include the Tabular List of Diseases, two supplemental classifications, and appendices, as outlined in Table 7-3.

Volume I: Tabular List of Diseases

The tabular list is a numerical listing of diseases, and it includes signs, symptoms, injury, illness, disease, or other reasons why the patient seeks health care. The listing is organized numerically in three-digit chapter classifications by condition (Table 7-3). For example, Chapter 1 represents Infectious and Parasitic Diseases, which are coded utilizing code range 001 to 139.

Within each chapter conditions and diseases are described with codes that are three to five digits. Figure 7-20 illustrates codes describing conditions of Blood and Blood Forming Organs listed in chapter 4. The ICD-9-CM provides instructions on code selection through the use of conventions, which will be discussed later in this chapter.

TABLE 7-3 ICD-9-CM Volume I: Tabular List of Diseases

Chapter	Heading	Range
1	Infectious and Parasitic Diseases	001–139
2	Neoplasms	140–239
3	Endocrine, Nutritional, and Metabolic Diseases and Immunity Disorders	240–279
4	Diseases of the Blood and Blood-Forming Organs	280–289
5	Mental Disorders	290–319
6	Diseases of the Nervous System and Sense Organs	320–389
7	Diseases of the Circulatory System	390–459
8	Diseases of the Respiratory System	460–519
9	Diseases of the Digestive System	520–579
10	Diseases of the Genitourinary System	580–629
11	Complications of Pregnancy, Childbirth, and the Puerperium	630–679
12	Diseases of the Skin and Subcutaneous Tissue	680–709
13	Diseases of the Musculoskeletal System and Connective Tissue	710–739
14	Congenital Anomalies	740–759
15	Certain Conditions Originating in the Perinatal Period	760–779
16	Symptoms, Signs, and Ill-Defined Conditions	780–799
17	Injury and Poisoning	800–999

Supplemental Classifications
1. Classification of Factors Influencing Health Status and Contact with Health Services: V01–V89
2. Classification of External Causes of Injury and Poisoning: E000–E999

Appendices*
Morphology of neoplasms
Glossary of mental disorders
Classification of drugs by American Hospital Formulary Service List Number and their ICD-9-CM equivalents
Classification of industrial accidents according to agency
List of three-digit categories

*Not all ICD-9-CM books contain the same appendices.

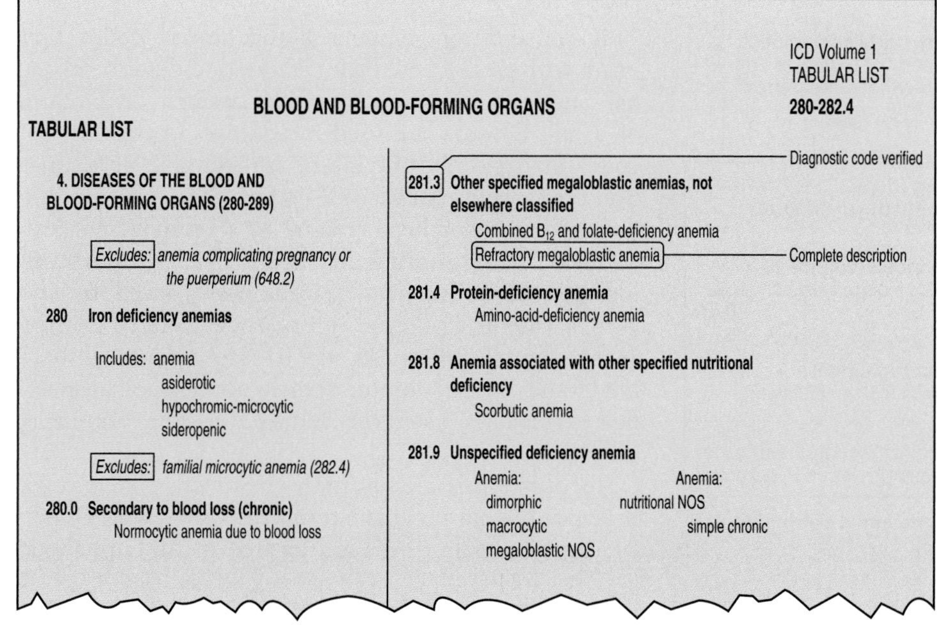

Figure 7-20 ICD-9-CM Volume I, Tabular List. *(From Fordney MT: Insurance handbook for the medical office, ed 11, St Louis, 2010, Elsevier.)*

Volume I: Supplemental Classifications

Volume I contains two supplemental classifications used to describe factors influencing health status and contact with health services and external causes of injury.

Classification of Factors Influencing Health Status and Contact with Health Services (V01 to V89)

This classification contains alphanumeric codes that begin with a V. These codes are used to describe reasons other than a condition, sign, symptom, injury, illness, or disease, that a patient seeks health care. An example of a situation that would require a V code is the admission of a patient for isolation, as illustrated in Figure 7-21. The record does not indicate any signs, symptoms, injury, illness, or diseases; therefore, code V07.0 "Need for isolation and other prophylactic measures" is assigned.

To utilize this classification effectively, coders must be aware of common main terms associated with V code assignment. Main terms are located in the alphabetic index in Volume II. Codes identified in the index are then referenced in the tabular list in Volume I to select the code that most adequately describes the situation. It is also important for coders to remember that not all V codes can be used as a first-listed or principal diagnosis as indicated in the ICD-9-CM manual (Figure 7-22).

Medical Record

Patient admitted to the hospital for quarantine (isolation) and screening for a seriously contagious disease. Patient states she has no signs or symptoms.

Admitting diagnosis:
isolation — exposure to unknown contagious disease.

Johnathan Sampson, M.D.

Admitting Diagnosis Code assignment: V07.0 "Need for isolation and other prophylactic measures"

Note: ICD-9-CM indicates this V code may be used as a principal diagnosis on Medicare Claims.

Coding Steps

Read the record; identify the main term
Isolation

Look up main term in index (Volume II)
The main term entry for isolation lists code(s)
V07.0
social V62.4

Refer to the tabular list (Volume I)
Review of V07.0 versus V62.4 verifies the correct code is

V07.0 "Need for isolation and other prophylactic measures"

Figure 7-21 Example of code assignment involving factors influencing health status V codes.

ICD-9-CM Volume I—Supplementary Classification of Factors Influencing Health Status and Contact with Health Services

I. Used to describe when patients seek health care for reasons other than injury, illness, or disease

II. Common main terms that describe these circumstances

Abnormal	Donor	Observation
Admission	Examination	Outcome (of delivery)
Aftercare	Exposure	Postoperative (status)
Attention to	Fitting (of)	Pregnancy
Checkup (Routine)	Follow-up	Screening
Counseling	Isolation	Status
Dialysis	History (of)	Supervision (of)

III. Steps to code factors influencing health status

Read the record
Identify the main term for the V code situation
Look the main term up in the index in Volume II
Identify possible codes to describe the situation in your record
Refer to the tabular section in Volume I to review codes identified and select the code that most accurately describes the circumstance recorded in the record

IV. Determine if the code can be used as a secondary or primary code

Note: V codes may be listed as the primary/principal diagnosis in specified circumstances as noted in the ICD-9-CM manual and in accordance with payer guidelines.

Figure 7-22 ICD-9-CM V code notes regarding main terms, steps to coding, and first-listed versus principal diagnosis.

BOX 7-13 ■ KEY POINTS

Classification of Factors Influencing Health Status and Contact with Health Services (V01–V89)

ICD-9-CM Alphanumeric Codes That Begin with a V

These codes are used to describe reasons patients seek health care services that are **other than** a condition, sign, symptom, injury, illness, or disease.

Classification of External Causes of Injury and Poisoning (E000 to E999)

This classification contains alphanumeric codes that begin with an E. These codes are used to describe external causes of injury, such as auto accident, explosion, or a fall. E codes are used in addition (secondary) to codes that describe the injury. An example of a situation that would require an E code is the admission of a patient for major head trauma as a result of an auto accident, as illustrated in Figure 7-23. The record indicates that the head trauma was caused by the auto accident. The head injury code would be listed as the admitting diagnosis, 959.01 "Head injury, unspecified," and E819.9 "Motor vehicle accident of unspecified nature" is listed in addition to the admitting diagnosis.

To utilize this classification effectively, coders must be aware of common main terms associated with E code assignment. Main terms are located in the alphabetic

Medical Record

Patient admitted to the hospital for major head trauma as a result of an auto accident.

Admitting diagnosis: head injury resulting from auto accident.

Johnathan Sampson, M.D.

Admitting Diagnosis Code assignment:
959.01 "Head injury, unspecified"
E819.9 "Motor vehicle accident of unspecified nature"

Note: E codes are never listed as the admitting or principal diagnosis.

Coding Steps for the External Cause of Injury

Read the record, identify the main term
Accident, motor vehicle

Look up main term in index to external causes of injury (Volume II)
The main term entry for accident, motor vehicle lists code(s) E819.9

Refer to the tabular list (Volume I)
Review of E819 verifies the correct code is

E819.9 "Motor vehicle traffic accident of unspecified nature"

Figure 7-23 Example of code assignment involving an external cause of injury, E codes.

ICD-9-CM Volume I—Supplementary Classification of External Causes of Injury and Poisoning

I. Used to describe the external cause of the injury or condition that is being treated

II. Common main terms that describe external causes of injury or condition

Abuse	Foreign body	Poisoning
Accident	Injury	Radiation
Adverse effect	Late effect	Reaction, abnormal
Assault	Malfunction	Submersion
Collision	Misadventure during surgical/medical care	Surgical procedure, complication
Effect (adverse)		Terrorism
Exposure		War operations
Fall	Object	

III. Steps to code external causes of injury
Read the record
Identify the main term for the external cause
Look the main term up in the index to external causes of injury (behind the drug table) in Volume II
Identify possible codes to describe the situation in your record
Refer to the tabular section in Volume I to review codes identified and select the code that most accurately describes the circumstance recorded in the record

Note: E codes should never be listed as a primary/principal diagnosis. Payer guidelines regarding when E codes should be submitted vary.

Figure 7-24 ICD-9-CM E code notes regarding main terms, steps to coding and first-listed condition versus principal diagnosis. E codes are a supplementary classification of external causes of injury and poisoning.

index to external causes of injury in Volume II. Codes identified in the index are then referenced in the tabular list in Volume I to select the code that most adequately describes the external cause. It is also important for coders to remember that E codes are never listed as the admitting, first-listed, or principal diagnosis (Figure 7-24).

BOX 7-14 ■ KEY POINTS

Classification of External Causes of Injury and Poisoning (E000–E999): E Codes

ICD-9-CM Alphanumeric Codes That Begin with an E

These codes are used to describe external causes of injury, such as auto accident, explosion, drug reaction, or a fall.

Volume I: Appendices

Appendices are generally located in the back of Volume I. The appendices are not used for the purpose of selecting codes; they are used for reference in various areas such as morphologies or mental disorders. Appendices listed in an ICD-9-CM book will vary as determined by the publisher. Examples of common appendices included in ICD-9-CM books are:

- Morphology of neoplasms
- Glossary of mental disorders
- Classification of drugs by American Hospital Formulary
- Service List Numbers and their ICD-9-CM equivalents
- Classification of industrial accidents according to agency
- List of three-digit categories.

Alphabetic Index to Diseases

- **Alphabetical listing** of signs, symptoms, injury, illness, disease, and other reasons that patients seek health care services.
- **Tables**
  Hypertension Table
  Neoplasm Table
  Table of Drugs and Chemicals
- **Alphabetic Index to External Causes of Injury**
  Alphabetic listing of external causes of injury

Figure 7-25 ICD-9-CM Volume II contents.

ICD-9-CM Volume II Content

Volume II is the alphabetic listing (index) to disease. It is generally located in the front of the ICD-9-CM book because it is the volume coders reference first. The content of Volume II consists of an alphabetic index to diseases, three tables, and an alphabetic index to external causes of injury, as outlined in Figure 7-25.

Volume II: Alphabetic Index to Diseases

Volume II contains an alphabetic listing of signs, symptoms, conditions, injuries, illnesses, diseases, and other reasons for which a patient seeks health care services organized by main term. The **main term** represents a sign, symptom, illness, injury, disease, condition, or other reason the patient is seeking health care. The coder will review the patient's medical record for the purpose of identifying the main term for all conditions treated and conditions that affect treatment. The coder then refers to the Volume II index, which is alphabetized according to main terms that represent signs, symptoms, illness, or injury, such as abscess, contusion, dermatitis, hypertension, lump, neoplasm, or pain. Indented below the main term are related subterms (Figure 7-26). All codes identified in Volume II must be verified in Volume I. Remember, ***NEVER*** use a code found in Volume II without verifying it in Volume I.

Volume II: Tables

Tables are utilized to effectively present information required to identify codes describing the patient's condition. The Volume II index contains three tables that are located alphabetically in the index: (1) Hypertension, (2) Neoplasm, and (3) Table of Drugs and Chemicals.

1. Hypertension Table

The hypertension table lists codes for malignant, benign, and unspecified hypertension and related conditions. The first column lists the condition hypertension with related conditions indented beneath. The remaining columns list codes for the hypertensive conditions that are malignant, benign, or unspecified, as outlined in Figure 7-27.

The following are definitions of terms required for coding hypertension:

BOX 7-15 ■ KEY POINTS

ICD-9-CM Tables: Tables Located in Volume II

Hypertension Table

Used to identify possible codes for hypertension and related conditions

Neoplasm Table

Used to identify possible codes for neoplasms

Table of Drugs and Chemicals

Used to identify possible codes for conditions related to poisoning and averse effects

BOX 7-16 ■ KEY POINTS

Hypertension versus High Blood Pressure

Hypertension Code Range 401

Hypertension is defined as high arterial blood pressure; various criteria for its threshold have been suggested, from 140 mm Hg systolic and 90 mm Hg diastolic to as high as 200 mm Hg systolic and 110 mm Hg diastolic. Hypertension is coded when the record indicates persistently high blood pressure at specified levels, at three consecutive visits.

Elevated Blood Pressure 796.2

Elevated blood pressure is coded when the patient presents with high blood pressure and there is no definitive diagnosis of hypertension recorded in the record.

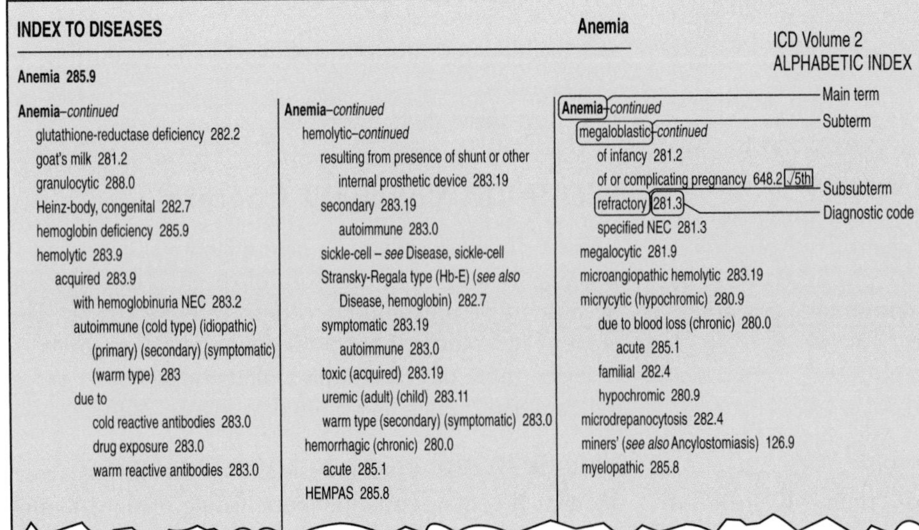

INDEX TO DISEASES — **Anemia**

Anemia 285.9

Anemia–*continued*
glutathione-reductase deficiency 282.2
goat's milk 281.2
granulocytic 288.0
Heinz-body, congenital 282.7
hemoglobin deficiency 285.9
hemolytic 283.9
acquired 283.9
with hemoglobinuria NEC 283.2
autoimmune (cold type) (idiopathic) (primary) (secondary) (symptomatic) (warm type) 283
due to
cold reactive antibodies 283.0
drug exposure 283.0
warm reactive antibodies 283.0

Anemia–*continued*
hemolytic–*continued*
resulting from presence of shunt or other internal prosthetic device 283.19
secondary 283.19
autoimmune 283.0
sickle-cell – *see* Disease, sickle-cell
Stransky-Regala type (Hb-E) (*see also* Disease, hemoglobin) 282.7
symptomatic 283.19
autoimmune 283.0
toxic (acquired) 283.19
uremic (adult) (child) 283.11
warm type (secondary) (symptomatic) 283.0
hemorrhagic (chronic) 280.0
acute 285.1
HEMPAS 285.8

Anemia–*continued*
megaloblastic–*continued*
of infancy 281.2
of or complicating pregnancy 648.2 √5th
refractory 281.3
specified NEC 281.3
megalocytic 281.9
microangiopathic hemolytic 283.19
micrycytic (hypochromic) 280.9
due to blood loss (chronic) 280.0
acute 285.1
familial 282.4
hypochromic 280.9
microdrepanocytosis 282.4
miners' (*see also* Ancylostomiasis) 126.9
myelopathic 285.8

Figure 7-26 ICD-9-CM Volume I Index to Diseases. *(From Fordney MT: Insurance Handbook for the medical office, ed 11, St Louis, 2010, Elsevier.)*

Hypertension, hypertensive

	Malignant	Benign	Unspecified
Hypertension, hypertensive (arterial) (arteriolar) (crisis) (degeneration) (disease) (essential) (fluctuating) (idiopathic) (intermittent) (labile) (low renin) (orthostatic) (paroxysmal) (primary) (systemic) (uncontrolled) (vascular)	401.0	401.1	401.9
with			
heart involvement (conditions classifiable to 429.0-429.3, 429.8, 429.9 due to hypertension) (*see also* Hypertension, heart)	402.00	402.10	402.90
with kidney involvement—*see* Hypertension, cardiorenal			
renal involvement (only conditions classifiable to 585, 586, 587) (excludes conditions classifiable to 584) (*see also* Hypertension, kidney)	403.00	403.10	403.90
renal sclerosis or failure	403.00	403.10	403.90
with heart involvement - *see* Hypertension, cardiorenal			
failure (and sclerosis)(*see also* Hypertension, kidney)	403.01	403.11	403.91
sclerosis without failure (*see also* Hypertension, kidney)	403.00	403.10	403.90
accelerated—(*see also* Hypertension, by type, malignant)	401.0	—	—
antepartum—*see* Hypertension, complicating pregnancy, childbirth, or the puerperium			
cardiorenal (disease)	404.00	404.10	404.90
with			
heart failure	404.01	404.11	404.91
and renal failure	404.03	404.13	404.93
renal failure	404.02	404.12	404.92
and heart failure	404.03	404.13	404.93
cardiovascular disease (arteriosclerotic) (sclerotic)	402.00	402.10	402.90
with			
heart failure	402.01	402.11	402.91
renal involvement (conditions classifiable to 403) (*see also* Hypertension, cardiorenal)	404.00	404.10	404.90

Figure 7-27 ICD-9-CM Volume II Hypertension table. *(Data from International classification of diseases, 9th revision, U.S. Department of Health and Human Services, Public Health Services, Centers for Medicare and Medicaid Services.)*

Hypertension is defined as high arterial blood pressure; various criteria for its threshold have been suggested from 140 mm Hg systolic and 90 mm Hg diastolic to as high as 200 mm Hg systolic and 110 mm Hg diastolic. Hypertension may have no known cause (essential) or be associated with other primary diseases (secondary). Hypertension is coded when the record indicates persistently high blood pressure over specified levels at three consecutive visits.

- **Essential hypertension** or primary hypertension means that there is no known underlying condition that is causing the blood pressure to increase.
- **Benign hypertension** is defined as mildly elevated arterial blood pressure. Benign hypertension may be indicated when blood pressure increases slightly over a long period of time.
- **Malignant hypertension** is a severe hypertensive state that is characterized by a diastolic pressure higher than 120 mm Hg, severe headaches, blurred vision, and confusion; it may result in fatal uremia, myocardial infarction, congestive heart failure, or a cerebrovascular accident.
- **Unspecified hypertension** is coded when the record does not indicate whether the hypertension is benign or malignant.

BOX 7-17 ■ KEY POINTS

Hypertension Terms

Hypertension
Essential hypertension
Benign hypertension
Malignant hypertension
Unspecified hypertension

2. Neoplasm Table

The neoplasm table lists codes for neoplasms according to behavior—malignant, benign, uncertain behavior, or unspecified as outlined in Figure 7-28. The first column lists the site or type of neoplasm. The remaining columns list codes for behavior of the specific neoplasm. The neoplasm table further identifies the neoplasm site as primary, secondary, and carcinoma in situ. The following are definitions of terms required for coding neoplasms:

Neoplasm is a new growth of tissue in which the growth is uncontrolled and progressive.

- **Benign neoplasm** is a growth that does not have properties of invasion, meaning it does not spread.

Index to Diseases

	Malignant					
	Primary	Secondary	Ca in situ	Benign	Uncertain Behavior	Unspecified
Neoplasm, neoplastic	199.1	199.1	234.9	229.9	238.9	239.9
abdomen, abdominal	195.2	198.89	234.8	229.8	238.8	239.8
cavity	195.2	198.89	234.8	229.8	238.8	239.8
organ	195.2	198.89	234.8	229.8	238.8	239.8
viscera	195.2	198.89	234.8	229.8	238.8	239.8
wall	173.5	198.2	232.5	216.5	238.2	239.2
connective tissue	171.5	198.89	—	215.5	238.1	239.2
abdominopelvic	195.8	198.89	234.8	229.8	238.8	239.8
accessory sinus — *see* Neoplasm, sinus						
acoustic nerve	192.0	198.4	—	225.1	237.9	239.7
acromion (process)	170.4	198.5	—	213.4	238.0	239.2
adenoid (pharynx) (tissue)	147.1	198.89	230.0	210.7	235.1	239.0
adipose tissue (*see also* Neoplasm, connective tissue)	171.9	198.89	—	215.9	238.1	239.2
adnexa (uterine)	183.9	198.82	233.3	221.8	236.3	239.5
adrenal (cortex) (gland) (medulla)	194.0	198.7	234.8	227.0	237.2	239.7
ala nasi (external)	173.3	198.2	232.3	216.3	238.2	239.2
alimentary canal or tract NEC	159.9	197.8	230.9	211.9	235.5	239.0
alveolar	143.9	198.89	230.0	210.4	235.1	239.0

Figure 7-28 ICD-9-CM Volume II Neoplasm table. *(Data from International classification of diseases, 9th revision, U.S. Department of Health and Human Services, Public Health Services, Centers for Medicare and Medicaid Services.)*

- **Malignant neoplasm** is a growth that has properties of invasion, meaning it can spread.
  - Primary—a growth that is in the original site.
  - Secondary—a growth that has spread to another site.
  - Carcinoma in situ: a growth that has properties of invasion but is confined within the margins.
  - Metastasis—to spread—the transfer of disease from one organ or part to another not directly connected with it.
  - Metastasize—the disease has spread to form a new focus of disease in a distant part by metastasis.
  - Metastatic—spread pertaining to or of the nature of metastasis.
- **Uncertain behavior** means that the pathology does not definitively indicate whether the growth is benign or malignant.
- **Unspecified** is used when the record does not indicate whether the growth is benign or malignant.

Coding the behavior of a neoplasm is performed using information from a pathology report found in the patient's medical record.

3. Table of Drugs and Chemicals

The table of drugs and chemicals list codes for poisoning and adverse reactions from chemicals and substances. The first column on the left lists the chemical or substance. The next column lists poison codes in the 900 range that describe poisoning involving specific chemicals and substances. E codes that describe external causes of the poisoning and E codes that describe the external cause for the adverse reaction are listed in the last five columns. The Table of Drugs and Chemicals is illustrated in Figure 7-29. The following are definitions of terms required for coding a poisoning or an adverse reaction:

Poisoning is a condition caused by the ingestion of a substance or chemical that is toxic. Poisoning can occur when a toxic substance is ingested or when a medication is taken that was not properly prescribed or administered. Codes from this column are selected when the record indicates poisoning.

- Accident—codes from this column are selected when the record indicates the poisoning was accidental, i.e., the substance was ingested by accident.

BOX 7-18 ■ KEY POINTS

Neoplasm Terms

Neoplasm
Benign neoplasm
Malignant neoplasm
  Primary
  Secondary
  Carcinoma in situ
  Metastasis
  Metastasize
  Metastatic
Uncertain behavior
Unspecified

Section 2 Alphabetic Index to Poisoning and External Causes of Adverse Effects of Drugs and Other Chemical Substances

		External Cause (E-Code)				
	Poisoning	Accident	Therapeutic Use	Suicide Attempt	Assault	Undetermined
1-propanol	980.3	E860.4	—	E950.9	E962.1	E980.9
2-propanol	980.2	E860.3	—	E950.9	E962.1	E980.9
2, 4-D (dichlorophenoxyacetic acid)	989.4	E863.5	—	E950.6	E962.1	E980.7
2, 4-toluene diisocyanate	983.0	E864.0	—	E950.7	E962.1	E980.6
2, 4, 5-T (trichlorophenoxyacetic acid)	989.2	E863.5	—	E950.6	E962.1	E980.7
14-hydroxydihydromorphinone	965.09	E850.2	E935.2	E950.0	E962.0	E980.0
ABOB	961.7	E857	E931.7	E950.4	E962.0	E980.4
Abrus (seed)	988.2	E865.3	—	E950.9	E962.1	E980.9
Absinthe	980.0	E860.1	—	E950.9	E962.1	E980.9
beverage	980.0	E860.0	—	E950.9	E962.1	E980.9
Acenocoumarin, acenocoumarol	964.2	E858.2	E934.2	E950.4	E962.0	E980.4
Acepromazine	969.1	E853.0	E939.1	E950.3	E962.0	E980.3
Acetal	982.8	E862.4	—	E950.9	E962.1	E980.9
Acetaldehyde (vapor)	987.8	E869.8	—	E952.8	E962.2	E982.8
liquid	989.89	E866.8	—	E950.9	E962.1	E980.9
Acetaminophen	965.4	E850.4	E935.4	E950.0	E962.0	E980.0

Figure 7-29 ICD-9-CM Volume II Table of drugs and chemicals. *(Data from International classification of diseases, 9th revision, U.S. Department of Health and Human Services, Public Health Services, Centers for Medicare and Medicaid Services.)*

- Suicide attempt—codes from this column are selected when the record indicates the ingestion of substance was self-inflicted.
- Assault—codes from this column are selected when the record indicates the poisoning was the result of an assault (inflicted by another person), for example, drugs slipped into a person's drink.
- Undetermined—codes from this column are selected when the record indicates the cause of the poisoning is undetermined.
- Unspecified—codes from this column are selected when the record does not indicate the cause of the poisoning.

Adverse reaction (adverse effect) is an unexpected condition that occurs in reaction to a medication that is properly prescribed and administered.

- Therapeutic—codes from this column are used when the record indicates the patient has had a reaction to a substance that was properly administered and taken.

BOX 7-19 ■ KEY POINTS

Poisoning versus Adverse Effect

Poisoning is a condition caused by the ingestion of a substance or chemical that is toxic. Poisoning can occur when a toxic substance is ingested or when a medication is taken that was not properly prescribed or administered.

Adverse effect is an unexpected condition that occurs in reaction to a medication that is properly prescribed and administered.

Alphabetic Index to External Causes of Injury

Coding external causes of injury requires the coder to identify the main term that describes the cause of the injury such as accident, fall, poisoning, adverse effect, or insect bite. The coder then refers to the Index to External Causes of Injury, which is the last section in Volume II, to find possible codes. Again, remember that all codes must be confirmed in Volume I, the Tabular List (Figure 7-30).

ICD-9-CM Volume III Content

ICD-9-CM Volume III is used by hospitals and other facilities to code significant procedures performed during the patient's hospital visit. It contains an alphabetic index and a tabular list of procedures and services (Figure 7-31).

Volume III: Alphabetic Index to Procedures

The ICD-9-CM Volume III alphabetic index is a listing of procedures outlined by main terms and subterms. The main term and subterm entries in Volume III represent procedures and services. This volume is sometimes referred to as the ICD-9-PC.

Volume III: Tabular List of Procedures

The tabular list of procedures is a numerical listing of procedures and services.

The focus of this chapter is diagnosis coding utilizing Volumes I and II. Volume III procedures will be discussed at length in the next chapter.

TEST YOUR *Knowledge* BOX 7-4

ICD-9-CM CONTENT

1. What providers are required to use the ICD-9-CM for coding conditions?
2. Provide a brief outline of the content of each of the following ICD-9-CM Volumes:
   A. Volume I
   B. Volume II
   C. Volume III.
3. How many chapters are in Volume I?
4. Explain how the codes listed in Volume I are categorized.
5. What are the V code and E code classifications in Volume I used for?
6. State the purpose of the appendices in Volume I.
7. Provide a brief description of the contents of Volume II.
8. Describe how a coder would utilize Volume II.
9. Is it true that a coder can use a code found in Volume II without having to refer to Volume I?
10. Name three tables listed in Volume II, and provide a brief explanation of each.
11. Is the hypertension table used to code high blood pressure?
12. Explain the difference between malignant hypertension and essential hypertension.
13. Provide an overview of the content of Volume III and what it is used for.
14. List the section of the ICD-9-CM in which a coder can look up main terms describing external causes of injury.
15. Explain the difference between a benign neoplasm and a malignant neoplasm.

INDEX TO EXTERNAL CAUSES — Collision

Collision (accidental)–*continued*
motor vehicle (on public highway) (traffic accident)–*continued*
and–*continued*
fallen–*continued*
tree E815
guard post or guard rail E815
inter-highway divider E815
landslide, fallen or not moving E815
moving E909
machinery (road) E815
nonmotor road vehicle NEC E813
object (any object, person, or vehicle off the public highway resulting from a noncollision motor vehicle nontraffic accident) E815
off, normally not on, public highway resulting from a noncollision motor vehicle traffic accident E816

Collision (accidental)–*continued*
motor vehicle (on public highway) (traffic accident)–*continued*
not on public highway, nontraffic accident–*continued*
and–*continued*
pedal cycle (moving) E822
stationary E823
pedestrian (conveyance) E822
person (using pedestrian conveyance) E822
railway rolling stock, train, vehicle (moving) E822
stationary E823
road vehicle (any) (moving) E822
stationary E823
tricycle (moving) E822
stationary E823
off-road type motor vehicle (not on public highway) E821

Figure 7-30 ICD-9-CM Volume II Index to External Causes of Injury. *(Data from* International classification of diseases, 9th revision, *U.S. Department of Health and Human Services, Public Health Services, Centers for Medicare and Medicaid Services.)*

ICD-9-CM Volume III Content

Alphabetic Index to Procedures

- **Alphabetical listing of procedures and services**

Tabular List of Procedures

- **Numerical listing of procedures**

Figure 7-31 ICD-9-CM Volume III contents.

ICD-9-CM CONVENTIONS

Convention is a term used to describe the special terms, punctuation marks, abbreviations, or symbols used as shorthand in a coding system to communicate special instructions efficiently to the coder. To code diagnoses effectively using ICD-9-CM Volumes I, II, and III, it is necessary to gain an understanding of the conventions used in Volumes I, II, and III.

BOX 7-20 ■ KEY POINTS

Conventions

Conventions are special terms, punctuation marks, abbreviations, or symbols, used as shorthand in a coding system to communicate special instructions efficiently to the coder.

ICD-9-CM Official Conventions

The ICD-9-CM Official Conventions published by the Department of Health and Human Services include abbreviations and symbols, instructional notes, and other conventions. Each of these conventions is used to communicate information or instructions to coders to assist them in understanding code ranges and for accurate code selection.

ICD-9-CM Official Abbreviations and Symbols

ICD-9-CM abbreviations and symbols are designed to communicate information to the coder, to assist with code selection. Figure 7-32 illustrates each of these conventions, as they appear in Volume I and/or Volume II of the ICD-9-CM.

- **NEC.** Not elsewhere classifiable is used in the index and tabular list to identify codes that are used when no other specific code for the patient's condition exists in the ICD-9-CM coding system. The coder may look in the patient's record to identify other main terms and related information that may be available for use in selecting a more specific code, for example, code 244.8 "Secondary hypothyroidism NEC."
- **NOS.** Not otherwise specified is used in the tabular list to tell the coder the code is not specific, similar to unspecified. A nonspecific code may be used when the documentation does not provide information required to select a more specific code. The coder should review the record and check with the provider to determine whether there is other information that can be utilized to select a more specific code. Code 281.2 "Folate-deficiency anemia" is an example of NOS.
- **Brackets [ ].** Brackets are found in the tabular list and enclose additional information about the code such as acronyms and synonyms, alternative terminology, or explanatory phrases. The coder can use the information enclosed in the brackets to understand the code further, for example, code 008.0 "*Escherichia*

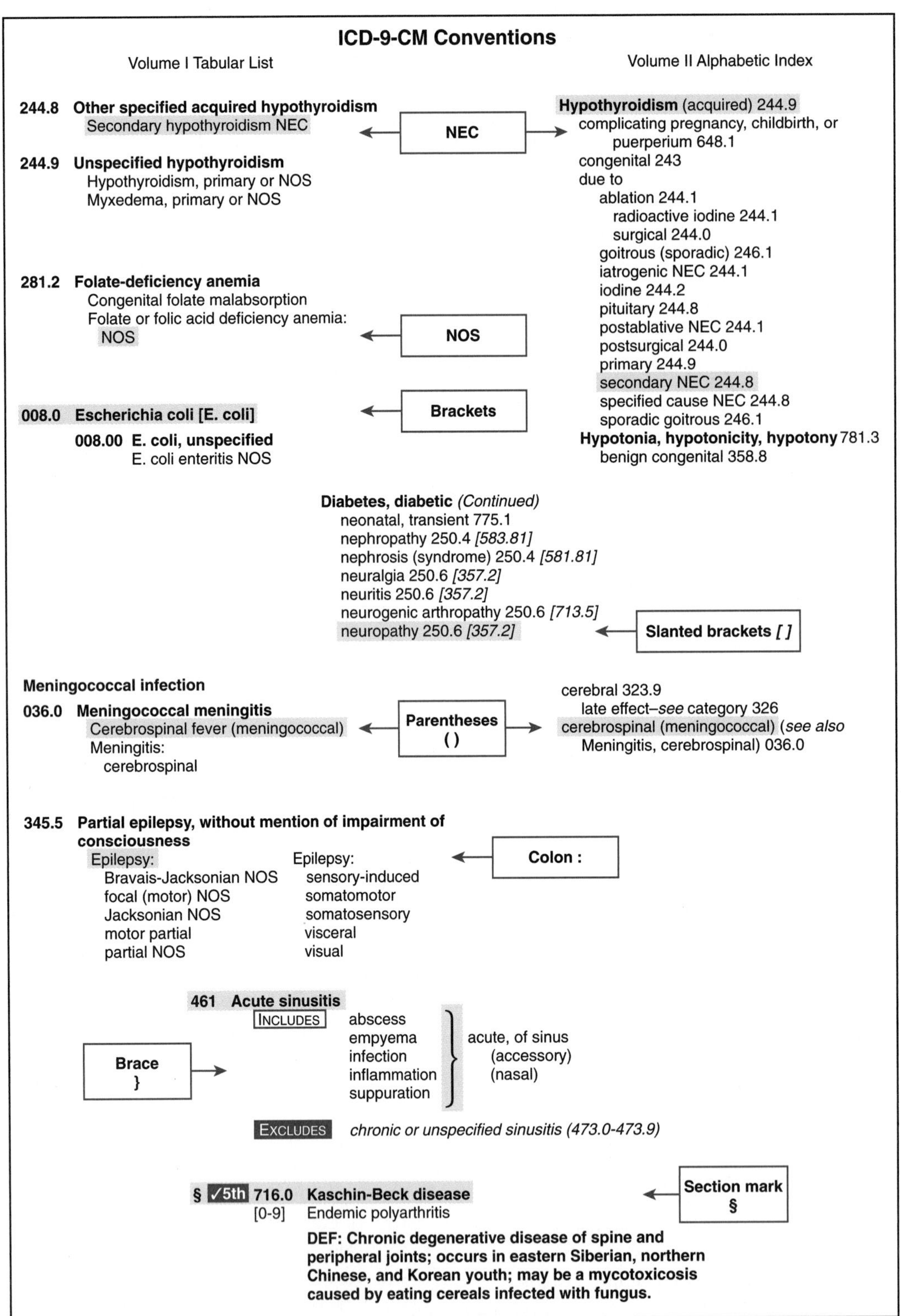

Figure 7-32 ICD-9-CM official abbreviations and symbols. *(Data from* International classification of diseases, 9th revision, *U.S. Department of Health and Human Services, Public Health Services, Centers for Medicare and Medicaid Services.)*

[*E. coli*]. The *E. coli* is listed in brackets to tell the coder *Escherichia coli* is also referred to as *E. coli*.

- **Slanted brackets *[ ]*.** Slanted brackets provide the coder with information about using multiple codes. The brackets are found in the alphabetic index, and they indicate codes that should be reported together to provide a complete picture of the patient's condition. The sequence in which the codes should be listed is also indicated. For example, slanted brackets in the index under Diabetes, neuropathy 250.6 *[*357.2*]* tells the coder the diabetes 250.6 is listed first and a code for neuropathy is listed in the slanted bracket to indicate the 357 code should be listed second. The documentation must indicate the conditions described in both codes; otherwise they should not be coded.
- **Parentheses ( ).** Parentheses are found in the tabular list and the alphabetic index. They are used to provide the coder with more information about the condition and the code such as modifying terms that help the coder understand what is in the code range. For example, the alternative word, meningococcal, is provided in parentheses for, cerebrospinal in the index and tabular list.
- **Colon :.** The colon placed after a description or term in the tabular list tells the coder that more information is listed such as modifying terms to help the coder understand the code range. For example, 345.5 "Partial epilepsy with impairment of consciousness" is followed by Epilepsy: partial, which tells the coder that the code range 345.5 does describe partial epilepsy.
- **Brace }.** The brace is used in the tabular list to tell the coder that information listed before the brace (on the left) will be modified by the information listed after the brace (on the right). Braces can include descriptions or terms. For example, code 461 "Acute sinusitis" provides a list of conditions included in the range. The description "acute, of sinus (accessory) (nasal)" is listed to the right, which tells the coder the conditions in the code range are acute and are in the nasal area.
- **Section mark §.** The section mark is used in the tabular listing to let the coder know there is information in a footnote that pertains to all codes in the section. For example, code 716.0 "Kaschin-Beck disease" and all codes in that range have a section mark. The footnote at the bottom of the page tells the coder a fifth digit is required and explains that valid digits are listed in brackets under each code.

ICD-9-CM Official Instructional Notes

ICD-9-CM Official Conventions are outlined in Table 7-4, including instructional notes that are designed to communicate instructions to the coder regarding code selection. Figure 7-33 illustrates each of these instructional notes as they appear in the ICD-9-CM coding manual.

- **Includes.** These notes are found in the tabular list to provide conditions that are included in the code range. For example, code range 801 "Fracture of base of skull" includes fractures of fossa and occiput bone.
- **Excludes.** These notes are used in the tabular list to tell the coder conditions that are not described in a code range. The excludes statement provides alternative code ranges to review for code assignment. For example, the excludes statement in code 876 range "Open wound of back" tells the coder that open wound into thoracic cavity is not included in this code range and that the coder should look at the code range 860.0 to 862.9 for code selection.
- **Use additional code.** This note is found in the tabular list under code ranges that require more information to describe the patient's condition accurately. The use additional code statement tells the coder that an additional code should be listed if the information is recorded in the medical record. For example, code 250.4 "Diabetes with renal manifestations" tells the coder that an additional code should be used to identify the manifestation such as nephrosis (581.81). The coder then must review the record to identify the manifestation to be coded.
- **Code first.** This note is found in the tabular list under a code that requires explanation of the underlying disease. It tells the coder to list the underlying disease first. For example, code 484.5 "Pneumonia in anthrax" tells the coder the underlying disease 022.1 "Pulmonary anthrax" should be coded first. The coder must review the record to identify the underlying disease for accurate code selection.
- **Code, if applicable, any causal condition first.** A statement used in the tabular list that tells the coder the condition can be used as a principal diagnosis when the cause is not applicable or not known. If the cause is known, it should be coded as the principal diagnosis. For example, code 707.1 "Ulcer of lower limbs, except pressure" indicates "Code, if applicable, any causal conditions first: atherosclerosis of the extremities with ulceration (440.23)."
- **And.** Code descriptions in the tabular section may contain the word "and" between two conditions, which tells the coder that if either condition is described in the record, the code may be assigned to describe the condition. For example, code 583 "Nephritis ***and*** nephropathy, not specified as acute or chronic" can be used to describe either nephritis or nephropathy. Interpret this convention to mean "and" or "or".
- **With.** Many code descriptions found in the tabular section contain the word "with" between two conditions, which tells the coder both conditions must be

TABLE 7-4 ICD-9-CM Official Abbreviations and Symbols

Conventions/Symbols	Coder's Notes
NEC	**Not elsewhere classifiable.** Codes with this symbol are used when no other specific code for the procedure/condition exists in the ***ICD-9-CM coding manual***. Check the medical record to see if there is additional information available to assign a more specific code.
NOS	**Not otherwise specified.** This symbol tells the coder the code is not specific, similar to unspecified. Check the medical record ***documentation*** to see if there is additional information available to assign a more specific code.
[ ]	**Brackets.** Terms enclosed in brackets are non-essential modifying terms, therefore, the terms do not need to be in the medical record. These terms are given to provide additional information about the code such as acronyms and synonyms, alternative terminology or explanatory phrases. The information enclosed does ***not change the code or intent of the code***.
[ ]	**Slanted brackets.** When brackets are found in the index the coder can ***identify multiple codes*** that should be reported together to provide a complete picture of the procedure/condition. Be sure to check the record to make sure the procedures are documented.
( )	**Parentheses.** Terms enclosed in parentheses are ***non-essential modifying terms***, therefore, the terms do not need to be in the medical record. These terms are given to provide the coder with more information about the procedure/condition and/or code.
:	**Colon.** The colon helps the coder to recognize when there is ***more information*** listed such as modifying terms to help the coder understand the code range.
Instructional Notes	
Conventions/Symbols	**Coder's Notes**
Includes	Includes notes are listed at the category level of a range. The note helps the coder to understand what kind of ***procedures or conditions are included*** in the code range.
Excludes	Excludes notes are listed at the category level of a range also and this note helps the coder to understand ***procedures or conditions that are not coded*** within the range.
Use additional code	A note that appears in the tabular list under code ranges to tell the coder more information is required to accurately describe the patient's condition. Review the record to identify ***other conditions*** that should be coded.
Code first	This note also appears in the tabular list under code ranges to tell the coder more information is required to accurately describe the patient's condition. Review the record to identify the ***underlying condition*** that should be coded.
Code, if applicable, any causal condition first	This statement is used in the tabular list to tell the coder the code with this designation can be used as a ***principal diagnosis*** when the cause it not applicable or not known.
And	This convention is to be interpreted as "***And/or***". It tells the coder that either condition/procedure is described in the record, the code may be assigned.
With	The "With" note tells the coder ***if both conditions are described in the record***, the code may be assigned.
See also See category See condition	These notes are ***references*** found in the alphabetic index to provide the coder with direction of other ways to look up the condition.

described in the record to assign the code. For example, code 582.9 "Chronic glomerulonephritis with unspecified pathological lesion in kidney" can only be used if both conditions are documented in the record.

- **See, See also, See category, See condition.** The "see" statements found in the alphabetic index are used to provide the coder with directions of other ways to look up the condition. For example, the main term Node(s) in the index indicates see also Nodules. The coder can cross-reference under Nodules to further identify possible code ranges that can be reviewed.

ICD-9-CM Official Other Conventions

- **Boldface type.** Boldface type is used in the alphabetic index to highlight main terms to help the coder to find main conditions identified in the patient record.

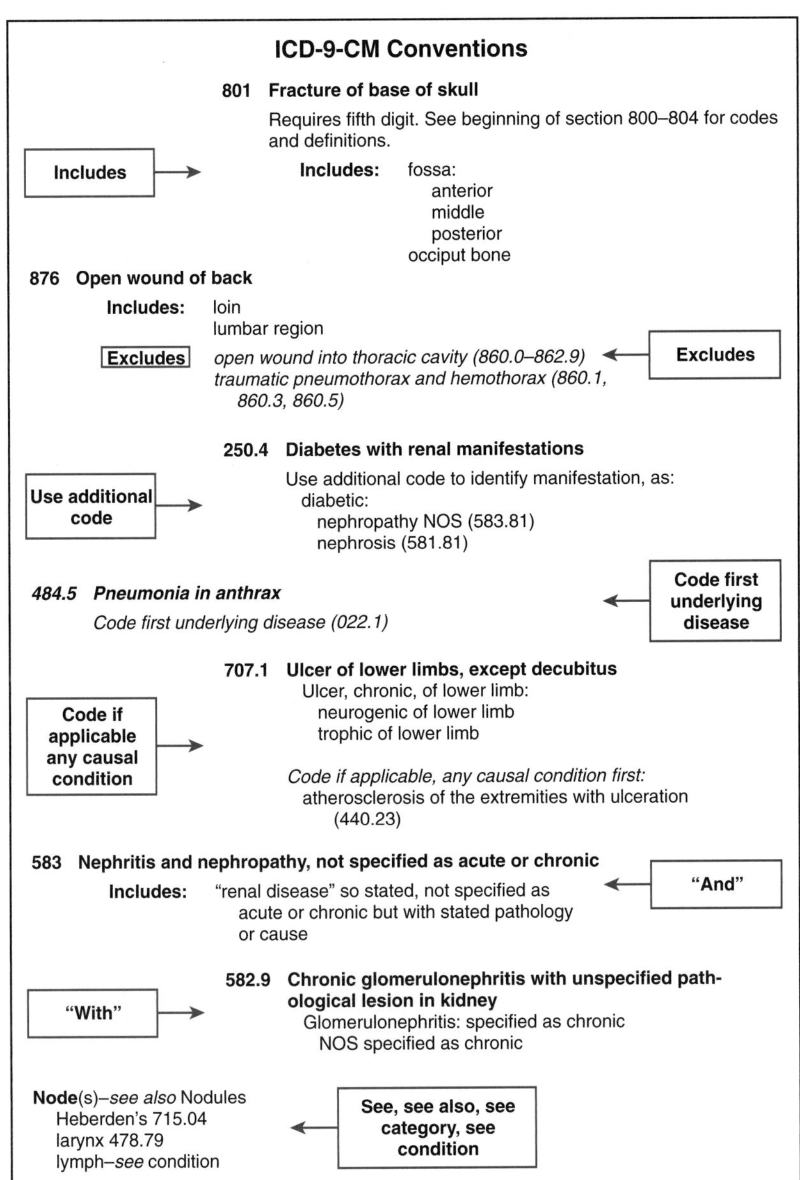

Figure 7-33 ICD-9-CM official instructional notes. *(Data from International classification of diseases, 9th revision, U.S. Department of Health and Human Services, Centers for Medicare and Medicaid Services.)*

For example, review of a record may tell a coder the patient's condition is a Migraine. The main term Migraine is listed in bold lettering in the index, and subterms are indented below.

- **Italicized type.** Italicized type is used in the tabular list to indicate conditions that are excluded in a range and also to indicate codes that should not be used as a primary diagnosis. For example, code 005.1 Botulism contains an excludes note in italicized type "*infant botulism (040.41)*". This tells the coder that range 005 does not describe infant botulism and that the coder should look at code 040.41.

The conventions listed above are the ICD-9-CM Official Conventions and therefore, publishers use them consistently. Other conventions found in the ICD-9-CM may not be identified in the same way in all ICD-9-CM books. The symbols and colors used to identify the conventions vary, as outlined in Table 7-5.

ICD-9-CM Conventions Variations

- **Age-specific** symbols are used by publishers to indicate specific conditions that are age specific.
- **The American Hospital Association (AHA)** publishes the Coding Clinic quarterly to provide information to coders that clarifies the intent of ICD-9-CM codes and coding guidelines. Many publishers include the abbreviation AHA or some other designation to indicate which publication of the Coding Clinic can be referred to for further information.
- **Complication** identifies conditions that are considered complications.
- **Definitions** of medical terms are included by many publishers in the tabular list.
- **Gender-specific** symbols are used by publishers to indicate specific conditions that are gender specific.
- **Medicare Code Edits**, used by some publishers, are numbers or symbols to identify various Medicare

TABLE 7-5 ICD-9-CM Other Conventions

Convention/Description	Various Symbols Used by Publishers
Age specific symbols are used by publishers to indicate conditions that are age specific.	Box with letter P, N, or A to designate age group Pediatric, Newborn, Adult
American Hospital Association publishes the coding clinic to provide information to coders that clarifies the intent of ICD-9-CM codes and coding guidelines. Many publishers include **AHA** or some other designation to indicate which publication of the coding clinic can be referred to for further information.	AHA
Complication or comorbidity designation tells the coder conditions that are considered complications.	CC
Definition abbreviations are used by some publishers to highlight the definition of a medical term in the tabular list for the coder.	DEF
Gender specific symbols are used by publishers to indicate conditions that are gender specific	♀ Female ♂ Male
Medicare Code Edits are identified by publishers, using use numbers or symbols to inform the coder of Medicare code edits such as invalid diagnosis or questionable admission.	May be indicated with color coding or with numbers
Medicare Secondary Payer tells the coder the code may indicate a trauma that may indicate another payer may be the primary payer.	MSP
New code identifies codes that are new to the ICD-9-CM book for the year.	• ◀
Nonspecific diagnosis symbols let the coder know the diagnosis is not specific.	Nonspecific PDx
Unacceptable principal diagnosis is used to tell the coder it is an unacceptable principal diagnosis for an inpatient submission.	Unacceptable PDx •
Revised code is used to tell the coder the code has been revised.	⇐ ▲
Revised text symbols are placed before and after new or revised text.	▶ ◀
Use additional digit tells the coder to code to the fourth or fifth digit.	√4 or √5 √4 or √5 •

code edits, such as invalid diagnosis or questionable admission.

- **Medicare secondary payer (MSP)** tells the coder the code describes a condition that may indicate another payer could be primary, such as head trauma.
- **New code** identifies codes that are new to the ICD-9-CM book for the year.
- **Nonspecific diagnosis** lets the coder know the diagnosis is not specific.
- **Primary/secondary diagnosis**, used by many publishers, utilizes symbols to indicate codes that can only be used as a primary or secondary diagnosis.
- **Revised code** is used to tell the coder the code has been revised.
- **Use additional digit** tells the coder to code to the highest level of specificity by using additional fourth or fifth digits.

Since there are so many variations of ICD-9-CM coding books, it is strongly recommended that hospital billing and coding professionals carefully review the guidelines in the introduction pages of the ICD-9-CM annually to gain an understanding of the conventions used. Accurate code selection is critical to ensuring that the patient's condition is described adequately and to establish medical necessity. An understanding of the conventions is critical to the code selection process.

BOX 7-21 ■ KEY POINTS

Basic Steps to Diagnosis Coding

Read the record; identify the main term for each condition treated and those that affect treatment.

Refer to the index in ICD-9-CM Volume II to identify all possible codes.

Refer to the tabular list in ICD-9-CM Volume I, review each code, and select the code that most adequately describes the condition recorded in the record.

Remember, ***NEVER*** *use a code found in Volume II without verifying it in Volume I.*

STEPS TO CODING DIAGNOSIS UTILIZING ICD-9-CM VOLUME I AND II

To code a diagnosis effectively, it is critical for a coder to gain an understanding of the content, conventions, and guidelines that apply to the ICD-9-CM Volumes I and II. The design, look, and conventions for ICD-9-CM may vary by publisher, as outlined above. The **first** thing a coder should do is read the guidelines to gain an understanding of the content and conventions specific to that version of ICD-9-CM.

The **second** thing a coder can do to ensure accurate and effective coding is to develop good coding habits and follow those habits in every coding situation. The development and application of good coding habits will help to prevent the coder from making mistakes that are very common.

With a good understanding of the content and conventions of the ICD-9-CM and development of good coding habits, you are ready to code effectively and efficiently. The basic steps involved in coding are as follows: read the record to identify the main terms of condition(s), refer to the index and look up all possible codes for the main terms, refer to the tabular section to select the code that adequately describes the diagnostic statement in the record, and sequence codes in accordance with claim form requirements (Figure 7-34).

BOX 7-22 ■ KEY POINTS

Golden Rule in Coding

Good Coding Habits

DO NOT ASSUME.
Identify all possible codes in the index (Volume II).
NEVER EVER code from the index (Volume II).
Review each code in the tabular list (Volume I).
Review all codes in the range.
WHEN IN DOUBT, ASK.
Never use an E code as the first-listed condition.

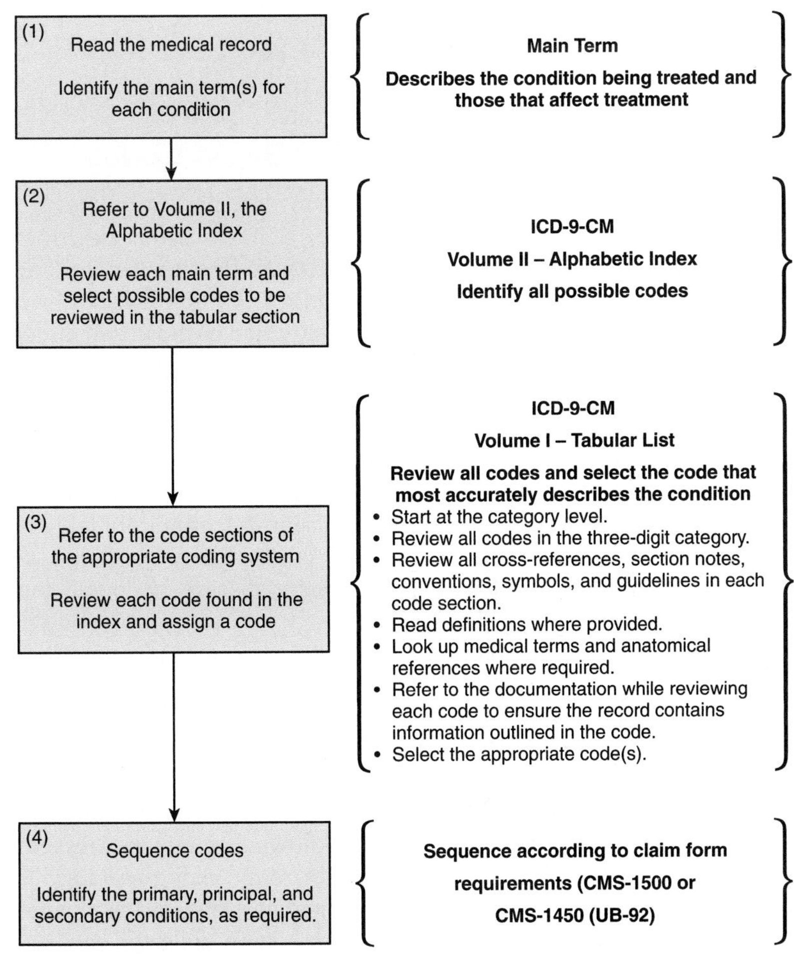
Basic Steps to Coding Diagnosis
(1) Read the medical record
Identify the main term(s) for each condition
Main Term
Describes the condition being treated and those that affect treatment
(2) Refer to Volume II, the Alphabetic Index
Review each main term and select possible codes to be reviewed in the tabular section
ICD-9-CM
Volume II – Alphabetic Index
Identify all possible codes
(3) Refer to the code sections of the appropriate coding system
Review each code found in the index and assign a code
ICD-9-CM
Volume I – Tabular List
Review all codes and select the code that most accurately describes the condition
• Start at the category level.
• Review all codes in the three-digit category.
• Review all cross-references, section notes, conventions, symbols, and guidelines in each code section.
• Read definitions where provided.
• Look up medical terms and anatomical references where required.
• Refer to the documentation while reviewing each code to ensure the record contains information outlined in the code.
• Select the appropriate code(s).
(4) Sequence codes
Identify the primary, principal, and secondary conditions, as required.
Sequence according to claim form requirements (CMS-1500 or CMS-1450 (UB-92)

Figure 7-34 Basic steps to coding diagnosis. Begins with reading the medical record.

Step 1: Read the Record

Carefully review the record or document used for coding. The document can be an operative report, encounter form, discharge summary from an inpatient medical record, or other record. It is critical to review the record carefully to identify the main term for each condition treated and for conditions that affect treatment. The main term represents the reason the patient received health care services or items. The main term may represent a sign, symptom, illness, injury, disease, or other reason for the visit. For example, the discharge summary in Figure 7-35 highlights the main term for the admitting diagnosis as dyspnea. The main terms for the discharge diagnoses are also highlighted in Figure 7-35 as failure and disease. Each main term identified in the record is reviewed in the alphabetic index.

Step 2: Refer to ICD-9-CM Volume II, Alphabetic Index

Refer to the alphabetic index to find possible codes for each of the main terms identified. Look up each identified main term alphabetically in the index (Volume II). The purpose of this step is to identify all possible code(s) to look at in the tabular list. Review subterms indented under the main term. Recognize conventions and notes in the index and follow the instructions indicated by them. Make note of each code identified. Do not try to decide which code to use while looking in the index; this should be done using the tabular list. Remember, ***NEVER*** use a code identified in the index (Volume II) without confirming the code in the tabular list. Figure 7-36 highlights index entries for the main terms identified in the record (dyspnea, failure, and disease). The next step is to review each of the codes in the tabular list (Volume I).

COMMUNITY GENERAL HOSPITAL
8192 South Street
Mars, Florida

Janice Beetlemeter, M.D.

Colegatson, Steven
MR#69745332

DISCHARGE SUMMARY

Date of Admission: 07/06/06
Date of Discharge: 07/07/06

ADMISSION DIAGNOSIS:
1. **Dyspnea**
main term

DISCHARGE DIAGNOSIS:
1. Respiratory **Failure**
main term
2. Chronic Obstructive Pulmonary **Disease** with acute exacerbation
main term

The patient arrived and wife explains he is having **difficulty breathing**. The patient was admitted with O2 saturation over 71 on room air, quite **dyspneic**. Patient went into **respiratory failure** and was then stabilized. He had been treated for bronchitis with antibiotics and was not getting any better.

Today's chest x-ray showed bilateral infiltrates with an advanced **COPD** pattern. White count was 4.95. This is increased to 9.1. Hgb was 15.4, now is 14.9, there was a shift to the left noted. Sodium 135, potassium 3.8, chloride 101, CO2 23, glucose 170, BUN 17, creatinine 0.9. Sodium 141, potassium 3.8, chloride 107, CO2 26, glucose 163, BUN 16, creatinine 0.9.

The patient was started on Zithromax and Levoquin, got minimally better and was started on Gentamicin as well and did get much better. The patient's pO2 now is 62, O2 saturation is between 91 and 90 degrees so there is some improvement. The patient is still quite weak and has quite a long way to go. He has been accepted by a Rehabilitation center where he will undergo extensive pulmonary rehabilitation. He and his wife understand this and are in full agreement of the plan. The patient will be discharged and transferred today to the Rehabilitation center by BLS.

Janice Beetlemeter, M.D.
Janice Beetlemeter, M.D.

Figure 7-35 Discharge summary illustrating main terms for patient conditions.

Step 3: Refer to ICD-9-CM Volume I, Tabular List

Refer to the tabular list (Volume I) to review each code identified in Volume II. Carefully review each code for the purpose of selecting the code that most accurately describes the diagnosis. The coder's review should include the following steps (Figure 7-37):

- Start at the category level (three-digit level).
- Review all codes in the three-digit category.
- Review all cross-references, section notes, conventions, symbols, and guidelines in each code section.
- Read definitions when provided.
- Look up medical terms and anatomical references when required.
- Refer back to the documentation while reviewing each code to ensure that the record contains information outlined in the code.
- Select the appropriate code(s).
- Sequence the codes.

Step 4: Sequence ICD-9-CM Codes

Sequencing is a term used to describe the process of listing the codes in an order that accurately describes conditions treated and those that affect treatment. The major most significant reason for the visit is listed first, followed by other conditions treated or those that affect treatment. Figure 7-38 illustrates the sequencing of diagnosis codes on the UB-04 for the Steven Colegatson case presented in the discharge summary. The UB-04 is utilized because it was an inpatient admission. The code for dyspnea (admitting diagnosis) is recorded in FL 69. The code for the principal diagnosis (respiratory failure) is recorded in FL 67. The co-morbidity condition of chronic obstructive pulmonary disease is coded and recorded in FL 67A.

The sequencing rules for physician and outpatient services reported on a CMS-1500 involve the first-listed condition and secondary diagnoses. Figure 7-39 illustrates how diagnosis codes would be sequenced on a CMS-1500 when the physician submits the claim form.

Coding utilizing ICD-9-CM requires knowledge of how to code. Additional knowledge in the areas of medical terminology and anatomy and physiology is also required. The development and application of good coding habits combined with coding skills and medical knowledge will provide a coder with information

TEST YOUR *Knowledge* BOX 7-5

ICD-9-CM CONVENTIONS

1. Provide a definition of convention.
2. Explain why conventions are used.
3. Are all conventions found in all three volumes of the ICD-9-CM?
4. What is the difference between the ICD-9-CM official conventions and other ICD-9-CM conventions?
5. Explain why a coder should review the introduction section of an ICD-9-CM manual.

Match each convention listed below with the description of what action a coder should take when the convention is identified.

1. And
2. Brace
3. Brackets
4. Code first underlying disease
5. Code, if applicable, any causal condition first
6. Colon
7. Excludes
8. Includes
9. NEC
10. NOS
11. Parentheses
12. See condition
13. Slanted brackets
14. Use additional code
15. With
    - A. To provide the coder with the directions for other ways to look up the condition.
    - B. Provide a list of conditions that are included in the code range.
    - C. They enclose additional information about the code such as acronyms and synonyms, alternative terminology, or explanatory phrases.
    - D. Symbol that is placed after a description or term in the tabulator list; tells the coder there is more information listed, such as modifying terms.
    - E. They indicate codes that should be reported together to provide a complete picture of the patient's condition. The sequence in which the codes should be listed is also indicated.
    - F. An additional code should be listed if the information is recorded in the medical record.
    - G. Tells the coder conditions that are not described in a code range.
    - H. The code is not specific, similar to unspecified.
    - I. They are used to provide the coder with more information about the condition and/or code, such as modifying terms that help the coder to understand what is in a code range.
    - J. The condition can be used as a principal diagnosis when the cause is not applicable or not known. If the cause is known it should be coded as the principal diagnosis.
    - K. Both conditions must be described in the record to assign the code.
    - L. Tells the coder that if either condition is described in the record; the code may be assigned to describe the condition.
    - M. To identify codes that are used when no other specific code for the patient's condition exists in the ICD-9-CM coding system.
    - N. The coder should list the underlying disease first.
    - O. That information listed before the symbol (on the left) will be modified by the information listed after the symbol (on the right).

- **Dysplasia** *(Continued)*
  - prostate *(Continued)*
    - intraepithelial neoplasia I [PIN I] 602.3
    - intraepithelial neoplasia II [PIN II] 602.3
    - intraepithelial neoplasia III [PIN III] 233.4
  - renal 753.15
  - renofacialis 753.0
  - retinal NEC 743.56
  - retrolental 362.21
  - spinal cord 742.9
  - thymic, with immunodeficiency 279.2
  - vagina 623.0
  - vocal cord 478.5
  - vulva 624.8
    - intraepithelial neoplasia I [VIN I] 624.8
    - intraepithelial neoplasia II [VIN II] 624.8
    - intraepithelial neoplasia III [VIN III] 233.3
    - VIN I 624.8
    - VIN II 624.8
    - VIN III 233.3
- **Dyspnea** (nocturnal) (paroxysmal) 786.09
  - asthmatic (bronchial) (*see also* Asthma) 493.9
    - with bronchitis (*see also* Asthma) 493.9
      - chronic 493.2
    - cardiac (*see also* Failure, ventricular, left) 428.1
  - cardiac (*see also* Failure, ventricular, left) 428.1
  - functional 300.11
  - hyperventilation 786.01
  - hysterical 300.11
  - Monday morning 504
  - newborn 770.89
  - psychogenic 306.1
  - uremic–*see* Uremia
- **Dyspraxia** 781.3
  - syndrome 315.4
- **Dysproteinemia** 273.8
  - transient with copper deficiency 281.4
- **Dysprothrombinemia** (constitutional) (*see also* Defect, coagulation) 286.3
- **Dysreflexia, autonomic** 337.3
- **Dysrhythmia**
  - cardiac 427.9
    - postoperative (immediate) 997.1
      - long-term effect of cardiac surgery 429.4
    - specified type NEC 427.89
  - cerebral or cortical 348.30
- **Dyssecretosis, mucoserous** 710.2
- **Dyssocial reaction, without manifest psychiatric disorder**
  - adolescent V71.02
  - adult V71.01
  - child V71.02
- **Dyssomnia NEC** 780.56
  - nonorganic origin 307.47
- **Dyssplenism** 289.4
- **Dyssynergia**
  - biliary (*see also* Disease, biliary) 576.8
  - cerebellaris myoclonica 334.2
  - detrusor sphincter (bladder) 596.55
  - ventricular 429.89
- **Dystasia, hereditary areflexic** 334.3

- **Failure, failed** *(Continued)*
  - prerenal 788.9
  - renal 586
    - with
      - abortion–*see* Abortion, by type, with renal failure
      - ectopic pregnancy (*see also* categories 633.0-633.9) 639.3
      - edema (*see also* Nephrosis) 581.9
      - hypertension (*see also* Hypertension, kidney) 403.91
      - hypertensive heart disease (conditions classifiable to 402) 404.92
        - with heart failure 404.93
        - benign 404.12
          - with heart failure 404.13
        - malignant 404.02
          - with heart failure 404.03
      - molar pregnancy (*see also* categories 630-632) 639.3
      - tubular necrosis (acute) 584.5
    - acute 584.9
      - with lesion of
        - necrosis
          - cortical (renal) 584.6
          - medullary (renal) (papillary) 584.7
          - tubular 584.5
        - specified pathology NEC 584.8
    - chronic 585
      - hypertensive or with hypertension (*see also* Hypertension, kidney) 403.91
    - due to a procedure 997.5
    - following
      - abortion 639.3
      - crushing 958.5
      - ectopic or molar pregnancy 639.3
      - labor and delivery (acute) 669.3
    - hypertensive (*see also* Hypertension, kidney) 403.91
    - puerperal, postpartum 669.3
  - respiration, respiratory 518.81
    - acute 518.81
    - acute and chronic 518.84
    - center 348.8
      - newborn 770.84
    - chronic 518.83
    - due to trauma, surgery or shock 518.5
    - newborn 770.84
  - rotation
    - cecum 751.4
    - colon 751.4
    - intestine 751.4
    - kidney 753.3
  - segmentation–*see also* Fusion
    - fingers (*see also* Syndactylism, fingers) 755.11
    - toes (*see also* Syndactylism, toes) 755.13
  - seminiferous tubule, adult 257.2
  - senile (general) 797
    - with psychosis 290.20
  - testis, primary (seminal) 257.2
  - to progress 661.2
  - to thrive
    - adult 783.7
    - child 783.41
  - transplant 996.80
    - bone marrow 996.85
    - organ (immune or nonimmune cause) 996.80
      - bone marrow 996.85
      - heart 996.83

- **Disease, diseased** *(Continued)*
  - pneumatic
    - drill 994.9
    - hammer 994.9
  - policeman's 729.2
  - Pollitzer's (hidradenitis suppurativa) 705.83
  - polycystic (congenital) 759.89
    - kidney or renal 753.12
      - adult type (APKD) 753.13
      - autosomal dominant 753.13
      - autosomal recessive 753.14
      - childhood type (CPKD) 753.14
      - infantile type 753.14
    - liver or hepatic 751.62
    - lung or pulmonary 518.89
      - congenital 748.4
    - ovary, ovaries 256.4
    - spleen 759.0
  - Pompe's (glycogenosis II) 271.0
  - Poncet's (tuberculous rheumatism) (*see also* Tuberculosis) 015.9
  - Posada-Wernicke 114.9
  - Potain's (pulmonary edema) 514
  - Pott's (*see also* Tuberculosis) 015.0 *[730.88]*
    - osteomyelitis 015.0 *[730.88]*
    - paraplegia 015.0 *[730.88]*
    - spinal curvature 015.0 *[737.43]*
    - spondylitis 015.0 *[720.81]*
  - Potter's 753.0
  - Poulet's 714.2
  - pregnancy NEC (*see also* Pregnancy) 646.9
  - Preiser's (osteoporosis) 733.09
  - Pringle's (tuberous sclerosis) 759.5
  - Profichet's 729.9
  - prostate 602.9
    - specified type NEC 602.8
  - protozoal NEC 136.8
    - intestine, intestinal NEC 007.9
  - pseudo-Hurler's (mucolipidosis III) 272.7
  - psychiatric (*see also* Psychosis) 298.9
  - psychotic (*see also* Psychosis) 298.9
  - Puente's (simple glandular cheilitis) 528.5
  - puerperal NEC (*see also* Puerperal) 674.9
  - pulmonary–*see also* Disease, lung
    - amyloid 277.3 *[517.8]*
    - artery 417.9
    - circulation, circulatory 417.9
      - specified NEC 417.8
    - diffuse obstructive (chronic) 496
      - with
        - acute bronchitis 491.22 ◄
        - asthma (chronic) (obstructive) 493.2 ◄
        - exacerbation NEC (acute) 491.21
    - heart (chronic) 416.9
      - specified NEC 416.8
    - hypertensive (vascular) 416.0
      - cardiovascular 416.0
    - obstructive diffuse (chronic) 496
      - with
        - acute bronchitis 491.22 ◄
        - asthma (chronic) (obstructive) 493.2
        - bronchitis (chronic) 491.20
          - with
            - exacerbation (acute) 491.21 ◄
            - exacerbation NEC (acute) 491.21 ◄
          - acute 491.22 ◄
        - exacerbation NEC (acute) 491.21 ◄
    - valve (*see also* Endocarditis, pulmonary) 424.3

Figure 7-36 ICD-9-CM index illustrating Dyspnea, Failure, and Disease and subterms that lead to identifying codes for those conditions. *(Data from* International classification of diseases, 9th revision, U.S. *Department of Health and Human Services, Public Health Services, Centers for Medicare and Medicaid Services.)*

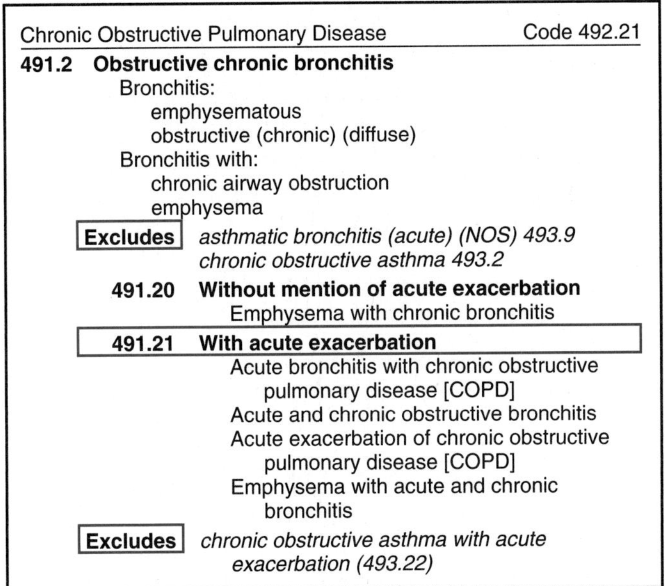

Chronic Obstructive Pulmonary Disease — Code 492.21

491.2 Obstructive chronic bronchitis
Bronchitis:
emphysematous
obstructive (chronic) (diffuse)
Bronchitis with:
chronic airway obstruction
emphysema

Excludes *asthmatic bronchitis (acute) (NOS) 493.9*
chronic obstructive asthma 493.2

491.20 Without mention of acute exacerbation
Emphysema with chronic bronchitis

491.21 With acute exacerbation
Acute bronchitis with chronic obstructive pulmonary disease [COPD]
Acute and chronic obstructive bronchitis
Acute exacerbation of chronic obstructive pulmonary disease [COPD]
Emphysema with acute and chronic bronchitis

Excludes *chronic obstructive asthma with acute exacerbation (493.22)*

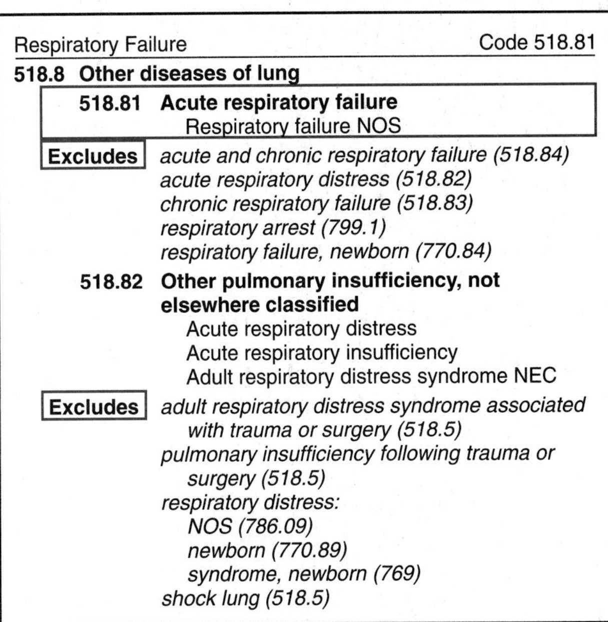

Respiratory Failure — Code 518.81

518.8 Other diseases of lung

518.81 Acute respiratory failure
Respiratory failure NOS

Excludes *acute and chronic respiratory failure (518.84)*
acute respiratory distress (518.82)
chronic respiratory failure (518.83)
respiratory arrest (799.1)
respiratory failure, newborn (770.84)

518.82 Other pulmonary insufficiency, not elsewhere classified
Acute respiratory distress
Acute respiratory insufficiency
Adult respiratory distress syndrome NEC

Excludes *adult respiratory distress syndrome associated with trauma or surgery (518.5)*
pulmonary insufficiency following trauma or surgery (518.5)
respiratory distress:
NOS (786.09)
newborn (770.89)
syndrome, newborn (769)
shock lung (518.5)

Figure 7-37 ICD-9-CM tabular list illustrating chronic obstructive pulmonary disease and respiratory failure. *(Data from* International classification of diseases, 9th revision, *U.S. Department of Health and Human Services, Public Health Services, Centers for Medicare and Medicaid Services.)*

CMS-1450 Sequencing Guidelines

Form Locator 67-72

67 PRIN. DIAG. CD.	67 A-Q OTHER DIAG. CODES				69 ADM. DIAG. CODE	72 E-CODE
518.81	491.21				786.09	

Discharge Summary
Steven Colegatson

Date of admission: 07/06/06
Date of discharge: 07/07/06
Admission diagnosis:
1. Dyspnea 786.09
Discharge diagnosis:
1. Respiratory failure 518.81
2. Chronic obstructive pulmonary disease 491.21

Figure 7-38 Principal and other diagnosis codes are recorded in FL 67a–q. Admitting diagnosis is recorded in FL 69. External cause of injury code is recorded in FL 72.

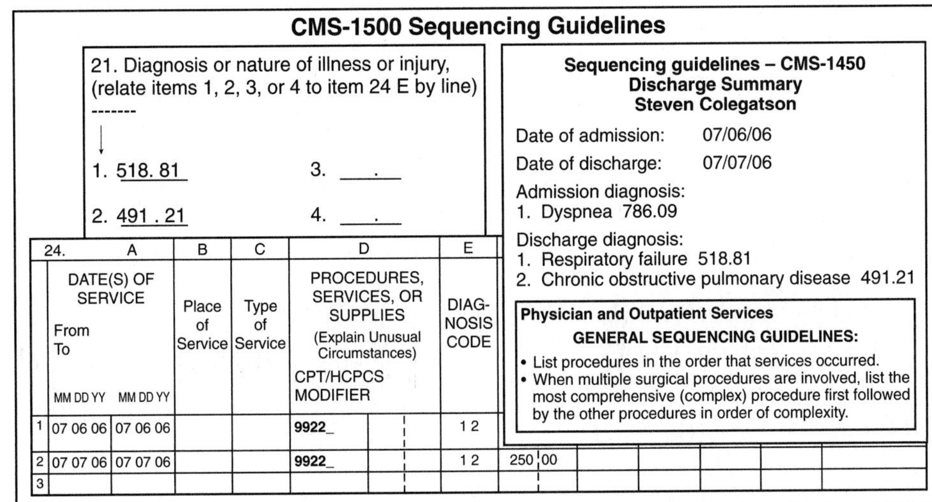

CMS-1500 Sequencing Guidelines

21. Diagnosis or nature of illness or injury, (relate items 1, 2, 3, or 4 to item 24 E by line)

1. 518. 81 3. ___ . ___
2. 491 . 21 4. ___ . ___

24. A DATE(S) OF SERVICE From To (MM DD YY MM DD YY)		B Place of Service	C Type of Service	D PROCEDURES, SERVICES, OR SUPPLIES (Explain Unusual Circumstances) CPT/HCPCS	MODIFIER	E DIAGNOSIS CODE	
1 07 06 06	07 06 06			9922_		1 2	
2 07 07 06	07 07 06			9922_		1 2	250 00
3							

Sequencing guidelines – CMS-1450
Discharge Summary
Steven Colegatson

Date of admission: 07/06/06
Date of discharge: 07/07/06
Admission diagnosis:
1. Dyspnea 786.09
Discharge diagnosis:
1. Respiratory failure 518.81
2. Chronic obstructive pulmonary disease 491.21

Physician and Outpatient Services
GENERAL SEQUENCING GUIDELINES:
- List procedures in the order that services occurred.
- When multiple surgical procedures are involved, list the most comprehensive (complex) procedure first followed by the other procedures in order of complexity.

Figure 7-39 Diagnosis codes on the CMS-1500. The first-listed condition is recorded in Block 21, on reference line 1. The secondary diagnosis is recorded in Block 21, on reference line 2. The diagnosis code that explains why the service was performed is linked to the procedure in 24E.

required to effectively and accurately code patient conditions.

ICD-9-CM OFFICIAL GUIDELINES

An integral part of learning to code using ICD-9-CM involves learning the guidelines on how to use the coding system and how to code various circumstances. The ICD-9-CM Official Guidelines for Coding and Reporting are provided by the Centers for Medicare and Medicaid Services (CMS), formerly the Health Care Financing Administration (HCFA), and the National Center for Health Statistics (NCHS). CMS and NCHS are agencies within the Department of Health and Human Services (DHHS). The ICD-9-CM guidelines were developed and approved by the Cooperating Parties for ICD-9-CM—the American Hospital Association, The American Health Information Management Association (AHIMA), CMS, and the NCHS. The guidelines published by the DHHS have also been published in the Coding Clinic for ICD-9-CM, published by the American Hospital Association.

The ICD-9-CM Official Guidelines for Coding and Reporting provides coders with critical information about how to use the ICD-9-CM and with instructions on how to code and report various clinical circumstances. The guidelines are broken down into the following sections:

- Section I: ICD-9-CM Conventions, General Coding Guidelines, and Chapter-Specific Guidelines.
- Section II: Selection of Principal Diagnosis(es) for Inpatient, Short-Term, Acute Care Hospital Records.
- Section III: Reporting Additional Diagnoses for Inpatient, Short-Term, Acute Care Hospital Records.
- Section IV: Diagnostic Coding and Report Guidelines for Outpatient Services.

ICD-9-CM guidelines will be discussed further in Chapter 9.

CHAPTER SUMMARY

Diagnosis coding is the process of translating written descriptions of the patient's signs, symptoms, illness, disease, injury, condition, or other reason for the hospital visit. The system utilized to code diagnosis is the International Classification of Diseases, 9th Revision, Clinical Modification (ICD-9-CM). Accurate diagnosis coding is critical to ensure patient conditions are described accurately and medical necessity is established. Payment for services is provided when they are medically necessary, as defined by the payer. Accurate coding is also required to ensure compliance with payer guidelines.

Data collected using the ICD-9-CM coding systems serves many purposes involving the retrieval, tracking, and researching of data. The data are used to track morbidity and mortality data, monitor procedures and outcomes, set standards of care, monitor health care costs, and predict health care trends. Reimbursement methods are developed and utilized through coding systems such as the ICD-9-CM.

It is important for coders to have knowledge of medical terminology, anatomy and physiology, and coding principles and guidelines. An effective coder must be able to read and understand a medical record, identify conditions that are treated and those that affect treatment, and find a code that adequately describes why the patient received the health care services provided. The ICD-9-CM coding system includes official coding guidelines that the coder must also understand. Diagnosis coding supports codes that provide descriptions of services and items provided. An in-depth discussion of coding procedures and items will be given in the next chapter.

TEST YOUR *Knowledge* BOX 7-6

STEPS TO CODING CONDITIONS UTILIZING ICD-9-CM VOLUME I AND II; ICD-9-CM GUIDELINES

1. Coders must have a good understanding of ______________, ______________, and ______________ to code effectively.

2. Explain why a coder should review the guidelines in the introduction section of the ICD-9-CM.

3. What can a coder do to ensure accurate and effective coding?

4. List four good coding habits and provide a brief explanation.

Explain the following basic steps in coding:

5. Coders must read the medical record for the purpose of ______________.

6. When coding diagnosis, a coder must identify codes for ______________ and ______________.

7. How does a coder use ICD-9-CM Volume I?

8. Coders should never select codes from the index (Volume II). They should always verify codes identified by referring to ______________, referred to as ______________.

9. The ICD-9-CM official guidelines for coding and reporting are provided by ________ and ________.

10. Explain how codes are sequenced on the CMS-1500 and the CMS-1450 (UB-04).

TEST YOUR *Knowledge* BOX 7-7

STEPS TO CODING CONDITIONS UTILIZING ICD-9-CM VOLUME I AND II

Follow the basic coding steps discussed in this chapter, read the following statements, and assign diagnosis code(s) for conditions treated and those that affect treatment.

Hospital Outpatient Cases

Hospital-Based Primary Care Office Visit

1. Mrs. Jones brings her 6-year-old son, Jason, to the office today because he stepped on a nail. A problem-focused history and examination was performed. The puncture in his heel is not very deep; we cleaned and bandaged it. A shot of tetanus and diphtheria was given intramuscularly.
2. Sam Goliath, a 42-year-old male established patient, presents today for a routine physical examination. At the end of the examination the patient noted he had a good-sized growth on his back that has been present for several months. Problem-focused history and examination reveals a 1-cm-diameter wart-type growth that is an actinic keratosis. A diagnostic shave biopsy of the growth was performed.
3. A 25-year-old female established patient presents today complaining of bouts of dizziness, and she has also noticed difficulty swallowing and getting food to go down. An expanded problem-focused examination was performed. She is currently on medication for hypothyroidism. Blood was drawn and sent out to the laboratory to check the TSH levels.

Emergency Department Visit

4. Patient presents to the Emergency Department with a severe burn on the left upper arm. Level I evaluation and management reveals a third-degree burn. Debridement of the small area was performed, and dressings were applied.
5. Mr. Johnston came to the Emergency Department with a hurt wrist resulting from a fall from a ladder. Dr. Fixit performed a problem-focused history and examination. X-ray, 2 views, was taken, and it revealed a Colles fracture. Dr. Fixit treated the closed fracture and applied a cast.

Ambulatory Surgery Cases

6. A 62-year-old male patient presents today for a lumbar puncture to determine the cause of his vascular headaches. Patient was prepped and draped in the normal fashion and local anesthesia administered. A #20 gauge needle was introduced into the subarachnoid space of the lumbar region. Five centimeters of crystal-clear fluid was obtained and sent to the laboratory for diagnostic studies. The patient tolerated the procedure well.
7. Patient arrived for scheduled arthroscopic surgery to determine the cause of pain in her right shoulder. While the nurse was obtaining information and consents, the patient indicated she was experiencing chest pain. The surgeon performed a detailed history and examination and an EKG that showed no findings. The operation was then performed and the patient tolerated the procedure well.

Inpatient Cases

8. A 28-year-old female is admitted with a malignant mass in the left breast. A biopsy was performed last week and pathology showed presence of carcinoma that has not spread outside the margins. The patient has hypertension and a family history of breast cancer. The surgeon performed a mastectomy including pectoralis muscle and the internal mammary and axillary nodes, and local excision of a benign mass from right breast for biopsy. Patient tolerated procedure well.
9. List the principal diagnosis for the following scenario.
10. List the other diagnoses for the following scenario.

A 67-year-old male was admitted to the hospital for a pancreatectomy after being diagnosed with cancer of the tail and body of the pancreas involving the left kidney and spleen. Pancreatectomy, distal was performed. A splenectomy and left nephrectomy was also performed. During the procedure the patient went into cardiac arrest due to the adverse effect of the general anesthetic.

CHAPTER REVIEW 7-1

True/False

1. One purpose of coding conditions is to establish medical necessity. T F
2. A coder does not need to refer to Volume I if codes are found in Volume II. T F
3. ICD-9-CM codes are selected based on written descriptions in the medical record of the patient's condition. T F
4. Only conditions treated are coded. T F
5. Payers will not pay for services rendered that are not considered medically necessary. T F

Fill in the Blank

6. The first step in coding is to read the record for the purpose of ____________________.
7. The standard coding system used to describe the patient's conditions is ____________________.
8. The process of translating written descriptions of the patient condition(s) is called ____________________.
9. Information utilized to code a condition is located in the patient's ____________________.
10. Diagnosis codes are used for several reasons, such as ____________________ and ____________________. Explain.
11. The ICD-9-CM allows for the collection of data regarding ____________________, ____________________ and ____________________.
12. The term found in the medical record that describes the main reason why the patient is seeking health care services is ____________________.
13. Inpatient claims require the coder to identify the ____________________, which is the condition determined after study.
14. Coding diagnosis for physician and outpatient services involves identifying and coding the ____________________ diagnosis.
15. Conditions that develop during the patient's stay in the hospital are referred to as ____________________.
16. Diagnosis codes are ____________________ to procedures codes on the CMS-1500 to explain why the service or procedure was medically necessary.

Match the Following Definitions With the Terms at Right

17. Numeric listing of patient signs, symptoms, injury, illness, disease, and other reasons for the visit.
18. Condition determined after study.
19. Location where diagnosis codes are listed on the CMS-1450.
20. Volumes of the ICD-9-CM that are used for coding diagnosis and inpatient procedures.
21. Term that describes special terms, punctuation marks, abbreviations, or symbols used as shorthand in a coding system to communicate special instructions efficiently to the coder.

A. Principal diagnosis
B. Volumes I, II, and III
C. Conventions
D. Volume I
E. FL 67, 69, 70, 72

Research Project

Use the Internet to find Medicare National Coverage Determinations (NCD). Identify a coverage determination for one procedure. Review the coverage determination and discuss the conditions for which Medicare will consider the procedure to be medically necessary.

CHAPTER REVIEW 7-1—*cont'd*

Diagnosis Coding

Follow the basic coding steps discussed in this chapter, read the following statements, and list the following for each problem: (1) main term(s), (2) diagnosis code(s), and (3) an indication of whether the diagnosis is first-listed condition, secondary, principal, or other diagnoses.

Hospital Outpatient Cases: Hospital-Based Primary Care Office Visit

1. Ms. Pertrivuti presents complaining of difficulty walking due to severe osteoarthritis in the hip. A problem-focused history and examination was performed with straightforward decision making. I prescribed medication to alleviate the pain and supplied her with a cane.
2. An established patient presents complaining of a sore throat for 4 days. A problem-focused evaluation and management service was performed, with automated CBC, automated differential WBC count. Antibiotics were prescribed for strep throat. Patient will be seen in 10 days for a follow-up.
3. Mr. Jamerstonig presents to the doctor's office complaining of a cough, dyspnea, and chest pain with respiration. An expanded problem-focused evaluation and management was performed. A chest X-ray, single view, was performed in the office and interpreted; findings were normal.

Emergency Department Visit

4. Patient presents to the Emergency Department with a 4.5-cm laceration on the left leg. A Level II evaluation and management service was performed. Debridement and complex repair of the wound was done. Disposable drug delivery system, flow rate of 5 mL per hour was utilized.
5. Patient arrived at the Emergency Department by ambulance, unconscious. Paramedics indicate the patient was found in his apartment not breathing. CPR was administered. The patient's roommate indicates he was drinking whisky heavily the night before and he found the patient in the morning and could not wake him up. A Level II evaluation and management was performed by the Emergency Room physician. The patient is currently in a coma. A drug screen for alcohol and opiates revealed high amounts of morphine and alcohol in his system. The roommate indicates he is on morphine and does not know how or why the patient took it.

Ambulatory Surgery Cases

6. Mr. Smith underwent an arthroplasty of the knee, condyle and plateau, medial compartment for aseptic necrosis of the bone. The procedure was performed in the Ambulatory Surgery Suite. Patient tolerated procedure well. Discharge instructions indicate non-weight bearing for 6 weeks. Patient was provided with a pair of crutches (adjustable with tips and handgrips).
7. Mrs. Hartenshogan arrived today for scheduled colonoscopy. Patient has been experiencing severe abdominal pain and nausea after eating. Scope, flexible, inserted for visualization proximal to splenic flexure revealed inflammation and infection of the peritoneal cavity. Sacs of mucous membrane are protruding through the muscular wall of the colon. The scope was withdrawn and the patient was moved to recovery.

Inpatient Cases

8. Mr. Fordmanston was admitted to the hospital with coronary atherosclerosis of native arteries, for a coronary bypass. Patient also has malignant hypertension. Three coronary vessels were bypassed during the procedure. Patient tolerated procedure well.
9. Patient with a malignant neoplasm of ureter was admitted to the hospital for an ureterectomy. Partial ureterectomy performed and formation of other cutaneous ureterostomy. Patient tolerated procedure well.
10. Patient JB was admitted to the hospital as he was experiencing severe chest pain. An EKG was performed, which showed arrhythmia. The patient underwent a right heart catheterization. Right heart cardiac catheterization showed no findings.

GLOSSARY

Admitting diagnosis The major most significant reason why the patient is being admitted.

Adverse reaction An unexpected condition that occurs in reaction to a medication that is properly prescribed and administered.

Benign hypertension Mildly elevated arterial blood pressure. Benign hypertension may be indicated when blood pressure increases slightly over a long period of time.

Benign neoplasm A growth that does not have properties of invasion, meaning it does not spread.

Chief complaint (CC) Term used to describe the main reason (problem) the patient is seeking health care services.

Coding The assignment of numeric or alphanumeric codes to all health care data elements of inpatient and outpatient care.

Complication A disease or condition that develops during the course of a hospital stay.

Co-morbidity A secondary condition that coexists with the condition for which the patient is seeking health care services.

Convention A term used to describe the special terms, punctuation marks, abbreviations, or symbols used as shorthand in a coding system to efficiently communicate special instructions to the coder.

Diagnosis coding The process of translating written descriptions of signs, symptoms, illnesses, injuries, diseases, conditions, or other reasons for health care services documented in the patient's medical record into codes.

Documentation A term utilized to describe information regarding the patient's condition, treatment, and response to treatment.

Essential Hypertension Also known as primary hypertension and it means that there is no known underlying condition that is causing the blood pressure to increase.

First-Listed Condition The major most significant reason why the patient is seeking health care services.

Hypertension Persistently high arterial blood pressure over specified levels at three consecutive visits.

International Classification of Diseases, 9th Revision, Clinical Modification (ICD-9-CM) Standard coding system currently utilized to describe patient's condition, injury, illness, disease, or other reasons the patient is receiving health care services.

International Classification of Diseases (ICD) A classification system that was utilized to collect data regarding causes of death for statistical purposes. It is a revised version of the International List of the Causes of Death classification. The ICD was published by the World Health Organization.

International List of the Causes of Death A classification of causes of death that was based on the London Bills of Mortality.

London Bills of Mortality Developed by John Graunt in an attempt to estimate the proportion of live-born children who died before reaching the age of six years. The London Bills of Mortality was the basis for development of the International Classification of Diseases (ICD).

Main term The term that represents the sign, symptom, illness, injury, disease, condition, or other reason the patient is seeking health care.

Malignant hypertension A severe hypertensive state, characterized by a diastolic pressure higher than 120 mm Hg, severe headaches, blurred vision, and confusion, that may result in fatal uremia, myocardial infarction, congestive heart failure, or a cerebrovascular accident.

Malignant neoplasm A growth that has properties of invasion, meaning it can spread.

Medical necessity A term used to describe procedures or services performed that are reasonable and medically necessary to address the patient's medical condition based on standards of medical practice.

Morbidity Refers to the patient's illness or disease.

Mortality Refers to death.

Neoplasm A new growth of tissue in which the growth is uncontrolled and progressive.

Poisoning A condition caused by the ingestion of a substance or chemical that is toxic. Poisoning occurs when a medication that is taken is not properly prescribed and administered.

Principal diagnosis The condition determined after study.

Sequencing A term utilized to describe the process of listing codes in an order that accurately describes conditions treated and those that affect treatment.

World Health Organization (WHO) Published the International Classification of Diseases (ICD) classification system utilized to collect data regarding causes of death for statistical purposes.

Chapter 8

Coding Procedures, Services, and Items (Procedure Coding)

The objective of this chapter is to provide an overview of the history and purpose of coding procedures, services, and items provided during a hospital visit. The previous chapter provided an overview of coding medical conditions (diagnosis) that explain why services and procedures were performed. This chapter focuses on coding procedures, services, and items, referred to as procedure coding. Hospital coding and billing professionals are required to have an understanding of procedure coding systems. The ability to understand and apply coding principles and guidelines is essential to ensure that procedures, services, and items provided are described accurately and to make sure the hospital is in compliance with coding guidelines. A discussion of how procedure coding relates to documentation, medical necessity, claim forms, and reimbursement will demonstrate the importance of procedure coding in the hospital. Variations in coding system utilization are outlined to illustrate appropriate code usage for outpatient, inpatient, and non-patient services. The content, format, and conventions of the Health Care Common Procedure Coding System (HCPCS) and the International Classification of Diseases, 9th Revision, Clinical Modification (ICD-9-CM), Volume III are reviewed to provide an overview of coding utilizing these systems. The chapter will close with a discussion on the basic steps to coding utilizing HCPCS and ICD-9-CM Volume III procedure codes.

Outline

Chapter Objectives

- Define terms, phrases, abbreviations, and acronyms related to coding procedures rendered during hospital visits.
- Demonstrate an understanding of the history and purpose of procedure coding systems.
- Discuss how procedure coding data are utilized for research, education, and administrative purposes.
- Demonstrate an understanding of coding utilizing the HCPCS and ICD-9-CM Volume III procedure coding systems.
- Explain the two levels of HCPCS.
- Provide an explanation of the relationship among procedure coding and documentation, medical necessity, claim forms, and reimbursement.
- List the content of the CPT coding system.

(*Continued*)

- Outline the content of the ICD-9-CM Volume III coding system.
- Demonstrate an understanding of the steps to coding.
- Discuss the relationship between procedure coding and diagnosis coding.
- Demonstrate an understanding of coding principles.

Key Terms

Abstracting
Convention
CPT Category I Codes
CPT Category II Codes
CPT Category III Codes
Current Procedural Terminology (CPT)
Documentation
Form locator (FL)
Health Care Common Procedure Coding System (HCPCS)
ICD-9-CM Volume III (ICD-9-PCS)
Inpatient services
Medical necessity
Medicare National Codes
Modifier
Non-patient services
Outpatient services
Principal procedure
Procedure coding
Sequencing
Significant procedure
Tabular list

Acronyms and Abbreviations

AHA—American Hospital Association
AMA—American Medical Association
APC—Ambulatory Payment Classifications
ASC—ambulatory surgery center
CDM—Charge Description Master or chargemaster
CIM—Coverage Issues Manual
CMS—Centers for Medicare and Medicaid Services
CPT—Current Procedural Terminology
DEF—Definition
DHHS—Department of Health and Human Services
E/M—evaluation and management
FL—form locator
HCFA—Health Care Financing Administration
HCPCS—Health Care Common Procedure Coding System
HIM—Health Information Management
HIPAA—Health Insurance Portability and Accountability Act
ICD-9-CM—International Classification of Diseases, 9th Revision, Clinical Modification
ICD-9-PCS—International Classification of Diseases, 9th Revision Clinical Modification, Volume III Procedure Coding System
LCD—Local Coverage Determination
LMRP—Local Medical Review Policy
Lt—left
NEC—not elsewhere classifiable
NOS—not otherwise specified
Rt—right
UB-04—CMS-1450 Universal Bill implemented in 2007.
UHDDS—Uniform Hospital Discharge Data Set

HISTORY AND PURPOSE OF PROCEDURE CODING

Procedure coding is a vital function in the hospital billing process. As discussed in Chapter 5, the complex process of billing includes coding procedures (Figure 8-1). **Procedure coding** is the process of translating written descriptions of procedures, services, supplies, drugs, and equipment from the patient's record into numeric or alphanumeric codes. As discussed in Chapter 6, coded health care data constitute the primary key to reimbursement and statistical analysis by hospitals, insurance companies, health care facilities, and other relevant businesses. Procedure codes are used to communicate with various payers regarding procedures, services, or items provided during a hospital visit. Payers determine reimbursement utilizing the procedures codes submitted.

Hospital coding professionals are responsible for coding patient procedures, services, and items for the purpose of describing charges submitted to payers. HIM professionals are responsible for maintenance of the Charge Description Master (CDM), which contains descriptions of hospital procedures, services, and items, each of which is associated with a procedure code (Figure 8-2). The CDM is also referred to as the chargemaster. The hospital coding professional should master an understanding and application of coding guidelines and principals to ensure that an accurate description of procedure(s) is given, compliance with coding guidelines is achieved, and proper reimbursement is obtained. Hospital billing professionals need to achieve a good understanding of coding procedures to ensure that coding guidelines are satisfied on the claim form and to communicate with payers regarding reimbursement issues.

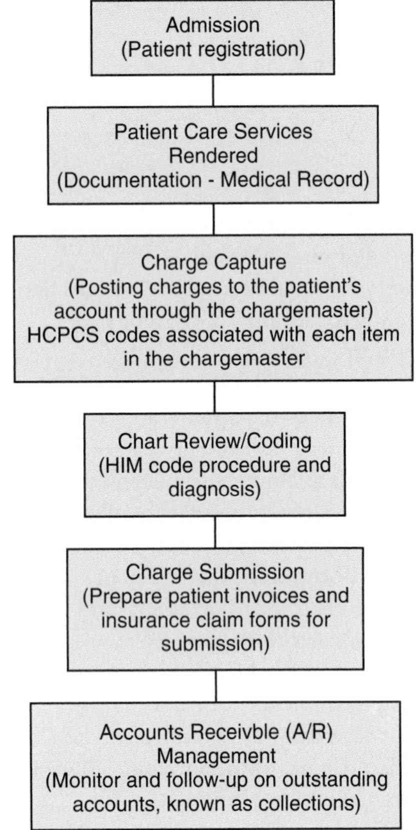

Figure 8-1 The hospital billing process involves all the functions required to prepare charges for submission to patients and third-party payers to obtain reimbursement.

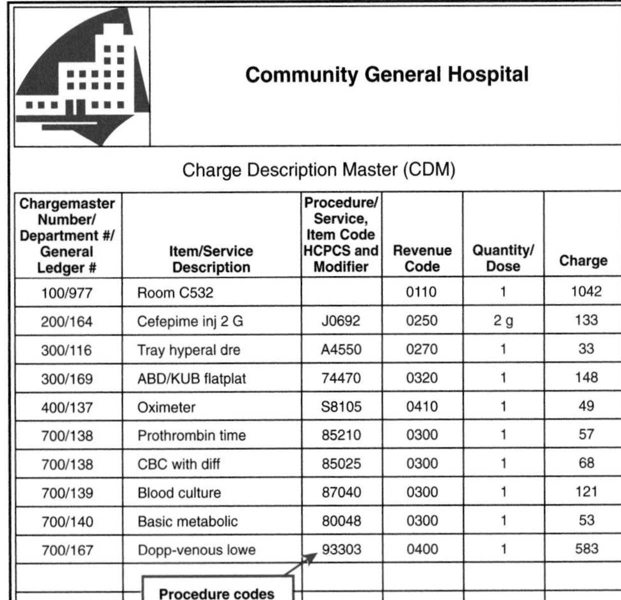

Community General Hospital

Charge Description Master (CDM)

Chargemaster Number/ Department #/ General Ledger #	Item/Service Description	Procedure/ Service, Item Code HCPCS and Modifier	Revenue Code	Quantity/ Dose	Charge
100/977	Room C532		0110	1	1042
200/164	Cefepime inj 2 G	J0692	0250	2 g	133
300/116	Tray hyperal dre	A4550	0270	1	33
300/169	ABD/KUB flatplat	74470	0320	1	148
400/137	Oximeter	S8105	0410	1	49
700/138	Prothrombin time	85210	0300	1	57
700/138	CBC with diff	85025	0300	1	68
700/139	Blood culture	87040	0300	1	121
700/140	Basic metabolic	80048	0300	1	53
700/167	Dopp-venous lowe	93303	0400	1	583
	Procedure codes				

Figure 8-2 Hospital Charge Description Master (CDM), also referred to as the chargemaster.

BOX 8-1 ■ KEY POINTS

Procedure Coding Defined

Coding is the assignment of numeric or alphanumeric codes to all health care data elements of outpatient and inpatient care.

Procedure coding involves assigning codes to written descriptions of procedures, services, and items.

BOX 8-2 ■ KEY POINTS

Procedure Coding and Hospital Coding and Billing Professionals

Hospital Coding Professionals

Must master coding principals and applications to describe services, procedures, and items accurately and to obtain proper reimbursement.

Hospital Billing Professionals

Must understand procedure coding to ensure compliance with coding guidelines and to obtain accurate reimbursement.

Procedure coding systems utilized to describe hospital procedures, services, and items are the Health Care Common Procedure Coding System (HCPCS) and the International Classification of Diseases, 9th Revision, Clinical Modification (ICD-9-CM), Volume III Procedures. Coding of procedures, services, and items is performed utilizing information from the patient's medical record, referred to as documentation. A discussion of coding guidelines is provided in this chapter. To understand the procedure coding systems utilized today, it is important to understand the evolution of various systems.

History of Procedure Coding Systems

The classification and coding of procedures, services, and items constitute a newer development than the coding of conditions, which began in the 17th century. Procedure coding systems were developed in the 1960s to provide a standardized system for providers to report procedures to third-party payers for reimbursement. The system also allows for collection of data to be utilized for statistical purposes. Historically, physicians and other providers submitted a written description of procedures and services rendered on the claim form to explain charges. Payers experienced difficulty in processing claims submitted with the written descriptions. Additionally, tracking, monitoring, and statistical analysis utilizing the written descriptions was a very complex process. The need for a standardized system of reporting procedures and services was addressed first when the

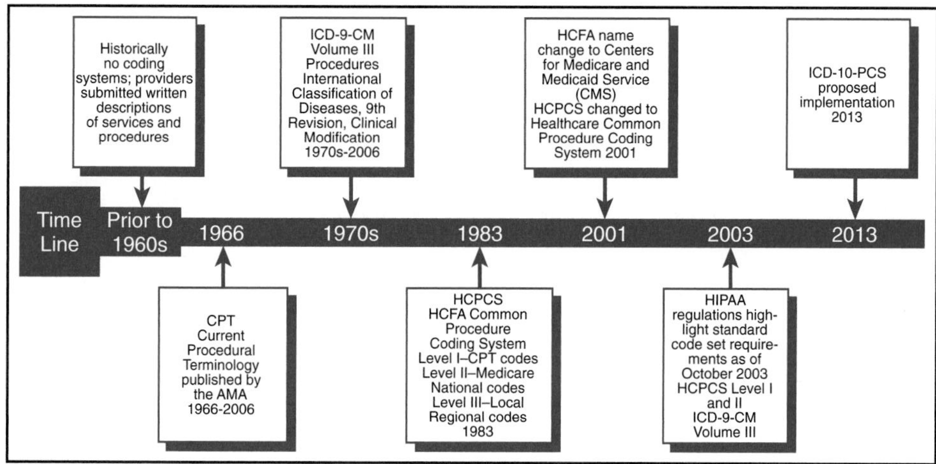

Figure 8-3 Evolution of procedure coding systems from the 1960s to today.

American Medical Association (AMA) developed the Current Procedural Terminology (CPT) coding system. Other procedure coding systems were later introduced such as the International Classifications of Diseases, 9th Revision, Clinical Modification (ICD-9-CM), Volume III procedure coding system and the HCPCS Medicare National coding system. These systems provided codes for procedures, services, supplies, equipment, and medications. The evolution of the CPT, Medicare National, and ICD-9-CM Volume III coding systems is illustrated in Figure 8-3.

> **BOX 8-3 ■ KEY POINTS**
>
> **History of Procedure Coding**
>
> Prior to the development of CPT in 1960, physicians and other providers submitted written descriptions of procedures and services to payers for reimbursement.
>
> ***Development of Procedure Coding Systems***
>
> The following procedure coding systems were developed to provide a standardized method of reporting procedures and services to payers for reimbursement:
>
> - Current Procedural Terminology (CPT)
> - Medicare National Codes
> - International Classification of Diseases, 9th Revision, Clinical Modification, Volume III Procedures

Current Procedural Terminology (CPT)

The American Medical Association (AMA) first published the Current Procedural Terminology (CPT) in 1966. **CPT** is a coding system that contains a set of codes, descriptions, and guidelines intended to describe procedures and services performed by physicians and other health care providers. The coding system contains a listing of procedures and services, and each is associated with a five-digit numeric code. The system also contains a listing of two-digit modifiers utilized to describe various circumstances not explained by the procedure code. The codes are used by providers to submit descriptions of charges to payers for reimbursement. During the period from 1966 to 1983, many providers elected to continue using written descriptions of procedures and services instead of the CPT codes. From 1966 to today, the AMA published the second through the fourth editions of the CPT manual. We are currently working with the 4th edition, CPT-4. This text will reference the current edition using the CPT acronymn.

> **BOX 8-4 ■ KEY POINTS**
>
> **Current Procedural Terminology (CPT)**
>
> Published by the AMA in 1966 to provide a standardized system for reporting procedures and services. The 4th edition of CPT is currently used for reporting.
>
> - CPT codes have five numeric or alphanumeric digits. Examples: 99204, 0037T, or 4009F
> - CPT contains two-digit modifiers. Examples: 25, 51, or 91

Medicare National Codes

Medicare National Codes were developed in the 1980s to provide a standardized system for reporting supplies, equipment, medications, and other items to Medicare carriers. Many payers provided coverage for various items, but there were no codes to describe these items. The CPT coding system primarily described procedures and services, with a few codes for supplies, vaccines, and toxoids. Medicare National codes were developed to provide codes for reporting of services and items not described in CPT on Medicare claims. Some payers adopted Medicare National codes, but not all. The coding system contains a listing of procedures, services, supplies, equipment, medications, and other items, and each is associated with a five-digit alphanumeric code. The system also contains a listing of two-digit modifiers utilized to describe various circumstances not explained by the procedure code. Medicare National codes are now called HCPCS Level II codes, as they were adopted by Medicare as part of the Health Care Common Procedure Coding System (HCPCS).

BOX 8-5 ■ KEY POINTS

Medicare National Codes, HCPCS Level II

Developed in the 1980s to provide a standardized system for reporting supplies, equipment, medications, and other items to Medicare carriers.
HCPCS Level II codes have five alphanumeric digits.
Examples: A4455 or J1610
HCPCS contains two-digit modifiers.
Examples: F1, GA, or TC

ICD-9-CM Volume III Procedure Codes

As discussed in Chapter 7, the International Classification of Disease (ICD) was the primary coding system for reporting conditions, illness, injury, diseases and other reasons for services, until the late 1970s. The ICD was revised many times over the years, and eventually a classification of hospital procedures was included, ICD-9-CM Volume III. **ICD-9-CM Volume III procedures** are used today for the reporting of significant procedures and services performed in the hospital or other facility. The coding system contains a listing of procedures and services, and each is associated with a two- to four-digit numeric code. ICD-9-CM Volume III procedures are commonly referred to as ICD-9-PCS.

BOX 8-6 ■ KEY POINTS

Evolution of ICD-9-CM Volume III Procedure Codes

↓

International Classification of Diseases (ICD)

Revised in the 1970s to include a classification of hospital procedures.

↓

International Classification of Diseases, 9th Revision, Clinical Modification, Volume III Procedures

Volume III Procedure codes are two to four digits.
Examples: 03, 03.0, and 03.09

Health Care Common Procedure Coding System (HCPCS)

Health Care Common Procedure Coding System (HCPCS) is the standard coding system adopted under the Health Insurance Portability and Accountability Act (HIPAA) for use in coding services, procedures, and items. HCPCS contains two levels of codes—Level I CPT and Level II Medicare National codes.

BOX 8-7 ■ KEY POINTS

HCPCS: Health Care Common Procedure Coding System

HCPCS adopted in 1983 by HCFA (CMS) for submission of claims to Medicare Carriers. The system included three levels of codes:
Level I CPT
Level II Medicare National codes
Level III Local Regional (eliminated in 2003)

In 1983 the Health Care Financing Administration (HCFA), now known as the Centers for Medicare and Medicaid Services (CMS), adopted the HCFA Common Procedure Coding System (HCPCS) for use when submitting claims to Medicare carriers. Other payers such as Blue Cross/Blue Shield followed suit and adopted HCPCS for claim submission. In 1983, HCPCS consisted of three levels of codes: Level I CPT codes; Level II Medicare National codes; and Level III Local Regional codes.

In June 2001, HCFA changed its name to the Centers for Medicare and Medicare Services (CMS), and the procedure coding system name was changed to the Health Care Common Procedure Coding System (HCPCS). Level III Local Regional codes were eliminated as of 2003.

Prior to 1983, more than 120 different coding systems were utilized in the United States.The billing process was extremely complex because of the variations in payers' guidelines, claim forms, and coding systems. This complex system of billing was costly for payers and providers. Since the government became a major payer of health care services, efforts to control costs have led to various levels of standardization in the administration of health care claims. Today, three procedure coding systems are utilized: HCPCS Level I CPT; HCPCS Level II Medicare National; and ICD-9-CM Volume III (Figure 8-4).

Legislative intervention such as the Health Insurance Portability and Accountability Act (HIPAA) of 1996 laid the foundation for the standardization of transactions. HIPAA regulations highlight HCPCS Levels I and

I.	HCPCS Level I CPT
II.	HCPCS Level II Medicare National Codes
III.	International Classification of Diseases, 9th Revision, Clinical Modification (ICD-9-CM) Volume III Procedure Codes

Figure 8-4 Procedure coding systems utilized today.

Health Insurance Portability and Accountability Act (HIPAA) of 1996 Title II Administrative Simplification Standard Code Sets

International Classification of Diseases, 9th Revision, Clinical Modification (ICD-9-CM) codes, Volumes I, II, and III	Volumes I and II utilized to report the reason services were rendered such as: sign, symptom, condition, disease, illness, injury or other reason for the visit. Volume III utilized to report significant procedures performed by a facility.
HCPCS Level I CPT	To report physician and outpatient services, procedures, and items.
HCPCS Level II Medicare National	To report services, procedures, and items when no CPT code provides adequate description or when the payer indicates Level II codes should be used instead of the Level I CPT codes.

Figure 8-5 HIPAA Title II–Standard Code Sets for reporting diagnosis and procedures. *(Modified from Burton BK:* Quick guide to HIPAA, *ed 1, St Louis, 2004, Saunders.)*

II and ICD-9-CM Volumes I, II, and III as the standard code set required for submission of claims to payers effective October 2003, as illustrated in Figure 8-5.

The content and format of the Health Care Common Procedure Coding Systems (HCPCS) and the ICD-9-CM Volume III coding systems will be discussed later in this chapter. Although procedure coding is used to describe procedures, services, and items, it is also utilized for collection of data. Each of the coding systems used today allows for the collection of specified data that are utilized for statistical purposes.

BOX 8-8 ■ KEY POINTS

HIPAA: Health Insurance Portability and Accountability Act of 1996

Title II administrative simplification outlines the following standard code sets adopted for reporting procedures and diagnoses:

- HCPCS Level I CPT
- HCPCS Level II Medicare National Codes
- International Classification of Diseases, 9th Revision, Clinical Modification, Volume III, Procedures

Purpose of Procedure Coding

As discussed in Chapter 7, coding systems are designed to provide a standardized system for describing and classifying data. Procedure codes are used to describe services provided during a patient hospital visit. Charges are submitted to third-party payers for reimbursement, and the charges are explained with procedure codes. Procedure code data are also utilized for statistical purposes.

BOX 8-9 ■ KEY POINTS

Purpose of Procedure Coding Systems

To provide a standardized system for providers to report procedures and services to third-party payers for reimbursement and for the collection of data utilized for statistical purposes.

Utilization of Procedure Code Data

Procedure coding systems allow for the collection of data regarding procedures and services performed and the various items utilized to provide services. The data gathered through the use of these coding systems can be monitored, tracked, and retrieved for various purposes such as research, education, and administration, as illustrated in Figure 8-6.

Research

Data from procedure coding systems are used to research various patterns in the diagnosis and treatment of conditions. Researchers can monitor the various treatments provided for specific conditions to determine those that result in the best patient outcomes. Research data are also used to identify ways to improve or invent new procedures and technology. Through monitoring of these data, researchers can identify various risk factors related to specific procedures, services, or items.

Education

Data from procedure coding systems can be utilized to educate health care professionals and the public. The education of health care professionals can be enhanced through knowledge gained by analyzing data from these coding systems. New treatments, supplies, and

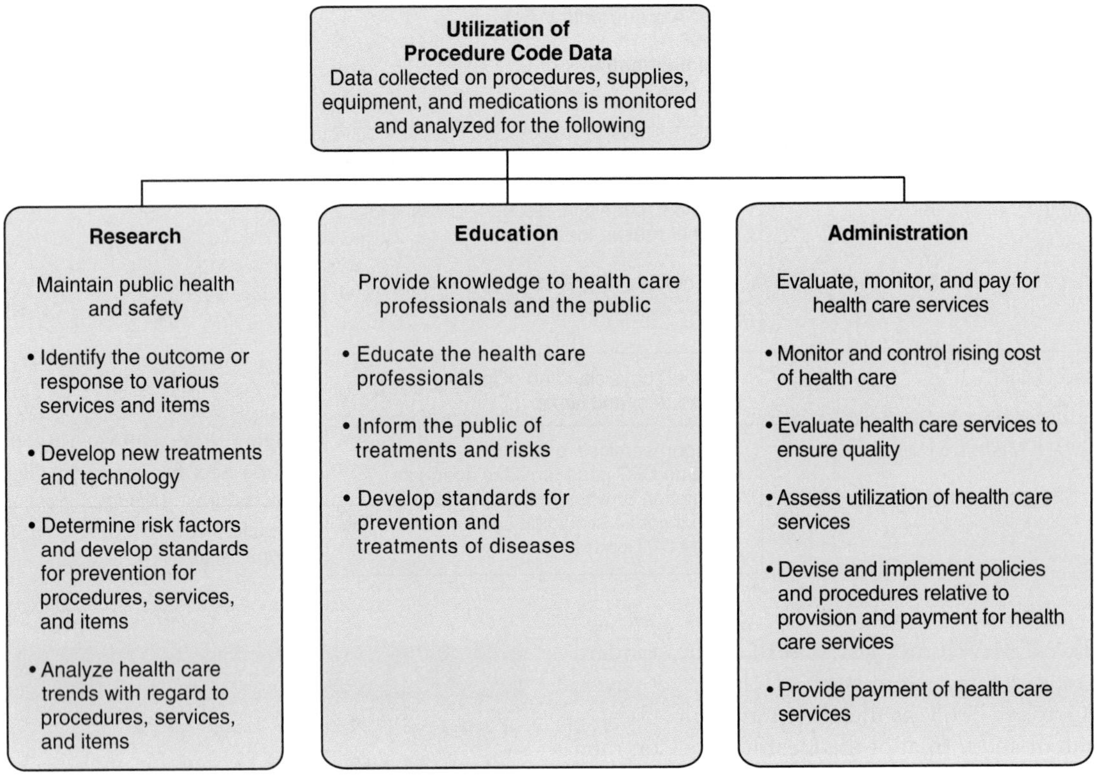

Utilization of Procedure Code Data
Data collected on procedures, supplies, equipment, and medications is monitored and analyzed for the following

Research

Maintain public health and safety

- Identify the outcome or response to various services and items
- Develop new treatments and technology
- Determine risk factors and develop standards for prevention for procedures, services, and items
- Analyze health care trends with regard to procedures, services, and items

Education

Provide knowledge to health care professionals and the public

- Educate the health care professionals
- Inform the public of treatments and risks
- Develop standards for prevention and treatments of diseases

Administration

Evaluate, monitor, and pay for health care services

- Monitor and control rising cost of health care
- Evaluate health care services to ensure quality
- Assess utilization of health care services
- Devise and implement policies and procedures relative to provision and payment for health care services
- Provide payment of health care services

Figure 8-6 Utilization of procedure code data.

medications can be monitored for the assessment of positive outcomes that show a decrease in mortality and morbidity. Educating the public on topics such as disease prevention is also enhanced through the use of procedure code data.

Administration

There are various administrative uses of data collected from procedure coding systems. Data can be used to evaluate, assess, monitor, and pay for health care services. Utilization of services is a major focus area to assess the quality of health care services. Many payers utilize data collected through these systems to develop and implement policies and procedures related to the provision of health care services. Procedure coding system data are also utilized by payers to develop reimbursement systems. Providers analyze procedure code data to assess and negotiate payer contracts.

BOX 8-10 ■ KEY POINTS

Procedure Code Data Utilization

Data collected through the use of procedure coding systems are utilized for:

- Research
- Education
- Administration

Procedure Coding Defined

As discussed previously, the definition of coding is the assignment of numeric or alphanumeric codes to all health care data elements of outpatient and inpatient care. Procedure coding is the process of translating written descriptions of procedures, services, supplies, drugs, and equipment from the patient's record into numeric or alphanumeric codes.

Procedure coding is an essential component of the billing process. The description of procedures, services, and items provided during a hospital visit is communicated to payers utilizing coding systems (Figure 8-7). The process begins when the patient presents at the hospital with a health care issue that requires attention, or for a service that involves health care status. The physician or other provider reviews the history, performs an examination, and prepares a plan of care. Patient care services are rendered in accordance with physician's orders and the plan of care. Written descriptions of health care services, procedures, and items are recorded in the patient's medical record. Charges are posted through the chargemaster by various departments. All procedures, services, and items listed in the chargemaster are associated with a code from the appropriate procedure coding system. HIM coders are involved in coding procedures, services, and items from the patient record that are not posted through the chargemaster and the patient's diagnosis (Figure 8-8). To code effectively, it is important to understand the relationship of procedure coding to documentation, medical necessity, claim forms, and reimbursement.

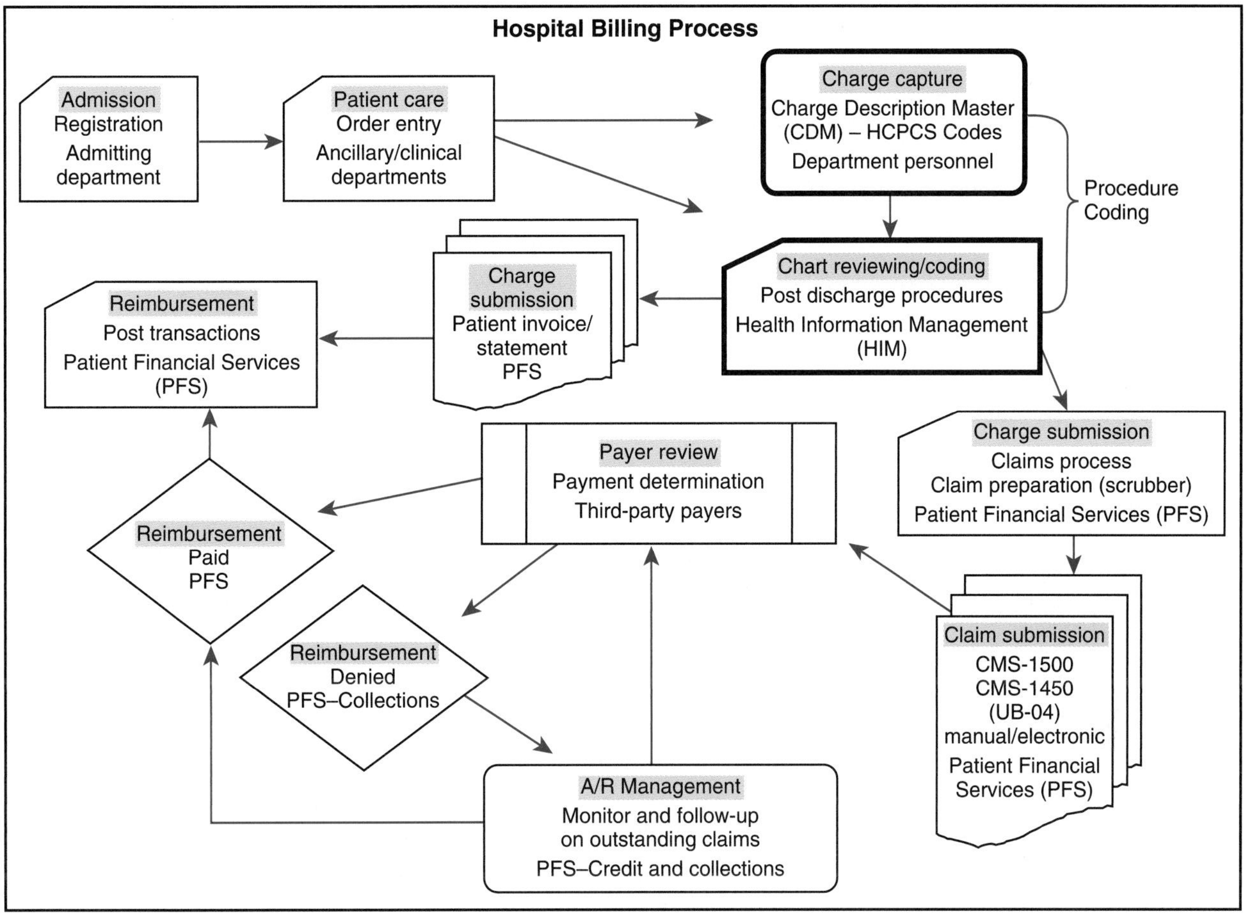

Hospital Billing Process

Admission
Registration
Admitting department

Patient care
Order entry
Ancillary/clinical departments

Charge capture
Charge Description Master (CDM) – HCPCS Codes
Department personnel

Procedure Coding

Chart reviewing/coding
Post discharge procedures
Health Information Management (HIM)

Charge submission
Patient invoice/ statement
PFS

Reimbursement
Post transactions
Patient Financial Services (PFS)

Charge submission
Claims process
Claim preparation (scrubber)
Patient Financial Services (PFS)

Payer review
Payment determination
Third-party payers

Reimbursement
Paid
PFS

Reimbursement
Denied
PFS–Collections

Claim submission
CMS-1500
CMS-1450 (UB-04)
manual/electronic
Patient Financial Services (PFS)

A/R Management
Monitor and follow-up on outstanding claims
PFS–Credit and collections

Figure 8-7 Hospital billing process highlighting an essential component of billing (procedure coding). *(Revision of illustration courtesy Sandra Giangreco.)*

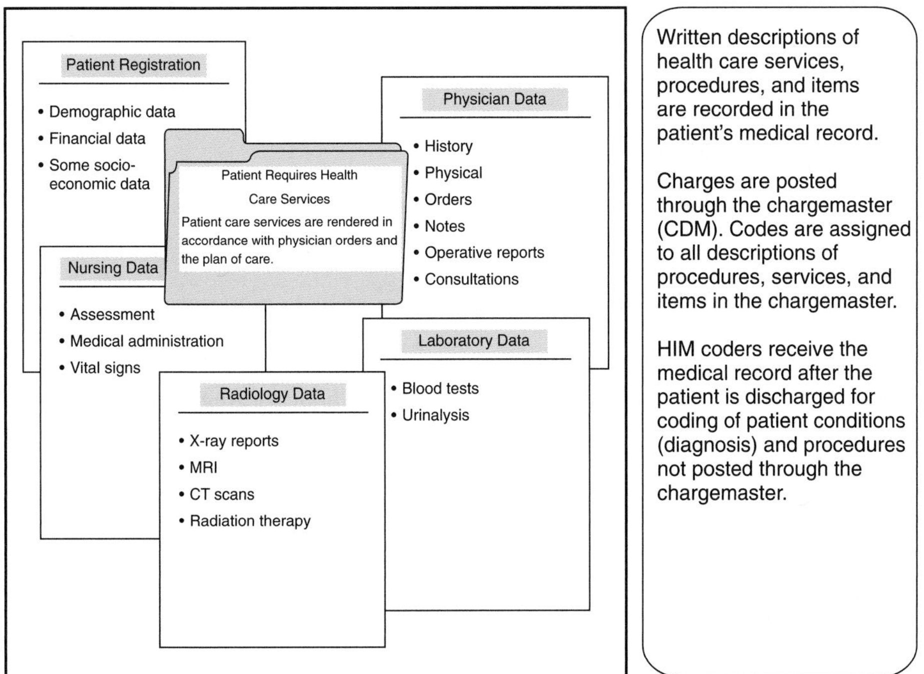

Figure 8-8 Information in the patient's medical record that is utilized for procedure coding.

TEST YOUR *Knowledge* BOX 8-1

HISTORY, DEFINITION, AND PURPOSE OF PROCEDURE CODING

1. Explain why procedure coding systems were developed.
2. State how providers communicated procedures and services performed to payers prior to the development of coding systems.
3. What coding system was published by the AMA and when?
4. List the two levels of the HCPCS Coding System.
5. Discuss when HCPCS was adopted, the organization that adopted HCPCS, and explain what HCPCS means.
6. Explain why HCPCS Level II codes were developed.
7. Provide a brief explanation of the difference between an HCPCS Level I CPT and ICD-9-CM Volume III procedure code.
8. Name three coding systems utilized to describe procedures, services, and items.
9. State the difference between an HCPCS Level I CPT and Level II code.
10. Provide a brief explanation of how HIPAA affected coding systems utilized today.
11. Explain the purpose of procedure coding systems.
12. Describe how data collected using procedure coding systems can be used for research purposes.
13. Describe how data collected using procedure coding systems can be used for education purposes.
14. Describe how data collected using procedure coding systems can be used for administrative purposes.
15. Define procedure coding.

BOX 8-11 ■ KEY POINTS

Procedure Coding: An Essential Component of Billing

- Procedures, services, and items are recorded in the patient's medical record
- Charges for services are posted through the chargemaster or by HIM professionals
- All charges are described utilizing a procedure coding system

PROCEDURE CODING SYSTEM RELATIONSHIPS

Procedure coding systems relate to other components of the billing process as highlighted previously. The process of procedure coding is dependent on information recorded in the medical record. Charges for services recorded in the medical record are described on the claim form utilizing procedure codes. Payers conduct medical necessity reviews and payment determination based on the procedure and diagnosis codes submitted. In essence, procedure coding is the key to obtaining reimbursement for services rendered. It is important for hospital coding and billing professionals to understand how procedure coding relates to documentation, medical necessity, claim forms, and reimbursement, as illustrated in Figure 8-9.

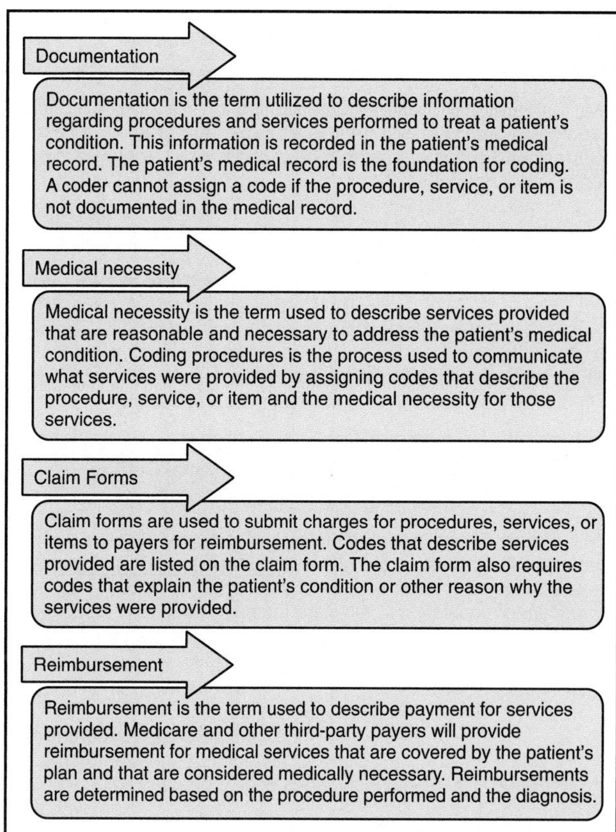

Documentation
Documentation is the term utilized to describe information regarding procedures and services performed to treat a patient's condition. This information is recorded in the patient's medical record. The patient's medical record is the foundation for coding. A coder cannot assign a code if the procedure, service, or item is not documented in the medical record.
Medical necessity
Medical necessity is the term used to describe services provided that are reasonable and necessary to address the patient's medical condition. Coding procedures is the process used to communicate what services were provided by assigning codes that describe the procedure, service, or item and the medical necessity for those services.
Claim Forms
Claim forms are used to submit charges for procedures, services, or items to payers for reimbursement. Codes that describe services provided are listed on the claim form. The claim form also requires codes that explain the patient's condition or other reason why the services were provided.
Reimbursement
Reimbursement is the term used to describe payment for services provided. Medicare and other third-party payers will provide reimbursement for medical services that are covered by the patient's plan and that are considered medically necessary. Reimbursements are determined based on the procedure performed and the diagnosis.

Figure 8-9 Procedure coding relationship to documentation, medical necessity, claim forms, and reimbursement.

BOX 8-12 ■ KEY POINTS

Golden Rule in Coding

IF IT IS NOT DOCUMENTED, DO NOT CODE IT

Documentation

Documentation is the term utilized to describe information recorded regarding patient conditions and procedures, services, supplies, equipment, and medications provided as part of the patient's care. This information is recorded in the patient's medical record. The patient's medical record is the foundation for coding. The golden rule in coding is "**IF IT IS NOT DOCUMENTED, DO NOT CODE IT**." When coding procedures, services, supplies, equipment, and medications it is necessary to read the record to identify the service or item that is to be coded for billing purposes. A code from the HCPCS or ICD-9-CM Volume III is assigned to provide a description that most closely matches that of the record. Figure 8-10 illustrates three short examples of coding from the medical record utilizing the HCPCS and ICD-9-CM Volume III.

1. Example 1 is assigned an HCPCS Level I CPT code 71010 "Radiologic examination, chest, and single view, frontal" because the record indicates that a chest X-ray was performed.
2. Example 2 is assigned an HCPCS Level II code E0100 "Cane, includes canes of all materials, adjustable or fixed, with tip" to describe the cane provided as recorded in the patient's record.
3. Example 3 is assigned an ICD-9-CM Volume III procedure code 36.13 "(Aorto) coronary bypass of three coronary arteries" to describe the bypass procedure performed during the inpatient stay.

Medical Necessity

Medical necessity is the term used to describe procedures and services that are considered reasonable and necessary to address the patient's condition, based on standards of medical practice. Medical necessity is determined by payers based on a review of procedure and diagnosis codes submitted. The diagnosis code must describe a medical reason for the service that meets medical necessity criteria. Medical necessity guidelines are generally determined based on standards of medical care, and they vary by payer. For example, Medicare and their fiscal intermediaries publish national coverage determinations or local medical review policies

Example 1 HCPCS Level I CPT Procedure Coding

Medical Record of Jon Jamerstonig

Mr. Jamerstonig presents complaining of a cough, dyspnea, and chest pain with respiration. An expanded problem-focused **history and exam** was performed. A chest **x-ray** single view was performed, normal findings.

Johnathan Sampson, M.D.

Procedure Code assignment:
99213 "Evaluation and Management"
71010 "Radiologic examination, chest; single view, frontal"

Diagnosis codes: 786.52, 786.00, 786.2
Painful Respiration, Dyspnea, and Cough

Example 2 HCPCS Level II Medicare National Coding

Medical Record of Jana Pertrivuti

Ms. Pertrivuti presents complaining of difficulty walking due to severe osteoarthritis in the hip. A **problem-focused history and exam** was performed with straightforward decision making. I prescribed medication to alleviate the pain and supplied her with a **cane**.

Johnathan Sampson, M.D.

Procedure Code assignment:
99213 "Evaluation and Management"
E0100 "Cane, includes canes of all materials, adjustable or fixed, with tip"

Diagnosis code: 715.15
Osteoarthritis

Example #3 Volume III Procedure Coding

Medical Record of Howard Fordmanston

Mr. Fordmanston was admitted to the hospital with coronary atherosclerosis of native arteries, for a coronary **bypass**. Patient also has malignant hypertension. Three coronary vessels were bypassed during the procedure. Patient tolerated the procedure well.

Johnathan Sampson, M.D.

Procedure Code assignment:
36.13 "(Aorto)coronary bypass of three coronary arteries"

Diagnosis codes: 414.01, 401.0
Atherosclerosis and Hypertension

Figure 8-10 Examples of coding procedures from the medical record.

outlining diagnosis codes that support medical necessity (Figure 8-11). Local medical review policies (LMRPs) were replaced with local coverage determinations (LCDs) in December, 2005. Payers will not provide reimbursement for services that are not medically necessary. It is critical for coders to assign codes that accurately describe information in the medical record.

BOX 8-13 ■ KEY POINTS

Medical Necessity

- Medically necessary services are those that are reasonable and medically necessary to address the patient's medical condition
- Medical necessity is determined based on standards of medical practice
- Procedure codes are submitted with diagnosis codes that explain the medical necessity for procedures, services, or items provided

Claim Forms

As discussed in Chapter 7, claim forms are used to submit charges for procedures, services, and items to payers for reimbursement. The CMS-1500 and CMS-1450 (UB-04) are the claim forms utilized to submit charges. Procedures, services, and items are reported on the appropriate claim form utilizing the HCPCS or ICD-9-CM Volume III procedure coding systems. Medical necessity for the services is explained using ICD-9-CM Volume I and II codes that describe the patient's condition; injury, illness, disease, or other reason the service or item was provided. Procedure coding systems vary based on the claim form used, as illustrated in Table 8-1.

CMS-1500

The CMS-1500 is utilized to submit charges for physician and outpatient services. Professional services provided in a hospital-based primary care office or other clinic, are also reported on the CMS-1500 when the physician is employed by, or under contract with, the hospital. Information regarding procedures, services, and items are recorded in Block 24A through 24D. Block 24 provides six lines and each line requires date of service, place of service, type of service, the appropriate HCPCS code, and a modifier where applicable. As discussed in Chapter 7, diagnosis codes are recorded in Block 21. Each procedure is linked to the diagnosis code that explains why the service or item was provided. Block 24E is used to link the procedure to a diagnosis, as discussed in Chapter 7. This tells the payer why the service or item was provided, as illustrated in Figure 8-12. Claim forms are carefully reviewed by the payer to identify potential reimbursement issues. Block 24 is compared against Block 21 to determine whether the service provided was medically necessary (Figure 8-12).

CMS-1450 (UB-04)

The UB-04 is utilized to submit facility charges for hospital outpatient, non-patient, and inpatient services provided by a hospital or other facility. Fields that require data on the UB-04 are referred to as **form locators (FL)**. The UB-04 contains 81 FLs. Codes represent-

MEDICARE PART A SAMPLE LOCAL COVERAGE DETERMINATION (LCD)			
CONTRACTOR NAME: Medicare Administrative Contractor **CONTRACTOR NUMBER:**		**CONTRACTOR TYPE:** MAC-Part A	
LCD ID#: L924358		**LCD TITLE:** Screening and Diagnostic Mammography	
INDICATIONS AND LIMITATIONS OF COVERAGE AND/OR MEDICAL NECESSITY: A screening mammography is performed when a woman presents without signs or symptoms of breast disease, for the purpose of early detection breast cancer, or a personal history. Medicare beneficiaries are allowed screening mammogram(s) (digital and non-digital) for the following indications:			
CPT/HCPCS CODES			
76082	Computer aided detection (computer algorithm analysis of digital image data for lesion detection) with further physician review for interpretations, with or without digitizationof film radiographic images; diagnostic mammography (List separately in addition to code for primary procedure		
76090	Mammography; unilateral		
76091	bilateral		
G0204	Diagnostic mammography, producing direct image, bilateral, all views		
G0206	Diagnostic mammography, producing direct image, unilateral, all views		
ICD-9-CM CODES THAT SUPPORT MEDICAL NECESSITY			
174.0	Malignant neoplasm of female breast, nipple, and areola	610.3	Fibrosclerosis of breast
174.1	Malignant neoplasm of female breast, central portion	610.4	Mammary duct ectasia
174.2	Malignant neoplasm of female breast, upper-inner quadrant	610.8	Other specified benign mammary dysplasias
174.3	Malignant neoplasm of female breast, lower-inner quadrant	611.0-611.8	Other disorders of breast
174.4	Malignant neoplasm of female breast, upper-outer quadrant	793.80-793.89	Nonspecific abnormal findings on radiological and other examination of breast
174.5	Malignant neoplasm of female breast, lower-outer quadrant	879.0	Open wound of breast, without mention of complication
174.6	Malignant neoplasm of female breast, axillary tail	879.1	Open wound of breast, complicated
174.8	Malignant neoplasm of other specified sites of female breast	996.54	Mechanical complications due to breast prothesis
175.0-175.9	Malignant neoplasm of male breast	V10.3	Personal history of malignant neoplasm, breast
610.0	Solitary cyst of breast	V15.89	Other specified personal history presenting hazards to health (Personal history of benign breast disease)
		V71.1	Observation for suspected malignant neoplasm
610.1	Diffuse cystic mastopathy		
610.2	Fibroadenosis of breast		

Figure 8-11 Example of a Local Medical Review Policy (LMRP) for mammography.

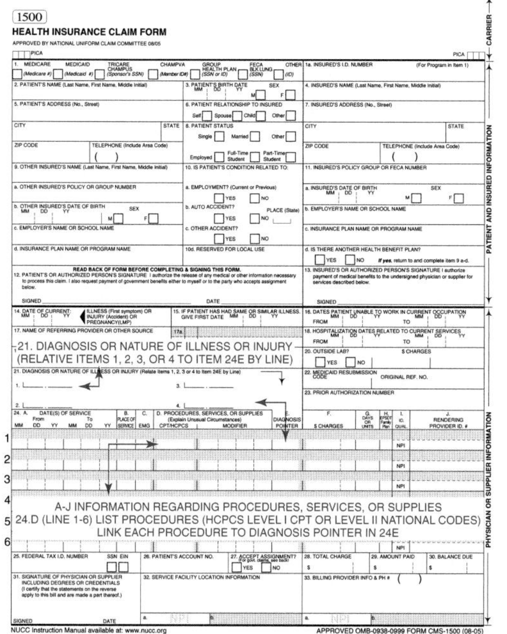
1500
HEALTH INSURANCE CLAIM FORM
21. DIAGNOSIS OR NATURE OF ILLNESS OR INJURY (RELATIVE ITEMS 1, 2, 3, OR 4 TO ITEM 24E BY LINE)
A-J INFORMATION REGARDING PROCEDURES, SERVICES, OR SUPPLIES
24.D (LINE 1-6) LIST PROCEDURES (HCPCS LEVEL I CPT OR LEVEL II NATIONAL CODES)
LINK EACH PROCEDURE TO DIAGNOSIS POINTER IN 24E
NUCC Instruction Manual available at: www.nucc.org
APPROVED OMB-0938-0999 FORM CMS-1500 (08-05)

Figure 8-12 CMS-1500 claim form illustrating Blocks 21, 24, and 24E used to record procedures and diagnosis.

ing procedures are listed in FL 44 and 74a–e. Codes representing the patient's condition are recorded in FL 67, 69, 70, 72. FL 44 is used to indicate the HCPCS code that describes the service or item. The appropriate HCPCS code and rate is listed in FL 44 for the service or item provided on an outpatient or non-patient basis. FL 74a–e is used to indicate the appropriate ICD-9-CM Volume III code representing significant procedures and services during an inpatient visit, as illustrated in Figure 8-13. These FLs require codes representing the principal procedure and other procedures that are considered *significant procedures*.

BOX 8-14 ■ KEY POINTS

CMS Claim Forms

CMS-1500

Physician and Outpatient Services
Procedure codes are recorded in Block 24D

CMS-1450 (UB-04)

Hospital services provided on outpatient, inpatient, and non-patient bases
Procedure codes are reported in FL 44 and/or FL 74a–e.

TABLE 8-1 **Claim Form Variations for Procedure Codes**

Procedure Coding	CLAIM FORMS: CMS-1500 Procedure Codes Blocks	CLAIM FORMS: CMS-1450 (UB-04) Procedures FL	Coding Systems and Guidelines
Procedure codes are used to report procedures, services, and items provided during the hospital visit (outpatient, inpatient, or non-patient).			
Physician and outpatient services			
Physician and Outpatient Services	Block 24D line 1–6		HCPCS Level I CPT Codes and guidelines HCPCS Level II Medicare National Codes and guidelines
Hospital based primary care office or other clinic			
Physician services*	Block 24D line 1–6		HCPCS Level I CPT codes and guidelines HCPCS Level II Medicare National codes and guidelines
Services performed in a hospital or other facility			
Procedures and items Categorized by Revenue Code utilizing HCPCS codes		FL 44 outpatient and non-patient services	HCPCS Level I CPT codes and guidelines HCPCS Level II Medicare National codes and guidelines
Significant procedures			
Principal procedure		FL 74 inpatient services	ICD-9-CM Volume III general coding guidelines ICD-9-CM Volume III coding guidelines for outpatient services or inpatient, short-term, acute care, and long-term care hospital records
Other procedures		FL 74a–e inpatient services	ICD-9-CM Volume III General Coding guidelines ICD-9-CM Volume III Coding guidelines for outpatient services or inpatient, short-term, acute care, and long-term care hospital records

*The hospital can bill physician services when the physician is employed by or under contract with the hospital.

Significant Procedure

A **significant procedure** is one that is: 1. surgical in nature, or 2. carries a procedural risk, or 3. carries an anesthetic risk, or 4. requires specialized training. This definition is stated in the Uniform Hospital Discharge Data Set (UHDDS), as published in the Federal Register in 1985.

- Infusions, catheterizations, and surgeries are examples of significant procedures.
- Electrocardiogram, complete blood count, and magnetic resonance imaging are not significant procedures.

Principal Procedure

The **principal procedure** is the one performed for definitive treatment of the principal diagnosis or the procedure that most closely relates to the principal diagnosis (Figure 8-14).

Other Procedures

Other significant procedures performed during the stay are recorded in FL 74a–e.

BOX 8-15 ■ KEY POINTS

Significant Procedure

The Uniform Hospital Discharge Data Set (UHDDS), as published in the *Federal Register*, Volume 50, Number 147, July 31, 1985, includes data items for reporting procedures. The definitions included can be used to determine which codes should be reported. Item 12 of UHDDS states that all significant procedures are to be reported and defines a significant procedure as one that is:

- surgical in nature, or
- carries a procedural risk, or
- carries an anesthetic risk, or
- requires specialized training.

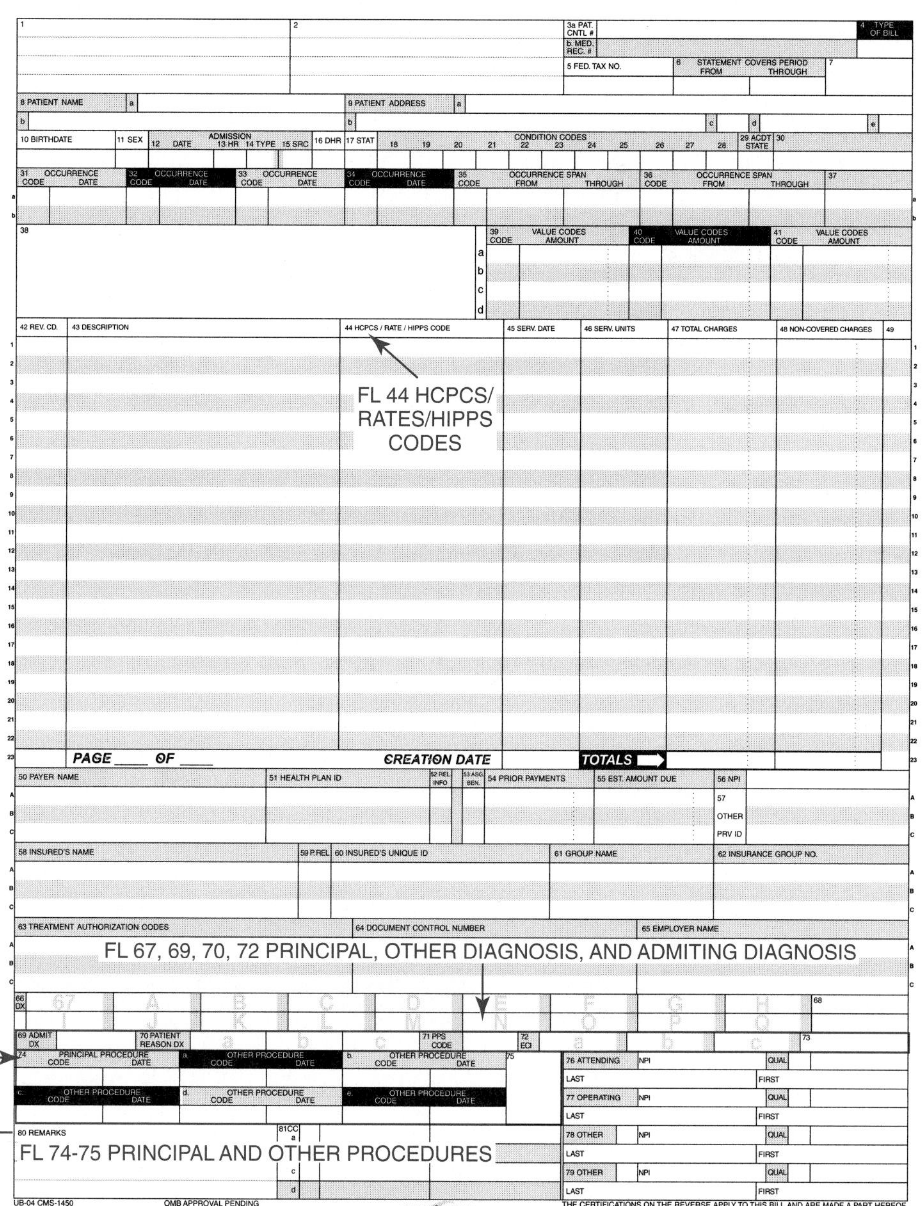

Figure 8-13 CMS-1450 (UB-04) claim form illustrating FL 67, 69, 70, 72 used to record the admitting, principal, and other diagnosis. FL 44 for HCPCS and FL 74a–e used to record the principal and other diagnosis to include FL 44 for HCPCS/Rates and FL 74a–e for principal and other procedures.

It is important to remember that the payer will carefully review and compare these fields to determine whether the service provided was medically necessary.

BOX 8-16 ■ KEY POINTS

Principal Procedure

The principal procedure is the one performed for definitive treatment of the principal diagnosis or the procedure that most closely relates to the principal

Reimbursement

Medicare and other third-party payers will provide reimbursement for medical services that are covered, in accordance with the patient's health care plan or policy;

Medical Record

Patient with a malignant neoplasm of ureter admitted to the hospital for a ureterectomy. Partial ureterectomy performed and formation of other cutaneous ureterostomy. Patient tolerated procedure well.

Johnathan Sampson, M.D.

Principal Procedure code assignment:
56.41 "Partial ureterectomy"
Other Procedure Code assignment:
56.61 "Formation of other cutaneous ureterostomy"

Principal diagnosis: 189.2 Malignant neoplasm of ureter

Note: The partial ureterectomy was performed to remove the malignant neoplasm, therefore, it is considered the principal procedure.

Figure 8-14 Example of coding a principal procedure.

however, they must be considered medically necessary. For example, a payer will not usually pay for a lung biopsy if the diagnosis codes do not represent a medical condition that would indicate the need for a biopsy such as a lung mass and family history of lung cancer.

BOX 8-17 ■ KEY POINTS

Reimbursement

- Procedure codes are submitted to payers for reimbursement utilizing a claim form.
- Reimbursement is payment from a third-party payer to a provider for services rendered.
- Reimbursement is provided when services are covered in accordance with the patient's plan and when the services are considered medically necessary.

PROCEDURE CODING SYSTEM VARIATIONS

Procedure coding systems are utilized to communicate with payers regarding services, procedures, and items provided. As discussed in the previous chapter, the ICD-9-CM diagnosis coding system is used to report the medical reason why procedures, services, or items are provided. The chapter also highlighted coding system variations based on service category, which illustrates ICD-9-CM diagnosis codes are used for all service categories (Table 8-2). Unlike diagnosis code usage, procedure code utilization varies by service category. Service categories include outpatient, non-patient, and inpatient. The following section presents procedure coding system variations based on services provided on an outpatient, inpatient, or non-patient basis (Figure 8-15).

TABLE 8-2 Coding System Variations

		PROCEDURES HCPCS			
Hospital Service Categories (Facility Charges)	**Diagnosis ICD-9-CM Volume I & II**	**Level I CPT**	**Level II Medicare National**	**Procedures ICD-9-CM Volume III**	**Variations**
Outpatient					
Ambulatory surgery	√	√	*	†	Some payers may require ICD-9-CM Volume III procedures for ambulatory surgery claim submitted on the CMS-1450 (UB-04)
Emergency Department	√	√	*	†	*
Ancillary Departments: Radiology Laboratory Physical, Occupational, and Speech Therapy	√	√	*	†	*
Other Outpatient Services: Infusion Therapy Observation	√	√	*	†	*
Durable medical equipment (provided on an outpatient or inpatient basis)	√	√	*	†	*
Hospital-based primary care office	√	√	*	†	*
Other hospital-based clinic	√	√	*	†	*
Inpatient					
Inpatient services Inpatient procedures are posted through the chargemaster utilizing HCPCS codes	√	√	*	√	ICD-9-CM Volume III procedure codes are utilized to reported significant procedures
Non-patient					
A specimen received and processed—the patient is not present	√	√	*		*

√ Coding procedure used.
*HCPCS Level I CPT codes are generally utilized to describe services and some items. HCPCS Level II Medicare National Codes are utilized when a CPT code cannot be found that adequately describes the service or item or when the payer requires a Level II code
†ICD-9-C M Volume III code usage varies by payer. Generally required to report significant procedures on the CMS-1450 (UB-04) claim form.

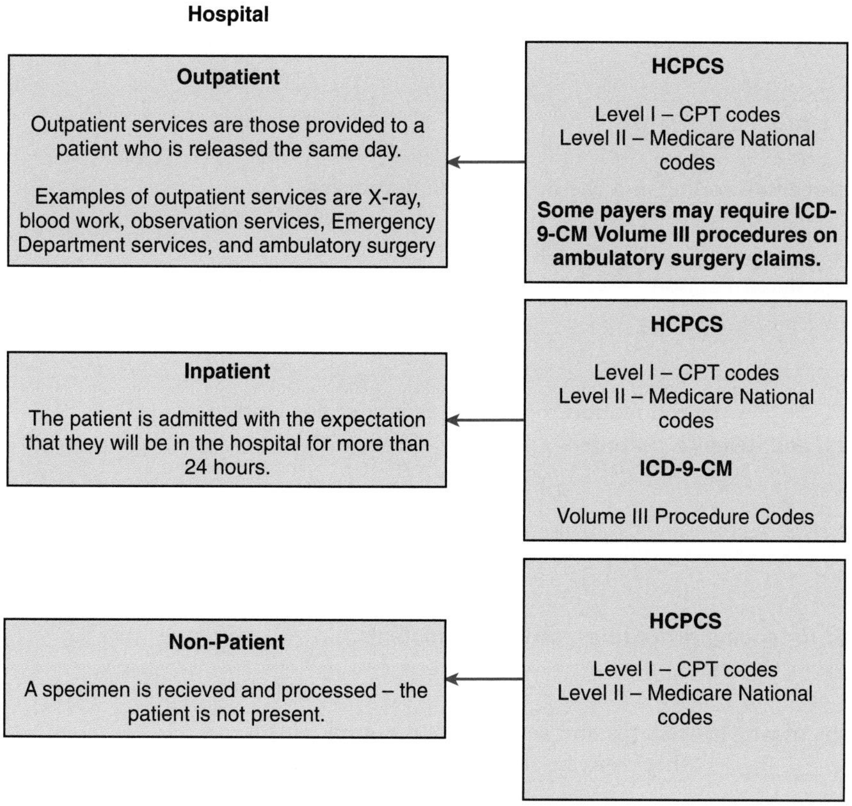

Hospital

Service category	Coding systems
Outpatient Outpatient services are those provided to a patient who is released the same day. Examples of outpatient services are X-ray, blood work, observation services, Emergency Department services, and ambulatory surgery	**HCPCS** Level I – CPT codes Level II – Medicare National codes **Some payers may require ICD-9-CM Volume III procedures on ambulatory surgery claims.**
Inpatient The patient is admitted with the expectation that they will be in the hospital for more than 24 hours.	**HCPCS** Level I – CPT codes Level II – Medicare National codes **ICD-9-CM** Volume III Procedure Codes
Non-Patient A specimen is recieved and processed – the patient is not present.	**HCPCS** Level I – CPT codes Level II – Medicare National codes

Figure 8-15 Coding system variations by service category.

BOX 8-18 ■ KEY POINTS

Hospital Service Categories

The procedure coding systems required vary based on the following hospital service categories:

- Outpatient
- Inpatient
- Non-patient

BOX 8-19 ■ KEY POINTS

Outpatient Procedure Code Requirements

Outpatient Services

Outpatient services are those provided on the same day the patient is released. HCPCS Level I CPT codes and HCPCS Level II Medicare National codes are required for reporting these services.

Some payers may require ICD-9-CM Volume III procedure codes on ambulatory surgery claims.

Outpatient Services

Outpatient services are those provided on the same day the patient is released. The patient does not stay overnight. Outpatient services include ambulatory surgery and ancillary department services such as radiology and the emergency room. HCPCS Level I and/or II codes are utilized for reporting procedures, services, and items provided on an outpatient basis. Some payers may require ICD-9-CM Volume III procedure codes in addition to HCPCS codes on ambulatory surgery claims. Most hospital outpatient services are reported on the UB-04 including ambulatory surgery. Professional services provided by a physician in a hospital-based primary care clinic or other clinic are reported by the hospital if the physician is employed by or under contract with the hospital. Professional services are reported utilizing HCPCS codes on the CMS-1500 (see Table 8-2).

HCPCS Level I CPT Coding System

HCPCS Level I CPT codes are accepted by all payers for reporting procedures and services. Coding guidelines indicate that procedures and services should be reported using Level I CPT codes unless there is no CPT code that adequately describes the procedure or service.

HCPCS Level II Medicare National codes describe supplies, equipment, medications, and some services. Coding guidelines indicate that if you are unable to locate a code that adequately describes the service or item in CPT, look for a Level II Medicare National code. Certain payers will require a Level II code and modifier as opposed to the CPT code and modifiers in certain circumstances.

TEST YOUR *Knowledge* BOX 8-2

PROCEDURE CODING SYSTEMS RELATIONSHIPS

1. Explain the relationship between procedure coding and the hospital billing process.

2. Payers conduct reviews and payment determination based on the ________________ and diagnosis codes submitted.

3. The __________ __________ __________ is the foundation for coding as it contains written descriptions of services, procedures, and items to be coded.

4. The Golden Rule in coding is ____________________.

5. Name three coding systems utilized for coding procedures, services, and items.

6. Providers must provide explanations of why procedures and services are required. This is accomplished utilizing __________ __________ that describe the patient's condition.

7. Payers will not pay for procedures, services, or items if they are not considered __________ __________.

8. Charges for services, procedures, and items are submitted utilizing two claim forms and they are ____________________ and ____________________.

9. Explain where procedure and diagnosis codes are reported on the CMS-1500.

10. State where HCPCS codes are reported on the CMS-1450 (UB-04).

11. Explain where the principal diagnosis and principal procedure are reported on the CMS-1450 (UB-04).

12. Other significant procedures are reported in what form locator on the CMS-1450 (UB-04)?

13. A significant procedure is one that is: __________, or __________, or __________, or __________.

14. The procedure that is performed for definitive treatment of the patient condition is the __________ __________.

15. Procedure codes are required to submit charges to payers and to obtain the appropriate __________.

As discussed previously, outpatient procedures, services, or items are recorded in the patient's medical record. Charges are posted through the chargemaster by the departments involved in the patient's care. The HIM Department receives the medical record after the patient is released to code procedures not posted through the chargemaster, to code the patient's diagnosis, and for APC assignment. The procedure and diagnosis code(s) are reported on the appropriate claim form. Figures 8-16, 8-17, and 8-18 illustrate coding systems and reporting on the claim form for the following outpatient services: an Emergency Department visit, ambulatory surgery visit, and a hospital-based primary care clinic visit.

Inpatient Services

Inpatient services are services provided to a patient who is admitted to the hospital for more than 24 hours. The patient is assigned a room/bed required for overnight accommodations. Procedures, services, and items provided during the inpatient stay are recorded in the patient's medical record. Inpatient services are reported on the UB-04 utilizing ICD-9-CM Volume III procedure codes.

Hospital facility charges for Emergency Department services.
Physician services are not billed by the hospital.

Form Locator 44

42 REV. CD.	43 DESCRIPTION	44 HCPCS/ RATES	45 SERV. DATE
0270	MEDICAL SURGICAL SUPPLIES AND DEVICES	A4306	11 27 2006
0450	EMERGENCY ROOM GENERAL	99281 25	11 27 2006
0450	EMERGENCY ROOM GENERAL	13121	11 27 2006

CMS-1450 (UB-04) Form Locator 67 A-Q

67 PRIN. DIAG. CD.	OTHER DIAG. CODES					
	67A CODE	B CODE	C CODE	D CODE	E CODE	F CODE
891.0						

Medical Record
Emergency Department Visit

Patient presents to the emergency department with a 4.5-cm laceration on the left leg. A Level II E/M performed. Debridement and complex repair of wound was done. Disposable drug delivery system, flow rate of 50 mL per hour was utilized.

Johnathan Sampson, M.D.

Procedure code assignments:
13121 "Repair, complex, legs 2.6 cm to 7.5 cm"
99282 "Emergency department visit", Level II
A4306 "Disposable drug delivery system, flow rate of 50 mL or less per hour"

Diagnosis code assignment:
891.0 "Open wound of leg without mention of complication"

Figure 8-16 Coding an Emergency Department visit for reporting on the CMS-1450 (UB-04).

Form Locator 44

42 REV. CD.	43 DESCRIPTION	44 HCPCS/ RATES	45 SERV. DATE
0293	MEDICAL/SURGICAL SUPPLIES GENERAL	E0110	07 27 2006
0490	AMBULATORY SURGICAL CARE GENERAL	27446	07 27 2006

CMS-1450 (UB-04) Form Locator 67 A-Q

67 PRIN. DIAG. CD.	OTHER DIAG. CODES					
	67A CODE	B CODE	C CODE	D CODE	E CODE	F CODE
733.49						

CMS-1450 (UB-04) Form Locator 74 A-E

74 PRINCIPAL PROCEDURE CODE	DATE	74 A-E OTHER PROCEDURE CODE	DATE
81.47	07 27 2006		
OTHER CODE			

ICD-9-CM Volume III codes are not required for Medicare ambulatory surgery claims, however, other payers may require a Volume III code.

Medical Record
Ambulatory Surgery

Mr. Smith underwent an arthroplasty of the knee, condyle and plateau; medial compartment due to asceptic necrosis of the bone.

The procedure was performed in the Ambulatory Surgery Suite. Patient tolerated procedure well. Discharge instructions indicate non weight bearing for six weeks. Patient was provided with a pair of crutches (adjustable with tips and handgrips).

Beatrice J. Peterson, M.D.

The ambulatory surgery charge is posted in Revenue Code category 0490. The crutches are reported in Revenue Code category 0270.

PROCEDURE AND DIAGNOSIS CODE ASSIGNMENT

HCPCS Level I CPT – Arthroplasty, knee condyle and plateau, medial or lateral compartment 27446
HCPCS Level II – Crutches, forearm adjustable complete with tips and handgrips E0110

Note: some payers may require ICD-9-CM Volume III Procedures reported on the CMS-1450
ICD-9-CM Volume III Procedure 81.47
"Other repair of joint, knee"
Diagnosis Code–Asceptic necrosis of bone, knee 733.49

Figure 8-17 Coding an ambulatory surgery visit for reporting on the CMS-1450 (UB-04).

CMS-1500 Block 21

21. Diagnosis or nature of illness or injury, (relate item

1. 041. 00 3. ___.___
2. ___.___ 4. ___.___

CMS-1500 Block 24

24. A		B	C	D		E
DATE(S) OF SERVICE From To MM DD YY	MM DD YY	Place of Service	Type of Service	PROCEDURES, SERVICES, OR SUPPLIES (Explain Unusual Circumstances) CPT/HCPCS	MODIFIER	DIAGNOSIS POINTER
1 06 09 06	06 09 06			99212		1
2 06 09 06	06 09 06			36415		
3 06 09 06	06 09 06			85025		

Medical Record

Established patient presents complaining of a sore throat for 4 days. Problem-focused evaluation and management service performed. An automated CBC performed with automated differential WBC count. Prescribed antibiotics. Will see patient in 10 days for a follow-up.

Diagnosis: Strep throat

Howard Fetterbeginn, M.D.

PROCEDURE AND DIAGNOSIS CODE ASSIGNMENT

Evaluation and Management HCPCS Level I CPT	**99212**
Venipuncture	**36415**
Complete Blood Count (CBC)	**85025**
Strep throat	**041.00**

Figure 8-18 Coding a hospital-based primary care visit for reporting on the CMS-1500.

BOX 8-20 ■ KEY POINTS

Inpatient Procedure Code Requirements

Inpatient Services

The patient is admitted with the expectation that he or she will be in the hospital for more than 24 hours (overnight). ICD-9-CM Volume III Procedure codes are required for reporting these services.

Note: Services, procedures, and items provided during an inpatient stay are posted through the chargemaster utilizing HCPCS codes.

ICD-9-CM Volume III Procedure Codes

ICD-9-CM Volume III procedure codes are utilized to code significant procedures performed during a hospital inpatient stay (see Table 8-2). The principal procedure is the significant procedure performed for definitive treatment of the principal diagnosis or the procedure that most closely relates to the principal diagnosis. Other significant procedures are also coded to explain the inpatient case further. Hospital inpatient services are submitted on the UB-04. ICD-9-CM Volume III procedure codes are reported in FL 74a–e on the claim form. The principal and other diagnosis are reported in FL 67, 69, 70, 72. It is important to remember that the payer will compare the principal and other procedures codes with the principal and other diagnosis codes to determine medical necessity (Figure 8-19).

Charges for services provided on an inpatient basis are posted through the chargemaster by the departments involved in the patient's care. Services and items listed in the chargemaster are associated with an HCPCS code. The inpatient claim is a summary claim that categorizes all charges in revenue code categories, and therefore HCPCS codes are not required on the claim form. After the patient is discharged, the medical record is forwarded to HIM for coding of diagnosis and other procedures not posted through the chargemaster and for MS-DRG assignment (see Figure 8-7).

Non-Patient Services

Non-patient services are those involving tests or procedures performed on a specimen when the patient is not present. Laboratory testing on a specimen sent to the hospital from the physician's office is an example of a non-patient service. Non-patient services are coded utilizing HCPCS Level I and Level II codes. Most hospital non-patient services are submitted utilizing the UB-04 (see Table 8-2). Department personnel post non-patient services through the chargemaster (Figure 8-20).

BOX 8-21 ■ KEY POINTS

Non-patient Procedure Code Requirements

Non-Patient Services

A specimen is received and processed and the patient is not present. HCPCS Level I CPT codes and HCPCS Level II Medicare National codes are required for reporting these services.

HCPCS LEVEL I—CURRENT PROCEDURAL TERMINOLOGY (CPT)

As outlined previously, HCPCS Level I CPT codes are utilized to code physician and outpatient services. Hospital services provided on an outpatient and non-patient basis are coded utilizing CPT codes. Procedures and services are also identified in the chargemaster and are associated with an HCPCS Level I CPT or Level II

Form Locator 44

42 REV. CD.	43 DESCRIPTION	44 HCPCS/ RATES	45 SERV. DATE	46 SERV. UNITS
0101	ALL INCL R & B	600.00		2
0481	CARDIAC CATH LAB			1
0620	MED SURG SUPPLIES			1
0730	EKG			

CMS-1450 (UB-04) Form Locator 67 A-Q, 69

67 PRIN. DIAG. CD.	OTHER DIAG. CODES				
	67A CODE	B CODE	C CODE	D-Q CODE	69 ADM. DIAG. CODES
427.9					786.50

CMS-1450 (UB-04) Form Locator 74 a-e

74 PRINCIPAL PROCEDURE CODE	DATE	74 A-E OTHER PROCEDURE CODE	DATE
37.21	05 16 06		
OTHER PROCEDURE CODE	DATE	OTHER PROCEDURE CODE	DATE

Medical Record
Inpatient Case

Patient JB was admitted to the hospital as he was experiencing severe chest pain. An EKG was performed, which showed arrhythmia. The patient underwent a right heart catheterization. Right heart cardiac catheterization showed no findings. One irrigation tray was used. The patient tolerated the procedure well. The patient was discharged two days later.

Dr. Howard Jones, M.D.

Charge Sheet–Charges posted through the chargemaster

REVENUE CODES/ DESCRIPTION		CHARGES	HCPCS CODE
0101	All inclusive Room & Board	1,200.00	
0730	EKG	95.00	93000
0481	Cardiac Cath Lab	4,733.00	93501
0620	Med Surg Supplies	124.00	A4320

HIM Coding Performed After Discharge

Admitting Diagnosis:	786.50	Chest Pain
Principal Diagnosis	427.9	Arrhythmia
Principal Procedure	37.21	Right Heart Catheterization

Figure 8-19 Coding an inpatient case for reporting on the CMS-1450 (UB-04).

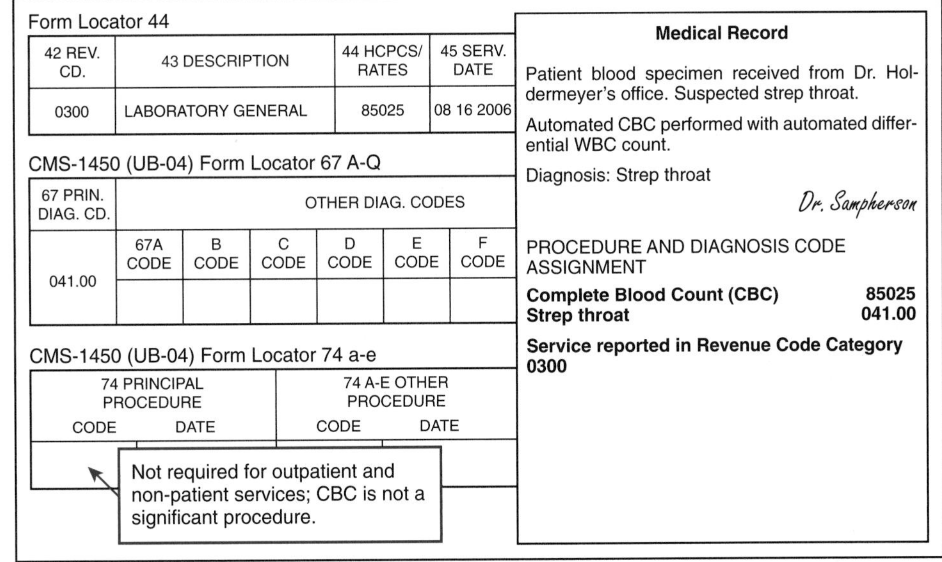

Form Locator 44

42 REV. CD.	43 DESCRIPTION	44 HCPCS/ RATES	45 SERV. DATE
0300	LABORATORY GENERAL	85025	08 16 2006

CMS-1450 (UB-04) Form Locator 67 A-Q

67 PRIN. DIAG. CD.	OTHER DIAG. CODES					
	67A CODE	B CODE	C CODE	D CODE	E CODE	F CODE
041.00						

CMS-1450 (UB-04) Form Locator 74 a-e

74 PRINCIPAL PROCEDURE CODE	DATE	74 A-E OTHER PROCEDURE CODE	DATE

Not required for outpatient and non-patient services; CBC is not a significant procedure.

Medical Record

Patient blood specimen received from Dr. Holdermeyer's office. Suspected strep throat.

Automated CBC performed with automated differential WBC count.

Diagnosis: Strep throat

Dr. Sampherson

PROCEDURE AND DIAGNOSIS CODE ASSIGNMENT

Complete Blood Count (CBC)	**85025**
Strep throat	**041.00**

Service reported in Revenue Code Category 0300

Figure 8-20 Coding a nonpatient case for reporting on the CMS-1450 (UB-04).

Medicare National code. A review of the content, format, and conventions of CPT will enhance our understanding of the coding system structure.

CPT Content

The CPT coding manual contains an introduction, six sections of codes with descriptions, appendices A–N, and an index (Figure 8-21).

Introduction

The introduction provides information about the content, format, and usage of the CPT coding manual. It outlines the section numbers, descriptions, and instructions for use. The instructions explain the format, terminology, and guidelines. It also contains information regarding conventions and code changes. The CPT coding system contains three categories of codes: Category I, Category II, and Category III codes.

TEST YOUR *Knowledge* BOX 8-3

PROCEDURE CODING SYSTEM VARIATIONS

1. Explain why procedure coding systems are utilized.

State what coding systems are used to report procedures, services, and items for the following service categories:

2. Hospital outpatient services.
3. Hospital ambulatory surgery.
4. Hospital inpatient services.

Explain what claim forms are used to submit charges for procedures, services, and items for the following service categories:

5. Hospital outpatient services.
6. Hospital ambulatory surgery.
7. Hospital inpatient services.

Describe each coding system and explain guidelines regarding when the system should be used:

8. HCPCS Level I CPT codes.
9. HCPCS Level II Medicare National codes.
10. ICD-9-CM Volume III procedure codes.

Category I Codes

CPT **Category I codes** describe services, procedures, and some items and they are listed in the Evaluation and Management, Anesthesia, Surgery, Radiology, Pathology/Laboratory and Medicine sections of CPT. Each section begins with guidelines that are specific to the section. The guidelines provide information regarding usage of the codes in the section, terminology, and instructions. The sections and code ranges are: Section I, Evaluation and Management (E/M) 99201 to 99499; Section II, Anesthesia 00100 to 01999; Section III, Surgery 10021 to 69990; Section IV, Radiology 70010 to 79999; Section V, Pathology and Laboratory 80047 to 89398; and Section VI, Medicine 90281 to 99607.

Category II Codes

CPT **Category II codes** are supplemental tracking codes developed for use in the measurement of performance

HCPCS LEVEL I CPT

Introduction

Category I Codes

Section I – Evaluation and Management	99201 - 99499
Section II – Anesthesia	00100 - 01999
Section III – Surgery	10021 - 69990
Section IV – Radiology	70010 - 79999
Section V – Patholgy and Laboratory	80048 - 89356
Section VI – Medicine	90281 - 99602
Category II Codes	0500F-4011F
Category III Codes	0003T-0088T

Appendices
- Appendix A – Modifiers
- Appendix B – Summary of Additions, Deletions, and Revisions
- Appendix C – Listing of Clinical Examples
- Appendix D – Summary of CPT Add-On codes
- Appendix E – Summary of CPT Codes Exempt from Modifier 51
- Appendix F – Summary of CPT Codes Exempt from Modifier 63
- Appendix G – Summary of CPT Codes That Include Conscious Sedation
- Appendix H – Alphabetic Index of Performance Measures by Clinical Condition or Topic
- Appendix I – Generic Testing Code Modifiers
- Appendix J – Electrodiagnostic Medicine Listing of Sensory, Motor and Mixed Nerves
- Appendix K – Product Pending FDA Approval
- Appendix L – Vascular Families
- Appendix M – Summary Crosswalked Deleted Codes
- Appendix N – Summary Resequenced CPT Codes

Index

Figure 8-21 HCPCS Level I CPT manual content. *(Data from AMA:* CPT 2010 professional edition, *Chicago, 2010, American Medical Association.)*

and they are listed after the Medicine section in the CPT manual. Category II codes reduce the administrative burden of performance measurement by minimizing the need for chart reviews. The codes are also intended to enhance data collection regarding quality of care by coding certain services and/or test results that support performance measures. The AMA outlines the following points regarding Category II codes:
- Use of Category II codes is optional.
- Category II codes are four numeric numbers followed by an alphabetic character such as 0012F.
- Some of the Category II codes may relate to compliance by the health care professional with state or federal law.
- Category II codes do not have a relative value associated with them, since the codes describe components that are typically included in an E/M service or test results that are part of the laboratory test or procedure. Code 2000F "Blood pressure, measured" is an example of a Category II code.
- These codes are released twice a year.

Category III Codes

CPT **Category III codes** are temporary codes used to describe emerging technologies, services, or procedures and they are listed after the Medicine section in the CPT manual. Historically, an unlisted code with an

CPT Category I Code Unlisted Procedure
Provides no detail regarding the procedure

37799 Unlisted procedure, vascular surgery

➲ *CPT Assistant Spring* 93:12, Fall 93:3, Feb 97:10, Sep 97:10, May 01:11

CPT Category III Code
Provides more detail regarding the emerging technology, service, or procedure

0051T Implantation of total replacement heart system (artificial heart) with recipient cardiectomy

Figure 8-22 HCPCS Level I CPT Category III code versus an unlisted code for vascular surgery. *(Data from AMA:* CPT 2006 professional edition, *Chicago, 2010, American Medical Association.)*

unspecified description from Category I would be used to describe a new procedure. Unlisted procedure codes are found in each section of the CPT manual, such as 37799 "Unlisted procedure, vascular surgery." Unlisted procedure codes from Category I provide no detail regarding the procedure and therefore a chart review is generally required. Category III codes address this problem as they describe new procedures. The category III code that would be used in place of 37799 is 0051T, which describes "Implantation of total replacement heart system (artificial heart) with recipient cardiectomy" (Figure 8-22). The AMA outlines the following points regarding Category III codes:
- Category III codes are four numeric numbers followed by an alphabetic character such as 0016T.
- Category III codes must be used instead of the Category I unlisted codes.
- Category III codes allow data collection for emerging technology, services, and procedures, which is critical for evaluating health care services and the development of public health policy.
- These codes may eventually receive a Category I CPT code.
- New Category III codes are released semi-annually.

BOX 8-22 ■ KEY POINTS

CPT Category Code Sections

Category I codes	
Section I: Evaluation and Management (E/M)	99201-99499
Section II: Anesthesia	00100-01999
Section III: Surgery	10021-69990
Section IV: Radiology	70010-79999
Section V: Pathology and Laboratory	80047-89398
Section VI: Medicine	90281-99607
Category II codes	0001F-7025F
Category III codes	0016T-0207T

Appendices

CPT contains information in various appendices to provide assistance with code selection, the update of internal systems, and modifier usage: A complete list is illustrated in Figure 8-21.

Index

The alphabetical index is generally in the last part of the CPT manual along with instructions on how to use the index. The index is an alphabetical list of main terms and subterms that represent services and procedures. Next to the main term and subterm are codes to review in the code section prior to selecting a code. The index is used to identify possible codes that describe the procedure or service recorded in the patient's record. Accurate code selection requires that all possible codes identified in the index be reviewed in the code section.

CPT Conventions and Format

Conventions are special terms, punctuation marks, abbreviations, or symbols used as shorthand in a coding system to efficiently communicate special instructions to the coder. It is critical for coding and billing professionals to understand what each of the following conventions is communicating to the coder, as illustrated in (Table 8-3).

CPT Conventions

Conventions included in the CPT coding system are semicolon, plus sign, modifier 51 exempt, bullet, revised code symbol, new or revised text symbols, conscious sedation, and the reference symbol.

- **Semicolon ;.** The semicolon is used in code descriptions to save space. It tells the coder that part of the description for the indented code is found in the description of the main code. All information to the left of the semicolon in the main code is part of the description for each of the indented codes below.
- **Plus Sign +.** The plus sign is used in code sections to tell the coder the procedure is considered an add-on procedure. Add-on procedures are those that are performed in addition to another procedure. Codes with the plus sign also indicate that a modifier 51 is not required for that code when reported with another procedure. This symbol has been deleted.
- **Modifier 51 Exempt ⃠.** The modifier 51 exempt symbol is used to tell the coder that the code does not require a modifier 51 when reported with another procedure. Modifier 51 is used to indicate multiple procedures performed at the same session by the same physician.
- **Bullet •.** The bullet is listed to the left a procedure code to indicate that the code is new for the current year. The first time a new code is published it will be designated with bullet.
- **Revised code symbol ▲.** The revised code symbol is found to the left of a procedure code to indicate that the procedure description has been altered substantially.
- **New or revised text symbols ▶ ◀.** The new or revised text symbols are placed around text that has been changed or added.

TABLE 8-3 HCPCS Level I: CPT Coding Conventions

Convention/Symbol	Coder's Notes
; Semicolon	Refer to the main code and include all of the description to the left of the semicolon in the description for each indented code.
⃠ Modifier 51 except	Procedures with this symbol do not require a modifier 51 when reported with another procedure. Appendix E lists all the codes that are modifier –51 exempt.
• Bullet	Helps you to identify codes that are new for the current year. Appendix B provides a summary of Additions, Deletions, and Revisions.
▲ Revised code	This symbol helps you to identify procedure descriptions that have been altered substantially, in the current year. Appendix B provides a summary of Additions, Deletions, and Revisions.
▶ ◀ New or revised text	Highlights text that has changed or has been added. Appendix B provides a summary of Additions, Deletions, and Revisions.
⊙ Conscious sedation	Conscious sedation is included in the procedure that has this symbol; do not code conscious sedation separately. Appendix G provides a list of codes that include conscious sedation.
➲ Reference	Refer to the reference (AMA's CPT Assistant newsletter or CPT Changes "An Insider's View) to gain an understanding of information regarding a particular code and its usage.

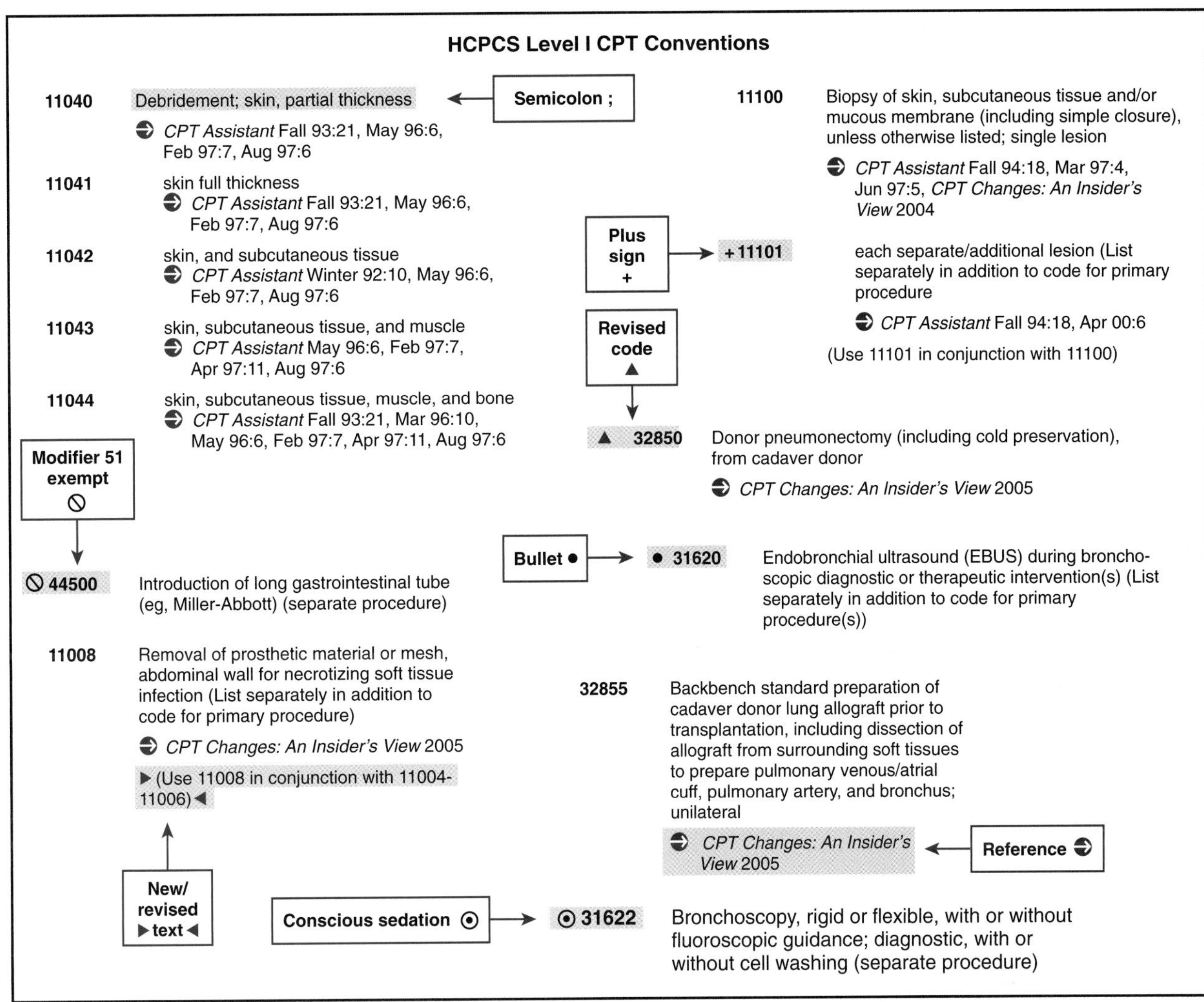

Figure 8-23 HCPCS Level I CPT coding conventions as displayed in the CPT manual. *(Data from AMA:* CPT professional edition, *Chicago, 2010, American Medical Association.)*

- **Conscious sedation ⊙.** The conscious sedation symbol is placed to the left of a CPT code to indicate that conscious sedation is included.
- **Reference symbol ➲.** The reference symbol is placed below a code description to provide the coder with a reference to the AMA's *CPT Assistant* newsletter or *CPT Changes: An Insider's View.* These publications contain material that provides explanations and information regarding a particular code and its usage.

Figure 8-23 illustrates examples of each the conventions as they are displayed in the CPT coding manual.

> **BOX 8-23 ■ KEY POINTS**
>
> **Conventions Defined**
>
> Special terms, punctuation marks, abbreviations, or symbols used as shorthand in a coding system to communicate special instructions to the coder efficiently.

The CPT code section and index format are designed utilizing various conventions to present procedures, services, and code descriptions in a manner that is easily recognized. The code section and index formatting conventions are illustrated in Tables 8-4 and 8-5.

> **BOX 8-24 ■ KEY POINTS**
>
> **HCPCS Level I CPT Conventions**
>
> Semicolon ;
> Modifier 51 exempt ⃠
> Bullet •
> Revised code symbol ▲
> New or revised text symbol ▶ ◀
> Conscious sedation ⊙
> Reference symbol ➲

TABLE 8-4 CPT Code Section Format

Convention	Surgery Section Outline	Evaluation and Management Section Outline
Section	Surgery	Evaluation and management (E/M)
Category	**Respiratory Systems**	**Office and Other Outpatient Services**
Subcategory	Nose	
Heading	Excision	New patient
Code and description	30100 Biopsy, intranasal	99201 Office and other outpatient visit
Notes	(For biopsy skin of nose, see 11100, 11101)	Counseling and/or coordination of care with other providers or agencies are provided.

Data from AMA: CPT professional edition, *Chicago, 2010, American Medical Association.*

TABLE 8-5 CPT Index Section Format

Convention	Index Outline	
	A	
Main term	A Vitamin	
Cross reference	See Vitamin, A	
	Abbe-Estlander Procedure	
	See Reconstruction; Repair, Cleft Lip	
Main term	Abdomen	
Subterm	Abdominal Wall	
Subterm of *Abdominal Wall*	Repair	
Subterm of *Repair*	Hernia	49491–49496, 49501,49507, 49521, 49590
Subterm of *Abdominal Wall*	Tumor	
Subterm of *Tumor*	Excision	22900
	Unlisted Services and Procedures	22999

Data from HCPCS 2010: level II national codes, *U.S. Department of Health and Human Services, Centers for Medicare and Medicaid Services.*
Possible codes to look up in the tabular list (code section) are listed to the right of the main term or subterm.

CPT Code Section Format

The CPT code section format is designed to assist the coder with the selection of codes that describe procedures. CPT code sections present code descriptions using the following formatting conventions:

- **Section.** CPT codes are divided into sections, and section descriptions are listed at the top of each page. The six sections are Evaluation and Management (E/M), Anesthesia, Surgery, Radiology, Pathology/Laboratory, and Medicine.
- **Category/Subcategory.** Codes within each section are further categorized based on type of service, site of service, or anatomical area of the procedure. For example, Office and Other Outpatient Services is a category under the E/M section. Respiratory System is a category under the Surgery section. Nose is a subcategory under Respiratory System section.
- **Headings.** Within each code range headings are used to list the subdivisions of codes under the categories and subcategories. For example, New Patient is a heading listed under the subcategory Office and Other Outpatient Services in the E/M section.
- **Codes and Description.** Codes are listed with descriptions under each heading in the section.
- **Notes.** Notes are provided where further clarification or information is given.

TEST YOUR *Knowledge* BOX 8-4

PROCEDURE CODING SYSTEM VARIATIONS; HCPCS LEVEL I CURRENT PROCEDURAL TERMINOLOGY (CPT)

Identify the HCPCS Level I CPT category of codes that matches each of the following descriptions. Provide an example of the code.

1. ____________________ codes are found in the Evaluation and Management, Anesthesia, Surgery, Radiology, Pathology/Laboratory, and Medicine sections. An example of this code is ____________________.

2. ____________________ codes are found after the Medicine section and they are supplemental tracking codes for performance measurement. An example of this code is ____________________.

3. ____________________ codes are found after the Medicine section and they represent new procedures or services or emerging technology. An example of this code is ____________________.

4. Explain the purpose of HCPCS Level I CPT conventions.

5. Discuss the purpose of modifier 51 exempt.

Provide the convention or symbol for each of the following descriptions:

6. Tells the coder a modifier 51 is not required.

7. Represents a procedure that is considered an add-on.

8. Indicates that the procedure code description has been revised substantially.

9. Used to advise the coder that part of the description on indented codes can be found in the main code description.

10. New codes are identified with this symbol.

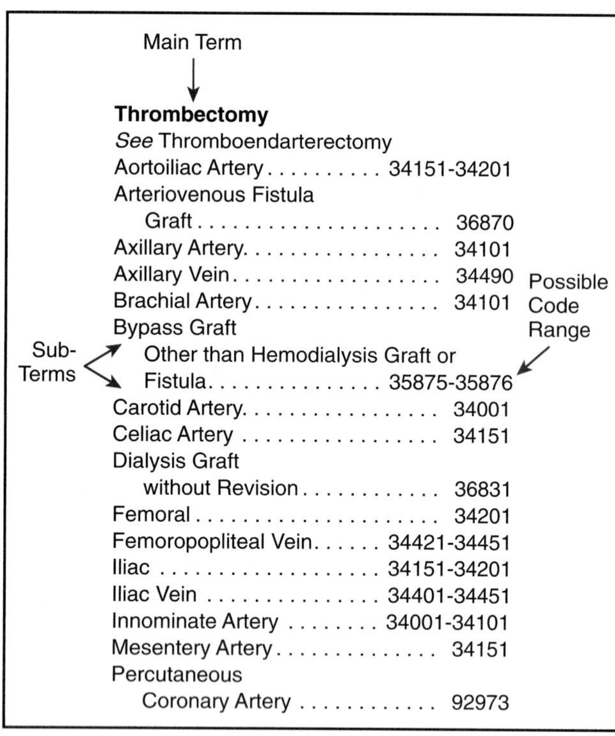
Main Term

Thrombectomy
See Thromboendarterectomy
Aortoiliac Artery 34151-34201
Arteriovenous Fistula
  Graft 36870
Axillary Artery 34101
Axillary Vein 34490
Brachial Artery 34101
Bypass Graft
  Other than Hemodialysis Graft or
  Fistula 35875-35876
Carotid Artery 34001
Celiac Artery 34151
Dialysis Graft
  without Revision 36831
Femoral 34201
Femoropopliteal Vein 34421-34451
Iliac 34151-34201
Iliac Vein 34401-34451
Innominate Artery 34001-34101
Mesentery Artery 34151
Percutaneous
  Coronary Artery 92973

Sub-Terms

Possible Code Range

Figure 8-24 HCPCS Level I CPT index entries illustrating main terms and subterms. *(Data from AMA:* CPT 2006 professional edition, *Chicago, 2010, American Medical Association.)*

CPT Index Format

The CPT index format is designed to assist the coder in finding possible codes to be reviewed and selected from the appropriate code section(s). The index is an alphabetical listing of procedures and services broken down into main terms and subterms (Figure 8-24).

- **Main Terms** are bolded terms listed at the margin in the index that represent procedures and services.
- **Subterms** are terms indented under the main term to further define procedures and services in the index.

Cross-references are used to provide the coder with additional terms to be used to look up a procedure or service. Possible codes to review in the code section are to the right of the main terms and subterms.

HCPCS LEVEL II—MEDICARE NATIONAL CODES

HCPCS Level II Medicare National codes are utilized by hospitals and other providers when a code that adequately describes the procedure, service, or item cannot be found in the CPT manual or when the payer requires a Level II code as opposed to a Level I code. Hospital services provided on an outpatient and non-patient basis are coded utilizing HCPCS Level I or Level II codes. Procedures, services, and items listed in the hospital chargemaster are associated with an HCPCS code. A review of the content, format, and conventions of HCPCS Level II will enhance our understanding of the coding system.

HCPCS LEVEL II
Medical National Code Manual Content

Introduction

Level II Modifiers

Procedure Coding System
  Code Sections — A0000-V5364
Table of Drugs

Index

Appendices
  Appendix A-Select Internet Only Manuals (IOM)

Updates
  New/Revised/Deleted Codes and Modifiers
  Administrative, Payment, and Miscellaneous Changes

Figure 8-25 HCPCS Level II Medicare National code manual content. *(Data from* HCPCS 2010: level II national codes, *U.S. Department of Health and Human Services, Centers for Medicare and Medicaid Services.)*

HCPCS Level II Content

The HCPCS Level II Medicare National coding system contains an introduction, index, table of drugs, and code sections with descriptions. These codes are utilized to report supplies, equipment, medications, and services to various payers. It is important to remember that the Level II codes are printed by various publishers, and therefore the content and conventions may vary by publisher (Figure 8-25).

Introduction

The introduction section of the HCPCS Level II manual provides information regarding the content and usage of the manual. It explains the effective date of codes, code sections, organization, and how to use the manual. It is important to review the introduction section of any coding manual to gain an understanding of the content, format, conventions, and how to use the manual.

Index

The index is an alphabetical list of procedures, services, equipment, medications, and other items. The index is used to locate possible codes that describe procedures, services, and items recorded in the patient's record. Codes found in the index must be reviewed in the code section for the purpose of assigning the code that most accurately describes the procedure, service, or item.

TABLE 8-6 HCPCS Level II Medicare National Codes Table of Drugs

Drug Name	Route of Administration	Unit/Dose	Code
A-HYDROCORT	IV, IM, SC	50 mg	J1710
A-METHAPRED	IM, IV	125 mg	J2930
ABBOKINASE	IV	5,000 IU vial	J3364
ABBOK1NASE, OPEN CATH	IV	250,000 IU vial	J3365
ACETAZOLAMIDE SODIUM	IM, IV	500 mg	J1120
ACETYLCYSTEINE, UNIT DOSE	INH	1 g	J7608
ACOVA	IV	5 mg	C9121
ACTH	IV, IM, SC	40 units	J0800
ACTHREL	IV	1 dose	Q2004
ACYCLOVIR SODIUM INJECTION	IV	50 mg	S0071

Data from HCPCS 2010: level II national codes, *U.S. Department of Health and Human Services, Centers for Medicare and Medicaid Services.*

Table of Drugs

Drugs may be found in the index; however, the HCPCS Level II manual contains a table of drugs, which includes a more comprehensive drug listing and possible codes to be reviewed in the code section. The table of drugs provides four columns indicating the drug name, route of administration, unit/dose, and code, as illustrated in Table 8-6. The table lists drugs by generic and trade name.

- **Drug Name.** The first column is an alphabetical listing of drug names by their generic or trade name.
- **Route of Administration.** The second column lists various routes of administration for the drug such as intramuscular, intravenous, or oral (Figure 8-26).
- **Unit/Dose.** The third column indicates the unit or dosage of a drug.
- **Code.** The last column lists possible codes to review in the J code section.

IA	Intraarterial administration
IM	Intramuscular administration
INH	Administration by inhaled solution
IT	Intrathecal
IV	Intravenous administration
OTH	Other routes of administration
ORAL	Orally administered
SC	Subcutaneous administration
VAR	Administered through various routes

Figure 8-26 HCPCS Level II routes of administration of drugs. *(Data from HCPCS 2010: level II national codes, U.S. Department of Health and Human Services, Centers for Medicare and Medicaid Services.)*

Code Sections

HCPCS Level II Medicare National codes are five alphanumeric characters. The first character is alphabetic, followed by four numeric characters. Procedures, services, and items are classified within the coding system by the first alphabetic character, such as A codes, B codes, and C codes, as outlined in Table 8-7.

Appendices

The HCPCS Level II manual contains appendices that include various information regarding codes and code selection. The number and content of appendices may vary based on the publisher. Some publishers number their appendices 1, 2, and 3, and others may label them A, B, and C. For example, two appendices listed in the *Saunders 2010 ICD-9-CM and HCPCS Level II* manual are Appendix A contains information from publication 100–internet-only manual.

Other publishers may list other appendices covering topics such as Modifiers, Abbreviations, and Acronyms, Table of Drugs, Medicare References, Companies Accepting HCPCS Level II Codes, HCPCS Codes for Which CPT Codes Should Be Reported, and New, Changed, and Deleted HCPCS Codes for the current year.

TABLE 8-7 **HCPCS Level II Medicare Code Sections**

Category	Description	Code Range
A Codes	Transportation codes	A0021-A0999
	Medical and surgical supplies	A4206-A9000
	Administrative, miscellaneous, and investigational services	A9150-A9999
B Codes	Enteral and parenteral therapy	B4034-B9999
C Codes	Temporary codes for use with CMS hospital outpatient payment system	C1000-C9999
D Codes	Dental procedures	D0120-D9999
E Codes	Durable medical equipment	E0100-E9999
G Codes	Procedures/professional services (temporary)	G0001-G9999
H Codes	Behavioral health and/or substance abuse treatment	H0001-H9999
J Codes	Drugs	J0100-J9999
K Codes	Temporary codes assigned to durable medical equipment regional carriers (DMERC)	K0001-K9999
L Codes	Orthotic procedures	L0100-L4999
	Prosthetic procedures	L5000-L9999
M Codes	Medical services	M0064-M0302
P Codes	Pathology and laboratory services	P2028-P9615
Q Codes	Procedures, services, and supplies on a temporary basis	Q0034-Q9967
R Codes	Diagnostic radiology services	R0070-R0076
S Codes	Temporary national codes (non-Medicare)	S0009-S9999
T Codes	Temporary national codes established for state Medicaid agencies	T1000-T9999
V Codes	Vision services	V0000-V2999
	Hearing, which also includes speech-language pathology services	

Data from HCPCS 2010: level II national codes, *U.S. Department of Health and Human Services, Centers for Medicare and Medicaid Services.*

BOX 8-25 ■ KEY POINTS

HCPCS Level II Medicare National Code Manual Content

Introduction
Modifiers
Code Sections
  A0000-V5364
Table of Drugs
Index
Appendices
Updates

HCPCS Level II Conventions and Format

HCPCS Level II conventions and format vary by publisher. Some include symbols to identify specific coding issues, and others may include symbols and/or color coding.

HCPCS Level II Conventions Variations

Common conventions outlined in HCPCS Level II coding manuals include symbols indicating new and revised codes, special coverage instructions, and designations indicating gender or age-specific procedures, quantity alerts and ASC groupings and status indicators. Table 8-8 highlights some of the common coding conventions used by various publishers. The symbols and abbreviations utilized to identify these conventions vary by publisher.

TABLE 8-8 **HCPCS Level II Medicare National Code Convention Variations**

Symbol	Convention/Description and Meaning
• or ▶	**New code symbol** indicates that the code designated with this symbol is new to the Level II manual for the current year.
▲ or ⇒	**Revised code symbol** tells the coder the code description has been revised.
✪	**Special coverage instructions designations** are used to identify codes that have special coverage instructions.
Color coded box	
CIM	
◆	**Not covered by or valid for Medicare designations** identifies codes that are not covered or valid for Medicare
Color coded box	
MCM	
*	**Carrier discretion designations** advise the coder that the carrier has discretion on payment determinations. The carrier should be contacted for clarification.
♀	**Gender-specific** symbols are used by publishers to tell coders that the code is gender specific for female.
♂	**Male only symbols** tell coders that the code is gender specific for male
☑	**Quantity alert symbols** advise coders to check the quantity indicated to ensure that the quantity reported is accurate.
❶ indicates group number	**ASC groupings** designate codes that are payable under ambulatory surgery groupings.
Box with various letters to indicate the status	**APC status indicators** identify codes that may or may not be paid under the Outpatient Prospective Payment System (Ambulatory Payment Classifications).
A	
P Pediatric	**Age designations** are used to indicate that the code may be considered inappropriate for specific age categories.
A Adult	
M Maternity	

Data from HCPCS 2010: level II national codes, *U.S. Department of Health and Human Services, Centers for Medicare and Medicaid Services.*

BOX 8-26 ■ KEY POINTS

HCPCS Level II Convention Variations

Conventions

New code symbol
Revised code symbol
Special coverage instructions
Not covered by or valid for Medicare designation
Carrier discretion
Gender-specific symbols
Quantity alert symbol
ASC groupings
ASC status indicators
Age designation

Note: The symbols and abbreviations utilized to identify these conventions vary by publisher.

HCPCS Level II Index Format

The HCPCS Level II index format is designed to assist the coder in finding possible codes to be reviewed and selected from the appropriate code section (Figure 8-27). The index is an alphabetical listing of procedures and services categorized by main terms and subterms.

- **Main Terms** are listed in bold print at the margin and they represent procedures, services, items, drugs, or equipment.
- **Subterms** are indented under the main term and they further define the procedure, service, or item described by the main term.

Cross-references are listed to provide the coder with additional terms to be used to look up the item or procedure. Possible codes to review are in the code section to the right of the main term and subterm.

HCPCS

A

Figure 8-27 HCPCS LEVEL II manual index format. *(Data from* HCPCS 2010: level II national codes, *U.S. Department of Health and Human Services, Centers for Medicare and Medicaid Services.)*

TABLE 8-9 HCPCS Level II Medicare National Code Tabular List Code Section Format

Convention	A Code Section Outline	M Code Section Outline
Section	MEDICAL SURGICAL SUPPLIES	MEDICAL SERVICES
Category	MISCELLANEOUS SUPPLIES	OTHER MEDICAL SERVICES
Code and description	A4206 Syringe with needle, sterile 1 cc, each	M0076 Cellular therapy
Notes	This code specifies a 1-cc syringe but is also used to report $^{3}/_{10}$ cc or $^{1}/_{2}$ cc syringes	The therapeutic efficacy of injecting foreign proteins has not been established.

Data from HCPCS 2010: level II national codes, *U.S. Department of Health and Human Services, Centers for Medicare and Medicaid Services.*

TABLE 8-10 HCPCS Level II Medicare National Code Tabular List Code Section Format

Convention	Index Outline
Main term	Abbokinase J3364, J3365 Abscess, incision and drainage D7510-D7520 Abdomen/abdominal
Subterm	dressing holder/binder A4462 pad, low profile L1270 Abdominal binder elastic A4462 Accessories ambulation devices E0153-E0159 artificial kidney and machine
Cross reference	(see also ESRD) E1510-E1699

Data from HCPCS 2010: level II national codes, *U.S. Department of Health and Human Services, Centers for Medicare and Medicaid Services.*
Possible codes to look up in tabular list code section are listed to the right of the main term or subterm.

HCPCS Level II Code Section Format

The HCPCS Level II code section is a numerical listing of codes and descriptions for items and services broken down by section and category. Each section begins with a letter, for example, A codes, B codes, and J codes. Within each section, codes are further categorized. Notes provide additional information for further clarification. HCPCS Level II formatting of the code sections and the index are illustrated in Tables 8-9 and 8-10.

- **Section.** Level II codes are divided into sections based on the type of service or item. The section description is listed on the top of each page to tell the coder what section of the HCPCS Level II manual they are in. There are 17 sections, each having a letter designation such as A codes for transportation, medical and surgical supplies, and administrative, miscellaneous, and investigation services.

TEST YOUR *Knowledge* BOX 8-5

HCPCS LEVEL II; MEDICARE NATIONAL CODES

1. Explain why HCPCS Level II codes were developed.

2. Explain how a coder determines whether to use an HCPCS Level I CPT or HCPCS Level II code.

3. The HCPCS level II coding system contains a(n) ___________, ___________, ___________, and ___________ ___________ with descriptions.

4. State the purpose of the table of drugs in the HCPCS Level II manual.

5. Provide a description of HCPCS Level II codes.

6. ___________ and other ___________ are found in HCPCS Level II code sections to communicate instructions and other information to the coder regarding the code listing.

7. ___________ ___________ found in the HCPCS Level II index are bolded and they represent services, procedures, and various items.

8. Discuss how services, procedures, and items are categorized in the HCPCS Level II coding manual.

Review the conventions in your HCPCS Level II manual and answer the following questions.

9. The symbol that designates a new code is the ___________.

10. The symbol that tells the coder that the terminology or rules of the code have been revised is the ___________.

- **Category.** Within each section, codes are divided by categories that further describe the services or items. For example, miscellaneous supplies are a category in Section A of the coding manual.
- **Code and Description.** Codes and their descriptions are listed under each heading within a section. For example, A4206 "Syringe with needle, sterile 1 cc or less each" is a code listed under miscellaneous supplies with the description of that code.
- **Notes.** Notes are utilized to provide the coder with instruction and clarification regarding the code. The note under A4210 refers you to "IOM: 100-03, 4, 280.1", in Appendix A.

ICD-9-CM VOLUME III PROCEDURES

ICD-9-CM Volume III procedure codes are utilized by hospitals and other facilities to report significant procedures or services performed during an inpatient stay, as discussed previously. Some payers may also require Volume III codes on ambulatory surgery claims. Vol-ume III procedure codes are reported on the UB-04 in the

ICD-9-CM

Volume III
(for hospitals and other facilities)
Content

Introduction

Alphabetic Index
Alphabetical listing of procedures and services

Tabular List of Procedures
Numerical listing of procedures and services

Figure 8-28 ICD-9-CM Volume III manual content and format. *(Data from* International classification of diseases, 9th revision, *U.S. Department of Health and Human Services, Public Health Service, Centers for Medicare and Medicaid Services.)*

FL 74a–e. The ICD-9-CM content, format, and conventions were reviewed in the previous chapter on ICD-9-CM diagnosis coding. This section will highlight conventions that are consistent through all three volumes and provide a review of conventions and format specific to Volume III.

Content and Format of ICD-9-CM Volume III

ICD-9-CM Volume III contains an alphabetical index of procedures and services and a tabular listing of procedures and services (Figure 8-28). The **tabular list** is a numerical listing.

Introduction

The introductory information for Volume III is in the front of the ICD-9-CM manual. It provides information regarding how to use Volume III, conventions, and coding guidelines. ICD-9-CM manuals vary by publisher; therefore it is critical to review the introductory section of the manual to gain an understanding of how to use the manual.

Tabular (Numeric) List

ICD-9-CM Volume III procedures and services are listed numerically in the tabular list. The tabular list of procedures and services consists of 17 chapters that list procedures and services based on body systems, as outlined in Figure 8-29.

Volume III codes are two to four digits. The two-digit level defines the type of procedure and/or body area, for example, code 01 describes "Incision and Excision of Skull, brain. . . . . ." The two-digit category code is followed by a decimal and one or two more digits. The third- and fourth-digit levels provide more detail regarding the procedure. The third and fourth digits differentiate between unilateral or bilateral procedures, surgical approach or technique, or by condition types such as indirect versus direct hernia. The format of the Volume III tabular list of procedures and services is illustrated in Tables 8-11 and 8-12.

ICD-9-CM Volume III

Chapter	Procedure/System	Code Range
00	Procedures and interventions, Not elsewhere classifiable	00 – 00.9
01	Nervous	01 – 05
02	Endocrine	06 – 07
03	Eye	08 – 16
04	Ear	18 – 20
05	Nose, Mouth, and Pharynx	21 – 29
06	Respiratory	30 – 34
07	Cardiovascular	35 – 39
08	Hemic and Lymphatic	40 – 41
09	Digestive	42 – 54
10	Urinary	55 – 59
11	Male Genital	60 – 64
12	Female Genital	65 – 71
13	Obstetrical Procedures	72 – 75
14	Musculoskeletal	76 – 84
15	Integumentary	85 – 86
16	Miscellaneous Diagnostic/ Therapeutic Procedures	87 – 99

Figure 8-29 ICD-9-CM Volume III chapters. *(Data from* International classification of diseases, 9th revision, *U.S. Department of Health and Human Services, Public Health Service, Centers for Medicare and Medicaid Services.)*

TABLE 8-11 ICD-9-CM Volume III Tabular List

Convention	Tabular List Outline
Chapter	1. Operation on the Nervous System (01-05)
Category (two digits) (code and description)	01 Incision and excision of skull, brain . . .
One or two digits beyond decimal point to differentiate between: Unilateral or bilateral Surgical approach or technique Condition types (indirect vs. direct hernia)	01.0 Cranial puncture 01.01 Cisternal Puncture

Data from International classification of diseases, 9th revision, *U.S. Department of Health and Human Services, Public Health Service, Centers for Medicare and Medicaid Services.*

Index Format

The index is an alphabetical listing of procedures or services that is designed to assist the coder in finding possible codes to be reviewed and selected from the tabular listing of codes and descriptions. The index outlines procedures by main terms and subterms.

TABLE 8-12 ICD-9-CM Volume III Alphabetic Index

Convention	Index Outline
Main term	Abbe Operation
Subterm	construction of vagina 70.61 intestinal anastomosis
Cross reference	see Anastomosis, intestine
Possible codes to look up in tabular list code section are listed to the right the main term or subterm	**Abciximab, infusion** 99.20 **Abdominouterotomy** 68.0 obstetrical 74.99 **Abduction, arytenoids** 31.69 **Ablation** biliary track (lesion) by ERCP 51.64 endometrial (hysteroscopic) 68.28

Data from International classification of diseases, 9th revision, *U.S. Department of Health and Human Services, Public Health Service, Centers for Medicare and Medicaid Services.*

- **Main Terms** are listed in bold print at the margin in the index and they represent procedures and services.
- **Subterms** are indented under the main term to further define a procedure or service described by the main term.

The index is used to identify possible codes to review in the tabular list and they are listed to the right of the main terms and subterms. The format of the alphabetical index of procedures is illustrated in Table 8-12.

BOX 8-27 ■ KEY POINTS

ICD-9-CM Volume III Manual Content

Introduction
Tabular List of Procedures
Alphabetic Index of Procedures

ICD-9-CM Volume III Official Conventions

Conventions are used in all coding systems and they consist of special terms, punctuation marks, abbreviations, or symbols used to provide the coder with instructions. To code effectively, using any coding system, it is necessary to gain an understanding of the conventions used.

ICD-9-CM Volume III Official Abbreviations and Symbols

The ICD-9-CM Official Conventions are published by the Department of Health and Human Services (DHHS), as discussed in the diagnosis coding chapter. Official conventions utilized in ICD-9-CM Volume III include NEC, NOS, brackets, slanted brackets, parentheses, colon, and brace as outlined in Table 8-13.

- **NEC.** Not elsewhere classifiable is used in the index to identify codes that are used when no other specific code for the procedure exists in the ICD-9-CM coding system. The coder may look in the patient's record to identify other main terms and related information that may be available for use in selecting a more specific code.
- **NOS.** Not otherwise specified is used in the tabular list to tell the coder the code is not specific, similar to unspecified. The coder should review the patient's record and check with the provider to identify related information that may be available for use in selecting a more specific code.
- **Brackets [ ].** Brackets are found in the tabular list and they enclose additional information about the code such as acronyms and synonyms, alternative terminology, or explanatory phrases. The coder can use the information enclosed in the brackets to understand the code further.
- **Slanted Brackets *[ ]*.** Slanted brackets provide the coder with information about using multiple codes. The brackets are found in the alphabetic index and they indicate codes that should be reported together to provide a complete picture of the procedures performed.
- **Parentheses ( ).** Parentheses are found in the tabular list and the alphabetic index. They are used to provide the coder with more information about the procedure, such as modifying terms, that help the coder understand what is in the code range.
- **Colon :.** A colon is placed after a description or term in the tabulator list to tell the coder there is more information listed, such as modifying terms, to help the coder understand the code range.

Figure 8-30 illustrates examples of each the conventions listed above as they are displayed in the ICD-9-CM coding manual.

ICD-9-CM Official Instructional Notes

Official Instructional Notes utilized in ICD-9-CM Volume III include: includes, excludes, code also synchronous procedure, and, with, omit code, and see also as outlined in Table 8-13:

- **Includes.** The includes statement is used in the tabular list to highlight procedures that are included in the code range.
- **Excludes.** The excludes statement is used in the tabular list to inform the coder about procedures that are not described in a code range. This statement includes alternative code ranges to review for code assignment.

TABLE 8-13 ICD-9-CM Official Abbreviations and Symbols

Convention/Symbols	Coder's Notes
NEC	**Not elsewhere classifiable.** Codes with this symbol are used when no other specific code for the procedure/condition exists in the ***ICD-9-CM coding manual***. Check the medical record to see if there is additional information available to assign a more specific code.
NOS	**Not otherwise specified.** This symbol tells the coder the code is not specific, similar to unspecified. Check the medical record ***documentation*** to see if there is additional information available to assign a more specific code.
[ ]	**Brackets.** Terms enclosed in brackets are non-essential modifying terms, therefore, the terms do not need to be in the medical record. These terms are given to provide additional information about the code such as acronyms and synonyms, alternative terminology or explanatory phases. The information enclosed does ***not change the code or intent of the code***.
[ ]	**Slanted Brackets.** When brackets are found in the index the coder can ***identify multiple codes*** that should be reported together to provide a complete picture of the procedure/condition. Be sure to check the record to make sure the procedures are documented.
( )	**Parentheses.** Terms enclosed in parentheses are ***non-essential modifying terms***, therefore, the terms do not need to be in the medical record. These terms are given to provide the coder with more information about the procedure/condition and/or code.
:	**Colon.** The colon helps the coder to recognize when there is ***more information*** listed such as modifying terms to help the coder understand the code range.
OFFICIAL INSTRUCTIONAL NOTES	
Conventions/Symbols	**Coder's Notes**
Includes	Includes notes are listed at the category level of a range. The note helps the coder to understand what kind of ***procedures or conditions are included*** in the code range.
Excludes	Excludes notes are listed at the category level of a range also and this note helps the coder to understand ***procedures or conditions that are not coded*** with the range.
Code also	Review medical record documentation to identify ***additional procedures*** that should be coded.
Code also synchronous	Review medical record documentation to identify ***other procedures*** that should be coded as individual components.
Valid OR	The Valid OR note tells the coder that the ***procedure coded is valid*** for MS-DRG assignment. If non-OR procedure is indicated the coder should review the record again to ensure accurate coding of the procedure is accomplished.
And	This convention is to be interpreted as "***And/Or***". It tells the coder that either condition/procedure is described in the record, the code may be assigned.
With	The "With" note tells the coder ***if both conditions are described in the record***, the code may be assigned.
Omit code	Tells the coder the a ***procedure is an integral part*** of a more comprehensive procedure and it should not be coded separately.

Data from International classification of diseases, 9th revision, *U.S. Department of Health and Human Services, Public Health Service, Centers for Medicare and Medicaid Services.*

- **Code also synchronous procedure.** Code also is found in the tabular list under a code that requires an additional code to be assigned to describe the procedure(s) fully. The coder must review the record to identify synchronous procedures performed and assign the appropriate code (s).
- **And.** Code descriptions in the tabular section may contain the word "And" between two conditions, which tells the coder that if either condition is described in the record, the code may be assigned to describe the condition. Interpret this convention to Mean "And" or "Or". For example, code 20.32 "Biopsy of middle and inner ear" can be used to describe biopsy of the middle ear and/or biopsy of the inner ear.
- **With.** Many code descriptions found in the tabular section contain the word "with" between two procedures, which tells the coder that both procedures must be described in the record to assign the code.
- **Omit code.** The omit code is used in Volume III to advise the coder that the procedure is an integral part

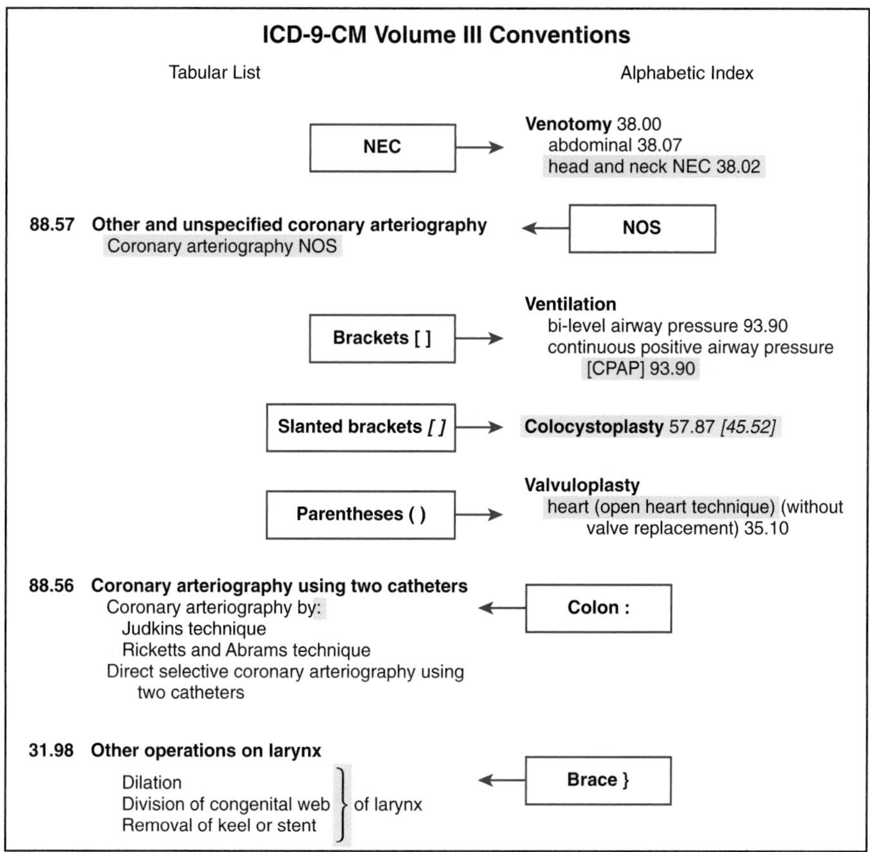

Figure 8-30 ICD-9-CM Volume III official abbreviations and symbols as displayed in the ICD-9-CM manual. *(Data from* International classification of diseases, 9th revision, *U.S. Department of Health and Human Services, Public Health Service, Centers for Medicare and Medicaid Services.)*

of a more comprehensive procedure and that it should not be coded separately.

- **Valid OR.** This instructional note is used to indicate a procedure is valid operating room procedure. MS-DRG assignment is determined in part based on whether a non-OR procedure or valid OR procedure is performed. A case involving a valid OR procedure will change the MS-DRG assignment to a higher level. MS-DRG assignment will be discussed further in Chapter 13.

BOX 8-28 ■ KEY POINTS

ICD-9-CM Volume III Official Conventions

NEC
NOS
Brackets
Slanted brackets
Colon
Brace
Includes
Excludes
Code also synchronous procedure
Omit code
See also

ICD-9-CM Official Other Conventions

- **Boldface type.** Boldface type is used in the alphabetic index to highlight main terms to help the coder find procedures identified in the patient record.
- **Italicized type.** Italicized type is used in the tabular list to indicate procedures that are excluded in a range.

Figure 8-31 illustrates examples of each these conventions listed as they are displayed in the ICD-9-CM coding manual.

The conventions listed above are the ICD-9-CM Official Conventions, and therefore publishers use them consistently. Other conventions found in the ICD-9-CM may not be identified in the same way in all ICD-9-CM manuals. The symbols and colors used to identify the convention may vary; however, the meaning is consistent. Variations in ICD-9-CM Volume III conventions include symbols utilized to indicate new or revised codes, revised text, additional digits required, omit code, synchronous procedures, gender- or age-specific procedures, and Valid, Nonspecific, or Non-OR procedures. Publishers may include various instructional statements such as DEF, for definition, or AHA, indicating guidelines published in the Coding Clinic. Table 8-14 highlights some of the different conventions utilized by publishers.

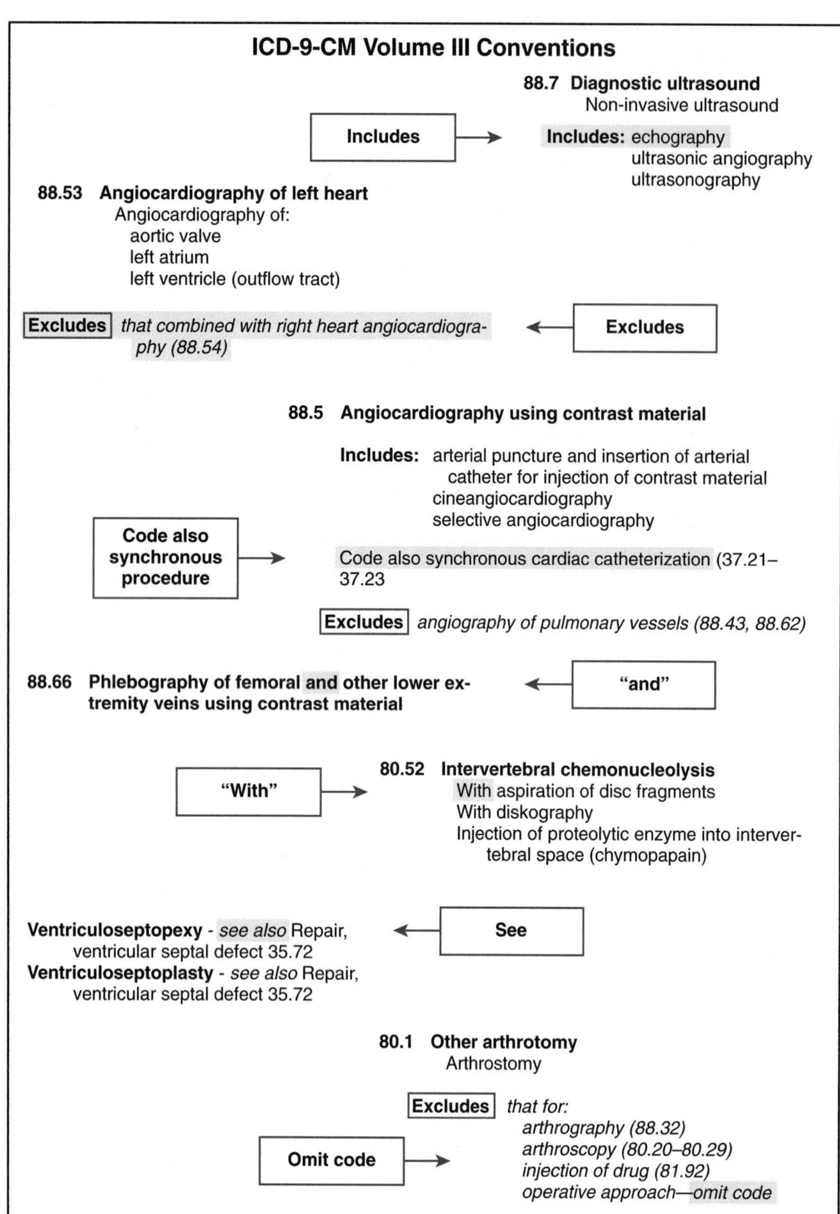

Figure 8-31 ICD-9-CM Volume III official instructional notes as displayed in the ICD-9-CM manual. *(Data from* International classification of diseases, 9th revision, *U.S. Department of Health and Human Services, Public Health Service, Centers for Medicare and Medicaid Services.)*

Since there are many variations of ICD-9-CM coding books, it is strongly recommended that hospital coding professionals carefully review the introduction pages of the ICD-9-CM to gain an understanding of the conventions used. An understanding of the conventions will ensure accurate assignment of codes. Accurate code selection is critical to ensuring that the procedures are described accurately and to establish medical necessity.

STEPS TO CODING UTILIZING HCPCS AND ICD-9-CM VOLUME III

Coding is the process of translating written descriptions of procedures and items into codes. The basic steps in coding are the same regardless of whether you are coding procedures, items, or conditions. The following review of the basic steps to coding includes: read the medical record, refer to the index, refer to the code section, identify modifier circumstances for HCPCS Level I and II procedure codes and sequence codes as outlined in Figure 8-32.

Step 1: Read the Medical Record

The written description of a procedure or item is found in the patient's medical record or other document such as an operative report, encounter form, laboratory slip, or radiology requisition. We will refer to all documents as a "record" for the purpose of reviewing the basic steps. Coding requires the coder to read the record and

TABLE 8-14 **ICD-9-CM Volume III Convention Variations**

Various Symbols Used by Publishers	Convention/Description
• or ▶	**New code** identifies codes that are new to the ICD-9-CM book for the year.
⇐ or ▲	**Revised code** is used to tell the coder the code has been revised.
▶ ◀	**Revised text** symbols are used to let the coder know the text has been revised.
√4 or • √4	**Additional digit required** tells the coder to code to the highest level of specificity (fourth or fifth digit) when documentation supports higher level.
× Valid OR procedure	**Valid OR procedure** affects DRG assignment.
Nonspecific OR procedure	**Nonspecific OR procedure** affects DRG assignment.
Non-OR procedure	**Non-OR procedure** affects DRG assignment.
DEF	**Definitions** of medical terms are included in the tabular list by many publishers.
AHA	**American Hospital Association** publishes the Coding Clinic to provide information to coders that clarifies the intent of ICD-9-CM codes and coding guidelines. Many publishers include **AHA** or some other designation to indicate which publication of the Coding Clinic can be referred to for further information.

Data from International classification of diseases, 9th revision, *U.S. Department of Health and Human Services, Public Health Service, Centers for Medicare and Medicaid Services.*

abstract pertinent information regarding services, procedures, and items to be billed. **Abstracting** is the process of identifying or pulling out specific information from the record. When coding procedures, the coder will abstract information regarding services and procedures performed and supplies, medications, equipment, and other items provided.

Identify the Main Term(s)

The first step involves a review of the medical record to identify the main term(s). The main term when coding services or procedures can be determined by asking "what procedure or service was performed?" Figure 8-33 illustrates that the main terms identified in Case 1 are: ***Urinalysis***, ***Cystourethroscopy***, and ***Fulgurated***. These main terms will be utilized to look up possible codes in the HCPCS Level I CPT manual. When coding items, the main term can be determined by asking, "what item was provided?" The main terms identified in Case 1 are: ***Lidocaine*** and ***Tubing.*** These main terms will be utilized to look up possible codes in the HCPCS Level II manual.

Now that the main terms have been identified, we can begin to look for codes in the index. To determine what coding systems to use, refer back to Case 1 to identify the service category for the case: outpatient, inpatient, or non-patient. This is an inpatient case, so the HCPCS Level I and II coding systems and the ICD-9-CM Volume III Procedures coding system are used. It is important to remember that charges incurred during an inpatient visit are posted through the chargemaster. Each item in the chargemaster has a HCPCS code associated with it. The HCPCS codes are not reported on the claim form for inpatient cases; however, they may print on the detailed itemized statement. The HIM coder will assign codes utilizing Volume III as well as codes for the patient's condition.

Step 2: Refer to the Alphabetic Index

This section outlines the process of utilizing the alphabetic index in the HCPCS and ICD-9-CM Volume III manuals to identify possible codes for main terms identified in the record.

HCPCS Level I CPT Coding System

Refer to the HCPCS Level I CPT index and identify possible codes for the main terms identified in Case 1. Remember, good coding habits are to identify *all possible codes* in the index and review all cross-references. Figure 8-34 illustrates the possible HCPCS Level I codes identified for Case 1: 81001 and 81003 for the urinalysis and 52234 to 52240 for the cystourethroscopy and fulguration.

HCPCS Level II Medicare National Coding System

Refer to the HCPCS Level II Medicare National code index and identify possible codes for the main terms identified in Case 1. Figure 8-35 illustrates the possible HCPCS Level II codes identified: A4355 for the tubing and J2001 for the lidocaine.

TEST YOUR *Knowledge* BOX 8-6

ICD-9-CM VOLUME III PROCEDURES

1. Explain what the ICD-9-CM Volume III coding system is used for.

2. What claim form(s) is used to submit Volume III procedures?

3. Indicate the form locator in which ICD-9-CM Volume III procedure codes are recorded.

4. The content of ICD-9-CM Volume III includes an alphabetic ____________ and a ____________ listing of procedures and services.

5. State how procedures and services are listed in the tabular listing of the ICD-9-CM Volume III manual.

6. Describe what Volume III procedure codes look like.

7. Main terms identified for ICD-9-CM Volume III procedure codes represent ____________ or ____________.

8. An ICD-9-CM convention found only in Volume III is ____________ ____________ ____________, and it tells the coder that other procedures should be reported as individual components.

9. The ____________ ____________ convention is found only in ICD-9-CM Volume III; it tells the coder that the procedure is an integral part of a more comprehensive procedure and it should not be coded separately.

10. Review each procedure or service listed below and mark a Y or N to indicate whether or not it is a significant procedure.
    a. MRI
    b. Heart catheterization
    c. Infusion therapy
    d. Craniotomy
    e. Comprehensive metabolic panel

ICD-9-CM Volume III Procedure Coding System

Refer to the ICD-9-CM Volume III index and identify possible codes for the main terms identified in Case 1. Figure 8-36 illustrates possible ICD-9-CM Volume III codes identified: 57.32 and 57.33 for the cystourethroscopy and 57.49 for the fulguration. Remember, when coding Volume III procedures only significant procedures are coded. The significant procedures to be coded are Cystourethroscopy and Fulgurated tumor. The urinalysis is not a significant procedure, and therefore it is not coded utilizing ICD-9-CM Volume III.

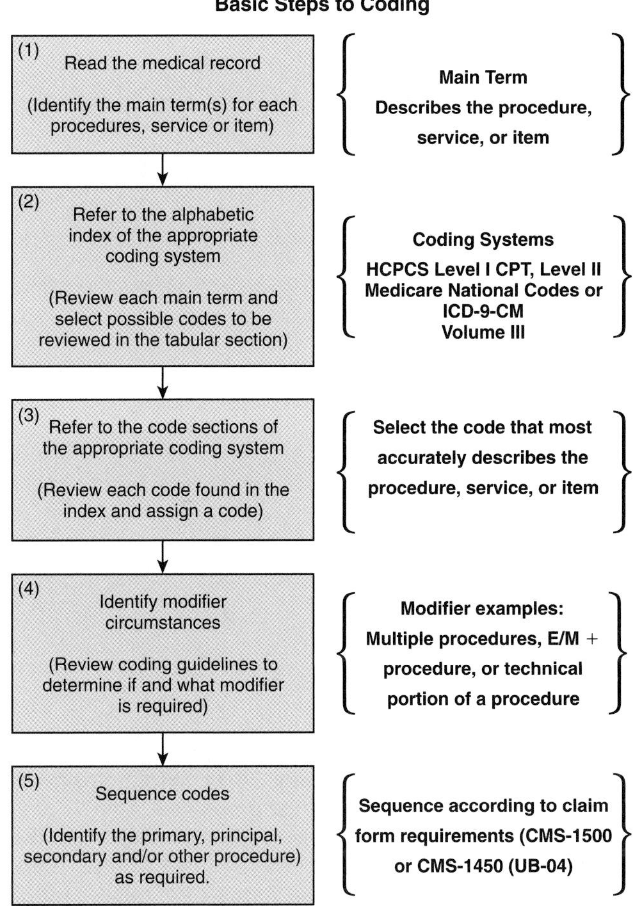

Figure 8-32 The first step in coding is to read the medical record and identify services provided and patient conditions for which those services were provided.

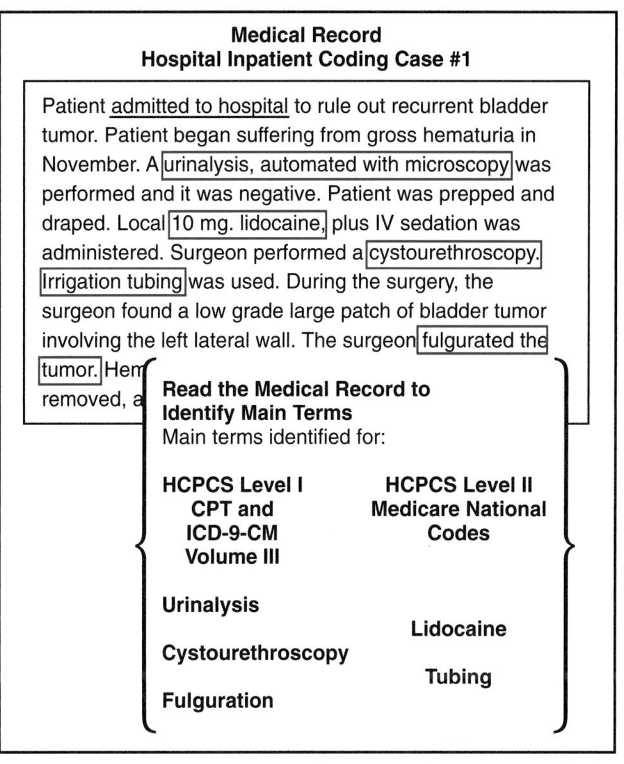

Figure 8-33 Basic steps to coding procedures: Step 1, highlighting main terms identified.

To this point, we have read the record, identified the main terms, and referred to the index to identify all possible codes. The next step is to review all possible codes in the tabular list and select the codes that most accurately describe what is in the record. All codes identified in the index must be reviewed in the tabular section. Remember good coding habits, and ***NEVER, EVER*** select a code from the index without verifying it in the tabular list (code section).

BOX 8-29 ■ KEY POINTS

Golden Rule in Coding

Good Coding Habits

- DO NOT ASSUME.
- Identify all possible codes in the index (Volume II).
- NEVER, EVER code from the index (Volume II).
- Review each code in the tabular list (Volume I).
- Review all codes in the range.
- WHEN IN DOUBT, ASK.
- Never use an E code as the first-listed condition.

Step 3: Refer to the Code Sections for Code Assignment

HCPCS Level I CPT Coding System

Refer to the HCPCS Level I CPT code sections to review and select the code for each procedure listed below from Case 1. Figure 8-37 illustrates the CPT code assignment for Case 1: 81001 "Urinalysis, automated with microscopy" and 52234 "Cystourethroscopy, with fulguration of tumor."

HCPCS Level II Medicare National Coding Systems

Refer to the HCPCS Level II Medicare National code sections to review and select the code for each item from Case 1. Figure 8-38 illustrates the HCPCS Level II code assignment for Case 1: J2001 "Lidocaine, 10 mg" and A4355 "Tubing, Irrigation."

ICD-9-CM Volume III Procedure Coding System

Refer to the ICD-9-CM Volume III tabular list to review and select the code for each significant procedure from Case 1. Figure 8-39 illustrates the ICD-9-CM Volume III code assignment for Case 1: 57.33 "Closed Biopsy of Bladder." Note that the fulgurated tumor is included in the code for the cystourethroscopy.

Medical Record
Hospital Inpatient Coding Case #1

Patient admitted to hospital to rule out recurrent bladder tumor. Patient began suffering from gross hematuria in November. A urinalysis, automated with microscopy, was performed and it was negative. Patient was prepped and draped. Local 10 mg Lidocaine plus IV sedation was administered. Surgeon performed a cystourethroscopy. Irrigation tubing was used. During the surgery the surgeon found a low grade large patch of bladder tumor involving the left lateral wall. The surgeon fulgurated the tumor. Hemostasis was controlled, the scope removed, and patient was sent to recovery.

Johnathan Sampson, M.D.

HCPCS Level I CPT

Main term and subterm	Codes identified in the index
Urinalysis, automated	81001, 81003
Cystourethroscopy with Fulguration, tumor	52234-52240
Fulguration Cystourethroscopy with, tumor	52234-52240

Fulguration
See Destruction
Bladder 51020
Cystourethroscopy with 52214
  Lesion 52224
  Tumor 52234-52240
Ureter 50957, 50976
Ureterocele
  Ectopic 52301
  Orthotopic 52300

Urinalysis 0041T, 81000-81099
Automated 81001, 81003
Glass Test 81020
Microalbumin 82043-82044
Microscopic 81015
Pregnancy Test 81025
Qualitative 81005
Routine 81002

Cystourethroscopy 52000, 52351, 52601, 52647-52648, 53500
Vasectomy
  Transurethral 52402
Vasotomy
  Transurethral 52402
with Direct Vision Internal
  Urethrotomy 52276
with Ejaculatory Duct
  Catheterization 52010
with Fulguration 52214, 52354
  Lesion 52224
  Tumor 52234-52240
with Internal Urethrotomy
  Female 52270
  Male 52275

Figure 8-34 Basic steps to coding procedures: Step 2, possible codes identified in the HCPCS Level I CPT Index. *(Data from AMA: CPT 2010 professional edition, Chicago, 2010, American Medical Association.)*

HCPCS Level II
Medicare National Codes

Main term and subterm	Codes identified in the index
Table of drugs	
Lidocaine, 10 mg	J2001
Index	
Tubing, irrigation	A4355

Tube/Tubing
  anchoring device, A5200
  blood, A4750, A4755
  drainage extension, A4331
  gastrostomy, B4087, B4088
  irrigation, A4355
  laryngectomy, A4622

Librium, see Chlordiazepoxide HCl	up to 100 mg	IM, IV	J1990
Lidocaine HCl	10 mg	IV	J2001
Lidoject-1, see Lidocaine HCl			
Lidoject-2, see Lidocaine HCl			
Lincocin, see Lincomycin HCl			
Lincomycin HCl	up to 300 mg	IV	J2010
Linezolid	200 mg	IV	J2020
Liquaemin Sodium, *see* Heparin sodium			

Figure 8-35 Basic steps to coding procedures: Step 2, possible codes identified in the HCPCS Level II Medicare National code index. *(Data from* HCPCS 2010: level II national codes, *U.S. Department of Health and Human Services, Centers for Medicare and Medicaid Services.)*

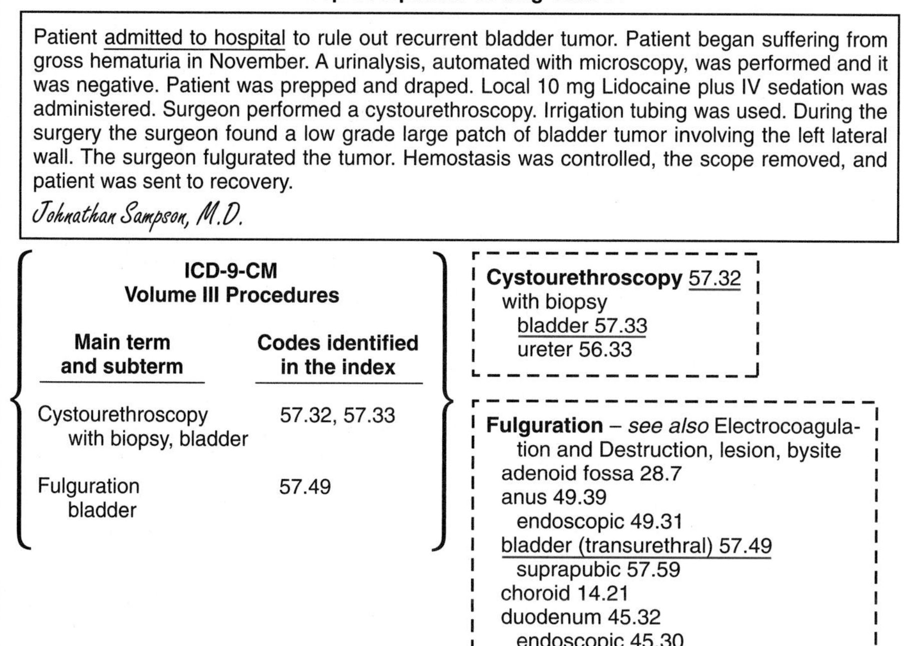

Medical Record
Hospital Inpatient Coding Case #1

Patient admitted to hospital to rule out recurrent bladder tumor. Patient began suffering from gross hematuria in November. A urinalysis, automated with microscopy, was performed and it was negative. Patient was prepped and draped. Local 10 mg Lidocaine plus IV sedation was administered. Surgeon performed a cystourethroscopy. Irrigation tubing was used. During the surgery the surgeon found a low grade large patch of bladder tumor involving the left lateral wall. The surgeon fulgurated the tumor. Hemostasis was controlled, the scope removed, and patient was sent to recovery.

Johnathan Sampson, M.D.

ICD-9-CM
Volume III Procedures

Main term and subterm	Codes identified in the index
Cystourethroscopy with biopsy, bladder	57.32, 57.33
Fulguration bladder	57.49

Cystourethroscopy 57.32
with biopsy
bladder 57.33
ureter 56.33

Fulguration – *see also* Electrocoagulation and Destruction, lesion, bysite
adenoid fossa 28.7
anus 49.39
endoscopic 49.31
bladder (transurethral) 57.49
suprapubic 57.59
choroid 14.21
duodenum 45.32
endoscopic 45.30

Figure 8-36 Basic steps to coding procedures: Step 2, possible codes identified in the, ICD-9-CM Volume III Procedure code index. *(Data from* International classification of diseases, 9th revision, *U.S. Department of Health and Human Services, Public Health Service, Centers for Medicare and Medicaid Services.)*

HCPCS Level I Code Selection

Urinalysis, Automated with Microscopy — Code 81001

81000	Urinalysis, by dip stick or tablet reagent for bilirubin, glucose, hemoglobin, ketones, leukocytes, nitrite, pH, protein, specific gravity, urobilinogen, any number of these constituents; non-automated, with microscopy ➲ *CPT Assistant* Winter 90-91:10, Fall 93:25, Aug 05:09
81001	automated, with microscopy
81002	non-automated, without microscopy ➲ *CPT Assistant* Mar 98:3, Apr 07:1
81003	automated, without microscopy ➲ CPT Assistant Apr 07:1

Cystourethroscopy, with fulguration of tumor — Code 52234

52234	Cystourethroscopy, with fulguration (including cryosurgery or laser surgery) and/or resection of; SMALL bladder tumor(s) (0.5 up to 2.0 cm) ➲ *CPT Assistant* May 01:5, Sep 01:1, Oct 02:12, Jan 03:19; *CPT Changes: An Insider's View* 2005
52235	MEDIUM bladder tumor(s) (2.0 to 5.0 cm) ➲ *CPT Assistant* May 01:5, Sep 01:1, Oct 02:12, Jan 03:19
52240	LARGE bladder tumor(s) ➲ *CPT Assistant* May 01:5, Sep 01:1

Figure 8-37 Basic steps to coding procedures: Step 3, code selection from HCPCS Level I CPT code section for Case 1. *(Data from AMA:* CPT 2010 professional edition, *Chicago, 2010, American Medical Association.)*

Figure 8-40 is provided to illustrate coding from all systems for Hospital Inpatient Case #1. The following section reviews identifying modifier circumstances and sequencing codes on the claim forms.

Step 4: Identify Modifier Circumstances

A **modifier** is a one- or two-digit code utilized with an HCPCS Level I or II procedure code to describe existing circumstances that are not explained in the procedure code description. An example of a modifier circumstance is when a procedure was performed bilaterally and the code describes a unilateral procedure. A modifier –50 or LT and RT is utilized in addition to the procedure code to explain that the procedure was performed bilaterally. HCPCS Level I and II contain modifiers. HCPCS Level I modifiers cannot be used with a HCPCS Level II code. They can only be used

HCPCS Level II Code Selection

Tubing, Irrigation	Code A4355
A4355	Irrigation tubing set for continuous bladder irrigation through a three-way indwelling Foley catheter, each MCM 2130

Lidocaine, Injection 10 mg	Code J2001
J2001	Injection, lidocaine HCL for intravenous infusion, 10 mg MCM 2049

Figure 8-38 Basic steps to coding procedures: Step 3, code selection from HCPCS Level II Medicare National Code Section. *(Data from* HCPCS 2010: level II national codes, *U.S. Department of Health and Human Services, Centers for Medicare and Medicaid Services.)*

ICD-9-CM Volume III Code Selection

Cystourethroscopy, with Biopsy of Tumor

Note: This code describes biopsy of tissue

57.3 Diagnostic procedures on bladder

- **57.31 Cystoscopy through artificial stoma**
- **57.32 Other cystoscopy**
  Transurethral cystoscopy
  Excludes *cystourethroscopy with ureteral biopsy (56.33)*
  retrograde pyelogram (87.74)
  that for control of hemorrhage (postoperative):
  bladder (57.93)
  prostate (60.94)
- **57.33 Closed [transurethral] biopsy of bladder**
- **57.34 Open biopsy of bladder**
- **57.39 Other diagnostic procedures on bladder**

Cystourethroscopy, with Fulguration of Tumor — Code 57.49

Note: This code describes fulguration of tumor

57.4 Transurethral excision or destruction of bladder tissue

- **57.41 Transurethral lysis of intraluminal adhesions**
- **57.49 Other transurethral excision or destruction of lesion or tissue of bladder**
  Endoscopic resection of bladder lesion
  Excludes *transurethral biopsy of bladder (57.33)*
  transurethral fistulectomy (57.83–57.84)

Figure 8-39 Basic steps to coding procedures: Step 3, code selection from ICD-9-CM Volume III Procedure code section for Case 1. *(Data from* International classification of diseases, 9th revision, *U.S. Department of Health and Human Services, Centers for Medicare and Medicaid Services.)*

Medical Record
Hospital Inpatient Coding Case #1

Patient admitted to hospital to rule out recurrent bladder tumor. Patient began suffering from gross hematuria in November. A urinalysis, automated with microscopy was performed and it was negative. Patient was prepped and draped. Local 10 mg. lidocaine, plus IV sedation was administered. Surgeon performed a cystourethroscopy. Irrigation tubing was used. During the surgery, the surgeon found a low grade large patch of bladder tumor involving the left lateral wall. The surgeon fulgurated the tumor. Hemostasis … was sent to …

Read the Medical Record to Identify Main Terms
Main terms identified for:

HCPCS Level I CPT and	**HCPCS Level II Medicare National Codes**
Urinalysis 81000	**Lidocaine A4355**
Cystourethroscopy with fulguration 52234	**Tubing J2001**
ICD-9-CM Volume III Procedures	
Cystourethroscopy with biopsy, bladder	**57.33**
Fulguration, bladder	**57.49**

Figure 8-40 Basic steps to coding procedures: Step 3, procedure codes assigned. *(Data from* HCPCS 2010: level II national codes, *U.S. Department of Health and Human Services, Centers for Medicare and Medicaid Services.)*

with a Level I CPT code. HCPCS Level II modifiers may be used with HCPCS Level I or Level II codes. They can be utilized with a CPT or Medicare National code. Modifier usage is determined by reviewing the record to identify coding situations that require a modifier. ***Coders must also know what modifiers are required. It is important to note that modifiers are not used with ICD-9-CM codes; they are only used with HCPCS Level I or II procedure codes.***

HCPCS Level I CPT Modifiers

HCPCS Level I modifiers are listed on the CMS-1500 in Block 24D. Payers may also require Level I modifiers on the UB-04 in FL 44 for outpatient and non-patient services. Modifier usage varies according to payer guidelines for specific service types and categories. For example, E/M modifiers are only used with E/M codes. HCPCS Level I CPT modifiers are found in Appendix A. Appendix A contains a detailed listing of CPT modifiers and descriptions. HCPCS Level I CPT modifiers approved for hospital outpatient use are outlined in Table 8-15.

TABLE 8-15 HCPCS Level I CPT Modifiers for Hospital Outpatient Use Modifier attached to the following codes

Modifier	Title of Modifier	E/M	Surgery	Radiology	Laboratory and Laboratory	Medicine
25	Significant, separately identifiable E/M Service by the same physician on the same day of the procedure or Other Service	X				
27	Multiple outpatient hospital E/M encounters on the same date	X				
50	Bilateral procedure					
52	Reduced services		X	X	X	X
58	Staged or related procedure or service by the same physician during the postoperative period		X			X
59	Distinct procedural service		X	X		X
73	Discontinued outpatient procedure prior to anesthesia administration		X			
74	Discontinued outpatient procedure after anesthesia administration		X			
76	Repeat procedure by the same physician		X	X		X
77	Repeat procedure by another physician		X	X		X
78	Return to the Operating Room for a related procedure during the postoperative period		X			X
91	Repeat clinical diagnostic laboratory test				X	

Data from AMA: CPT 2006 professional edition, *Chicago, 2010, American Medical Association.*

HCPCS Level II Medicare National Code Modifiers

HCPCS Level II modifiers are also listed on the CMS-1500 in Block 24D. Payers may also require Level II modifiers on the UB-04 in FL 44 for outpatient and non-patient services. Level II modifiers are generally found in an appendix or introduction of a Level II manual. Level II modifiers were designed to describe particular circumstances to Medicare carriers, and there are more than 200 Level II modifiers available for use when submitting Medicare claims. Many payers accept Level II modifiers; however, Level II modifier usage is payer specific. It is important to remember that Level II modifiers can be attached to a CPT code, but CPT modifiers cannot be attached to a Level II code. Table 8-16 outlines HCPCS Level II modifiers approved for hospital outpatient use.

Step 5: Sequence Codes

Sequencing is the process of listing codes in an order that accurately describes conditions treated and those that affect treatment. When listing procedure codes on the claim form, the sequence may need to be carefully determined. Sequencing rules are determined by the following service categories and the type of claim form submitted. Figure 8-41 illustrates the following general sequencing rules:

CMS-1500 Physician and Outpatient Services

General sequencing rules for the CMS-1500 indicate that procedures are generally listed in the order in which services occurred. When multiple surgical procedures are performed, list the most comprehensive (complex) procedure first, followed by other procedures in order of complexity.

CMS-1450 (UB-04) Hospital Outpatient and Non-Patient Services

The UB-04 outpatient and non-patient claim requirements indicate that services identified with HCPCS codes should be grouped into revenue code categories; therefore, the sequencing is in the order of the revenue code. Revenue code categories will be discussed later in this text.

TABLE 8-16 HCPCS Level II Medicare National Code Modifiers for Hospital Outpatient Use

Modifier	Description of Modifier	Modifier	Description of Modifier
CR	Catastrophe/disaster related		
E1	Upper left, eyelid	QM	Ambulance service provided under arrangement by a provider of services
E2	Lower left, eyelid	QN	Ambulance service furnished directly by a provider of services
E3	Upper right, eyelid	RC	Right coronary artery
E4	Lower right, eyelid	RT	Right side
FA	Left hand, thumb	TA	Left foot, great toe
F1	Left hand, second digit	T1	Left foot, second digit
F2	Left hand, third digit	T2	Left foot, third digit
F3	Left hand, fourth digit	T3	Left foot, fourth digit
F4	Left hand, fifth digit	T4	Left foot, fifth digit
F5	Right hand, thumb	T5	Right foot, great toe
F6	Right hand, second digit	T6	Right foot, second digit
F7	Right hand, third digit	T7	Right foot, third digit
F8	Right hand, fourth digit	T8	Right foot, fourth digit
F9	Right hand, fifth digit	T9	Right foot, fifth digit
GA	Waiver of liability on file		
LC	Left circumflex, coronary artery		
LD	Left anterior descending coronary artery		
LT	Left side		

Data from HCPCS 2010: level II national codes, *U.S. Department of Health and Human Services, Centers for Medicare and Medicaid Services.*

CMS-1450 (UB-04) Inpatient Services

The UB-04 claim requirements for inpatient services indicate that ICD-9-CM Volume III procedure codes describing significant procedures are recorded in FL 74a–e. The principal procedure is listed in FL 74. Other significant procedures are recorded in FL 74a–e.

BOX 8-30 ■ KEY POINTS

Basic Steps to Procedure Coding

1. Read the medical record. Identify the main terms that represent procedures, services, and items.
2. Refer to the alphabetic index of the appropriate coding system. Look up each main term and identify possible codes.
3. Refer to the tabular (numerical) list. Look up each code identified in the index and select the code that most accurately describes the service or item.
4. Identify modifier circumstances.
5. Sequence the codes

CHAPTER SUMMARY

Procedure coding involves translating written descriptions of procedures and services recorded in the patient's medical record into HCPCS Level I CPT, HCPCS Level II Medicare National, or ICD-9-CM Volume III procedure codes. Supplies, equipment, medications, and other items provided are also coded using the HCPCS Level II Medicare National codes. Hospital billing and coding professionals must have an understanding of the conventions and format of the coding systems used in the hospital in order to ensure that patient services and items are described accurately on the claim forms. The coding system used is determined by the service category. Outpatient services, physician services, and items are represented using HCPCS Level I and II codes. The service category also indicates what claim form is used. Significant procedures for inpatient and ambulatory surgery services are coded and reported using

CMS-1500 Block 24

24.	A		B	C	
	DATE(S) OF SERVICE From To MM DD YY	MM DD YY	Place of Service	Type of Service	PROC SERV SUR (Explai Circum CPT/HCP MODIFIE
1	09 27 06	09 27 06	11		**99212**
2	09 27 06	09 27 06	11		**10060**
3					

CMS-1500 **Physician and Outpatient Services**

Case Example:
Established patient presents with a cyst. Problem-focused office visit performed. Incision and drainage of cyst performed.

General Sequencing Guidelines:

- List procedures in the order that services occurred
- When multiple surgical procedures are involved, list the most comprehensive (complex) procedure first followed by the other procedures in order of complexity

CMS-1450 (UB-04) Form Locator 44

42 REV. CD.	43 DESCRIPTION	44 HCPCS/ RATES
0101	ALL INCL R & B	
0293	MED/EQUIP USED	E0720
0490	AMBU SURG	27447

CMS-1450 (UB-04) **Hospital Outpatient and Non-Patient Services**

FL 44 is used to report outpatient and non-patient procedures as required

Case Example:	Hospital charge information:
Room and Board	Rev Code 0101
Ambulatory Surgery	Rev Code 0490 HCPCS Code 27447
Medical Equipment	Rev Code 0293 HCPCS Code E0720

General Sequencing Guidelines:

- Procedure codes are grouped into revenue code categories
- Payers provide guidelines regarding specific requirements for reporting procedures in FL 44

CMS-1450 (UB-04) Form Locator 74

74 PRINCIPAL PROCEDURE CODE	DATE	CO
81.54	09 27 2006	
OTHER PROCEDURE		

Note:
Some payers may require FL 74 a-e to be completed for ambulatory surgery claims.

CMS-1450 (UB-04) **Hospital Inpatient Services**

Case Example:
Patient admitted for total knee replacement. Patient tolerated procedure well.

General Sequencing Guidelines:

- Principal procedure is listed first in FL 74
  The principal procedure is performed for definitive treatment of the principal diagnosis or the one that most closely relates to the principal diagnosis
- Other procedures are listed in order of complexity in FL 74 A-E

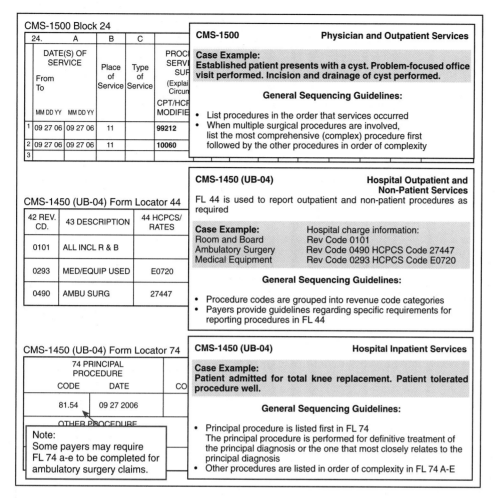

Figure 8-41 General Sequencing rules for the CMS-1500 and CMS-1450 (UB-04).

ICD-9-CM Volume III procedures. It is important for coders to have knowledge of medical terminology, anatomy, and physiology, as well as coding principles and guidelines. An effective coder must be able to read and understand a medical record and identify the procedures, services, and items that are to be billed.

The claim form used to report services and items varies based on service category—outpatient, non-patient, or inpatient basis. Charges are submitted to payers utilizing the HCFA-1500 or the CMS-1450 (UB-04) claim forms. The HCFA-1500 is used to report physician and outpatient services. The UB-04 is used to report facility charges for services provided in the hospital. Accurate completion of the claim form requires that hospital billing and coding professionals have an understanding of payer specifications regarding the claim forms. Now that we have an understanding of coding systems and claim form usage, we will continue on to coding applications and guidelines in Chapter 9 and claim forms in Chapter 10.

TEST YOUR *Knowledge* BOX 8-7

ICD-9-CM VOLUME III PROCEDURES

Steps to coding are consistent no matter what coding system is used. Review the following questions and provide an answer that applies to each of the coding systems discussed in this chapter.

1. ____________ is the process of identifying or pulling out specific information from the record.

2. The first step in coding is to read the record and identify the ________ ________ for each procedure, service, or item.

3. A coder utilizes the main terms to identify possible codes by referring to the ________.

4. A review of each code found in the ____________ is conducted and the code that most adequately ____________ the procedure, service, or item is selected from the ____________.

5. Codes found in the index are never utilized without confirming them in the ____________ ____________.

6. When all the codes involving the HCPCS Level I and II coding systems are selected, the coder must then review the record to identify circumstances that require the use of a ____________.

7. The ________________ procedure coding system does not utilize modifiers.

8. Explain the difference between HCPCS Level I modifiers and HCPCS Level II modifiers.

9. State the general sequencing rules for the CMS-1500.

10. Describe the general sequencing guidelines for the CMS-1450 (UB-04).

CHAPTER REVIEW 8-1

True/False

1. Coding is not necessary to submit a claim. T F
2. Coding can be accomplished without documentation. T F
3. Conventions are used to communicate information and instructions to the coder. T F
4. ICD-9-CM Volume III procedures are required for inpatient claims. T F
5. HCPCS Level II codes are used for physician and outpatient services. T F

Fill in the Blank

6. The coding systems used to report physician and outpatient services are _______________ and _______________.
7. The coding system used to report significant procedures is _______________.
8. HCPCS consists of two levels of codes, which are _______________ and _______________.
9. Modifiers are used to _______________.
10. Codes used to describe emerging technologies, services, or procedures are _______________.

Match the Following Definitions With the Terms at Right

11. ____ The procedure performed for definitive treatment of the principle diagnosis.
12. ____ A procedure that is surgical in nature, or carries a procedural risk, or carries an anesthetic risk, or requires specialized training. This definition is stated in the Uniform Hospital Discharge Data Set (UHDDS), as published in the *Federal Register* in 1985.
13. ____ Codes developed in the 1980s to provide a standard system for reporting supplies, equipment, medication, and other items to Medicare carriers.
14. ____ Procedures that are considered to be reasonable and necessary to treat the patient's condition.
15. ____ The process of assigning codes to written descriptions of procedures, services, or items.

A. HCPCS Level II Medicare National codes
B. Principal procedure
C. Procedure coding
D. Significant procedure
E. Medically necessary

Research Project

Follow the basic coding steps discussed in this chapter, read the following statements, and list the following for each problem: (1) main term(s) for procedures and items, and (2) HCPCS or ICD-9-CM Volume III code(s) as indicated. Remember, only significant procedures are coded utilizing ICD-9-PCS.

Hospital Outpatient Cases: Hospital-Based Primary Care Office Visit

Review each case and assign the appropriate procedure codes.

1. Mrs. Jones brings her 7-year-old son Jason, an established patient, to the office today because he stepped on a nail. A problem-focused history and exam is performed. The puncture in his heel is not very deep; we cleaned and bandaged it. A shot of tetanus and diphtheria was given intramuscularly.

2. Sam Goliath, a 42-year-old male established patient, presents today for a routine physical exam. At the end of the exam the patient noted he had a good-sized growth on his back that has been present for several months. Problem-focused history and exam reveals a 1-cm-diameter wart-type growth that is an actinic keratosis. A diagnostic shave biopsy of the growth was performed.

CHAPTER REVIEW 8-1—*cont'd*

3. This 25-year-old female, an established patient, presents today, for the first time in 5 years, complaining of bouts of dizziness, and she has also noticed difficulty swallowing and getting food to go down. An expanded problem-focused history and exam was performed. She is currently on medication for hypothyroidism. Blood was drawn and sent out to the lab to check the TSH levels.

Emergency Department Visit

4. Patient presents to the Emergency Department with a severe burn on the left upper arm. Level I E/M reveals a third-degree burn. Debridement of the small area was performed and dressings were applied.
5. Patient arrived at the Emergency Department by ambulance, unconscious. Paramedics indicate the patient was found in his apartment not breathing. CPR was administered. The patient's roommate indicates he was drinking whisky heavily the night before and he found the patient in the morning and could not wake him up. The emergency room physician performed a Level IV E/M. The patient is currently in a coma. A drug screen for alcohol and opiates revealed high amounts of morphine and alcohol in his system. The roommate indicates he is on morphine and does not know how or why the patient took it.

Ambulatory Surgery Cases

6. A 62-year-old male patient presents today for a lumbar puncture to determine the cause of his vascular headaches. Patient was prepped and draped in the normal fashion and local anesthesia administered. A 20-gauge needle was introduced into the subarachnoid space of the lumbar region. Five centimeters of crystal-clear CSF was obtained and sent to the laboratory for diagnostic studies. The patient tolerated the procedure well. Provide a CPT code and an ICD-9-CM Volume III procedure code for this procedure. Select a code for a surgical tray.
7. Mrs. Hartenshogan arrived today for scheduled colonoscopy. Patient has been experiencing severe abdominal pain and nausea after eating. Scope, flexible, inserted for visualization proximal to splenic flexure revealed inflammation and infection of the peritoneal cavity. Sacs of mucous membrane are protruding through the muscular wall of the colon. The scope was withdrawn and the patient was moved to recovery. Select the appropriate CPT code(s).

Inpatient Cases

8. A 28-year-old female is admitted with a malignant mass in the left breast. A biopsy was performed last week and pathology showed presence of carcinoma that has not spread outside the margins. The patient has hypertension and a family history of breast cancer. The surgeon performed a mastectomy including pectoralis muscle and the internal mammary and axillary nodes. Local excision of a benign mass excised from right breast for biopsy. Patient tolerated procedure well. List the Volume III and CPT procedure code(s) that describe the principal and other procedures.
9. List the Volume III procedure code that describes the principal procedure for the following scenario.
10. List the Volume III procedure code(s) for other significant procedures for the following scenario.

A 67-year-old male was admitted to the hospital for a pancreatectomy due to severe abdominal pain. A CT scan revealed a mass in the tail and body of the pancreas involving the left kidney and spleen. Pancreatectomy, distal was performed. A splenectomy and left nephrectomy were also performed. During the procedure the patient went into cardiac arrest due to the adverse effect of the general anesthetic.

GLOSSARY

Abstracting The process of identifying or pulling out specific information from the record.

Convention Special terms, punctuation marks, abbreviations, or symbols, used as shorthand in a coding system to communicate special instructions to coders efficiently.

Current procedural terminology (CPT) A coding system published by the American Medical Association (AMA) in 1966 that contains a set of codes, descriptions, and guidelines intended to describe procedures and services performed by physicians and other health care providers. The CPT, 4th edition is currently used today and may be referred to as CPT-4.

CPT Category I Codes Codes that describe services, procedures, and some items and they are listed in the Evaluation and Management, Anesthesia, Surgery, Radiology, Pathology/Laboratory, and Medicine sections of CPT.

CPT Category II Codes A set of supplemental tracking codes developed for use in the measurement of performance. Category II codes are listed after the Medicine section I the CPT manual.

CPT Category III Codes Codes are temporary codes used to describe emerging technologies, services, or procedures. Category III codes are listed after the Medicine section in the CPT manual.

Documentation A term utilized to describe information recorded regarding patient conditions and procedures, services, supplies, equipment, and medications provided as part of the patient's care.

Form locator (FL) Fields that require data on the CMS-1450 (UB-04) are referred to as form locators (FL). There are 81 form locators on the UB-04.

Health Care Common Procedure Coding System (HCPCS) The standard coding system adopted under the Health Insurance Portability and Accountability Act (HIPPA) for use in coding services, procedures, and items. HCPCS contains two levels of codes: Level I CPT and Level II Medicare National codes.

ICD-9-CM Volume III (ICD-9-PCS) Procedure coding system used for reporting of significant procedures and services performed in the hospital or other facility. The coding system contains a listing of procedures and services and each is associated with a 2-to 4-digit numeric code.

Inpatient services Services provided to a patient who is admitted to the hospital for more than 24 hours.

Medical necessity A term used to describe procedures or services that are considered reasonable and medically necessary to address the patient's medical condition, based on standards of medical practice.

Medicare National Codes A coding system developed in the 1980s to provide a standardized system for reporting supplies, equipment, medication and other items to Medicare carriers. Medicare National codes are now called HCPCS Level II codes, as they were adopted by CMS as part of the Health Care Common Procedure Coding System (HCPCS).

Modifier One-or two-digit code utilized with a procedure code to describe circumstances that exist that are not explained in the procedure code description. The HCPCS Level I and Level II coding systems contain modifiers.

Non-patient services A service involving tests or procedures performed on a specimen when the patient is not present.

Outpatient services Services provided on the same day the patient is released. The patient does not stay overnight.

Principal procedure The procedure is one that is performed for definitive treatment of the principal diagnosis or the procedure that most closely relates to the principal diagnosis.

Procedure coding The process of translating written descriptions of procedures, services, supplies, drugs, and equipment from the patient's record into numeric or alphanumeric codes.

Sequencing The process of listing codes in an order that accurately describes conditions treated and those that affect treatment.

Significant procedure A significant procedure is one that is: 1. surgical in nature, or 2. carries a procedural risk, or 3. carries an anesthetic risk, or 4. requires specialized training. This definition is stated the Uniform Hospital Discharge Data Set (UHDDS), as published in the *Federal Register* in 1985.

Tabular list A term used to describe a numerical listing.

Chapter 9

Coding Guidelines and Applications

The objective of this chapter is to provide a basic understanding of coding guidelines for diagnosis and procedure coding in the hospital setting. Coding principles and guidelines vary by provider, category of service, and payer type. The challenge for hospital coding and billing professionals is to understand those variations and effectively apply the principles and guidelines applicable to coding patient care services rendered by providers. Hospital coding and billing professionals must also understand the relationship between billing and coding. This relationship is significant because coding describes diagnostic and therapeutic services provided and the medical conditions for which those services were provided. Concepts on documentation, diagnosis and procedure coding, the billing process, payer processing, and accounts receivable management were covered in previous chapters. This chapter will provide a brief review of those concepts, demonstrating the relationship between coding and billing. The chapter will then explore diagnosis and procedure coding guidelines and their appropriate application. Abstracting and the basic steps to coding conditions and procedures will be revisited to assist with the application of coding guidelines, using case scenarios for outpatient, non-patient, and inpatient cases.

Chapter Objectives

- Define terms, phrases, abbreviations, and acronyms related to coding guidelines and applications.
- Explain the relationship between billing and coding.
- Discuss variations in coding systems utilized for inpatient and outpatient services.
- Provide an outline of the basic steps to abstracting from the medical record.
- Apply coding guidelines for inpatient and outpatient cases.
- Demonstrate an understanding of coding principles and guidelines.

Outline

Key Terms

Correct Coding Initiative (CCI)
Facility charges
First Listed Condition
Global procedure
Medicare Code Editor (MCE)
Medicare Outpatient Code Editor (OCE)
Payer edits
Phantom billing
Principal diagnosis
Principal procedure
Professional component
Significant procedure
Surgical package
Technical component
Unbundling
Upcoding

Acronyms and Abbreviations

AHA—American Hospital Association
AMA—American Medical Association
APC—Ambulatory Payment Classification
CCI—Correct Coding Initiatives
CDM—Charge Description Master
CIM—Coverage Issues Manual
CPT—Current Procedural Terminology
CMS—Centers for Medicare and Medicaid Services
E/M—evaluation and management
HCPCS—Health Care Common Procedure Coding System
HIM—Health Information Management
ICD-9-CM—International Classification of Diseases, 9th Revision, Clinical Modification
IPPS—Inpatient Prospective Payment System
MCE—Medicare Code Editor
MCM—Medicare Carrier Manual
MS-DRG—Medicare Severity Diagnosis Related Groups
NCCI—National Correct Coding Initiatives
NCHS—National Center for Health Statistics
OCE—Medicare Outpatient Claim Editor
OPPS—Outpatient Prospective Payment System
PPS—Prospective Payment System
RBRVS—resource-based relative value scale
UB-04—CMS-1450 Universal Bill implemented in 2007.
UHDDS—Uniform Hospital Discharge Data Set

RELATIONSHIP BETWEEN BILLING AND CODING

To maintain financial stability, hospitals must bill patients and third-party payers for services rendered and obtain reimbursement in a timely manner. Billing is the process of submitting charges for services, procedures, and items to patients and third-party payers. The hospital billing process is complex, and it involves all functions required to bill for services rendered, as illustrated in Figure 9-1. Functions of the billing process are interrelated as various departments within the hospital complete them.

Each function in the process can be thought of as an individual step contributing to the completion of patient statements and claim forms. As discussed in previous chapters, the function of coding is integral to the billing process. The relationship between coding and billing is simply that coding is required to bill for services rendered. Codes are used on claim forms to describe diagnostic and therapeutic services, procedures, and items. Codes are also used to describe the patient's condition(s) and explain why the services were required. Figure 9-2 illustrates the relationship between coding and billing and the significance of documentation and claim forms in obtaining reimbursement for services provided.

As discussed in previous chapters, the billing process begins when the patient is received at the hospital for outpatient services or an inpatient admission. Patient care services are rendered and documented in the patient's medical record. Facility charges for services, procedures, and items are posted through the Charge Description Master (CDM), also referred to as the chargemaster, by various departments including the Health Information Management (HIM) Department. **Facility charges** represent the cost and overhead (technical component) of providing patient care services, including space, equipment, supplies, drugs and biologicals, and technical staff. All items listed in the chargemaster are associated with the appropriate procedure code that describes it (Figure 9-3). Professional services provided in a hospital-based clinic or primary care office are posted to the patient's account utilizing an encounter form. Charges for professional services represent the **professional component** of services that involves the physician or other non-physician provider's work in performing a service, such as administering anesthesia, performing surgery, or supervision and interpretation of a radiology procedure. The patient's medical record is reviewed to identify and code services rendered during the patient visit and the medical reason(s) why services were required.

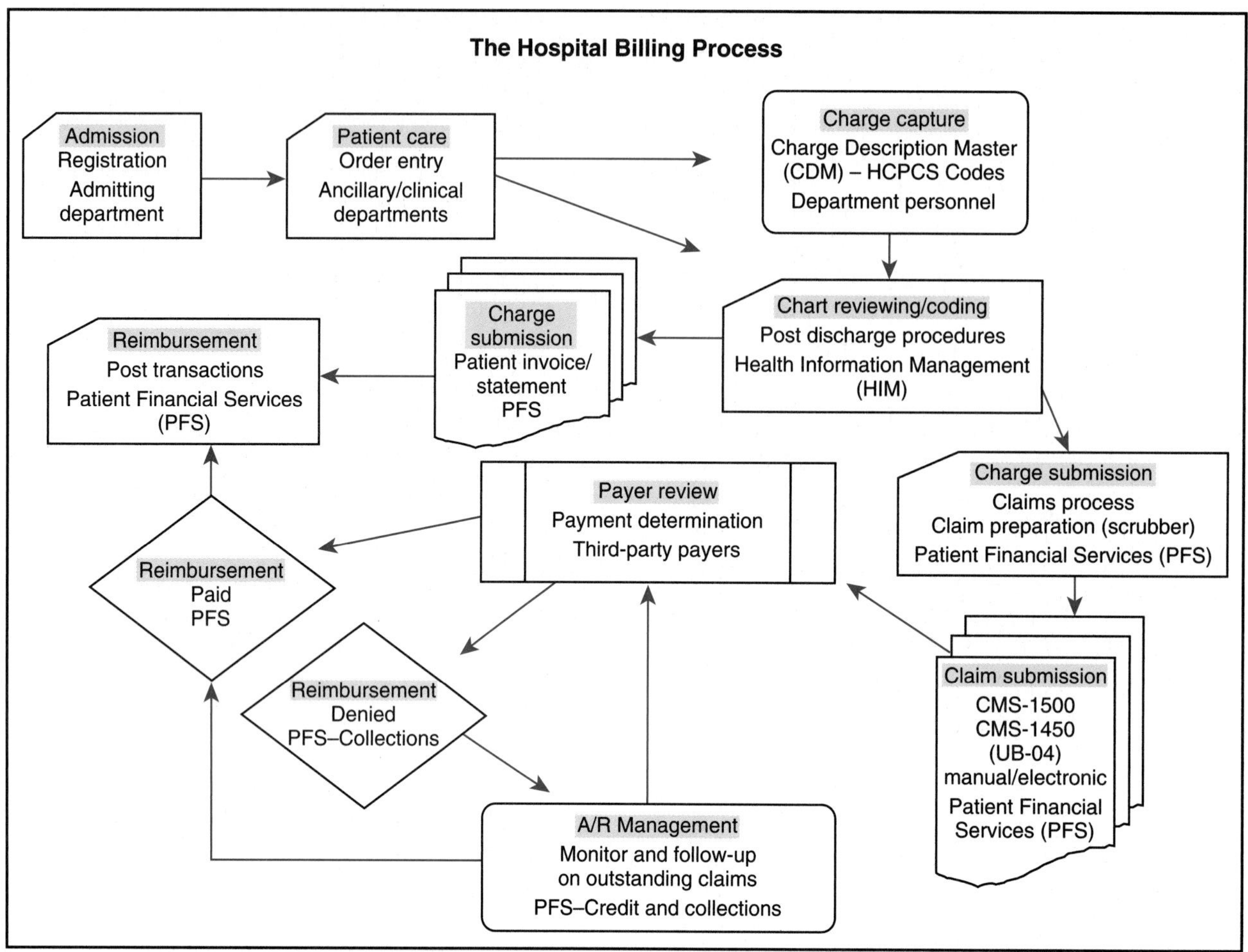

Figure 9-1 The hospital billing process illustrating functions required to bill for services rendered. *(Revision of illustration courtesy Sandra Giangreco.)*

BOX 9-1 ■ KEY POINTS

Relationship between Billing and Coding

Codes are used on claim forms to describe diagnostic and therapeutic services, procedures, and items. Codes are also used to describe the patient condition(s), explaining why the services were required.

ACCURATE CODING
plus
ACCURATE BILLING
helps to ensure receipt of
APPROPRIATE REIMBURSEMENT.

BOX 9-2 ■ KEY POINTS

Charge Description Master (CDM)

Chargemaster

Hospital charges are posted through the chargemaster. All services, procedures, and items listed in the chargemaster are associated with a HCPCS Level I CPT or Level II Medicare National Code.

Documentation and Coding

Documentation is a critical element in the coding and billing process because the medical record contains information regarding patient care services and the medical reason for services provided. The written descriptions of services, procedures, items, and patient conditions are translated into procedure or diagnosis codes as discussed in Chapters 7 and 8. Coders commonly refer to medical record documentation as source documents. Hospital source documents found in the medical record include the admission summary, history and physical, physician's orders, progress notes, ancillary department reports, medication records, and the discharge summary, as discussed in Chapter 4 (Figure 9-4). Other source documents may be an encounter form, a requisition, or an Emergency Department record. Documentation supports the charges submitted. Remember the Golden Rule in coding: **"IF IT IS NOT DOCUMENTED, DO NOT CODE IT."**

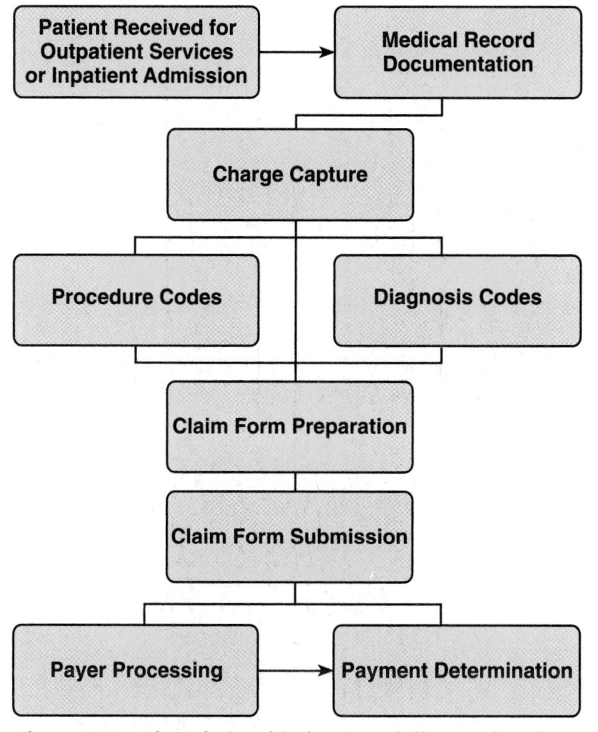

Figure 9-2 The relationship between billing and coding.

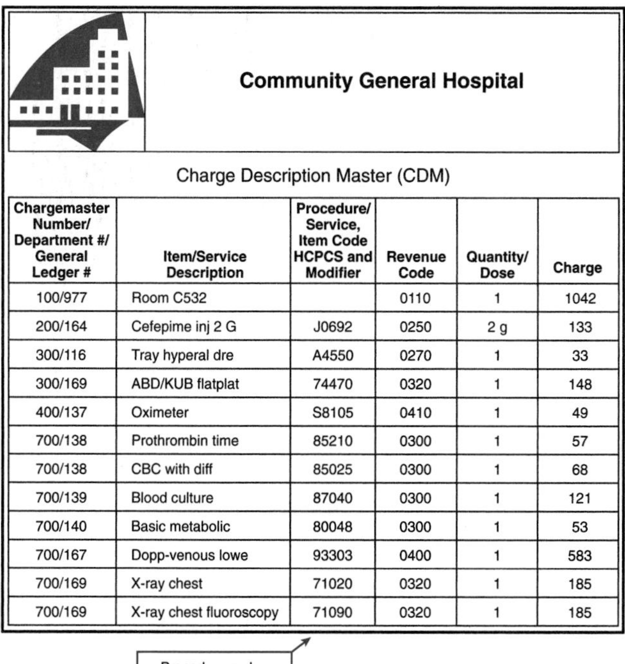

Community General Hospital

Charge Description Master (CDM)

Chargemaster Number/ Department #/ General Ledger #	Item/Service Description	Procedure/ Service, Item Code HCPCS and Modifier	Revenue Code	Quantity/ Dose	Charge
100/977	Room C532		0110	1	1042
200/164	Cefepime inj 2 G	J0692	0250	2 g	133
300/116	Tray hyperal dre	A4550	0270	1	33
300/169	ABD/KUB flatplat	74470	0320	1	148
400/137	Oximeter	S8105	0410	1	49
700/138	Prothrombin time	85210	0300	1	57
700/138	CBC with diff	85025	0300	1	68
700/139	Blood culture	87040	0300	1	121
700/140	Basic metabolic	80048	0300	1	53
700/167	Dopp-venous lowe	93303	0400	1	583
700/169	X-ray chest	71020	0320	1	185
700/169	X-ray chest fluoroscopy	71090	0320	1	185

Procedure codes

Figure 9-3 Hospital Charge Description Master (CDM) commonly referred to as the chargemaster.

BOX 9-3 ■ KEY POINTS

Documentation Supports Charges Submitted

The Golden Rule in coding is:
"IF IT IS NOT DOCUMENTED, DO NOT CODE IT"

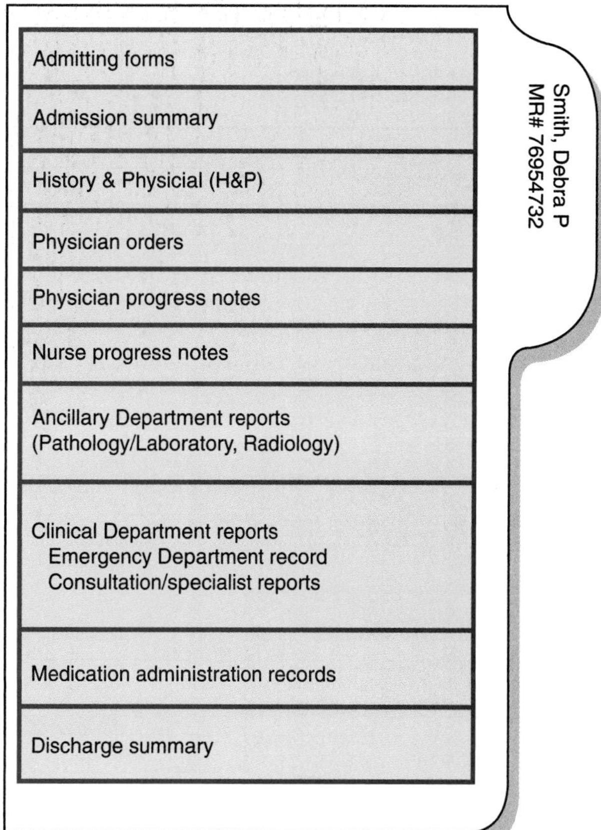

Figure 9-4 Source documents found in the patient's medical record.

BOX 9-4 ■ KEY POINTS

Coding and Claim Form Submission

Services, procedures, and items are coded. Codes are submitted on the claim form to explain charges and the medical reason for services rendered.

Claim Form Submission and Coding

Claim forms are prepared for submission of charges to third-party payers. Procedure and diagnosis codes are reported on the claim form to describe the services rendered and the medical reason (medical necessity) for them. Hospitals utilize two claim forms to submit charges (Figure 9-5). The CMS-1500 is used to submit charges for physician and outpatient professional services. The CMS-1450 (UB-04) is used to submit facility charges for outpatient, non-patient, and inpatient services. Health Care Common Procedure Coding System (HCPCS) Level I and II and International Classification of Diseases, 9th Revision, Clinical Modification (ICD-9-CM) Volume III procedure codes are reported in the appropriate fields on the claim form to describe services and items provided. ICD-9-CM Volume I and

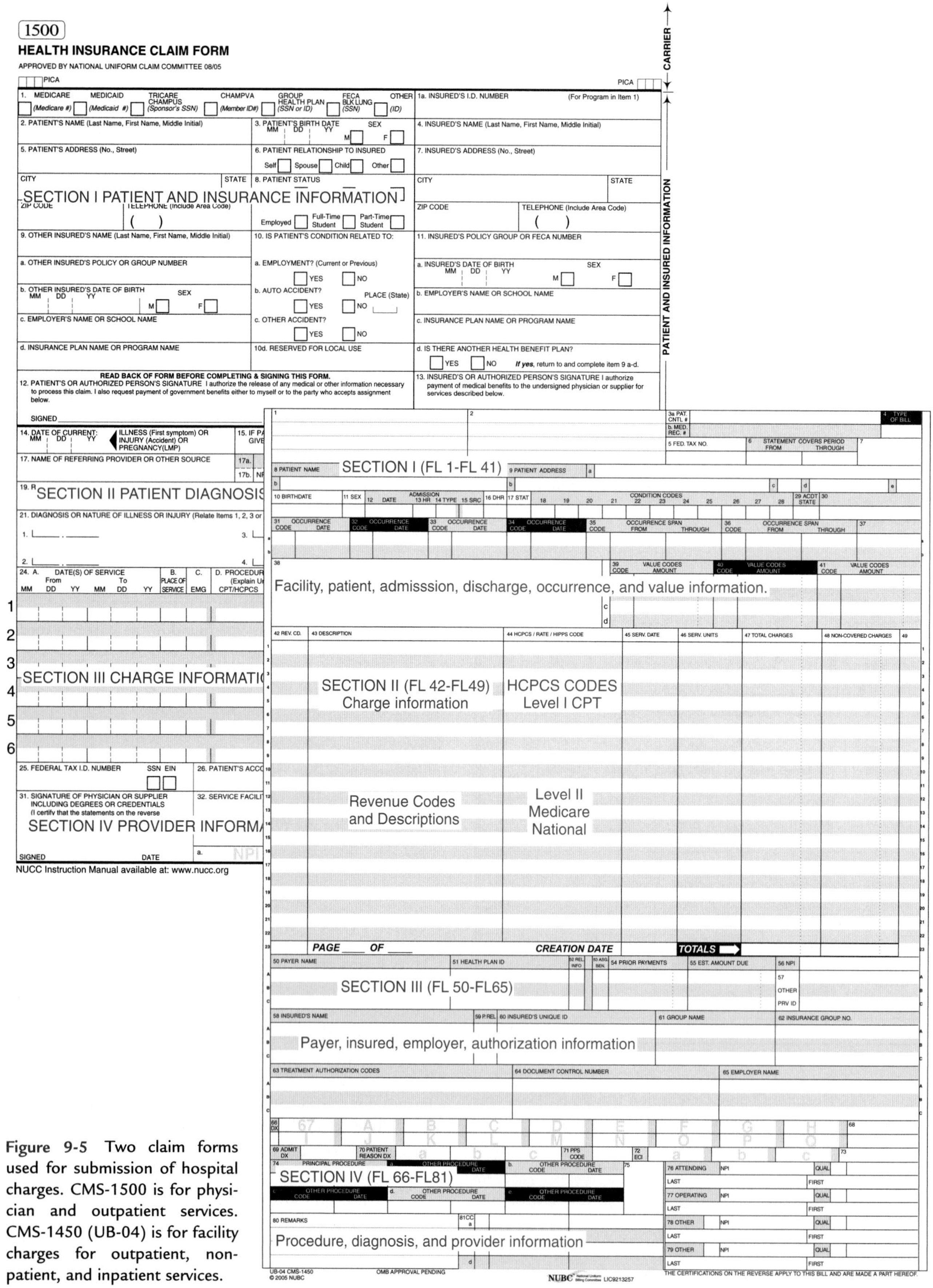

1500

HEALTH INSURANCE CLAIM FORM

APPROVED BY NATIONAL UNIFORM CLAIM COMMITTEE 08/05

PICA — PICA — CARRIER

1. MEDICARE (Medicare #) MEDICAID (Medicaid #) TRICARE CHAMPUS (Sponsor's SSN) CHAMPVA (Member ID#) GROUP HEALTH PLAN (SSN or ID) FECA BLK LUNG (SSN) OTHER (ID) | 1a. INSURED'S I.D. NUMBER (For Program in Item 1)

2. PATIENT'S NAME (Last Name, First Name, Middle Initial) | 3. PATIENT'S BIRTH DATE MM DD YY SEX M F | 4. INSURED'S NAME (Last Name, First Name, Middle Initial)

5. PATIENT'S ADDRESS (No., Street) | 6. PATIENT RELATIONSHIP TO INSURED Self Spouse Child Other | 7. INSURED'S ADDRESS (No., Street)

CITY STATE | 8. PATIENT STATUS | CITY STATE

SECTION I PATIENT AND INSURANCE INFORMATION

ZIP CODE TELEPHONE (Include Area Code) ( ) | Employed Full-Time Student Part-Time Student | ZIP CODE TELEPHONE (Include Area Code) ( )

9. OTHER INSURED'S NAME (Last Name, First Name, Middle Initial) | 10. IS PATIENT'S CONDITION RELATED TO: | 11. INSURED'S POLICY GROUP OR FECA NUMBER

a. OTHER INSURED'S POLICY OR GROUP NUMBER | a. EMPLOYMENT? (Current or Previous) YES NO | a. INSURED'S DATE OF BIRTH MM DD YY SEX M F

b. OTHER INSURED'S DATE OF BIRTH MM DD YY SEX M F | b. AUTO ACCIDENT? PLACE (State) YES NO | b. EMPLOYER'S NAME OR SCHOOL NAME

c. EMPLOYER'S NAME OR SCHOOL NAME | c. OTHER ACCIDENT? YES NO | c. INSURANCE PLAN NAME OR PROGRAM NAME

d. INSURANCE PLAN NAME OR PROGRAM NAME | 10d. RESERVED FOR LOCAL USE | d. IS THERE ANOTHER HEALTH BENEFIT PLAN? YES NO *If yes*, return to and complete item 9 a-d.

PATIENT AND INSURED INFORMATION

READ BACK OF FORM BEFORE COMPLETING & SIGNING THIS FORM.
12. PATIENT'S OR AUTHORIZED PERSON'S SIGNATURE I authorize the release of any medical or other information necessary to process this claim. I also request payment of government benefits either to myself or to the party who accepts assignment below.
13. INSURED'S OR AUTHORIZED PERSON'S SIGNATURE I authorize payment of medical benefits to the undersigned physician or supplier for services described below.

SIGNED

14. DATE OF CURRENT: MM DD YY ILLNESS (First symptom) OR INJURY (Accident) OR PREGNANCY(LMP) | 15. IF PA... GIVE...

17. NAME OF REFERRING PROVIDER OR OTHER SOURCE | 17a. | 17b. NP...

19. R... SECTION II PATIENT DIAGNOSIS

21. DIAGNOSIS OR NATURE OF ILLNESS OR INJURY (Relate Items 1, 2, 3 or ...

1. 3. 2. 4.

24. A. DATE(S) OF SERVICE From MM DD YY To MM DD YY | B. PLACE OF SERVICE | C. EMG | D. PROCEDUR... (Explain U... CPT/HCPCS

1 2 3 4 5 6

SECTION III CHARGE INFORMATI...

25. FEDERAL TAX I.D. NUMBER SSN EIN | 26. PATIENT'S ACC...

31. SIGNATURE OF PHYSICIAN OR SUPPLIER INCLUDING DEGREES OR CREDENTIALS (I certify that the statements on the reverse ... | 32. SERVICE FACILI...

SECTION IV PROVIDER INFORM...

SIGNED DATE | a. NPI

NUCC Instruction Manual available at: www.nucc.org

---

1 | 2 | 3a PAT. CNTL # | b. MED. REC. # | 4 TYPE OF BILL

5 FED. TAX NO. | 6 STATEMENT COVERS PERIOD FROM THROUGH | 7

8 PATIENT NAME — SECTION I (FL 1-FL 41) — 9 PATIENT ADDRESS

10 BIRTHDATE | 11 SEX | ADMISSION 12 DATE 13 HR 14 TYPE 15 SRC | 16 DHR | 17 STAT | CONDITION CODES 18 19 20 21 22 23 24 25 26 27 28 | 29 ACDT STATE | 30

31 OCCURRENCE CODE DATE | 32 OCCURRENCE CODE DATE | 33 OCCURRENCE CODE DATE | 34 OCCURRENCE CODE DATE | 35 OCCURRENCE SPAN CODE FROM THROUGH | 36 OCCURRENCE SPAN CODE FROM THROUGH | 37

38 | 39 VALUE CODES CODE AMOUNT | 40 VALUE CODES CODE AMOUNT | 41 VALUE CODES CODE AMOUNT

Facility, patient, admisssion, discharge, occurrence, and value information.

42 REV. CD. | 43 DESCRIPTION | 44 HCPCS / RATE / HIPPS CODE | 45 SERV. DATE | 46 SERV. UNITS | 47 TOTAL CHARGES | 48 NON-COVERED CHARGES | 49

SECTION II (FL 42-FL49) Charge information

HCPCS CODES Level I CPT

Revenue Codes and Descriptions

Level II Medicare National

PAGE ___ OF ___ CREATION DATE TOTALS

50 PAYER NAME | 51 HEALTH PLAN ID | 52 REL INFO | 53 ASG BEN. | 54 PRIOR PAYMENTS | 55 EST. AMOUNT DUE | 56 NPI | 57 OTHER PRV ID

SECTION III (FL 50-FL65)

58 INSURED'S NAME | 59 P.REL | 60 INSURED'S UNIQUE ID | 61 GROUP NAME | 62 INSURANCE GROUP NO.

Payer, insured, employer, authorization information

63 TREATMENT AUTHORIZATION CODES | 64 DOCUMENT CONTROL NUMBER | 65 EMPLOYER NAME

66 DX | 67 A B C D E F G H I J K L M N O P Q | 68

69 ADMIT DX | 70 PATIENT REASON DX a b c | 71 PPS CODE | 72 ECI a b c | 73

74 PRINCIPAL PROCEDURE CODE DATE | a. OTHER PROCEDURE CODE DATE | b. OTHER PROCEDURE CODE DATE | 75 | 76 ATTENDING NPI QUAL LAST FIRST

SECTION IV (FL 66-FL81)

c. OTHER PROCEDURE CODE DATE | d. OTHER PROCEDURE CODE DATE | e. OTHER PROCEDURE CODE DATE | 77 OPERATING NPI QUAL LAST FIRST

80 REMARKS | 81CC a b c d | 78 OTHER NPI QUAL LAST FIRST | 79 OTHER NPI QUAL LAST FIRST

Procedure, diagnosis, and provider information

UB-04 CMS-1450 © 2005 NUBC | OMB APPROVAL PENDING | NUBC National Uniform Billing Committee LIC9213257 | THE CERTIFICATIONS ON THE REVERSE APPLY TO THIS BILL AND ARE MADE A PART HEREOF.

Figure 9-5 Two claim forms used for submission of hospital charges. CMS-1500 is for physician and outpatient services. CMS-1450 (UB-04) is for facility charges for outpatient, nonpatient, and inpatient services.

TABLE 9-1 **Coding System Variations**

Hospital Service Categories (Facility Charges)	Diagnosis ICD-9-CM Volume I & II	PROCEDURES HCPCS Level I CPT	Level II Medicare National	Procedures ICD-9-CM Volume III	Variations
Outpatient					
Ambulatory surgery	√	√	*	†	
	Note: Some payers may require ICD-9-CM Volume III procedures for ambulatory surgery claim submitted on the CMS-1450 (UB-04)				
Emergency Department	√	√	*	†	*
Ancillary Departments:	√	√	*	†	*
Other Outpatient Services:	√	√	*	†	*
Durable medical equipment	√	√	*	†	*
Hospital-based primary care cffice	√	√	*	†	*
Other hospital-based clinic	√	√	*	†	*
Inpatient					
Inpatient services Inpatient procedures	√		*	√	ICD-9-CM Volume III procedure codes are utilized to reported significant procedures
Non-patient					
A specimen processed when the patient is not present	√	√	*		*

Data from Medicare 2005, Physician Fee Schedule.
√Coding procedure used.
*HCPCS Level I CPT codes are generally utilized to describe services and some items. HCPCS Level II Medicare National Codes are utilized when a CPT code cannot be found that adequately describes the service or item or when the payer requires a Level II code.
†ICD-9-C M Volume III code usage varies by payer. Generally required to report significant procedures on the CMS-1450 (UB-04) claim form.

II diagnosis codes are reported in the appropriate fields on the claim form to describe the medical reason for services provided. Table 9-1 illustrates coding system variations by service category for the UB-04 and CMS-1500.

Coding and Payer Processing

Third-party payer claim processing includes a detailed review of the claim form, as discussed in previous chapters (Figure 9-6). Payment determination is performed after the claim is reviewed.

Payer Edits

The payer's review of a claim includes computer edits of claim data. **Payer edits** involve a computer process designed to check data on the claim against the payer's data file and to check the codes submitted to identify problems related to services billed, such as coding errors or issues involving medical necessity. Data submitted on the claim is also reviewed against the payer's files to confirm eligibility and determine coverage. The codes submitted on the claim form are reviewed and compared to other clinical and demographic data to ensure the services billed are appropriate and to identify coding errors, as discussed in previous chapters. Computerized edits vary by payer. For example, Medicare's edits are referred to as the Medicare Code Editor (MCE) and the Outpatient Code Editor (OCE). Payer edits for outpatient services generally include the Medicare National Correct Coding Initiatives (CCI).

Medicare Code Editor (MCE)

The **Medicare Code Editor (MCE)** is a computerized program that incorporates various Medicare edits designed to check inpatient claim data to identify problems related to services billed, such as coding errors or issues involving medical necessity. All inpatient claims

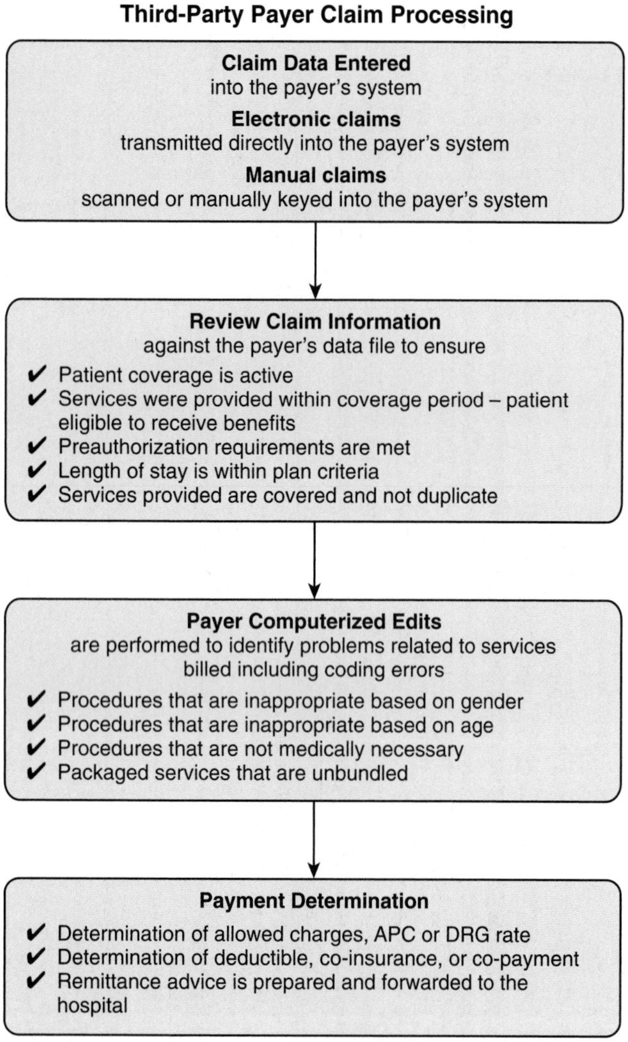

Third-Party Payer Claim Processing

Claim Data Entered
into the payer's system
Electronic claims
transmitted directly into the payer's system
Manual claims
scanned or manually keyed into the payer's system

↓

Review Claim Information
against the payer's data file to ensure
- ✔ Patient coverage is active
- ✔ Services were provided within coverage period – patient eligible to receive benefits
- ✔ Preauthorization requirements are met
- ✔ Length of stay is within plan criteria
- ✔ Services provided are covered and not duplicate

↓

Payer Computerized Edits
are performed to identify problems related to services billed including coding errors
- ✔ Procedures that are inappropriate based on gender
- ✔ Procedures that are inappropriate based on age
- ✔ Procedures that are not medically necessary
- ✔ Packaged services that are unbundled

↓

Payment Determination
- ✔ Determination of allowed charges, APC or DRG rate
- ✔ Determination of deductible, co-insurance, or co-payment
- ✔ Remittance advice is prepared and forwarded to the hospital

Figure 9-6 Phases of third-party payer claims processing includes entering data, review of claim information, computerized edits, and payment determination.

Medicare Outpatient Code Editor (OCE)	Medicare Code Editor (MCE)
Coding Edits ✔ Inpatient only procedure ✔ Invalid diagnosis or procedure code ✔ Age conflict ✔ Sex conflict ✔ Correct coding initiative edits **Coverage Edits** ✔ Non-covered procedures ✔ Questionable covered procedure **Clinical Edits** ✔ Invalid age ✔ Invalid sex **Claim Edits** ✔ Invalid date ✔ Date out of range ✔ Units of service edits ✔ Observation edits	**Inpatient Coding Edits** ✔ Invalid diagnosis or procedure code ✔ Invalid fourth or fifth digit for diagnosis codes ✔ E code used as a principal diagnosis ✔ Duplicate of the principal diagnosis ✔ Age conflict ✔ Sex conflict ✔ Manifestation code as principal diagnosis ✔ Nonspecific principal diagnosis ✔ Questionable admission ✔ Unacceptable principal diagnosis **Coverage Edits** ✔ Non-covered procedures ✔ Limited coverage ✔ Open biopsy ✔ Medicare secondary payer (MSP) alert **Inpatient Clinical Edits** ✔ Bilateral procedure ✔ Invalid age ✔ Invalid sex ✔ Invalid discharge status

Figure 9-7 Examples of edits incorporated in the Medicare Code Editor (MCE) for inpatient claims and the Outpatient Code Editor (OCE) for Medicare outpatient claims.

are processed through the MCE as required by the Centers for Medicare and Medicaid Services (CMS). The MCE includes inpatient coding edits, coverage edits, and inpatient clinical edits as outlined in Figure 9-7.

Medicare Outpatient Code Editor (OCE)

The **Medicare Outpatient Code Editor (OCE)** is a computerized program designed to check outpatient claim data to identify problems related to services billed, such as coding errors or issues involving medical necessity. OCE incorporates the National Correct Coding Initiatives (CCI) and other Medicare edits. All outpatient claims are processed through the OCE as required by CMS. The OCE includes edits related to HCPCS Level I and Level II codes. OCE has over 60 edits used to identify coding, coverage, clinical, and other claim issues.

Correct Coding Initiative (CCI)

The **Correct Coding Initiative (CCI)** was developed by the Centers for Medicare and Medicaid Services (CMS) to establish correct coding practices nationwide that would help to eliminate improper coding. The CCI is also referred to as the National Correct Coding Initiatives (NCCI). Implemented as a result of federal legislation, the CCI is designed to

> . . . ensure that uniform payment policies and procedures were followed by all carriers. The goal of the Correct Coding Initiative was to develop correct coding methodologies based on the coding conventions in the American Medical Association's Physicians' Current Procedural Terminology (CPT) book, national and local policies and edits, coding guidelines developed by national societies, analysis of standard medical and surgical practices, and review of current coding practices.*

The CCI was implemented in 1996 and it has been updated quarterly since its implementation. The CCI includes edits that provide explanation of coding situations that may be inappropriate and they are built into

*Medicare National Correct Coding Guide, Eden Prairie, Minn., Ingenix Inc.

National Correct Coding Initiatives Edits

Symbol ■ Comprehensive versus component code
Misuse of column 2 with column 1

Column 1	Column 2	Explanation
20605	J2001	**Procedures that would not typically be performed with other services but may be construed to represent other services are identified and paired with Column 1. Codes in Column 2 are generally not reported with a code from Column 1.** Code 20605 "Arthocentesis, aspiration and/or injection; major joint or bursa" should not be reported with J2001 "Injection, lidocaine HCl for intravenous infusion". The reasoning is that the injection of lidocaine is considered to be part of performing the arthrocentesis.

Symbol ▼ Most extensive procedure

Column 1	Column 2	Explanation
43632	43605	**Procedures that are the same but qualified by an increased level of complexity; the less extensive procedure is included in the more extensive procedure.** Code 43632 "Gastrectomy" and 43605 "Biopsy of Stomach" should not be reported together. Based on the most comprehensive procedure rule, 43605 is considered part of the "Gastrectomy" or a less complex procedure, therefore only the most comprehensive code 43632 should be reported.

Symbol ✓ Mutually exclusive procedures

Column 1	Column 2	Explanation
76856	76801	**Procedures that are generally not performed during the same session as they generally cannot be performed in the same session.** Code 76856 "Ultrasound, pelvic" and code 76801 "Ultrasound, pregnant uterus" would not be reported together as they are not typically performed in the same session.

Symbol ✚ CPT/HCPCS coding manual guideline

Column 1	Column 2	Explanation
87177	87015	**Coding instructions are provided in accordance with coding manual guidelines.** In accordance with CPT guidelines, code 87177 "Ova and parasites, direct smears" and code 87015 "Concentration (any type) for infectious agents" should not be reported together. CPT guidelines read "(Do not report 87177 in conjunction with 87105)".

Symbol ○ CPT separate procedure definition

Column 1	Column 2	Explanation
91032	91000	**Separate procedure definition states that when procedure is part of a more complex comprehensive service, it should not be reported separately.** Code 91032 "Esophagus, acid reflux test" and code 91000 "Esophageal intubation and collection of washings for cytology" should not be reported together as 91000 has a separate procedure designation.

Symbol ◆ CPT/HCPCS procedure code definitions

Column 1	Column 2	Explanation
99218	99217	**Code descriptions and instructions indicate correct coding relationships.** Code 99218 "Initial observation care" should not be reported with code 99217 "Observation care discharge" since the code reads "to report all services provided to a patient on discharge from "Observation status".

Symbol ❄ Standards of medical/surgical practice

Column 1	Column 2	Explanation
G0101	99201	**Procedures "activities" considered integral to performing another service.** Code G0101 "Cervical or vaginal cancer screening" can be performed by itself. When performed with a new patient office visit code 99201, standards of medical care, indicate the screening is part of the office visit and therefore code G0101 should not also be reported.

Figure 9-8 Examples of edits included in the National Correct Coding Initiatives, commonly referred to as the CCI. *(From Ingenix, Inc.: Medicare correct coding guide, Eden Prairie, Minn., Ingenix, Inc.)*

many billing software programs. CCI edits are published quarterly and applied based on the date of service. They can be obtained in manual format or they can be incorporated into some billing programs to ensure appropriate usage of codes and guidelines. Some of the most common CCI edits are outlined in Figure 9-8. The CCI provides edits for most all HCPCS Level I CPT codes and many of the HCPCS Level II National codes.

Payment Determination

When a claim satisfies all payer edits, payment determination is performed. Procedure and diagnosis codes submitted have a direct impact on reimbursement. The amount of reimbursement for outpatient services, procedures, or items is determined by the procedure code submitted. For example, hospital services provided to a Medicare patient are reimbursed under the Outpatient Prospective Payment System (OPPS), Ambulatory Payment Classification (APC). The APC reimbursement method assigns a payment amount based on the procedure code(s) submitted. Professional services provided to Medicare patients are reimbursed in accordance with the Medicare fee schedule that is based on the resource-based relative value scale (RBRVS). Table 9-2 illustrates a sample Medicare physician fee schedule. Services provided to Medicare patients on an inpatient basis are reimbursed under the Inpatient Prospective Payment System (IPPS), Medicare Severity Diagnosis Related Groups (MS-DRG). The MS-DRG reimbursement method assigns payment amounts for each MS-DRG. The MS-DRG is determined based on the diagnosis code(s) submitted in addition to the procedures and other clinical factors such as the age of the patient and discharge status. Prospective Payment Systems (PPS) will be discussed further in Chapter 13.

Submission of procedure or diagnosis codes that are incorrect will result in incorrect reimbursement, as illustrated in Figure 9-9. In accordance with the Medicare fee schedule, reimbursement for the code, submitted 99211, "Office or other outpatient Evaluation and Management (E/M) service," is $20.60. The record in this example supports a 99212 "Problem Focused E/M," and the reimbursement for this code is $36.82.

BOX 9-5 ■ KEY POINTS

Payment Determination

Impact of Coding

Procedure and diagnosis codes have a direct impact on payment determination because the payer calculates reimbursement based on codes submitted.

- Payer fee schedules list approved amounts by procedure code.
- The Outpatient Prospective Payment System (OPPS), APC payment rate is determined based on the procedure code submitted.
- The Inpatient Prospective Payment System (IPPS), MS-DRG rate is determined based on the diagnosis code(s) and procedure code(s) submitted and other clinical factors.

TABLE 9-2 Medicare Participating Physician Fee Schedule (Locality 01-04 Florida)

HCPCS Code and Modifier	LOC 01/02	LOC 03	LOC 04
17000	58.91	62.33	64.81
29822	567.93	609.93	650.83
37720	377.74	402.19	426.91
72010	63.22	68.34	72.36
72010-26	23.99	25.18	26.53
72020	23.27	25.09	26.44
72020-26	7.84	8.17	8.54
72040-TC	23.09	25.48	27.15
99201	35.41	37.14	38.48
99202	63.6	66.89	69.75
99203	94.68	99.67	104.13
99211	20.6	21.84	22.66
99212	36.82	38.66	40.06
99213	51.63	54.3	56.47
G0101	37.93	40.13	41.61
G0106	139.65	151.06	159.50
J0130	513.01	513.01	513.01
J0275	18.76	18.76	18.76

It is critical to understand the significance of coding. Coding describes what was done and why. Accurately describing information in the patient's record through the use of codes is essential to securing the appropriate reimbursement. The submission of inaccurate information that is not supported in the patient's record can cause delayed or reduced reimbursement. Submission of inaccurate information may also lead to investigations for fraud and abuse.

BOX 9-6 ■ KEY POINTS

Inaccurate Coding

Inaccurate coding can result in:
- Incorrect reimbursement.
- Payment denial.
- Third-party audit.
- Fraud or abuse investigation.

CODING SYSTEM VARIATIONS

The first step to accurate coding is to understand what coding system is required for submission of charges to payers. The coding system required varies based on the category of service. Four categories of service discussed in this text are outpatient, non-patient, professional, and inpatient services, as illustrated in Figure 9-10.

Coding and Reporting for a Hospital-Based Primary Care Visit

CMS-1500 Block 21
ICD-9-CM Diagnosis codes are reported on reference line 1-4

21. Diagnosis or nature of illness or injury, (relate item 1, 2, 3, or 4 to Item 24E by line) -------

1. 041.00 3. ___ . ___
2. ___ . ___ 4. ___ . ___

CMS-1500 Block 24
HCPCS Codes are reported on lines 1-6
ICD-9-CM Diagnosis code is linked to each procedure in 24E

24.	A DATE(S) OF SERVICE From	To	B Place of Service	C Type of Service	D PROCEDURES, SERVICES, OR SUPPLIES (Explain Unusual Circumstances) CPT/HCPCS	MODIFIER	E DIAGNOSIS CODE
	MM DD YY	MM DD					
1	06 09 06	06 09 06		11	99211		1
2	06 09 06	06 09 06		11	36415		1
3	06 09 06	06 09 06		11	85025		1

Medical Record

Established patient presents complaining of a sore throat for 4 days. Problem-focused evaluation and management service performed. Automated CBC performed with automated differential WBC count. Prescribed antibiotics. Will see patient in 10 days for a follow-up.

Diagnosis: Strep throat

Howard Fetterbeginn, M.D.

PROCEDURE AND DIAGNOSIS CODE ASSIGNMENT

Evaluation and Management HCPCS Level I CPT **99212**
Venipuncture **36415**
Complete Blood Count (CBC) **85025**

DIAGNOSIS CODE FROM LAST CHAPTER
Strep throat **041.00**

Figure 9-9 Example of incorrect code submission.

TEST YOUR *Knowledge* BOX 9-1

RELATIONSHIP BETWEEN BILLING AND CODING

1. The billing process is critical to hospitals maintaining ______________.

2. ______________ is the process of submitting charges for services, procedures, and items to patients and third-party payers.

3. Services provided in a hospital-based clinic or primary care office are posted to the ______________ utilizing an ______________ ______________.

4. Provide a brief explanation of the relationship between coding and billing.

5. State the relationship between procedure codes and the Charge Description Master.

6. Define coding.

7. Source documents used for coding are found in the medical record. List other source documents utilized by coders in addition to documents in the patient's medical record.

8. Explain why documentation is a critical element in the coding and billing process.

9. What is the Golden Rule in coding?

10. State the relationship between diagnosis codes and medical necessity.

11. Two claim forms utilized to submit charges to third-party payers are the ______________, used to submit charges for physician and outpatient services, and the ______________, used to submit facility charges.

12. Discuss the purpose of payer edits.

13. The codes submitted on the claim form will be reviewed and compared to other clinical and demographic data to ensure the services billed are ______________, and to ______________.

14. Provide a description of how payment is determined for Medicare inpatient services.

15. Explain how procedure codes relate to reimbursement for outpatient services.

TEST YOUR *Knowledge* BOX 9-1

RELATIONSHIP BETWEEN BILLING AND CODING—*cont'd*

16. Explain the difference between the Medicare Code Editor (MCE) and the Medicare Outpatient Code Editor (OCE).

17. The OCE has over 60 edits used to identify ______________, ______________, ______________, and other claim issues including the Correct Coding Initiatives.

18. Discuss the goal of CCI.

19. Explain how CCI edits are obtained, and how CCI is used.

20. MS-DRG reimbursement for inpatient services is based on ______________ codes, procedures, and other clinical factors.

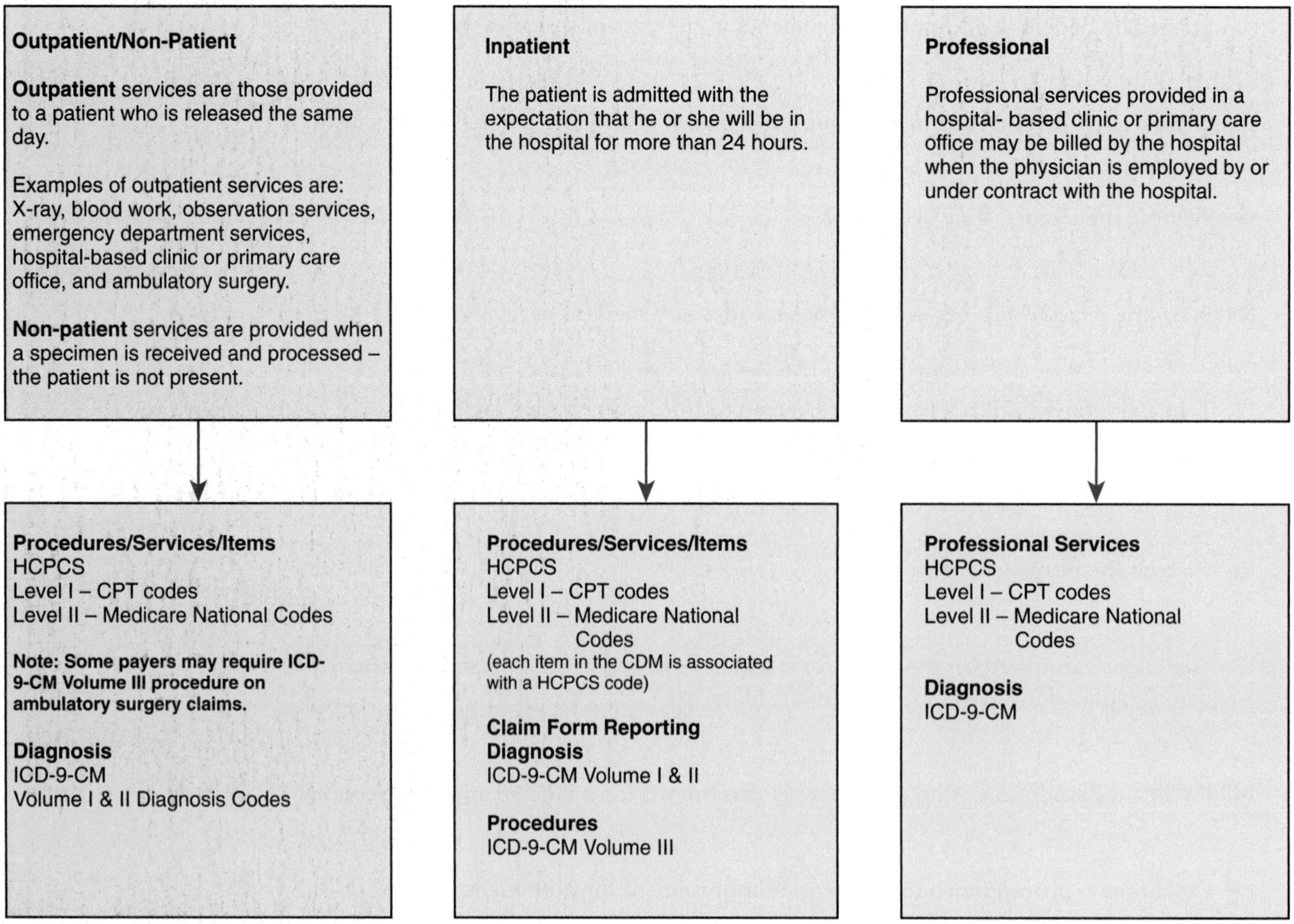

Outpatient/Non-Patient

Outpatient services are those provided to a patient who is released the same day.

Examples of outpatient services are: X-ray, blood work, observation services, emergency department services, hospital-based clinic or primary care office, and ambulatory surgery.

Non-patient services are provided when a specimen is received and processed – the patient is not present.

↓

Procedures/Services/Items
HCPCS
Level I – CPT codes
Level II – Medicare National Codes

Note: Some payers may require ICD-9-CM Volume III procedure on ambulatory surgery claims.

Diagnosis
ICD-9-CM
Volume I & II Diagnosis Codes

Inpatient

The patient is admitted with the expectation that he or she will be in the hospital for more than 24 hours.

↓

Procedures/Services/Items
HCPCS
Level I – CPT codes
Level II – Medicare National Codes
(each item in the CDM is associated with a HCPCS code)

Claim Form Reporting
Diagnosis
ICD-9-CM Volume I & II

Procedures
ICD-9-CM Volume III

Professional

Professional services provided in a hospital- based clinic or primary care office may be billed by the hospital when the physician is employed by or under contract with the hospital.

↓

Professional Services
HCPCS
Level I – CPT codes
Level II – Medicare National Codes

Diagnosis
ICD-9-CM

Figure 9-10 Coding system variations by service category.

BOX 9-7 ■ KEY POINTS

Coding System Variations for Outpatient and Non-Patient

Services, Procedures, and Items

HCPCS Level I CPT Codes
HCPCS Level II Medicare National Codes

Diagnosis

ICD-9-CM Volume I and II Diagnosis Codes
Note: Some payers may require ICD-9-CM volume III procedure code (s) for ambulatory surgery claims.

Outpatient and Non-Patient Services

Coding system and claim form requirements for outpatient and non-patient services are outlined in Figure 9-11. Hospital outpatient and non-patient facility charges are submitted for services provided by various departments within the hospital. Outpatient and non-patient services include ambulatory surgery, emergency room, observation, radiology, and pathology/laboratory. These facility charges are generally reported in form locator (FL) 44 on the UB-04, as required by the payer. The coding systems utilized are HCPCS Level I CPT and Level II National procedure codes. ICD-9-CM Volume I and II diagnosis codes are used to report patient conditions in FL 67, 69, 70, 72. An example of outpatient and non-patient coding and claim form reporting is illustrated in Figures 9-12 and 9-13.

Outpatient Professional Services

Coding system and claim form requirements for professional services are outlined in Figure 9-14. Hospitals may submit charges for professional services performed

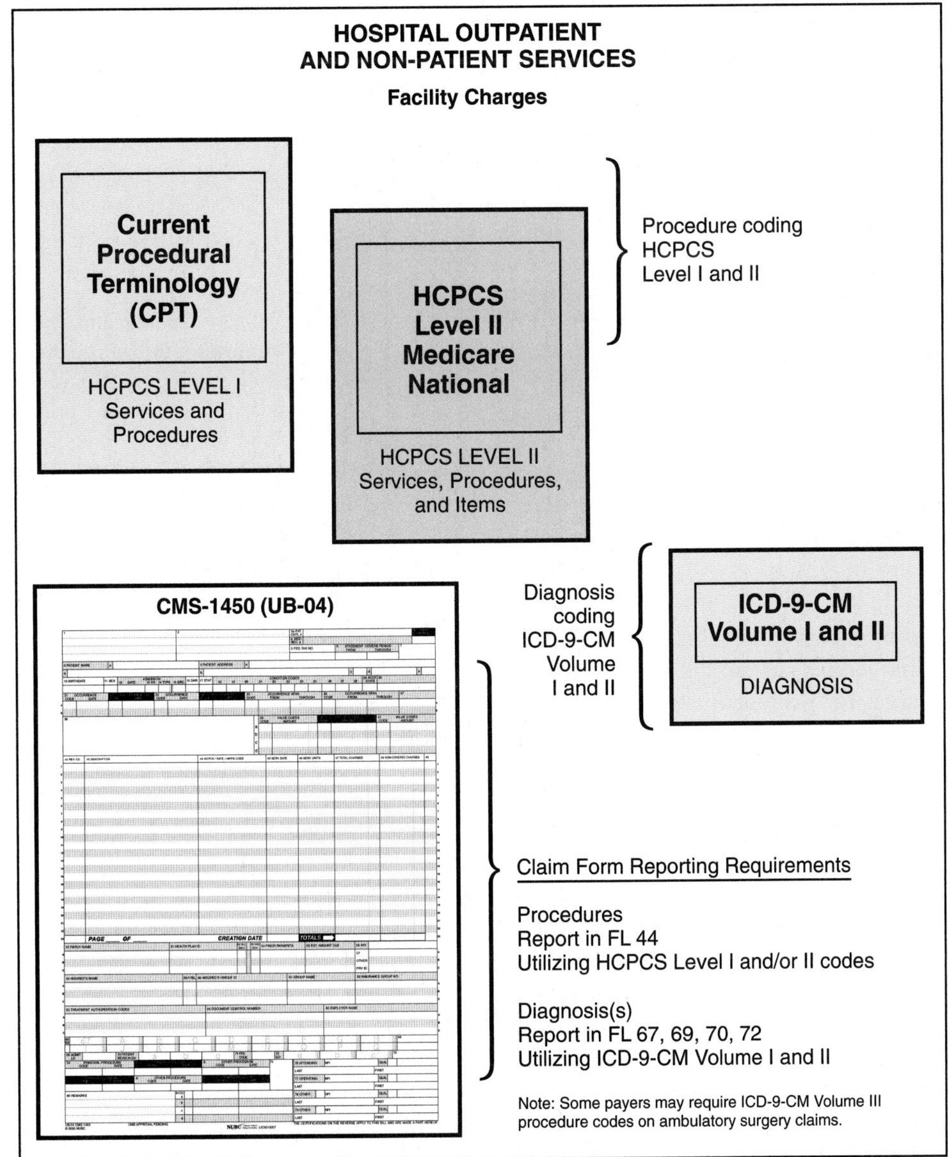

Figure 9-11 Coding and claim form requirements, outpatient and non-patient services.

Hospital Outpatient Services

CMS-1450 (UB-04)
Services are grouped into revenue code categories and reported in FL 42-49
HCPCS Level I and II codes are recorded in FL 44

42 REV. CD.	43 DESCRIPTION	44 HCPCS/ RATES
0270	Medical surgical supplies and devices	A4306
0450	Emergency room general	99281 25
0450	Emergency room general	13121

ICD-9-CM Volume I and II diagnosis codes are recorded in FL 67, 69, 70, 72

67 PRIN. DIAG. CD.	OTHER DIAG. CODES			69 ADM. DIAG. CODE	72 E-CODE
	67A CODE	B CODE	C-Q CODE		
891.0				733.99	

Medical Record
Emergency Department Visit

Patient presents to the emergency department with a 4.5 cm laceration on the left leg. A Level II E/M performed. Debridement and complex repair of wound was done. Disposable drug delivery system, flow rate of 5 mL per hour was utilized.

Johnathan Sampson, M.D.

PROCEDURE CODE ASSIGNMENTS
13121 "Repair, complex, legs 2.6 cm to 7.5 cm"
99282 "Emergency department visit", Level II
A4306 "Disposable drug delivery system, flow rate of 5 mL or less per hour"

DIAGNOSIS CODE ASSIGNMENT
891.0 "Open wound of leg without mention of complication"

Services are reported in revenue code categories 0270 and 0450

Figure 9-12 Coding and claim form reporting for outpatient services illustrating HCPCS codes recorded in FL 44 and the principal and admitting diagnoses recorded in FL 67 and FL 69 on the CMS-1450 (UB-04).

Hospital Non-Patient Services

CMS-1450 (UB-04)
Services are grouped into revenue code categories and reported in FL 42-49
HCPCS Level I and II codes are recorded in FL 44

42 REV. CD.	43 DESCRIPTION	44 HCPCS/ RATES
0300	LABORATORY–GENERAL	80525

ICD-9-CM Volume I and II diagnosis codes are recorded in FL 67, 69, 70, 72

67 PRIN. DIAG. CD.	OTHER DIAG. CODES			69 ADM. DIAG. CODE	72 E-C
	67A CODE	B CODE	C-Q CODE		
041.00				041.00	

Medical Record
Non-patient Service

Patient blood specimen received from Dr. Holdermeyer's office. Suspected strep throat. Automated CBC performed with automated differential WBC count. Diagnosis: Strep throat

Dr. Sampherson

PROCEDURE CODE ASSIGNMENT
80525 "Complete Blood Count (CBC)"

DIAGNOSIS CODE ASSIGNMENT
041.00 "Strep throat 041.00"

Services are reported in Revenue Code Category 0300

Figure 9-13 Coding and claim form reporting for non-patient services illustrating HCPCS codes recorded in FL 44 and the principal and admitting diagnoses recorded in FL 67 and FL 69 on the CMS-1450 (UB-04).

by physicians in a hospital-based physician office or clinic when the physician is employed by or under contract with the hospital. The charges for professional services are reported on the CMS-1500. The patient's diagnosis is reported utilizing ICD-9-CM Volume I and II diagnosis codes in Block 21. Services and items are described utilizing HCPCS Level I and II procedure codes that are reported in Block 24D. Each procedure is linked with a diagnosis by indicating a reference line number from Block 21 in Block 24E. An example of coding and claim form reporting for hospital professional charges is illustrated in Figure 9-15.

Inpatient Services

Coding and claim form requirements for hospital inpatient services are outlined in Figure 9-16. Hospitals submit facility charges for inpatient services on the UB-04. All services provided during the patient stay are grouped into revenue code categories that are listed on an individual line in FL 42-49. The services are posted through the chargemaster by various hospital departments including the HIM Department. Each item in the chargemaster is associated with an HCPCS code. HCPCS codes are not required in FL 44 for inpatient claims, however, they are printed on the detailed itemized statement. ICD-9-CM Volume I and II diagnosis codes are used to report the admitting, principal, and other diagnoses in FL 67, 69, 70, 72. Significant procedures performed during the visit are reported using ICD-9-CM Volume III codes and they are reported in FL 74a-e. An example of coding systems and claim form requirements for hospital inpatient services are outlined in Figure 9-17.

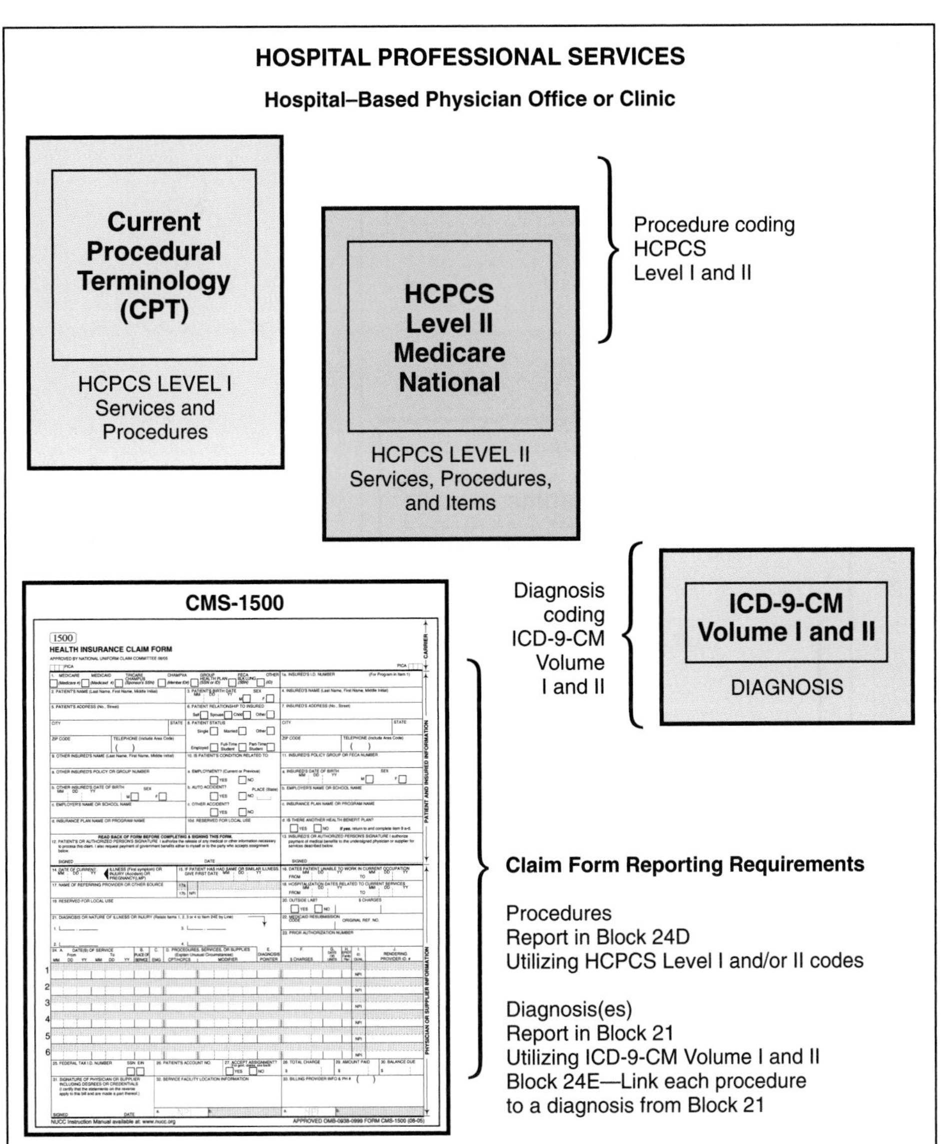

Figure 9-14 Coding system and claim form requirements for professional services.

Hospital Professional Services

CMS-1500

ICD-9-CM Diagnosis Codes are Recorded in Block 21 (lines 1-4)

21. Diagnosis or nature of illness or injury, (relate item 1, 2, 3, or 4 to Item 24E by line)

1. 041.00 3. ___.___

2. ___.___ 4. ___.___

Medical Record
Hospital Based Primary Care Office

Established patient presents complaining of a sore throat for 4 days. Problem-focused evaluation and management service performed. Automated CBC performed with automated differential WBC count. Prescribed antibiotics. Will see patient in 10 days for a follow-up.

Diagnosis: Strep throat

Howard Fetterbeginn, M.D.

PROCEDURE CODE ASSIGNMENT

Evaluation and Management	**99212**
Venipuncture	**36415**
Complete Blood Count (CBC)	**85025**

DIAGNOSIS CODE ASSIGNMENT

Strep throat	**041.00**

HCPCS Level I and II codes are recorded in Block 24D (lines 1-6)
Each procedure is linked with a diagnosis from 21

24.	A DATE(S) OF SERVICE From MM DD YY	To MM DD YY	B Place of Service	C Type of Service	D PROCEDURES, SERVICES, OR SUPPLIES (Explain Unusual Circumstances) CPT/HCPCS	MODIFIER	E DIAGNOSIS POINTER
1	06 09 06	06 09 06		11	99212		1
2	06 09 06	06 09 06		11	36415		1
3	06 09 06	06 09 06		11	85025		1

Figure 9-15 Coding and claim form reporting for professional services illustrating diagnosis codes recorded in Block 21, HCPCS codes recorded in Block 24D, and the diagnosis code linked to the procedure code in 24E.

Hospital Inpatient Services
Facility Charges
Cost and overhead of providing patient care services in the hospital: accommodations (room and board/operating and recovery rooms), medical/surgical supplies, instruments, equipment, pharmacy, and ancillary services.
ICD-9-CM Volume III
PROCEDURES
ICD-9-CM Volume III required on the CMS-1450 (UB-04)
Diagnosis coding ICD-9-CM Volume I and II
ICD-9-CM Volume I and II
DIAGNOSIS
CMS-1450 (UB-04)
Claim Form Reporting Requirements
Procedures
Report significant procedures in FL 74a-e
Utilizing HCPCS ICD-9-CM
Volume III procedure codes
Diagnosis(es)
Report in FL 67, 69, 70, 72
Utilizing ICD-9-CM Volume I and II
diagnosis codes

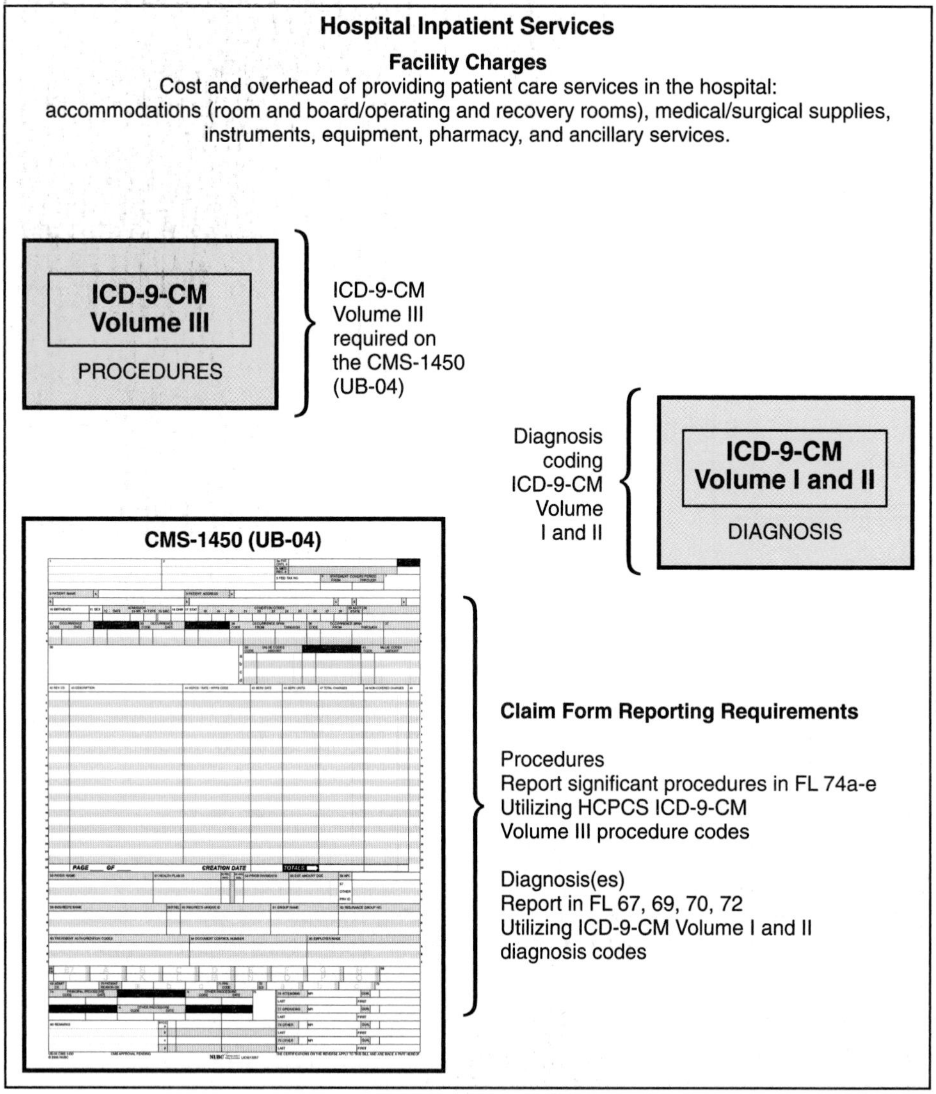

Figure 9-16 Coding system and claim form requirements for inpatient services.

BOX 9-8 ■ KEY POINTS

Coding System Variations for Inpatient

Services, Procedures, and Items

Listed in the chargemaster associated with the appropriate

- HCPCS Level I CPT Code or
- HCPCS Level II Medicare National Code
- HCPCS codes are not required on inpatient claims

ICD-9-CM Volume III Procedure Codes are reported on the claim form

Diagnosis

ICD-9-CM Volume I and II Diagnosis Codes

To ensure accurate and effective coding, coders should develop good coding habits such as "never code from the index" and "if it is not documented, do not code." A coder must be consistent in the process he or she follows to assign a code, and a coder must follow those good coding habits in every coding situation (Figure 9-18).

Accurate coding requires knowledge of coding system formats, content, and principles. Knowledge of coding guidelines is also essential to accurate coding. Coding guidelines vary according to the category of service performed, as discussed previously. To gain an understanding of the variations, we will explore outpatient and inpatient coding guidelines utilizing ICD-9-CM Volume I and II diagnosis codes, HCPCS, and ICD-9-CM Volume III procedure codes.

ICD-9-CM OFFICIAL DIAGNOSIS CODING GUIDELINES

Diagnosis coding guidelines are developed for the purpose of providing instruction and clarification to coding and billing professionals. Guidelines used for outpatient services vary from those used when coding

Hospital Inpatient Services

CMS-1450 (UB-04)

FL 42 – Services are grouped in revenue code categories

FL 44 – HCPCS Level I and II codes are not required in FL 44 on an inpatient claim

42 REV. CD.	43 DESCRIPTION	44 HCPCS/ RATES	45 SERV. DATE	46 SERV. UNITS	47 TOTAL CHARGES
0101	ALL INCL R & B	600.00		2	1,200.00
0481	CARDIAC CATH LAB			1	4,733.00
0620	MED SURG SUPPLIES			1	124.00
0730	EKG			1	95.00

FL 67, 69, 70, 72 ICD-9-CM Diagnosis Codes

67 PRIN. DIAG. CD.	OTHER DIAG. CODES					
	67A CODE	B CODE	C CODE	D-Q CODE	69 ADM. DIAG. CODE	72 E CODE
427.9					786.50	

FL 74 A-E ICD-9-CM Volume III Procedure Codes

74 PRINCIPAL PROCEDURE CODE	DATE	74a OTHER PROCEDURE CODE	DATE
37.21	05 17 06		
OTHER PROCEDURE CODE	DATE	OTHER PROCEDURE	

Medical Record
Inpatient Visit

05/17/06

Patient JB was admitted to the hospital as he was experiencing severe chest pain. An EKG was performed which showed arrhythmia. The patient underwent a right heart catheterization. Right heart cardiac catheterization showed no findings. One irrigation tray was used. The patient tolerated the procedure well. The patient was discharged two days later.

Dr. Howard Jones, M.D.

Charge Sheet–Charges posted through the charge master

REVENUE CODES/ DESCRIPTION		CHARGES	HCPCS CODE
0101	All inclusive Room & Board	1,200.00	
0730	EKG	95.00	93000
0481	Cardiac Cath Lab	4,733.00	93501
0620	Med Surg Supplies	124.00	A4320

HIM Coding Performed After Discharge

Admitting Diagnosis:	786.50	Chest Pain
Principal Diagnosis	427.9	Arrhythmia
Principal Procedure	37.21	Right Heart Catheterization

Figure 9-17 Coding and claim form reporting for inpatient services illustrating principal, other, and admitting diagnosis codes recorded in FL 67, 69, 70, 72. and the principal procedure is reported using ICD-9-CM Volume III procedure codes in FL 74a-e.

Good Coding Habits

✓ **If it is not documented, DO NOT CODE IT**

✓ **Never code only from the INDEX**

✓ **Review all codes in the CODE RANGE**

✓ **When in doubt ASK**

✓ **E codes NEVER FIRST-LISTED**

✓ **CONSISTENCY is critical**

Figure 9-18 Good coding habits. *(Modified illustration courtesy Laurie Maurhoff.)*

BOX 9-9 ■ KEY POINTS

Facility versus Professional Charges

Facility Charges

Charges that represent the cost and overhead for providing patient care services, which include space, equipment, supplies, drugs and biologicals, and technical staff. Facility charges represent the technical component of services.

Professional Charges

Charges that represent the portion of a procedure that involves the physician or other non-physician provider's work in performing a service, such as administering anesthesia, performing surgery, or supervision and interpretation of a radiology procedure. Professional charges represent the professional component of services.

inpatient services. The official guidelines provide instruction for specific outpatient and inpatient coding when the ICD-9-CM manual does not provide clarification. The ICD-9-CM manual also contains general coding guidelines that are applicable to coding for all health care settings.

Official guidelines for coding utilizing ICD-9-CM Volume I and II diagnosis codes are provided by the CMS and the National Center for Health Statistics (NCHS). It is recommended that the guidelines be used in addition to the ICD-9-CM coding manual. The guidelines for coding and reporting diagnoses have been approved by the cooperating parties for ICD-9-CM: the American Hospital Association, American Health Information Management Association, Centers for Medicare and Medicaid Services, and National Center for Health Statistics (Figure 9-19). The guidelines are published by the Department of Health and Human Services (DHHS) and have also been referenced in the *Coding Clinic for ICD-9-CM*, published by the American Hospital Association (AHA). The guidelines have been developed to assist coders in reporting situations for which the ICD-9-CM manual does not provide direction. The official guidelines are broken down into the following four sections:

I. ICD-9-CM conventions, general coding guidelines, and chapter-specific guidelines. These guidelines are applicable to all health care settings.
II. Selection of principal diagnosis for inpatient, short-term acute care hospital records.

TEST YOUR *Knowledge* BOX 9-2

CODING SYSTEM VARIATIONS

1. Services performed on a specimen when the patient is not present are ______________ services.

2. What claim form is used to report hospital outpatient and non-patient services?

3. Coding systems used to report hospital outpatient and non-patient services are ______________, ______________ and ______________.

4. Explain when a hospital may bill for professional services.

5. Charges for professional services are reported using the ______________ claim form.

6. ____________, ____________, ____________ are coding systems used to report professional services.

7. Discuss how procedures are linked with diagnoses on the CMS-1500.

8. Facility charges for inpatient services are reported on the ______________ claim form.

9. What coding systems are reported on the CMS-1450 (UB-04) for inpatient claims?

10. Each HCPCS code is associated with each item in the ______________.

11. Diagnosis codes are reported in Block ______________ and procedure codes are reported in Block ______________ on the CMS-1500.

12. HCPCS Level I and II codes are reported in FL ______________ on the CMS-1450 (UB-04) for hospital outpatient services.

13. All services provided are grouped by revenue code category and listed on an individual line in FL ______________.

14. Coding systems used to submit charges to third party payers vary based on the ______________.

15. ______________ services are those that are performed on the same day the patient is released.

TEST YOUR *Knowledge* BOX 9-2

CODING SYSTEM VARIATIONS—*cont'd*

Explain what claim form and procedure coding systems hospitals use to report the following services:

16. Emergency Department

17. Ambulatory surgery

18. Doctor visit at a hospital-based clinic

19. Inpatient

20. Laboratory test performed when the patient is not present.

ICD-9-CM Coordination and Maintenance Committee

Organization	Responsibilities
American Hospital Association (AHA)	• Maintains Central Office on ICD-9-CM • Approves official coding guidelines • Publishes *Coding Clinic*
American Health Information Management Association (AHIMA)	• Certifies coders • Provides coding education • Sponsors Council on Coding and Classification and the Society for Clinical Coding • Approves official coding guidelines
Centers for Medicare and Medicaid Services (CMS)	• Maintains the procedure classification • Approves official coding guidelines
National Center for Health Statistics (NCHS)	• Maintains the disease classification • Approves official coding guidelines

Figure 9-19 ICD-9-CM cooperating parties. *(Modified from Abdelhak M, Grostick S, Hanken MA, Jacobs E:* Health information: management of a strategic resource, *ed 2, St Louis, 2001, Saunders.)*

III. Reporting additional diagnoses for inpatient, short-term acute care hospital records.
IV. Diagnostic coding and report guidelines for outpatient services.

The complete ICD-9-CM Official Guidelines for Reporting are outlined in the front of most ICD manuals. As outlined in the official guidelines, there are variations in reporting diagnoses for outpatient versus inpatient services. This section provides an overview of some of the more significant guidelines for outpatient and inpatient services.

ICD-9-CM General Diagnosis Coding Guidelines

The ICD-9-CM general coding guidelines include good coding habits and they must be applied accurately when coding diagnostic statements from the patient's medical record. Coders must master an understanding and effective application of ICD-9-CM guidelines to ensure that accurate descriptions of the patient's conditions and procedures performed are submitted on the claim and that proper reimbursement is received. These

BOX 9-10 ■ KEY POINTS

ICD-9-CM Official Diagnosis Coding Guideline Sections

I. ICD-9-CM Conventions, General Coding Guidelines and Chapter-Specific Guidelines. These guidelines are applicable to all health care settings.
II. Selection of Principal Diagnosis for Inpatient, Short-Term, Acute Care Hospital Records.
III. Reporting Additional Diagnoses for Inpatient, Short-Term, Acute Care Hospital Records.
IV. Diagnostic Coding and Report Guidelines for Outpatient Services.

ICD-9-CM General Diagnosis Coding Guidelines

- Code only conditions that are treated (or managed), have an affect on treatment, or extend the patient's stay, including complications and co-morbidities.
- Code only conditions that are recorded in the patient's medical record.

Remember the Golden Rule in coding

"IF IT IS NOT DOCUMENTED, DO NOT CODE IT"

- Always use the ICD-9-CM Volume II alphabetic index and the Volume I tabular section to identify and select codes.
- Code to the highest level of specificity.
- Codes that describe symptoms and signs, as opposed to diagnoses, are acceptable for reporting purposes when a related definitive diagnosis has not been established.
- When the patient presents with problems other than signs, symptoms, injury, illness, or disease, code the reason for the visit utilizing ICD-9-CM code ranges V01 through V89 (Supplemental Classification of Factors Influencing Health Status and Contact with Health Services).
- A single condition may require multiple coding. Codes may describe conditions that are due to an underlying cause. The underlying condition is listed first.
- Acute and chronic conditions may be recorded in the patient record. If the same condition is described as both acute (subacute) and chronic, and separate subentries exist in the Alphabetic Index at the same indentation level, code both and sequence the acute (subacute) code first.
- A patient condition may be a Late Effect. A late effect is the residual effect (condition produced) after the acute phase of an illness or injury has terminated. Two codes are generally required. The condition or nature of the late effect is sequenced first. The late effect code is sequenced second.

Figure 9-20 ICD-9-CM general diagnosis coding guidelines. *(Data from* International classification of diseases, 9th revision, *U.S. Department of Health and Human Services, Public Health Service, Centers for Medicare and Medicaid Services.)*

guidelines provide instruction to coders regarding what conditions should be coded, how to use the coding system, and other specific instructions regarding code selection. ICD-9-CM general coding guidelines are outlined in Figure 9-20 and include the following:

- Code only conditions that are treated (or managed), have an effect on treatment, or extend the patient's stay, including complications and co-morbidities.
- Code only conditions that are recorded in the patient's medical record.
- Always use the ICD-9-CM Volume II alphabetic index and Volume I tabular section to identify and select codes.
- Code to the highest level of specificity.
- Codes that describe symptoms and signs, as opposed to diagnoses, are acceptable for reporting purposes when a related definitive diagnosis has not been established.
- When the patient presents with problems other than signs, symptoms, injury, illness, or disease, code the reason for the visit utilizing ICD-9-CM code ranges V01 through V89 (Supplemental Classification of Factors Influencing Health Status and Contact with Health Services).
- A single condition may require multiple coding. Codes may describe conditions that result from an underlying cause. The underlying condition is listed first.
- Acute and chronic conditions may be recorded in the patient record. If the same condition is described as both acute (subacute) and chronic, and separate subentries exist in the alphabetic index at the same indentation level, code both and sequence the acute (subacute) code first.
- A patient condition may be a late effect. A late effect is the residual effect (condition produced) after the acute phase of an illness or injury has terminated. Two codes are generally required. The condition or nature of the late effect is sequenced first. The late effect code is sequenced second.

BOX 9-11 ■ KEY POINTS

ICD-9-CM Official Outpatient Diagnosis Coding Guidelines

I. Selection of the first-listed condition (primary diagnosis).
II. Uncertain diagnoses are not coded.
III. Diagnostic tests require the reason for test or the definitive diagnosis documented in the record.
IV. Ambulatory surgery requires the postoperative diagnosis to be coded if it is different from the preoperative diagnosis.

ICD-9-CM Diagnosis Coding Guidelines for Outpatient Services

The ICD-9-CM official outpatient guidelines are applicable to all outpatient services including non-patient and professional services. The ICD-9-CM general coding guidelines are also applicable to coding outpatient services.

ICD-9-CM official guidelines for outpatient services include guidelines for selection of the first-listed condition (primary diagnosis), coding uncertain diagnoses, and coding diagnoses for diagnostic, therapeutic, preoperative, and ambulatory surgery services, as outlined in Figure 9-21. Several of these guidelines are outlined below.

- Identify and code the first-listed condition (primary diagnosis). The primary diagnosis is the major most significant reason for the visit. Identify and code other conditions documented in the record that are treated or affect treatment. For example:

ICD-9-CM Official Diagnosis Coding Guidelines

- Identify and code the first-listed condition (primary diagnosis)
- Identify and code all other conditions documented in the medical record that coexist at the time of the encounter/visit, and require or affect patient care treatment or management.
- **Do not code** Uncertain diagnosis qualified as "probable", "suspected," "likely," "questionable," "possible," or "still to be ruled out." Code the symptoms documented instead of qualified diagnoses.
- For a patient receiving diagnostic services only, sequence first the diagnosis, condition, problem, or other reason for the encounter/visit. Codes for other diagnoses may be sequenced as additional diagnosis.

  For outpatient encounters for diagnostic tests that have been interpreted by a physician, and the final report is available at the time of coding, code any confirmed or definitive diagnosis(es) documented in the interpretations. Do not code related signs and symptoms as additional diagnoses.
- For patients receiving therapeutic services only, sequence first the diagnosis, condition, problem or other reason for the encounter/visit to be chiefly responsible for the outpatient services provided. The only exception to this rule is that when the primary reason for the encounter is chemotherapy, radiation therapy, or rehabilitation, the appropriate V code for the services is listed first and the diagnosis or problem for which the service is being performed is listed second.
- For patients receiving preoperative evaluations only, sequence a code from the Category V72.8, Other specified examinations, to describe the preoperative service. Assign a code for the condition to describe the reason for the surgery as an additional diagnosis. Code also any findings related to the preoperative evaluation.
- For ambulatory surgery, code the diagnosis for which the surgery was performed. If the postoperative diagnosis is different from the preoperative diagnosis, select the postoperative diagnosis for coding, since it is the most definitive.

Figure 9-21 ICD-9-CM diagnosis coding guidelines for outpatient services. *(Data from* International classification of diseases, 9th revision, *U.S. Department of Health and Human Services, Public Health Service, Centers for Medicare and Medicaid Services.)*

Patient presents to the office with lower back pain and ankle pain that resulted from a fall. History and exam reveals the patient has a herniated disk, lumbar and a sprained ankle.

First Listed Condition	Herniated Disk	722.10
Secondary Diagnosis	Sprain, Ankle	845.00
Other Diagnosis	External Cause, Fall, unspecified	E888.9

"In the outpatient setting, the term first-listed condition (primary diagnosis) is recorded."*

- Uncertain diagnoses qualified as probable, suspected, likely, questionable, possible or rule-out *are not coded*. Review the record to identify and code other reasons for the visit, such as a sign, symptom, or other reason. For example:

Patient presents to the hospital based clinic complaining of a painful breast lump. The patient has a family history of breast cancer. A biopsy was taken and is to be tested to rule out malignancy.

First Listed Condition	Lump, breast	611.72
Secondary Diagnosis	Family history of breast cancer	V16.3

- When diagnostic tests are performed, sequence first the reason for the diagnostic service as documented in the patient record. If a definitive or confirmed diagnosis is documented, code the definitive or confirmed diagnosis. Do not code related signs and symptoms as additional diagnoses. The following is an example of this guideline.

Patient presents to the hospital radiology department for a chest x-ray. Indications for this exam are chest pain. The radiology exam reveals bronchitis.

First Listed Condition	Bronchitis	490

Note: If the patient record did not indicate a definitive diagnosis of bronchitis, code 786.59 "chest pain" would be recorded.

- For ambulatory surgery, code the diagnosis for which the surgery was performed. If the postoperative diagnosis is different from the preoperative diagnosis, select the postoperative diagnosis for coding, since it is most definitive. The following is an example of this guideline.

Patient admitted to the hospital ambulatory surgery center for exploratory surgery for a suspected malignant neoplasm in the pancreas. The patient was prepped and draped in the usual fashion. A tumor was identified and removed. Pathological findings: Islet cell tumor.

Postoperative diagnosis	Islet Cell Tumor	211.7
Preoperative diagnosis	Observation for Suspected Malignant Neoplasm	V71.1

Note: The postoperative diagnosis (islet cell tumor) is selected as the principal diagnosis.

BOX 9-12 ■ KEY POINTS

ICD-9-CM Official Inpatient Diagnosis Coding Guidelines

I. Select the principal diagnosis (condition determined after study).
II. Select additional other diagnoses that were treated or affect treatment.
III. Uncertain diagnosis is coded as if it existed or was established.
IV. Complications of surgery or medical care should be coded.

*National Center for Health Statistics: ICD-9-CM Official Guidelines 2005 web page www.cdc.gov/nchs/data/Icd9/ cdguide.pdf.

ICD-9-CM Official Diagnosis Coding Guidelines

Selection of the Principal Diagnosis

- Identify and code the principal diagnosis
  The condition determined after study to be chiefly responsible for the admission is coded and sequenced as the principal diagnosis. When two or more conditions meet the definition of principal diagnosis, either condition may be sequenced first as the principal diagnosis.
- Uncertain diagnosis – "probable," "suspected"
  If the diagnosis documented at the time of discharge is qualified as "probable," "suspected," "likely," "questionable," "possible," or "still to be ruled out," code the condition as if it existed or was established, except with HIV (only code HIV when diagnosis is confirmed)
- Two or more interrelated conditions
  If both conditions meet the definition of principal diagnosis, either may be sequenced as the principal diagnosis, unless the circumstances of the admission, the therapy provided, the Tabular List, or the Alphabetic Index indicate otherwise.
- Two or more comparative or contrasting conditions.
  If two or more comparative or contrasting conditions are documented as "either/or" (or similar terminology), they are coded as if the diagnosis were confirmed and the diagnoses are sequenced according to the circumstances of the admission.
- Symptom followed by contrasting/comparative diagnosis
  The symptom code is sequenced first as the principal diagnosis. All the contrasting/ comparative diagnoses should be coded as additional diagnoses.
- Complications of surgery or other medical care
  When the admission is for treatment of a complication of surgery or other medical care, the complication code is sequenced as the principal diagnosis. If the complication is classified to the 996-999 series, an additional code for the specific complication may be assigned.

Selection of Other Diagnoses

- Identify and code other diagnoses – Other diagnoses are conditions that require clinical evaluation, therapeutic treatment, diagnostic procedures, extended length of hospital stay, or increased nursing care and or monitoring
- Previous Conditions
  Resolved conditions or diagnoses and status-post procedures from previous admission that have no bearing on the current stay should not be reported and are coded only if required by hospital policy. History codes (V10-V19) may be used as secondary codes when the history has an impact on current care or influences treatment.
- Abnormal Findings
  Abnormal findings are not coded and reported unless the physician indicates their clinical significance.

Figure 9-22 ICD-9-CM diagnosis coding guidelines for inpatient services. *(Data from* International classification of diseases, 9th revision, *U.S. Department of Health and Human Services, Public Health Service, Centers for Medicare and Medicaid Services.)*

ICD-9-CM Diagnosis Coding Guidelines for Inpatient Services

Official diagnostic coding guidelines for inpatient services provide information regarding the selection of the principal diagnosis and other diagnoses, as outlined in Figure 9-22. Accurate coding requires knowledge of these guidelines and the ability to apply them. Hospital coders should utilize these guidelines when coding principal and other diagnoses. The following section provides an overview of several official guidelines related to the selection of principal and other diagnoses as outlined in the ICD-9-CM official coding guidelines.

Selection of the Principal Diagnosis

The **principal diagnosis** is defined in the Uniform Hospital Discharge Data Set (UHDDS) as "that condition established after study to be chiefly responsible for the admission of the patient to the hospital for care." Condition after study refers to the diagnosis made after an examination and/or diagnostic tests are performed.

Identify and Code the Principal Diagnosis

Signs, symptoms, and other ill-defined conditions recorded in the patient's record should not be coded as the principal diagnosis unless a definitive diagnosis is not noted in the patient's record. When two or more conditions meet the definition of principal diagnosis, either condition may be sequenced first as the principal diagnosis. The following is an example of this guideline.

> Patient is admitted to the hospital with chest pain, rapid heartbeat, and shortness of breath. Examination and further studies reveal the patient has an acute coronary occlusion.
>
> | Principal Diagnosis | Acute Coronary Occlusion | 411.81 |
> |---|---|---|
>
> Note: The symptom chest pain is not coded because there is a definitive diagnosis in the patient's record.

Two or More Interrelated Conditions

A patient medical record may indicate two or more interrelated conditions that meet the definition of a principal diagnosis. Select either condition as the principal diagnosis, unless the circumstances of the admission indicate otherwise. For example:

> Patient admitted to the hospital with suspected neoplasm of the glands. Further testing and workup reveal the patient has a malignant neoplasm on the adrenal gland and the pituitary gland.
>
> Principal Diagnosis:
>
> | Malignant Neoplasm of the Adrenal Gland | 194.0 |
> |---|---|
> | Malignant Neoplasm of the Pituitary Gland | 194.3 |
>
> Note: Either condition may be used as the principal diagnosis.

Two or More Comparative or Contrasting Conditions

There may be a case where the record indicates two or more comparative or contrasting conditions documented as "either/or." The guidelines indicate the conditions should be coded as if the diagnoses were confirmed and sequenced according to the circumstances of the admission. If a determination cannot be made regarding which diagnosis should be the principal diagnosis, *either condition may be listed*.

The following is an example of this guideline.

Patient is admitted with nausea, vomiting, and recurrent abdominal pain. Patient has a history of diverticula. Admitting physician recorded the patient's diagnosis as cholecystitis or diverticulitis of the small intestine. Patient scheduled for abdominal series and HIDA scan tomorrow.

Principal diagnosis:	
Cholecystitis	575.0
Diverticulitis	562.01

Note: Either condition may be used as the principal diagnosis because the physician stated "cholecystitis or diverticulitis."

Symptom Followed by a Contrasting or Comparative Diagnosis

When a symptom is recorded in the record followed by a contrasting or comparative diagnosis, the symptom is sequenced first as the principal diagnosis. List the contrasting or comparative diagnosis as an additional diagnosis. For example:

The patient is admitted for chronic pain in the wrist, numbness, and tingling. No fall or other injury is noted. The attending physician notes the patient has either tendonitis or carpal tunnel syndrome. Tests are performed. The final diagnosis recorded is wrist pain due to tendonitis versus carpal tunnel syndrome.

Principal diagnosis	Pain, wrist	719.43
Other Diagnosis	Tendonitis	726.4
	Carpal Tunnel Syndrome	354.0

Note: The symptom is coded as the principal diagnosis in this problem because the physician states the final diagnosis is "***pain*** due to tendonitis ***versus*** carpal tunnel syndrome."

Complications of Surgery or Other Medical Care

When a patient is admitted for treatment of a complication of surgery or other medical care, the code describing the complication should be listed as the principal diagnosis. An additional code describing the complication may be assigned when the complication is classified to 996-999. For example:

Patient admitted to the hospital with a postoperative infection as a result of failure or rejection of a kidney transplant.

Principal diagnosis	Complication of transplanted organ	996.81

Note: Use an additional to code to explain the infection.

Uncertain Diagnosis

When a patient's inpatient record lists uncertain diagnoses such as "probable," "suspected," "rule-out," ICD-9-CM guidelines state "code the condition as if it existed or were established. The basis for this guideline is that diagnostic workup and arrangements for further workup, observation, or therapies are the same whether treating the confirmed condition or ruling the condition out. This is because hospitals are paid a lump sum MS-DRG amount for each hospitalization for Medicare patients, so the facility resources used are averaged across the entire patient stay in the hospital.*

MS-DRG reimbursement will be discussed further in Chapter 13. The following is an example of this guideline.

Patient admitted to the hospital complaining of confusion occurring over several weeks. The patient has inability to remember recent events and there has been a decline in appearance or cleanliness. The family indicates there has also been a drastic personality change. CT scan shows atrophy and infarct. The attending physician's notes indicate cerebral artery occlusion with possible Alzheimer's disease.

Principal Diagnosis	Cerebral artery occlusion, unspecified	434.9
Other Diagnosis	Alzheimer's Disease	331.0

Selection of Other Diagnoses

Identifying and Coding Other Diagnoses

Identifying and coding other diagnoses requires the coder to understand the definition for "other diagnoses" as outlined in the official guidelines. "Other diagnoses" is interpreted as additional conditions that affect patient care in terms of requiring any of the following:

- Clinical evaluation
- Therapeutic treatment
- Diagnostic procedures
- Extended length of hospital stay
- Increased nursing care and/or monitoring

The following is an example of identifying and coding other diagnoses.

Patient admitted to the hospital for repair of a femoral hernia with obstruction. During the patient visit the diabetic patient required an insulin shot and close monitoring of his malignant hypertension.

Principal Diagnosis	Femoral hernia with obstruction	552.00
Other Diagnoses	Diabetes	250.00
	Hypertension	401.0

Note: Diabetes and Hypertension are coded as they required clinical evaluation and treatment.

*National Center for Health Statistics: ICD-9-CM Official Guidelines web page www.cdc.gov/nchs/data/Icd9/cdguide.pdf.

ICD-9-CM Guidelines for Outpatient versus Inpatient Diagnosis Coding

A comparison of ICD-9-CM diagnosis coding guidelines for outpatient versus inpatient services is outlined in Figure 9-23. Two significant differences in coding outpatient and inpatient services involve identifying and coding the principal versus the first-listed condition (primary diagnosis) and coding unqualified diagnoses.

> **BOX 9-13 ■ KEY POINTS**
>
> ICD-9-CM Diagnosis Coding Guidelines: Outpatient versus Inpatient
>
> Two major differences in coding guidelines for outpatient and inpatient services are:
> Primary versus principal diagnosis
> Coding uncertain diagnosis

Outpatient First-Listed Condition

The first-listed condition (primary diagnosis) is used for coding the patient's diagnosis for physician and outpatient services rather than the principal diagnosis. The fist-listed condition is the major most significant reason the patient is seeking health care services. The official guidelines for primary diagnosis are referred to as "Selection of First-Listed Condition."

> Patient presents to the hospital based clinic for a routine annual exam. On exam the patient indicates she is always tired and feeling run down. Further testing reveals the patient has pernicious anemia.

First Listed Condition	Routine Exam Annual	V70.0
Secondary Diagnosis	Pernicious Anemia	281.0

ICD-9-CM Diagnosis Coding Guidelines

Outpatient Diagnosis Coding

- Identify and code the first-listed condition (primary diagnosis). The primary diagnosis is the condition that is the major most significant reason for the visit. Each service or procedure must have a supporting diagnosis code.
- Identify and code other conditions treated or those that affect treatment including co-morbidities and factors that affect health status.
- **Do Not Code** Uncertain diagnosis qualified as "probable," "suspected," "likely," "questionable," "possible," or "still to be ruled out." Code symptoms instead of qualified diagnoses.
- Outpatient Diagnostic Services only
  Sequence first the diagnosis, condition, problem, or other reason for the encounter/visit. Codes for other diagnoses may be sequenced as additional diagnosis.

  Code the confirmed or definitive diagnosis(es) documented in the interpretation when the tests have been interpreted by a physician, and the final report is available at the time of coding. Do not code related signs and symptoms as additional diagnoses.
- Outpatient Therapeutic Services only
  Sequence first the diagnosis, condition, problem, or other reason for the encounter/visit to be chiefly responsible for the outpatient services provided.

  The only exception to this rule is that when the primary reason for the encounter is chemotherapy, radiation therapy, or rehabilitation, the appropriate V code for the services is listed first and the diagnosis or problem for which the service is being performed is listed second.
- Preoperative Evaluations only
  Sequence a code from the Category V72.8, Other specified examinations, to describe the pre-operative service. Assign a code for the condition to describe the reason for the surgery as an additional diagnosis. Code also any findings related to the preoperative evaluation.
- Abnormal findings
  Abnormal findings (laboratory, X-ray, pathologic, and other diagnostic results) are not coded and reported. Code the confirmed diagnosis or the signs and symptoms if a definitive diagnosis is not recorded in the record.

Inpatient Diagnosis Coding

- Identify and code the principal diagnosis (the condition determined after study) to be chiefly responsible for the admission. The principal and other diagnosis are reported to explain the reason for the hospital admission.
- Identify and code additional diagnoses including complications and co-morbidities. Additional diagnoses are defined as conditions that require clinical evaluation, therapeutic treatment, diagnostic procedures, extended length of hospital stay, or increased nursing care or monitoring
- **Code** uncertain diagnosis – if the diagnosis documented at the time of discharge is qualified as "probable," "likely," "suspected," "questionable," "possible," or "still to be ruled out," code the condition as if it existed or was established, except with HIV (only code HIV when diagnosis is confirmed)
- Two or more interrelated conditions
  If both conditions meet the definition of principal diagnosis either may be sequenced as the principal diagnosis, unless the circumstances of the admission, the therapy provided, the Tabular List, or the Alphabetic Index indicate otherwise.
- Two or more comparative or contrasting conditions.
  If two or more comparative or contrasting conditions are documented as "either/or" (or similar terminology), they are coded as if the diagnosis were confirmed and the diagnoses are sequenced according to the circumstances of the admission.
- Symptom followed by contrasting/comparative diagnosis
  The symptom code is sequenced first as the principal diagnosis. All the contrasting/comparative diagnoses should be coded as additional diagnoses.
- Complications of surgery or other medical care
  When the admission is for treatment of a complication of surgery or other medical care, the complication code is sequenced as the principal diagnosis. If the complication is classified to the 996-999 series, an additional code for the specific complication may be assigned.
- Abnormal findings
  Abnormal findings (laboratory, X-ray, pathologic, and other diagnostic results) are not coded and reported unless the provider indicates their clinical significance.

Figure 9-23 Comparison of ICD-9-CM diagnosis coding guidelines for outpatient versus inpatient services. *(Data from* International classification of diseases, 9th revision, *U.S. Department of Health and Human Services, Public Health Service, Centers for Medicare and Medicaid Services.)*

Inpatient Principal Diagnosis

The principal diagnosis is the condition determined after study to be the reason for the visit. The principal diagnosis is used on claims for inpatient and ambulatory surgery services submitted on the UB-04.

> Patient presents to the hospital with severe neck pain. The pain is sharp in the shoulders and arms when moving his head. The admitting physician performs an exam and orders diagnostic tests. The condition determined after study is ruptured disk.
>
> | Principal Diagnosis | Ruptured Cervical Disk | 722.0 |
> |---|---|---|
>
> Note: The principal diagnosis is: "that condition established after study to be chiefly responsible for occasioning the admission of the patient to the hospital for care."

Coding Uncertain Diagnosis

Uncertain diagnoses are handled differently when coding an outpatient case versus coding an inpatient case. Official coding guidelines indicate the following.

Outpatient Services

"Do not code diagnoses qualified as 'probable,' 'suspected,' 'likely' 'questionable,' 'possible', or 'still to be ruled out." "Rather, code the conditions(s) to the highest degree of certainty for that encounter/visit, such as symptoms, signs, or other reason for the visit.*

Inpatient Services

If the diagnosis documented at the time of discharge is qualified as 'probable,' 'suspected,' 'likely,' 'questionable,' 'possible,' or 'still to be ruled out,' code the condition as if it existed or was established. The basis for these guidelines is that the diagnostic workup, arrangements for further workup or observation, and initial therapeutic approach that correspond most closely with the established diagnosis.†

This review of ICD-9-CM diagnosis coding guidelines does not cover all the guidelines provided. This section covered some of the general and official coding guidelines for the purpose of providing an understanding of the significance of information provided in the guidelines. A complete listing of the ICD-9-CM coding guidelines is located in the front of most ICD-9-CM manuals.

*,†National Center for Health Statistics: ICD-9-CM Official Guidelines web page www.cdc.gov/nchs/data/Icd9/ cdguide.pdf.

ICD-9-CM VOLUME III PROCEDURE CODING GUIDELINES

ICD-9-CM Volume III procedure codes are used to report significant procedures performed during an inpatient visit. Some payers also require ICD-9-CM Volume III procedure codes for ambulatory surgery claims. As discussed in Chapter 8, Volume III procedure codes are listed on the UB-04 in FL 74a-e to describe the significant procedures performed during the visit. ICD-9-CM Volume III procedure coding guidelines are developed to provide instructions and clarification to coding professionals regarding coding ICD-9-CM Volume III procedures. Coders should follow applicable ICD-9-CM general guidelines when coding utilizing Volume III procedure codes. Official ICD-9-CM Volume III guidelines include instructions regarding the selection of principal and other procedures, as illustrated in Figure 9-24.

BOX 9-14 ■ KEY POINTS

ICD-9-CM General Procedure Coding Guidelines

Always use ICD-9-CM Volume III index and tabular section for code selection
Code to the highest level of specificity
ICD-9-CM Volume III codes are 2 to 4 digits
Seek clarification when documentation does not provide information required for code selection

ICD-9-CM Volume III Official Coding Guidelines

General Guidelines

- Always use the alphabetic index and the tabular section to identify and select codes.
- Code to the highest level of specificity
  Volume III lists procedures with codes that are two to four digits. Codes should be selected from the highest level when the documentation outlines specific information for code selection.
  Seek clarification from the provider when the documentation does not provide specific information required to select a code.

Selection of Principal and Other Procedure

- Identify and code only significant procedures
  Significant procedures are those that are invasive or surgical in nature, carry procedural or anesthesia risk, or require special training.
- Identify and code the principal procedure
  The principal procedure is the procedure that was performed for definitive treatment of the principal diagnosis or the procedure that most closely relates to the principal diagnosis. The principal procedure is listed first.
- Identify and code other significant procedures that were performed during the stay.
- Sequencing of procedures
  List the principal procedure first. List other significant procedures after the principal procedure.

Figure 9-24 Official coding guidelines for reporting procedures utilizing ICD-9-CM Volume III procedure codes. *(Data from* International classification of diseases, 9th revision, *U.S. Department of Health and Human Services, Public Health Service, Centers for Medicare and Medicaid Services.)*

TEST YOUR *Knowledge* BOX 9-3, A

ICD-9-CM DIAGNOSIS CODING GUIDELINES

1. ICD-9-CM official guidelines provide instructions that are specific to ________ and ________ coding.

2. ICD-9-CM general guidelines are applicable to all ____________ ____________.

3. List the agencies that provide the ICD-9-CM Official Diagnosis Coding Guidelines.

4. The AHA, AHIMA, CMS, and Center for Health Statistics are the ____________ ____________ that approve the ICD-9-CM guidelines.

5. The ICD-9-CM guidelines are published by the ____________.

6. List four sections of the ICD-9-CM guidelines.

7. State two major service categories for which the ICD-9-CM official guidelines differ.

8. ICD-9-CM general coding guidelines state that only conditions that are ____________, ____________, or ____________ should be coded.

9. ICD-9-CM general guidelines state coders should always code to the ____________ ____________ of ____________.

10. ICD-9-CM guidelines applicable to ____________ services instruct the coder to identify and code the first listed condition (primary diagnosis).

11. Define first listed condition.

12. Discuss the ICD-9-CM outpatient coding guidelines related to uncertain diagnosis.

13. ICD-9-CM guidelines for inpatient services indicate that the coder should identify and code the ____________ ____________, which is the condition determined after study to be chiefly responsible for the patient care services provided.

14. An uncertain diagnosis can be coded as if the condition existed or was established according to the ICD-9-CM guidelines for ____________ services.

15. The ICD-9-CM guidelines state that other diagnosis are conditions that require ____________, ____________, ____________, ____________, or ____________.

TEST YOUR *Knowledge* BOX 9-3, B

CLINICAL SCENARIOS: CODING GUIDELINES AND APPLICATION

ICD-9-CM DIAGNOSIS CODING GUIDELINES

Review the following case and refer to the ICD-9-CM Official Diagnosis Coding Guidelines to answer the questions below.

Patient Case 1

A patient arrives at the hospital clinic complaining of severe ear pain, hearing loss, and fever. The physician, who is an employee of the hospital, performs an initial visit detailed history and exam with straightforward medical decision making. The exam includes an otoscopy, which reveals the presence of a fluid-filled middle ear. The doctor diagnoses the patient with acute suppurative otitis media and prescribes antibiotics. A follow-up exam is scheduled to take place in 2 weeks.

1-1. Explain what first listed condition will be coded for this case

1-2. List the diagnosis code(s) for this case, in the appropriate order.

1-3. What claim form will be used to submit charges for this visit?

1-4. Name the field where diagnosis code(s) for this visit are listed on the claim form.

1-5. Will the hospital bill for professional services performed by the physician?

Patient Case 2

A patient arrives at the hospital complaining of severe headaches, nausea, and vomiting. The patient also notes he is currently being treated for chronic sinusitis. The physician conducts a comprehensive exam. An EEG is done and a CT scan is performed. The results on the CT scan show an intracranial abscess. The patient is admitted and antibiotics are administered intravenously. The doctor will assess the patient later to determine if the abscess will require draining.

2-1. Explain what first listed condition will be coded for this case.

2-2. Provide a diagnosis code for all conditions to be reported for this case. List the principal diagnosis first.

2-3. List one of the ICD-9-CM official guidelines used to code this case.

2-4. State which claim form will be used to submit charges for this case.

2-5. Explain where the principal and other diagnosis codes will be reported on the claim form.

ICD-9-CM Volume III General Procedure Coding Guidelines

- Always use the ICD-9-CM Volume III alphabetic index to identify possible procedure codes. Refer to the ICD-9-CM Volume III tabular list to verify all codes found in the index.
- Code to the highest level of specificity. Volume III lists procedures with codes that are two to four digits. The two-digit codes are listed as the category headings. The category is further specified at the 3rd and 4th digit level of the category. Codes should be selected from the highest level when the documentation outlines specific information for code selection.
- Seek clarification from the provider when the documentation does not provide specific information required to select a code.

BOX 9-15 ■ KEY POINTS

ICD-9-CM Volume III Procedure Coding Guidelines

- Selection of principal procedure
- Selection of other procedures
- Sequence procedures

BOX 9-16 ■ KEY POINTS

ICD-9-CM Volume III Significant Procedure

Significant procedure is defined in the Uniform Hospital Discharge Data Set (UHDDS), as published in the *Federal Register*, as one that is:

- surgical in nature, or
- carries a procedural risk, or
- carries an anesthetic risk, or
- requires specialized training.

Examples

Infusions
Catheterization
Surgery

BOX 9-17 ■ KEY POINTS

ICD-9-CM Volume III Principal Procedure

The significant procedure that was performed for definitive treatment of the principal diagnosis

Or

The significant procedure that most closely relates to the principal diagnosis

ICD-9-CM Volume III Guidelines for Selection of Principal and Other Procedures

- **Identify and code all significant procedures.** The UHDDS, as published in the *Federal Register*, Volume 50, Number 147, July 31, 1985, includes data items for reporting procedures. The definitions included can be used to determine which codes should be reported. Item 12 of UHDDS states that all significant procedures are to be reported. UHDDS defines a **significant procedure** as one that is: 1. surgical in nature, or 2. carries a procedural risk, or 3. carries an anesthetic risk, or 4. requires specialized training.
- **Identify and code the principal procedure.** The **principal procedure** is the significant procedure that was performed for definitive treatment of the principal diagnosis or the significant procedure that most closely relates to the principal diagnosis. When the record indicates more than one principal procedure, select the procedure that most closely relates to the principal diagnosis. If both are equally related to the principal diagnosis, list the most comprehensive or complex procedure as the principal procedure. The following is an example of this guideline.

  Patient is admitted with nausea, vomiting, and recurrent abdominal pain. Patient has a history of diverticula. An abdominal series and HIDA series are performed and reveal severe chronic cholecystitis. Patient undergoes a cholecystectomy. Patient tolerated the procedure well.

Principal procedure	Cholecystectomy	51.22

  Note: The abdominal series and HIDA scan are not considered significant procedures, therefore, an ICD-9-CM Volume III procedure is not assigned to those procedures.

- **Identify and code all other significant procedures.** Other significant procedures performed during the patient's stay are identified and reported. For example:

  Patient is admitted to the hospital with severe chest pain, rapid heartbeat, and shortness of breath. Patient is taken to the cath lab for a catheterization. Combined right and left heart catheterization is performed. Combined right and left angiography reveals coronary artery occlusive disease. Patient undergoes a percutaneous transluminal coronary angioplasty. The patient tolerates the procedure well.

Principal Procedure	PTCA	00.66
Other Procedures	Combined Right and Left Cardiac Catheterization	37.23
	Combined Right and Left Heart Angiocardiography	88.54

Note: The catheterization and angiocardiography are assigned an ICD-9-CM Volume III procedure code because the catheterization is a surgical procedure. The symptom "chest pain" is not coded because there is a definitive diagnosis in the patient's record.

- **Sequence the procedures.** List the principal procedure first. Other significant procedures are sequenced after the principal procedure.

This review of ICD-9-CM procedure coding guidelines does not cover all the guidelines provided. This section covered some of the general and official coding guidelines for the purpose of providing an understanding of the significance of information provided in the guidelines. A complete listing of ICD-9-CM coding guidelines is located in the front of most ICD-9-CM manuals. The next section provides a review of HCPCS coding guidelines.

HEALTH CARE COMMON PROCEDURE CODING SYSTEM (HCPCS) CODING GUIDELINES

HCPCS codes are used to describe services, procedures, and items when submitting claims to third-party payers. HCPCS consists of Level I CPT codes and Level II National codes, and both include coding guidelines. Third-party payers develop policies that define coverage criteria for specific services, procedures, and items. Procedure coding has become very complex and requires knowledge of universal coding guidelines in addition to payer-specific guidelines. Inaccurate coding can have many negative consequences, such as incorrect reimbursement or payment denial. Incorrect coding may also trigger a third-party audit resulting in an investigation of fraud or abuse. The depth and magnitude of all the procedure coding guidelines is too involved to review in this text. This section will focus on general correct coding guidelines for HCPCS Level I and II procedure coding.

BOX 9-18 ■ KEY POINTS

Health Care Common Procedure Coding System (HCPCS)

Level I CPT procedure codes
Level II Medicare National procedure codes

Procedure Coding Guidelines

Procedure coding is the process of translating written descriptions of services, procedures, and items into codes. All services, procedures, and items are recorded in the patient's medical record. Personnel in departments providing patient care services post charges through the chargemaster. Each item in the chargemaster is associated with a HCPCS code. The chargemaster lists procedure codes and revenue code categories for all services and items, as discussed in previous chapters. Other procedures are coded by HIM personnel. Regardless of where the coding occurs in the facility, it is essential that the codes accurately describe services, procedures, and items that are recorded in the patient's medical record. General coding guidelines should be followed regardless of the coding system used or where the coding is performed in a hospital. Figure 9-25 outlines the following general procedure coding guidelines.

General Procedure Coding Guidelines

- Always use the alphabetic index to identify possible codes and refer to the code section to confirm code selection.
- Never code services, procedures, and items that are not documented in the medical record. This is referred to as **phantom billing** and is considered fraudulent.
- Code to the highest level of specificity. The goal is to submit codes that accurately describe what is in the patient's record. If the record does not provide information required to code specific procedures or items, check with the provider.

HCPSC General Procedure Coding Guidelines

- Always use the alphabetic index to identify possible codes and refer to the code section to confirm code selection
- Never code services, procedures, and items that are not documented in the medical record. This is referred to as phantom billing and it is considered fraud.
- Code to the highest level of specificity
  The goal is to submit codes that accurately describe what is in the patient's record. If the record does not provide information required to code specific procedures or items, check with the provider.
- Coding multiple procedures
  It is critical to carefully review coding when multiple codes are used to be sure one procedure is not an integral part of another procedure. This is referred to as unbundling and it may be considered fraud or abuse.
- Code procedure at the level recorded in the patient's medical record. Carefully review the record to ensure the procedure or item coded matches the documentation. When the record does not provide specific information required to select a code, check with the provider. Coding procedures at a higher level is referred to as upcoding or creeping and it can be considered fraud or abuse.
- Medical necessity
  Services, procedures, and items must be medically necessary for treatment of the patient's condition. Accurate diagnosis coding will help to establish medical necessity.
- Modifier usage
  Modifiers are used to describe circumstances regarding the procedure performed that are not explained in the procedure code. When using modifiers it is important to understand what circumstance is explained by the modifier.

Figure 9-25 HCPCS general procedure coding guidelines apply to all providers utilizing HCPCS codes. *(Data from* HCPCS level II national codes, *U.S. Department of Health and Human Services, Centers for Medicare and Medicaid Services.)*

TEST YOUR *Knowledge* BOX 9-4, A

ICD-9-CM VOLUME III PROCEDURE CODING GUIDELINES

1. ICD-9-CM Volume III procedure codes are used to report ______________ ______________ performed during a(n) ______________ visit.

2. Some payers may require ICD-9-CM Volume III procedure codes on ______________ ______________ claims.

3. ICD-9-CM Volume III procedures are reported in what form locator on the CMS-1450 (UB-04)?

4. ICD-9-CM Volume III procedure codes are identified in the alphabetic index and they must be verified in the ______________ ______________.

5. Official guidelines state coders should code to the highest level of specificity. Explain what this means when coding utilizing ICD-9-CM Volume III procedure codes.

6. What should a coder do when information in the record is not specific enough to select a procedure code?

The UHDDS defines a significant procedure as one that is:

7. ______________, or 8. ______________, or 9. ______________, or 10. ______________.

11. Identify which procedures listed below are significant procedures.
    A. Kidney transplant
    B. EKG
    C. Infusion therapy
    D. Liver profile
    E. Heart catheterization

12. The procedure that is performed for definitive treatment of the principal diagnosis is the ______________ procedure.

13. When the record indicates more than one principal procedure, the coder should select the procedure that ______________.

14. Explain what procedure is listed first when sequencing procedures.

15. All other ______________ ______________ should be sequenced after the principal procedure.

TEST YOUR *Knowledge* BOX 9-4, B

CLINICAL SCENARIOS: ICD-9-CM VOLUME III PROCEDURE CODING GUIDELINES

Review the following cases and refer to the ICD-9-CM Procedure Guidelines to answer the questions below:

Patient Case 1

A patient presents today at the hospital ambulatory surgery unit for a gastroscopy. The patient has been experiencing epigastric pain, indigestion, and recently found blood in the stool. A gastroscopy is performed through artificial stoma with brushings and washing for biopsy. The patient tolerates the procedure well and is sent to the recovery room. The patient has bile induced gastritis, which appears to be bile induced. Medications are prescribed and the patient is discharged the same day.

1-1. Identify and code the principal procedure.

1-2. List the principal diagnosis and procedure.

1-3. What claim form will be used to submit charges for this visit?

1-4. Name the field where the principal procedure code for this visit will be listed on the claim form.

1-5. Will the hospital bill for professional services performed by the physician?

Patient Case 2

A patient is admitted to the hospital experiencing severe abdominal pain, vomiting, high fever, and discomfort. The referring physician suspects appendicitis. On exam, pain is noted in the right lower quadrant, where there is extreme tenderness. A CBC and urinalysis are performed. The diagnosis of appendicitis is confirmed. The patient is taken to the operating room for a laparoscopic appendectomy. Patient tolerates the procedure well.

2-1. Identify and code the principal procedure and diagnosis that will be listed for this case.

2-2. Explain why the CBC and urinalysis is not recorded as a principal or other procedure.

2-3. List one of the ICD-9-CM official guidelines used to code this case.

2-4. State what claim form will be used to submit charges for this case.

2-5. Explain where diagnosis and procedures codes will be listed on the claim form.

- When coding multiple procedures, it is critical to carefully review the codes to be sure one procedure is not an integral part of another procedure. This is referred to as unbundling and it may be considered fraud or abuse. **Unbundling** is the process of utilizing more than one code to describe a service that should be represented with a single code.
- Code procedures at the level recorded in the patient record. Carefully review the record to ensure the procedure or item coded matches the documentation. When the record does not provide specific information required to select a code, check with the provider. Utilizing a higher level code to describe a service or procedure that is not supported by the documentation is called **upcoding**. Upcoding is also referred to as "creeping."
- Services, procedures, and items must be medically necessary for treatment of the patient's condition. Accurate diagnosis coding will help to establish medical necessity.
- Modifiers are used to describe circumstances regarding the procedure performed that are not explained in the procedure code. When using modifiers it is important to understand what circumstance the modifier explains.

BOX 9-19 ■ KEY POINTS

General Procedure Coding Guidelines

Phantom Billing

Billing for services, procedures, or items that were not rendered. There is no supporting documentation.

Unbundling

Assigning multiple codes to a service, procedure or item when only one code should be assigned. For example, assigning multiple codes for a comprehensive metabolic panel.

Upcoding

Coding a service or procedure at a higher level than what is documented. For example, coding a complex fracture when the record indicates a simple fracture was performed.

Health Care Common Procedure Coding System Level I CPT Coding Guidelines

HCPCS Level I CPT codes are used to report services, procedures, supplies, and products to third-party payers for services rendered. CPT coding guidelines and instructions are outlined in the beginning of each section of the CPT manual and throughout the code sections. Specific information regarding code selection is also listed at the category and subcategory level. Figure 9-26 outlines the section guidelines. The CPT guidelines in each of the sections are used for reporting the services described in that section. There are some variations in these guidelines for hospital reporting of the technical portion of services, as explored subsequently.

HCPSC Level I CPT Procedure Coding Guidelines

The following CPT Guidelines are outlined at the beginning of each section of the CPT coding manual. Hospital-specific guidelines are outlined below.

- Evaluation and Management (E/M) Section
  Terminology, Components of E/M, and Selection of Levels of E/M
  Guidelines for reporting the technical portion of evaluation and management services have not been developed. CMS guidelines state that hospitals should develop criteria for the assignment of the E/M levels based on resource utilization and cost of providing E/M services. Hospitals utilize CPT E/M codes to report the technical portion of evaluation and management services provided in areas such as the Emergency Department and observation unit.
- Anesthesia Section
  Time reporting, Separate and Multiple Procedures, Anesthesia Modifiers, and Qualifying Circumstances
  Hospitals report the technical portion of anesthesia services, which includes space, equipment, and other hospital resources utilized. Hospitals also report anesthesia services in time increments.
- Surgery Section
  Surgical Package Definition, Follow-up Care, and Reporting More Than One Procedure or Service
  Hospitals do not apply the surgical package guidelines since the concept of preoperative and postoperative services does not apply in the hospital outpatient environment, except in a clinic or primary care office. Payer guidelines define services that are packaged for surgeries performed.
- Radiology Section
  Global Procedure, Technical Component, and Professional Component
  Hospitals submit facility charges for the technical portion of radiology procedures, which includes space, equipment, and technical staff.
- Pathology and Laboratory Section
  Separate or Multiple procedures, Special Report, and Unlisted Service or Procedure
  Hospitals submit facility charges for the technical portion of a pathology/laboratory procedures.
- Medicine Section
  Multiple Procedures, Add-on Codes, Separate Procedures, Unlisted Procedures, Special Report, and Materials Supplied by Physician
  Hospitals submit facility charges for the technical portion of medicine procedures. The professional portion of services may be reported by the hospital when the physician is employed by or under contract with the hospital.

Figure 9-26 The CPT Manual contains guidelines in the beginning of each section that apply to coding from that section only. *(Data from AMA:* CPT 2010 professional edition, *Chicago, 2010, American Medical Association.)*

BOX 9-20 ■ KEY POINTS

HCPCS Level I CPT Coding Guidelines

CPT coding guidelines and instructions are located in the CPT manual and in the *CPT Assistant* monthly newsletter published by the American Medical Association (AMA).

HCPCS Level I CPT codes are also used for reporting services performed in the hospital including those performed in hospital-based clinics or primary care offices. Hospital services are posted through the chargemaster. All items listed in the chargemaster are associated with the appropriate HCPCS code. CPT code usage and application of guidelines vary for hospitals. The American Medical Association (AMA) publishes a CPT manual that specifically addresses procedure coding for outpatient hospital services called the *Outpatient Services CPT*, a specifically annotated version for use in hospital outpatient settings. As discussed previously, Medicare reimbursement for hospital outpatient services is based on the APC Prospective Payment System. Therefore, the manual includes APC status indicators. Prospective Payment Systems (PPS) will be discussed in depth in Chapter 13. This section outlines CPT guidelines that vary in the hospital setting.

BOX 9-21 ■ KEY POINTS

HCPCS Level I CPT Coding Guideline Sections

- Evaluation and Management (E/M)
- Anesthesia
- Surgery
- Radiology
- Pathology/Laboratory
- Medicine

Evaluation and Management (E/M) Section Guidelines

Evaluation and management (E/M) section guidelines provide definitions of terms utilized in coding E/M services and instructions for the selection of a level of E/M service. These guidelines are followed for the professional portion of an E/M service performed by physicians and other non-physician providers, such as a physician assistant. Guidelines for reporting the technical portion of E/M services have not been developed. CMS guidelines state that hospitals should develop criteria for the assignment of the E/M levels based on resource utilization and cost of providing E/M services. Hospitals utilize CPT E/M codes to report the technical portion of E/M services provided in areas such as the Emergency Department.

Anesthesia Section Guidelines

Anesthesia section guidelines provide information regarding time reporting, physician services, materials supplied, separate or multiple procedures, special report, anesthesia modifiers, and qualifying circumstances.

Time reporting Time reporting describes when anesthesia time starts and ends. Anesthesia time starts when the anesthesiologist starts preparing to administer anesthesia and ends when the anesthesiologist stops attending to the patient. Hospitals report the technical portion of anesthesia services, which includes space, equipment, and other hospital resources utilized. Hospitals also report anesthesia services in time increments.

Surgery Section Guidelines

Surgery section guidelines provide information regarding the surgical package, follow-up care for diagnostic and therapeutic surgical procedures, materials supplied by the physician, reporting more than one procedure or service, and modifiers. The **surgical package** describes services that are included when performing surgical procedures: simple anesthesia, one E/M after the decision for surgery, writing orders, evaluating the patient after anesthesia, and normal, uncomplicated postoperative care. Hospitals do not apply the surgical package guidelines since the concept of preoperative and postoperative services does not apply in the hospital outpatient environment, except in a clinic or primary care office. Payer guidelines define services that are packaged for surgeries performed. For example, Medicare APC reimbursement guidelines outline services that are packaged, including all the components of care, as illustrated in Figure 9-27.

Radiology Section Guidelines

Radiology section guidelines provide information regarding separate procedures, special services, supervision and interpretation, and administration of contrast materials. One of the most common coding errors in radiology involves professional versus technical component. It is important for the coder to identify and code the appropriate component of a service professional, technical, or the global procedure.

Global procedure The **global procedure** represents the technical and professional portion of a procedure or service. CPT procedure codes represent the global procedure (service) unless otherwise stated. The global procedure is coded when the technical and professional

Hospital Outpatient Prospective Payment System (HOPPS)

Facility Resources Included in APC Payments

For those services that are under APC, typically all of the components of care are bundled with, or considered part of, the service. The following resources (costs) are directly related and integral to the performance of a procedure or service on an outpatient basis for Medicare beneficiaries and therefore, are included in the APC group payment rate. The following services and items are not separately payable:

- Use of an operating suite, procedure room, or treatment room or area
- Use of the recovery room
- Use of an observation bed (other than in the specific situation discussed in the text)
- Drugs, biologicals, and other pharmaceuticals; medical and surgical supplies and equipment; surgical dressings, splints, casts, and other devices used for reduction of fractures or dislocations
- Supplies and equipment used for administering and monitoring anesthesia or sedation
- Intraocular lenses (IOL) and several other designated implants

Figure 9-27 Facility resources included in the APC packaged components of care in accordance with provisions of the HOPPS. *(Data from Ingenix:* Outpatient billing expert, *Eden Prairie, Minn., Ingenix.)*

component of a procedure or service is performed and the physician or other non-physician provider is employed by or under contract with the hospital.

Technical component The **technical component** represents the cost and overhead of procedures performed, such as the equipment, technician, and supplies. Facility charges for the technical component of services are submitted by the entity that owns the equipment, employs the technician, and provides the materials and supplies. The technical portion is identified using a TC (technical component) modifier with the appropriate radiology code.

Professional component The **professional component** represents the portion of a procedure that involves the physician or other non-physician provider's work in performing a service, such as administering anesthesia, performing surgery, or supervision and interpretation of a radiology procedure. The professional component is identified using a modifier-26 with the appropriate radiology code. Hospitals may submit charges for the professional component of services when the physician is employed by or under contract with the hospital.

Pathology and Laboratory Section Guidelines

Pathology and laboratory section guidelines outline information regarding services in pathology and laboratory, separate or multiple procedures, special report, and unlisted service or procedure. Hospitals generally submit facility charges for the technical portion of pathology/ laboratory procedures, which include space, equipment, and technical staff.

Medicine Section Guidelines

Medicine section guidelines provide information regarding multiple procedures, add-on codes, separate procedures, unlisted procedures, special reports, and materials supplied by the physician. Hospitals submit facility charges for the technical portion of procedures in the medicine section, which includes space, equipment, and technical staff. The professional portion of medicine procedures may be reported by the hospital when they are performed in a hospital-based clinic or primary care office and the physician is employed by or under contract with the hospital.

BOX 9-22 ■ KEY POINTS

HCPCS Level II Medicare National Coding Guidelines

HCPCS Level II National codes were developed by the Centers for Medicare and Medicaid Services (CMS). CMS HCPCS Level II guidelines are published in the HCPCS Level II manual. Select internet-only manuals (IOM) are senerally included in the HCPCS manual.

It is essential for coders to have a good understanding of the CPT coding guidelines. The *CPT Assistant* is a publication from the AMA that coders can use to obtain updated information and to clarify the appropriate usage of CPT codes.

Health Care Common Procedure Coding System (HCPCS) Level II Medicare National Coding Guidelines

HCPCS Level II National codes are utilized to report services, procedures, items, equipment, drugs and biologicals to third-party payers. HCPCS Level II Medicare National codes were developed by the CMS, formerly known as Health Care Financing Administration (HCFA), for reporting of services and items. HCPCS Level II codes are used when a code that describes the service or item cannot be found in the HCPCS Level I CPT manual, or when the payer requires the use of a HCPCS Level II code instead of a HCPCS Level I CPT code. CMS guidelines published in the HCPCS Level II manual are outlined in the introduction and also at the category and subcategory level of codes.

Medicare guidelines state specific policies regarding coverage. Many HCPCS Level II manuals include a supplement to the codes in an appendix that references various Medicare issues. These references are referred to as internet-only manuals. Policies regarding payment conditions and coverage are outlined in these references. Most payers accept HCPCS Level II codes; how ever, their guidelines may vary from Medicare guidelines. Coding personnel should obtain guidelines and information regarding usage of HCPCS Level II codes from each payer. General coding guidelines discussed earlier in this chapter that apply to the HCPCS Level II Medicare National coding system are outlined below.

- Always use the alphabetic index to identify possible codes and refer to the code section to confirm code selection.
- Never code services, procedures, and items that are not documented in the medical record. This is referred to as phantom billing and is considered abuse or fraud.
- Code to the highest level of specificity. The goal is to submit codes that accurately describe what is in the patient's record. If the record does not provide information required to code specific procedures or items, check with the provider.
- Services, procedures, and items must be medically necessary for treatment of the patient's condition. Accurate diagnosis coding will help to establish medical necessity.
- When using modifiers it is important to apply the correct modifier and the impact of that modifier usage on billing.

Procedure Coding
Hospital Outpatient Services

- Code only procedures that are recorded in the patient's medical record.
- Identify and code procedures performed during the visit, using HCPCS Level I CPT and Level II Medicare National codes.
- Review code assignments and apply appropriate HCPCS modifier as required.
- Review coding assignments to ensure compliance with guidelines as outlined in CPT and the CCI manual.
- Review coding assignments to identify inpatient-only procedures.
- HCPCS procedures are reported on the CMS-1500 in Block 24 D and on the CMS-1450 (UB-04) in FL 44.

Procedure Coding
Hospital Inpatient Services

- Code only procedures that are recorded in the patient's medical record.
- Identify and code only significant procedures performed during the hospital visit, utilizing ICD-9-CM Volume III procedure codes.
- Identify and code the principal procedure, which is the procedure performed to treat the principal diagnosis or the procedure most closely related to the principal diagnosis.
- Identify and code other significant procedures recorded in the patient's medical record.
- HCPCS Level I CPT and Level II Medicare National codes are associated with items in the chargemaster, however, they are not reported on inpatient claims.
- ICD-9-CM Volume III procedures are reported on the CMS-1450 (UB-04) in FL 74 a-e.

Figure 9-28 Procedure coding guidelines for outpatient versus inpatient.

Procedure Coding Guidelines for Outpatient versus Inpatient Services

It is important to understand procedure coding guidelines required for outpatient versus inpatient services. Figure 9-28 illustrates some basic procedure coding guideline variations for outpatient versus inpatient services.

Coding is a highly complex process of translating written descriptions of services, procedures, and items into codes. Information is obtained from the patient's medical record. Abstracting is a critical part of coding. Abstracting is the process of reading the patient's record and identifying information necessary to select the appropriate codes. Before we begin applying coding guidelines we will review the basic steps to coding utilizing HCPCS and ICD-9-CM, as outlined in Figure 9-29.

BASIC STEPS TO CODING UTILIZING HCPCS AND ICD-9-CM

Coding is the process of translating written descriptions of services, procedures, items, and patient conditions into codes. To effectively code, the coder must read the record or other source document and abstract pertinent information regarding services and the patient's conditions for which the services were provided. Hospital source documents utilized by coders include various documents from the medical record such as the admission summary, history and physical, physician's orders, progress notes, ancillary department reports, medication records, discharge summary, encounter form, requisition, or an emergency room record. A coding worksheet may be utilized to abstract information regarding services provided and patient conditions from the medical record, as illustrated in Figure 9-30. The basic steps in coding are the same regardless of whether procedures, items, or conditions are being coded. The following is an outline of the basic steps to coding procedures or items.

BOX 9-23 ■ KEY POINTS

Basic Steps to Coding

Follow good coding habits.

1. Read the medical record and identify main terms.
2. Refer to the alphabetic index, look up main terms, and identify possible codes.
3. Refer to the code sections and review all codes identified in the index. Select the code that most accurately describes the service, procedure, item, or condition.
4. Review code assignment and record to identify circumstances that require a modifier.
5. Sequence code(s) appropriately.

Step 1: Read the Medical Record and Identify the Main Terms

The coder must identify the main terms for all services and conditions to be coded. The main term when coding services or procedures can be determined by asking, "what item was provided or procedure or service performed?" The main term for diagnoses can be determined by asking, "why was the item provided or procedure (service) provided?" Main terms and other relative information identified in the medical record are recorded on the coding worksheet.

Step 2: Refer to the Alphabetic Index

Step 2 is performed to identify possible codes that may describe the service or condition in the patient's record. Look up each main term abstracted from the patient's record in the index of the appropriate coding system. Identify all possible codes for services, items, and diagnosis. Possible codes are recorded on the coding worksheet.

Step 3: Refer to the Code Sections

Carefully review each code identified from the index in the code section for the service, item, and diagnosis. Select the code(s) that best describes the service, item, and diagnosis listed in the patient's record. As discussed in previous chapters, coders may utilize an encoder program to assign codes.

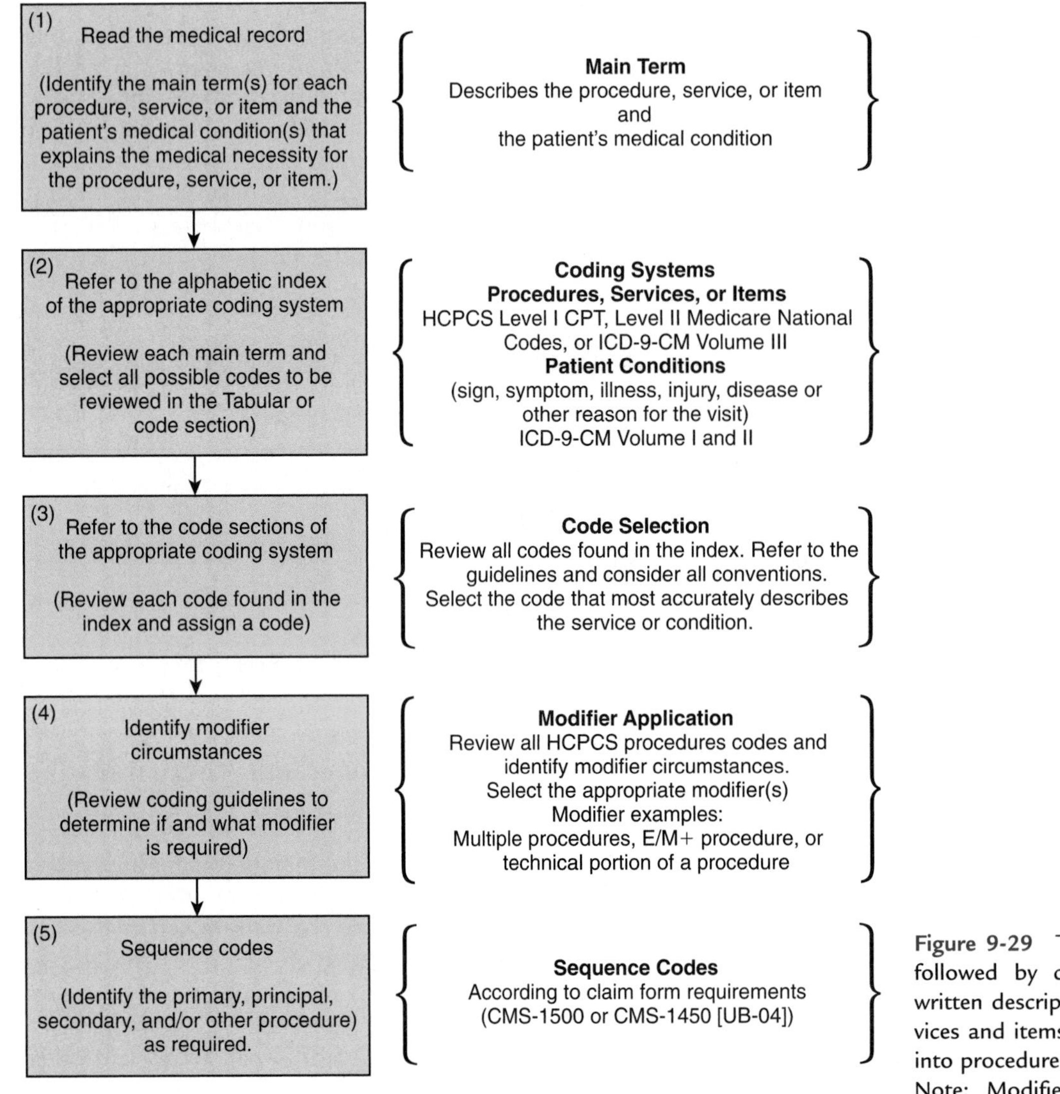

Basic Steps to Coding
(1) Read the medical record
(Identify the main term(s) for each procedure, service, or item and the patient's medical condition(s) that explains the medical necessity for the procedure, service, or item.)
Main Term
Describes the procedure, service, or item and the patient's medical condition
(2) Refer to the alphabetic index of the appropriate coding system
(Review each main term and select all possible codes to be reviewed in the Tabular or code section)
Coding Systems
Procedures, Services, or Items
HCPCS Level I CPT, Level II Medicare National Codes, or ICD-9-CM Volume III
Patient Conditions
(sign, symptom, illness, injury, disease or other reason for the visit) ICD-9-CM Volume I and II
(3) Refer to the code sections of the appropriate coding system
(Review each code found in the index and assign a code)
Code Selection
Review all codes found in the index. Refer to the guidelines and consider all conventions. Select the code that most accurately describes the service or condition.
(4) Identify modifier circumstances
(Review coding guidelines to determine if and what modifier is required)
Modifier Application
Review all HCPCS procedures codes and identify modifier circumstances. Select the appropriate modifier(s) Modifier examples: Multiple procedures, E/M+ procedure, or technical portion of a procedure
(5) Sequence codes
(Identify the primary, principal, secondary, and/or other procedure) as required.
Sequence Codes
According to claim form requirements (CMS-1500 or CMS-1450 [UB-04])
Note: Modifiers are only used with HCPCS Level I and Level II codes.

Figure 9-29 These basic steps can be followed by coders when translating written descriptions of procedures, services and items, and patient conditions into procedure and diagnosis codes. Note: Modifiers are only used with HCPCS Level I and Level II codes.

Step 4: Identify Modifier Circumstances

When coding is completed, the coder must review the codes to identify circumstances that require a modifier. Modifiers describe circumstances that exist that are not explained in the code description. Coding bilateral procedures is an example of a modifier circumstance. The code may describe a unilateral procedure. When the procedure is performed bilaterally, the coder must attach a modifier-50 or -LT/-RT to indicate the procedure was done bilaterally. The modifiers assigned are also recorded on the coding worksheet.

Diagnosis codes, procedure codes, and modifiers recorded on the coding worksheet are entered into a grouper program along with other clinical information for the appropriate APC or MS-DRG assignment.

BOX 9-24 ■ KEY POINTS

Sequencing Codes on the CMS-1500 Claim Form

Diagnosis codes are listed in block 21 (reference lines 1-4).

- The first listed condition is listed in reference line 1.
- Other diagnoses are listed in reference lines 2-4
  Procedure codes are listed in block 24D (line 1-6).
- List in order the procedures were performed, *unless reporting multiple surgeries*
- List multiple surgical procedure codes in order of complexity (most comprehensive first), followed by less complex procedures
  Link procedures with a diagnosis from block 21, record the
- Reference line number in 24E.

TEST YOUR *Knowledge* BOX 9-5

HCPCS CODING GUIDELINES CONCEPTS

1. Procedure coding is the process of ______________ into codes.

2. Most hospital services, procedures, and items are posted through the ______________ by department personnel. Some services, procedures, and items are coded and posted by ______________ personnel.

3. Coders should never report a code for services, procedures, or items that are not documented in the patient record. This is referred to as ______________.

4. What should a coder do when information in the record is not specific enough to select a specific code?

5. When coding multiple procedures, it is important to ensure that more than one code is not used to report services that should be reported with a single code. This is known as ______________ .

6. When a coder uses a code that describes a higher level of service than the service documented in the patient record, they are ______________. This is also referred to as ______________.

7. What is the purpose of a modifier?

8. HCPCS Level I CPT coding guidelines and code-specific instructions can be found at the ______________ and throughout each ______________.

9. CPT coding and application of guidelines vary in reporting ______________ services and the ______________ portion of services.

10. CPT codes are used for reporting the ______________ of evaluation and management (E/M) services. The guidelines for E/M code assignment are developed by the ______________.

11. Explain the variation in CPT guidelines for hospitals related to the surgical package.

12. Indicate whether facility charges for the following services represent the technical or professional component.
    A. Surgical procedures
    B. Hospital-based clinic (evaluation and management service)
    C. Radiology service
    D. Pathology/Laboratory service
    E. Services found in the Medicine section

TEST YOUR *Knowledge* BOX 9-5

HCPCS CODING GUIDELINES CONCEPTS—*cont'd*

13. Discuss how the coder determines whether to use HCPCS Level I CPT or HCPCS Level II codes.

14. Guidelines for HCPCS Level II codes are developed by ______________.

15. Many HCPCS Level II manuals include a supplement to the codes in an appendix that references various Medicare issues. These references are referred to as the ______________ and the ______________.

HEALTH INFORMATION MANAGEMENT
CODING WORKSHEET

DEMOGRAPHICS		
Medical Record Number:	**Bill Type#:**	
Patient Name: Last, First, Middle Init:	Admit Hour Code:	Discharge Hour Code:
	Admit Type Code:	Discharge Status Code:
	Admit Source Code:	
Condition Code (s)	Occurrence Span Code and Date	Value Code and Amount

ADMISSION INFORMATION	
Type of Admission: ER Facility Physician Referral Other Unknown	
Admitting Diagnosis	**HIM Code(s)**
Principal Diagnosis (Including complications and co-morbidities if applicable)	**HIM Code**
Other Secondary Diagnoses (Including complications and co-morbidities if applicable)	**HIM Code(s)**
Principal Procedure (Significant procedure performed for definitive treatment or that most closely relates to the principal diagnosis) **Date:**	**HIM Code**
Other Significant Procedure(s) **Date:**	**HIM Code(s)**
Medications, supplies, equipment or other item (s) **Date:**	**HIM Code(s)**

DISCHARGE INFORMATION				
Home	Facility	AMA	Deceased	Other

DRG ASSIGNMENT		APC ASSIGNMENT		
MDC:	Surgical/Medical:			

CONTRIBUTING FACTORS:				
Age	Sex	Discharge Status	Complications/Comorbidities	Birthweight

Questions/Need Clarification:

Figure 9-30 HIM coders often utilize a coding worksheet to abstract from the medical record and assign codes.

Step 5: Sequence Codes

When listing diagnosis and procedure codes on the claim form, the sequence must be carefully determined. The sequencing of procedures and diagnoses is different on the CMS-1500 than on the UB-04.

Sequencing on the CMS-1500

Diagnosis codes are reported in Block 21. List the major most significant diagnosis in reference line 1. The major most significant diagnosis is referred to as the first-listed condition (primary diagnosis). List other diagnoses in order of severity in reference lines 2-4.

Procedure codes are reported in Block 24A-K. Procedures can be listed in the order they were performed, with the exception of surgeries. When multiple surgical procedures are performed, a modifier 51 or 59 may be attached to the additional procedures. When utilizing modifier 51, it is critical to list the most extensive procedure first, followed by the lesser procedures. Most extensive procedures can be determined by reviewing the relative value units (RVU) for the procedures. The procedure with the highest RVU is listed first. Payer reimbursement is based on the multiple procedure rule, and payment is made at a reduced rate for additional procedures.

Sequencing on the CMS-1450 (UB-04)

Diagnoses and procedures should be sequenced according to how they will be listed on the claim form. The principal diagnosis is listed in form locator (FL) 67. Other diagnoses are listed in order of severity in FL 67A-Q. The admitting diagnosis is listed in FL 69.

BOX 9-25 ■ KEY POINTS

Sequencing Codes on the CMS-1450 (UB-04) Claim Form

Diagnosis codes are listed as follows:

- The principal diagnosis is listed in FL 67
- Other diagnoses are listed in FL 67A-Q
- The admitting diagnosis and related E code is listed in FL 69 and FL 72.

Procedure codes are listed in FL 74a-e.

- List the principal procedure in FL 74.
- List other significant procedures in FL 74a-e.

Services procedures, and items are listed by revenue code categories in FL 42-49. HCPCS are listed in FL 4L on outpatient claims.

The principal procedure is listed in FL 74 and other procedures are listed in FL 74a-e. Other procedures should be listed in order of complexity.

APPLICATION OF CODING GUIDELINES

The application of coding guidelines varies according to the coding system used. Each coding system provides specific guidelines. To code accurately, it is necessary to understand the guidelines for each coding system and how to use coding resources.

Coding Resources

Several resources can be utilized as a reference for coding. The International Classification of Diseases, 9th Revision, Clinical Modification (ICD-9-CM) provides guidelines specific to inpatient and outpatient coding. Guidelines for ICD-9-CM coding are the ICD-9-CM Official Coding Guidelines, found in the ICD-9-CM manual and the *Coding Clinic* published by the American Hospital Association. Guidelines for Current Procedural Terminology (CPT) coding are found in the CPT manual and in the *CPT Assistant*, published by the AMA (Figure 9-31). Guidelines for HCPCS Level II Medicare National codes can be found in most HCPCS Level II manuals in the appendix, in sections referred to as the Medicare Carrier Manual (MCM) and Coverage Issues Manual (CIM). CMS provides information and guidelines regarding coding on their Web site. Table 9-3 illustrates various coding guideline resources available.

It is critical for coders to have the most current information regarding billing and coding guidelines in

TABLE 9-3 Coding Guidelines Resources and Associations

Resources	Website
ICD-9-CM Official Coding Guidelines	
ICD-9-CM coding guidelines are published in the *Coding Clinic*. The *Coding Clinic* is published quarterly by the American Hospital Association (AHA).	www.aha.org
ICD-9-CM coding guidelines are approved by the cooperating parties: The National Center for Health Statistics (NCHS).	www.cdc.gov/nchs
The American Health Information Management Association (AHIMA).	www.ahima.org
The Centers for Medicare and Medicaid Services (CMS).	www.cms.hhs.gov
HCPCS Level I CPT Coding Guidelines	
CPT coding guidelines are published in the CPT manual. The CPT manual is published annually by the American Medical Association (AMA). The American Medical Association (AMA) also publishes a monthly newsletter, the *CPT Assistant*, which provides information regarding guidelines and procedure code selection. CPT code errata sheets that outline current code changes can also be viewed on the AMA Web site.	www.ama-assn.org
HCPCS Level II Medicare National Coding Guidelines	
HCPCS Level II coding guidelines are published in the HCPCS manual. The HCPCS manual is published annually by various publishers.	
Coding guidelines and updates can be viewed on the CMS Web site.	www.cms.hhs.gov/medicare/hcpcs/default.asp
The American Hospital Association publishes a *Coding Clinic* for the HCPCS Level II coding system.	www.aha.org
Associations	
American Academy of Professional Coders (AAPC)	www.aapc.com
American Association of Healthcare Administration Management (AAHAM)	www.ahima.org
American Health Information Management Association (AHIMA)	
American Medical Billing Association (AMBA)	www.ambanet.net/AMBA

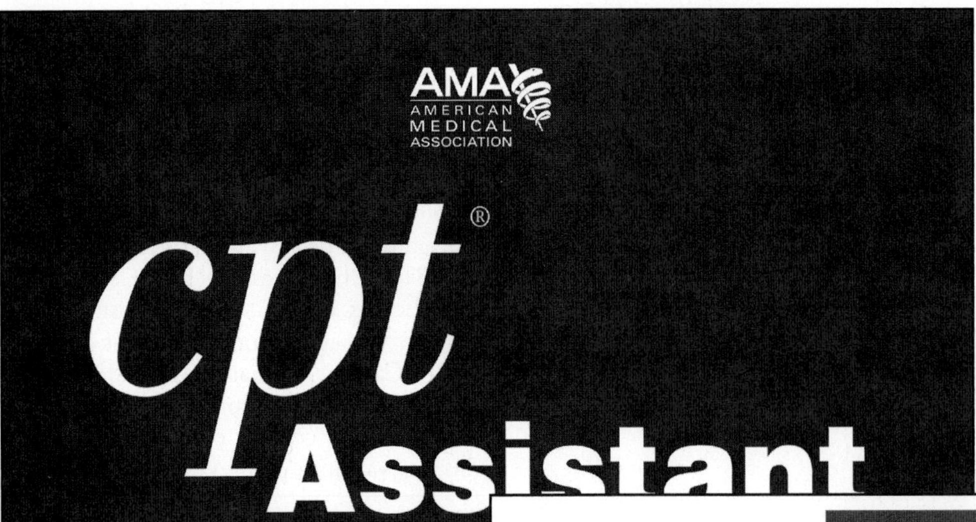

Your Practical

February 2006 / Volume 16, Issue 2

At Issue This Month

Changes to the 2006 Categor

The Category III section of the CPT codeboo
CPT 2006, the Category III section has 14 ne
codes. These changes include methods to re
testing, inert gas rebreathing, and extracorp
new series on medication therapy managem
reporting for these procedures.

AHA
Coding Clinic®
for ICD-9-CM

A quarterly publication of the Central Office on ICD-9-CM

Volume 22 **Fourth Quarter**
Number 4 **2005**

In this issue

New/Revised Codes

New codes contained in this issue effective with discharges October 1, 2005. Other coding advice or code assignments contained in this issue effective with discharges November 18, 2005.

Figure 9-31 Two primary coding resources are the AMA's *CPT Assistant* and the AHA's *Coding Clinic*. *(Courtesy American Medical Association,* CPT Assistant. *Used with permission. Courtesy American Hospital Association,* Coding Clinic. *Used with permission.)*

order to ensure compliance with those guidelines and to ensure that appropriate reimbursement is received. Application of coding guidelines varies according to the category of service, as discussed previously. Categories of services discussed in this text are outpatient, non-patient, and inpatient services. The claim form used for submission of charges for these services also varies. The CMS-1500 is utilized for physician and outpatient services. The UB-04 claim form is used to submit facility charges for hospital services.

TEST YOUR *Knowledge* BOX 9-6

STEPS TO CODING UTILIZING HCPCS AND ICD-9-CM: ABSTRACTING/CODING APPLICATIONS

Following the basic steps to coding, identify and code diagnosis(es) and procedure code(s) utilizing HCPCS and ICD-9-CM as outlined below.

Hospital Coding Case 1

Patient presented at the hospital Emergency Department with numbness down one side of the body, dizziness, dysphasia and confusion. A Level IV physical exam was performed. MRI and 12-lead EKG were performed which showed transient ischemic attack. The patient was admitted. Heparin was ordered 5,000 units SUBQ two times in the day. Arteriogram of the brain was performed the next day which showed carotid stenosis. A carotid endarterectomy was performed. The patient tolerated the procedure well.

1. Identify and code the principal diagnosis.

2. What procedures are not significant procedures?

3. Identify and code all non-significant procedures.

4. Identify and code the principal procedure for reporting on the claim form.

5. Select the appropriate CPT procedure code that describes the principal procedure.

6. Select and code any medications and supplies.

7. What claim form will be used to report these services?

8. List the field on the claim form where the principal diagnosis is reported.

9. List the field on the claim form where the principal procedure(s) is reported.

10. Explain how the emergency room services will be reported and on what claim form.

CHAPTER SUMMARY

This chapter provides an overview of the relationship between billing and coding to provide an understanding of the significance of coding in the billing process. Accurate coding is essential in order to obtain appropriate reimbursement and ensure compliance with guidelines. Concepts on documentation, diagnosis and procedure coding, the billing process, payer processing, and accounts receivable management were covered in previous chapters. This chapter provides a brief review of those concepts to further demonstrate how all elements are critical components to effective coding and billing.

Coding guidelines vary by provider, category of service, and payer type. The challenge for hospital coding and billing professionals is to understand those variations and effectively apply the principles and guidelines applicable to coding patient care services rendered by the provider. This chapter explored general diagnosis and procedure coding guidelines and their appropriate application. Abstracting and the basic steps to coding conditions and procedures was reviewed to assist with the application of coding guidelines, using case scenarios for outpatient, ambulatory surgery, and inpatient cases.

CHAPTER REVIEW 9-1

True/False

1. Coding represents the written description of a service provided and the diagnosis that explains why the service was provided, as recorded in the patient's medical record. T F
2. HCPCS and ICD-9-CM Volume III procedure codes are used to code services and conditions on all claims. T F
3. Claims received by payers undergo a computerized review of the claim, which is commonly referred to as edits. T F
4. The CMS-1450 (UB-04) is used to submit facility charges for inpatient services. T F
5. Coding systems utilized vary based on the category of service. T F

Fill in the Blank

6. Ambulatory surgery service charges represent the ____________________ component of performing the surgery.
7. The coding system used to report significant procedures is ____________________.
8. HCPCS consists of two levels of codes and they are ____________________ and ____________________.
9. The CMS-1450 (UB-04) requires reporting of significant procedures in form locators ____________________ and ____________________.
10. The CMS-1450 (UB-04) requires reporting of admitting, principal, and other diagnoses in form locators ____________________, ____________________, and ____________________ ____________________ through ____________________.

Match the Following Definitions With the Terms at Right

11. ___ The procedure performed for definitive treatment of the principal diagnosis.
12. ___A procedure that is surgical in nature, or carries a procedural risk, or carries an anesthetic risk, or requires specialized training as defined in the Uniform Hospital Discharge Data Set (UHDDS), published in the *Federal Register*, Volume 50, Number 147, July 31, 1985.
13. ___ The condition determined after study is called?
14. ___ Codes developed in the 1980s to provide a standard system for reporting supplies, equipment, medication and other items to Medicare carriers.
15. ___ The process of assigning codes to written descriptions of procedures, services, or items.

A. HCPCS Level II Medicare National codes
B. Principal procedure
C. Procedure coding
D. Significant procedure
E. Principal diagnosis

CHAPTER REVIEW 9-2: CODING CLINICAL SCENARIOS

The following outpatient, ambulatory surgery, and inpatient coding scenarios are designed to provide application of abstracting, coding, and claim form usage guidelines. Read each case carefully and utilize concepts reviewed in this chapter and appropriate HCPCS and ICD-9-CM manuals to code the case and answer the questions.

Coding Outpatient Cases

The following patient care services were performed at various hospital clinics or departments. The physician is an employee of the hospital in these cases. Review each case and assign appropriate diagnosis and procedure codes. Indicate what claim form will be used to submit charges and note in which fields on the claim form the diagnosis and procedures codes will be recorded.

Outpatient Case 1: OB/GYN Clinic Visit—Hospital Based

Report professional services

A new patient presents at the clinic complaining of occasional vaginal spotting and discharge and painful urination. Patient also notes she has been diagnosed with pernicious anemia and requires a B12 shot. The doctor performs a detailed history and exam, with low complexity decision making, which reveals cervicitis. Patient is given an IM shot of B12, 1000 μg. The doctor performs a colposcopy with biopsy of the cervix. Inflammation of the endothelial lining is present. Specimen is sent out for pathology exam.

1-1. List diagnosis code(s) for this case in the appropriate sequence.
1-2. List the appropriate procedure code(s).
1-3. Indicate what claim form will be used to submit charges for this visit.
1-4. State what field(s) on the claim form the diagnosis code(s) will be recorded in.
1-5. State what field(s) on the claim form the procedure code(s) will be recorded in.

Outpatient Case 2: Laboratory Visit—Hospital

A Medicare patient presents at the hospital laboratory department with a physician order for hepatitis A antibody, hepatitis B core antibody, hepatitis B surface antigen and hepatitis C antibody studies. Indications for the laboratory procedures are chronic flu-like symptoms and jaundice coloring of patient. Blood was drawn and studies performed which indicate viral hepatitis A. Lab report sent to physician.

2-1. List diagnosis code(s) for this case in the appropriate sequence.
2-2. List the appropriate procedure code(s).
2-3. Indicate what claim form will be used to submit charges for this visit.
2-4. State what field(s) on the claim form the diagnosis code(s) will be recorded in.
2-5. State what field(s) on the claim form the procedure code(s) will be recorded in.

Outpatient Case 3: Walk In Clinic Visit—Hospital

Report Professional Services

A 45-year-old woman presents with shortness of breath. Patient feels severe tightness in the chest. Patient states episodes of SOB happen more frequently. Expanded problem-focused history reveals the patient is under considerable amount of stress as result of family issues. Patient is a smoker and drinks occasionally.

An expanded problem-focused exam is performed with moderate complexity decision making which reveals the patient is experiencing severe atypical anxiety attacks.

3-1. List diagnosis code(s) for this case in the appropriate sequence.
3-2. List the appropriate procedure code(s).
3-3. Indicate what claim form will be used to submit charges for this visit.
3-4. State what field(s) on the claim form the diagnosis code(s) will be recorded in.
3-5. State what field(s) on the claim form the procedure code(s) will be recorded in.

CHAPTER REVIEW 9-2: CODING CLINICAL SCENARIOS—*cont'd*

Outpatient Case 4: Radiology Visit—Hospital

Patient presents at the hospital radiology department with a physician requisition for a chest X-ray, PA and lateral. Indication for exam: shortness of breath. Two views of the chest are taken. Radiologist findings indicate the lungs are clear and the cardiac and mediastinal silhouettes are of normal size and contour. The central pulmonary vasculature appears normal. No abnormalities indicated. Impression: Negative chest examination.

4-1. List diagnosis code(s) for this case in the appropriate sequence.
4-2. List the appropriate procedure code(s).
4-3. Indicate what claim form will be used to submit charges for this visit.
4-4. State what field(s) on the claim form the diagnosis code(s) will be recorded in.
4-5. State what field(s) on the claim form the procedure code(s) will be recorded in.

Outpatient Case 5: Primary Care Visit—Hospital Based

Report Professional Services

Patient presents with a multitude of skin problems. Patient has had long history of sun exposure. New patient expanded problem-focused history and exam reveals three scaling, erythematous, actinic keratotic plaques located two on the left temple and one on the right temple; each measures 5 mm in diameter. All three lesions were treated with liquid nitrogen cryosurgical destruction using the CryAc unit, D-tip, 3-second freeze thaw without complication. The patient's second problem is a centrally ulcerated pearly papule of the right mid bridge of the nose measuring 8 mm. Biopsy reveals primary basal cell carcinoma. Referred patient to surgeon for consultation.

5-1. List diagnosis code(s) for this case in the appropriate sequence.
5-2. List the appropriate procedure code(s).
5-3. Indicate what claim form will be used to submit charges for this visit.
5-4. State what field(s) on the claim form the diagnosis code(s) will be recorded in.
5-5. State what field(s) on the claim form the procedure code(s) will be recorded in.

Coding Outpatient Ambulatory Surgery Cases

The following patient care services were performed at the hospital's ambulatory surgery center (ASC). This hospital ASC is not an independent center therefore, Medicare reimbursement will be made based on the PPS APC. The physicians are not employees of the hospital in these cases. Review each case and assign appropriate diagnosis and procedure codes. Indicate which claim form will be used to submit charges and note in which fields on the claim form the diagnosis and procedures code will be recorded.

Ambulatory Surgery Case 1: Discharge Summary

Patient has been experiencing a severe cough, coughing spasms with thick sputum, shortness of breath, and chest pain. Patient was draped and prepped in the usual fashion, general anesthesia was administered. The fiber optic bronchoscope was introduced through the nostril and upper airways, vocal cords, trachea, and the right and left side of the bronchial trees. The right middle lobe and its subsegments, and the right lower lobe and its subsegments showed bronchitis. The left side of the left upper and lower lobe lingula and subsegment showed bronchitis with plenty of mucus plugging and a significant amount of inflammation and friability especially in the left lower lobe. Bronchomalacia was noted in the left lower lobe. Brushings, washings, and biopsy were done from the left lower lobe. The scope was removed and the patient was sent to recovery.

1-1. List the preoperative, postoperative, and other diagnoses.
1-2. List the procedure code(s) for this surgery.
1-3. Indicate what claim form will be used to submit charges for this case.
1-4. State what field(s) the diagnosis code(s) will be recorded in on the claim form.
1-5. State what field(s) the procedure code(s) will be recorded in on the claim form.

(*Continued*)

CHAPTER REVIEW 9-2: CODING CLINICAL SCENARIOS—*cont'd*

Ambulatory Surgery Case 2

Patient presented for scheduled excision of a centrally ulcerated papule on the right mid bridge of nose measuring 8 cm in diameter. Patient was prepped and draped in normal fashion and general anesthesia was administered. A full-thickness incision was made through the skin in an elliptical shape around the lesion. The lesion with a normal margin was removed, measurement 1.1-2. Pathology revealed squamous cell carcinoma. Skin from forehead was prepared and transferred to the defect area. The patient tolerated the procedure well. Patient provide with wound cleanser and six, 8-sq-in gauze, non-impregnated sterile pads without adhesive border for home care.

2-1. List diagnosis code(s) for this case in the appropriate sequence.
2-2. List the procedure code(s) for this surgery.
2-3. Provide codes for any items supplied and non-significant procedures
2-4. Indicate what claim form will be used and where the diagnosis code(s) will be recorded on the claim form.
2-5. State where HCPCS Level I and Level II codes will be recorded on the claim form.

Ambulatory Surgery Case 3

Patient arrived for scheduled arthroscopy. Indications for procedure include: Left knee chondromalacia, medial femoral condyle, and medial meniscus tear. Patient brought to OR; given IV sedation followed by general anesthesia. Tourniquet applied to left lower extremity and inflated. Portals, medial and lateral of the patella femoral were made. Scope introduced and knee was inspected revealing Grade II chondromalacia of the patella femoral joint. A complex meniscus tear was visualized in the medial compartment. Performed a partial medial meniscectomy and chondroplasty, medial femoral condyle. Patient tolerated procedure well. Patient given a set of aluminum crutches and instructed to use crutches for 5 days.

3-1. List diagnosis code(s) for this case in the appropriate sequence.
3-2. List the code(s) for procedure(s) performed during this visit.
3-3. Provide codes for any items supplied
3-4. Indicate what claim form will be used and where the diagnosis code(s) will be recorded on the claim form.
3-5. State where HCPCS Level I and Level II codes will be recorded on the claim form.

Ambulatory Surgery Case 4

Patient arrived to the emergency room with an injury and open fracture to the middle phalanx. X-ray of the hand, three views revealed an open fracture, middle phalanx and dislocation of the proximal interphalangeal joint, middle finger. Patient taken to the OR. Patient was prepped and draped in the normal fashion. Open treatment of interphalangeal dislocation of the joint was performed. Attention was turned to the fracture. Open treatment of the phalangeal fracture was performed. Incision made in the overlying skin fully exposing the fracture, the bones were reapproximated. A wire was placed for internal fixation. The incision was closed in sutured layers and the hand was splinted. Patient was given an injection of hydromorphone, 4 mg for pain. Patient was discharged the same day.

4-1. List diagnosis code(s) for this case in the appropriate sequence.
4-2. List the procedure codes(s) for procedures performed.
4-3. Provide codes for any items supplied.
4-4. Indicate what claim form will be used to report these services and where the diagnosis code(s) will be recorded on the claim form.
4-5. State where HCPCS Level I and Level II codes will be recorded on the claim form.

Ambulatory Surgery Case 5

Patient presented for scheduled cystoscopy. Indications for surgery include: elevated PSA, blood in urine and inability to control urination. Patient was draped and prepped in the normal fashion and general anesthesia administered. Cystocope was introduced through the urethra. The urethra was dilated and the scope advanced into the bladder where a needle biopsy was performed. The scope was removed and the patient was discharged.

5-1. List diagnosis code(s) for this case in the appropriate sequence.
5-2. List the procedure code(s) for this surgery.
5-3. Indicate what claim form will be used to report these services.
5-4. List where the diagnosis code(s) will be recorded on the claim form.
5-5. State where HCPCS Level I and Level II codes will be recorded on the claim form.

Coding Inpatient Cases

The following cases represent inpatient cases at the hospital. The physicians are not employees of the hospital in these cases. Review each case and assign appropriate diagnosis and procedure codes. Indicate which claim form will be used to submit charges and note in which fields on the claim form the diagnosis and procedures codes will be recorded.

Inpatient Case 1

Patient admitted for shortness of breath, dyspnea on exertion, sweats, and myalgias. CT scan showed a mass and massive pericardial effusion on the right side. Drainage of the pericardium was performed. A bronchoscopy with biopsy revealed adenocarcinoma of lung. Patient underwent chemotherapy. Diagnosis: Chronic obstructive pulmonary disease and acute malignant pericardial effusion due to the carcinoma.

1-1. List the admitting, principal, and other diagnosis code(s)
1-2. List the principal and other procedure code(s).
1-3. Indicate what claim form will be used to submit charges for this case.
1-4. State what field(s) on the claim form the diagnosis code(s) will be recorded in.
1-5. State what field(s) on the claim form the procedure code(s) will be recorded in.

Inpatient Case 2

Patient admitted for evaluation of longstanding history of gastroesophageal reflux disease and esophagitis. CBC and urinalysis performed. Barium swallow testing detected gross changes and erosion of the esophagus. Laparoscopic fundoplication (Nissen Procedure) performed under general anesthesia. Laparoscope was introduced into the abdomen. The fundus was then released and stayed in position. Several interrupted sutures were placed to close down the hiatal hernia. Interrupted sutures were used to anchor the fundic wrap to the stomach wall as well as the esophagus. Instruments were removed and the wound was closed. The patient tolerated the procedure well.

2-1. List the admitting, principal and other diagnosis code(s)
2-2. List the principal and other significant procedure code(s).
2-3. Indicate what claim form will be used to submit charges for this case.
2-4. State what field(s) on the claim form the diagnosis code(s) will be recorded in.
2-5. State what field(s) on the claim form the procedure code(s) will be recorded in.

(*Continued*)

CHAPTER REVIEW 9-2: CODING CLINICAL SCENARIOS—*cont'd*

Inpatient Case 3

Patient admitted with a pathologic compression fracture at L2 for surgery. Patient has also been diagnosed with severe lumbar stenosis. The surgeon performed bilateral laminotomies and foraminotomies with exploration and decompression of L2, L3, L4 and L5. Pedicle screws were placed at L1 through L4 with rods from L1 to L5. Fusion was performed posterolateral from L1 to L5.

3-1. List the admitting, principal and other diagnosis code(s)
3-2. List the principal and other procedure code(s).
3-3. Indicate what claim form will be used to submit charges for this case.
3-4. State what field(s) on the claim form the diagnosis code(s) will be recorded in.
3-5. State what field(s) on the claim form the procedure code(s) will be recorded in.

Inpatient Case 4

Patient admitted to undergo a cervical diskectomy. Patient is a 40-year-old male with severe and persistent pain involving his neck and left upper extremity unresponsive to conservative treatment. MRI scan showed displacement of cervical intervertebral disc without myelopathy at C5-6. Patient underwent a complete diskectomy C5-6 with removal of spondylitic bars C5-6. Anterior cervical fusion C5-6 using fibular strut graft and Orion plate under fluoroscopy control. Patient tolerated procedure well.

4-1. List the admitting, principal and other diagnosis code(s)
4-2. List the principal and other procedure code(s).
4-3. Indicate what claim form will be used to submit charges for this case.
4-4. State what field(s) on the claim form the diagnosis code(s) will be recorded in.
4-5. State what field(s) on the claim form the procedure code(s) will be recorded in.

Inpatient Case 5

Patient presents with symptoms of severe vertigo involving spinning and imbalance, nausea, and vomiting. The patient is experiencing these symptoms more frequently and in some cases the patient indicates it seems like he goes into shock for a brief period. The patient also states he is experiencing extreme hearing loss. After diagnostic testing the patient was diagnosed with active vestibular Meniere's disease. Treatment options were discussed with the patient's family. Due to the extreme hearing loss the patient decided to have surgery. The next day the patient was draped and prepped in the usual fashion. Anesthesia was administered. An incision was made anterior to the auricle and carried down to the temporalis muscle. The muscle was divided. Craniotomy performed and the skull removed exposing the dura over the temporal lobe of the brain. The bone over the flora of the middle fossa was drilled and the facial nerve was identified and followed to the internal auditory canal. The canal was decompressed and the vestibular nerves were opened. The vestibular nerves were cut while preserving the facial and cochlear nerves. A muscle graft was placed over the internal auditory canal, and the bone was replaced in the skull defect. The incision was sutured and dressing applied. The patient tolerated the nerve section procedure well.

5-1. List the admitting, principal and other diagnosis code(s).
5-2. List the principal and other procedure code(s).
5-3. Indicate what claim form will be used to submit charges for this case.
5-4. State what field(s) on the claim form the diagnosis code(s) will be recorded in.
5-5. State what field(s) on the claim form the procedure code(s) will be recorded in.

GLOSSARY

Correct Coding Initiatives (CCI) Outlines correct coding methodologies based on CPT coding conventions and guidelines and national and local policies and edits. The CCI is also referred to as the Medicare National Correct Coding Initiatives (NCCI).

Facility charges Charges that represent the cost and overhead for providing patient care services, including space, equipment, supplies, drugs and biologicals, and technical staff. Facility charges represent the technical component of the services.

Global procedure Represents the technical and professional portion of a procedure. CPT procedure codes represent the global procedure (service) unless otherwise stated.

Medicare Code Editor (MCE) A computerized program that incorporates various Medicare edits designed to check inpatient claim data to identify problems related to services billed, such as coding errors or issues involving medical necessity.

Medicare Outpatient Code Editor (OCE) A computerized program designed to check Medicare outpatient claim data to identify problems related to services billed, such as coding errors or issues involving medical necessity. OCE incorporates the National Correct Coding Initiatives (CCI) and other Medicare edits.

Payer edits A computer process designed to check data on the claim against the payer's data file and to check the codes submitted to identify problems related to services billed, such as coding errors or issues involving medical necessity.

Phantom billing Billing for services that are not recorded in the medical record documentation (not performed).

Primary diagnosis The major most significant reason why the patient is seeking health care services.

Principal diagnosis The patient's condition established after study to be chiefly responsible for the admission of the patient to the hospital for care. Condition after study refers to the diagnosis made after the examination and/or diagnostic tests are performed.

Principal procedure The significant procedure performed for definitive treatment of the principal diagnosis or the significant procedure that most closely relates to the principal diagnosis.

Professional component Represents the portion of a procedure that involves the physician or other non-physician provider's work in performing a service, such as administering anesthesia, performing surgery, or supervision and interpretation of a radiology procedure.

Significant procedures A significant procedure is one that is: 1. surgical in nature, or 2. carries a procedural risk, or 3. carries an anesthetic risk, or 4. requires specialized training. This definition is stated in the Uniform Hospital Discharge Data Set (UHDDS), as published in the *Federal Register* in 1985.

Surgical package Describes services that are included when performing surgical procedures such as simple anesthesia, one E/M after the decision for surgery, writing orders, evaluating the patient after anesthesia, and normal uncomplicated postoperative care. The surgical package is commonly referred to as the global surgical package and it is defined in the CPT guidelines.

Technical component Represents the cost and overhead of procedures performed such as the equipment, technician, and supplies. Facility charges for the technical component of services are submitted by the entity that owns the equipment, employs the technician, and provides the materials and supplies.

Unbundling The process of utilizing more than one code to describe a service that should be represented with a single code.

Upcoding Utilizing a higher-level code to describe a service or procedure that is not supported by the documentation. Upcoding is also referred to as "creeping".

SECTION FOUR

Claim Forms

Chapter 10

Claim Forms

The purpose of this chapter is to provide a basic understanding of claim forms utilized by hospital facilities to submit charges to payers for reimbursement. A discussion of the purpose of a claim form is followed by a review of manual and electronic claim submission. The provider, payer, and type of service determine claim form usage. A review of claim form variations will describe two forms utilized for submitting charges to payers: the CMS-1500 and the CMS-1450 (UB-04). Previous chapters have outlined information regarding the claims process, coding diagnoses and procedures, and the relationship between billing and coding. This chapter will illustrate how those elements relate to claim forms. Although hospitals utilize both claim forms to submit charges, the CMS-1450 (UB-04) is the primary claim form used for submission of charges for most services, procedures, and items. For this reason an overview of the CMS-1500 is provided but then is followed by an in-depth discussion on claim form completion requirements for the CMS-1450 (UB-04). The UB-04 claim form was implemented by May 22, 2007. This chapter will close with an overview of the UB-04 claim form.

Outline

Chapter Objectives

- Define terms, phrases, abbreviations, and acronyms related to claim forms.
- Explain the purpose of claim forms.
- Describe manual and electronic claim submission and discuss advantages and disadvantages of each submission method.
- Explain the difference between the CMS-1500 and CMS-1450 (UB-04) and outline when they are used.
- Discuss variations in claim form usage and coding systems utilized for each of the claim forms.
- Demonstrate an understanding of data requirements and completion instructions for the CMS-1500 and CMS-1450 (UB-04).

Key Terms

Assignment of benefits
Attending physician
Batch
Clearinghouse
Electronic data interchange (EDI)
Electronic media claim (EMC)
Form locator (FL)
Insurance claim form
Medical record number (MRN)
National Provider Identifier (NPI)
National Uniform Billing Committee (NUBC)
North American Industry Classification System (NAIC) Code
Optical scanning
Paper claim
Provider
Reimbursement
Revenue codes
State Uniform Billing Committee (SUBC)
Tertiary payer
Timely filing
Unique Provider Identification Number (UPIN)

Acronyms and Abbreviations

AMA—American Medical Association
CMS—Centers for Medicare and Medicaid Services
CMS-1450 (UB-04)—Uniform Bill Revised 2004
EDI—electronic data interchange
EIN—employer identification number
EMC—electronic media claim
ER/ED—emergency room, emergency department
FL—form locator
HCPCS—Health Care Common Procedure Coding System
HIAA—Health Insurance Association of America
HIPAA—Health Insurance Portability and Accountability Act
HIPPS—Health Insurance Prospective Payment System
HRN—health record number
ICD-9-CM—International Classification of Diseases, 9th Revision, Clinical Modification
MRN—medical record number
NAIC—North American Industry Classification System Code
NPI—National Provider Identifier
NUBC—National Uniform Billing Committee
OCR—optical character recognition
PoA—Present on Admission
RA—remittance advice
SUBC—State Uniform Billing Committee
UB-04—CMS-1450 Universal Bill implemented in 2007.
UPIN—Unique Provider Identification Number

PURPOSE OF CLAIM FORMS

An **insurance claim form** is a form that is completed by providers for the purpose of submitting charges for medical services and supplies to various third-party payers. Claim forms contain fields for recording data about the provider, insured, date of service, and charges. A **provider** is an individual or entity that provides medical services and/or supplies to patients. Examples of providers are physician, physician assistant, nurse practitioner, certified registered nurse anesthetist, clinic, laboratory, radiology center, hospital, ambulatory surgery center, rehabilitation facility, skilled nursing facility, home health agency, or durable medical equipment company. When a provider completes a patient encounter, charges for that encounter are coded and submitted to the patient or third-party payer for reimbursement. Charges are sent to patients on an invoice or patient statement. Charges are submitted to third-party payers utilizing claim forms. **Reimbursement** is a term used to describe the payment received from a third-party payer for services rendered by the provider to a patient. Third-party reimbursement for medical services or supplies is determined based on the information reported on the claim form. Claim form information is also utilized by various organizations and agencies for research, education, and administrative purposes, as discussed in previous chapters.

BOX 10-1 ■ KEY POINTS

Claim Form Submission Methods

Manual

Paper claim, typed or computer generated, sent by mail

Electronic Media Claim (EMC)

Transmitted through electronic data interchange (EDI)

CLAIM FORM SUBMISSION

Claim forms can be submitted to third-party payers manually on paper or by electronic transmission. A manual claim is a paper claim that is typed or computer generated on paper and sent by mail. This is referred to as manual claim submission. An **electronic media claim (EMC)** is a claim that is transmitted through electronic data interchange (EDI). **Electronic data interchange (EDI)** is the process of sending data from one computer to another by telephone line or cable. EDI requires data to be in a specific format, and both computers must be set up to send and receive data in the required format.

Today, claim forms are primarily computer generated. Two universal claim forms are utilized to submit charges to all payers, the CMS-1500 and CMS-1450 (UB-04). Although these claim forms are universal, the guidelines for completion vary by payer. The edits performed on the claims also vary by payer. These variations are addressed by setting up a computer template of required information by payer type. A computer template defines all the information required on the claim for the payer, and specific payer edits can also be programmed. Hospital personnel responsible for setting up these computer templates must have in-depth knowledge of various payer specifications for completion of the claim form. The payer-specific knowledge is beyond the scope of this text; however, an overview of general claim form completion requirements is provided. Hospital billing and coding professionals should have payer specifications available when setting up computer templates and submitting claims to various payers. The following review of manual versus electronic claim submission highlights the advantage of electronic claim submission, as illustrated in Figure 10-1.

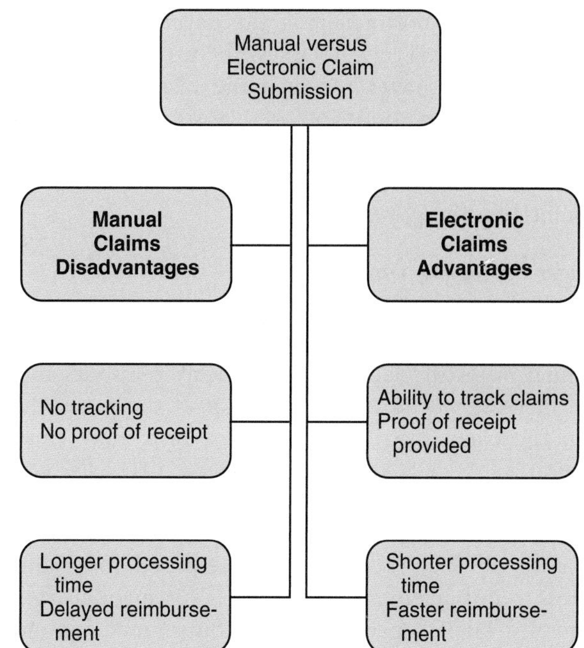

Figure 10-1 Disadvantages and advantages of manual versus electronic claim submission.

> **BOX 10-2 ■ KEY POINTS**
>
> **Universally Accepted Claim Forms**
>
> ***CMS-1500***
>
> Physician and outpatient services
>
> ***CMS-1450 (UB-04)***
>
> Hospital facility charges for outpatient, nonpatient, and inpatient services

Manual Claim Submission

Manual claim submission involves paper claims that are sent to third-party payers by mail or, in some cases, by fax. Many payers no longer allow fax transmission of claims. Historically, all claims were submitted on paper and manually processed by third-party payers. Today, claim forms are designed to be scanned and read utilizing optical character recognition (OCR) technology. **Optical scanning** is a process whereby the claim form is scanned and data on the claim are transferred into a computer system. Claim forms are outlined in red, which allows the scanner to pick up only data in the fields. Optical scanning replaces the process of having to input data manually from the claim form into a computer system. This technology has improved the efficiency of processing claims for third-party payers. **Paper claims** are prepared and sent to various payers primarily by mail. The payer manually inputs or scans the data from the claim form into their computer system. The claim data are then subject to computer edits. When the claim successfully passes through the computer edits, payment determination can be made. An advantage of the paper claim is the ability to review the paper claim before submission; however, there are many disadvantages for providers.

Disadvantages of Paper Claim Submission

A paper claim requires transfer of the data from the claim form to the payer's computer system. The transfer of data may be accomplished through data entry or scanning. Scanning the claim form does improve the time required for payers to process a claim; however, there are still many disadvantages to the submission of paper claims.

No Tracking

Paper claims can be lost in the mail. The claim could also have been lost or misplaced after the payer received it. From the time the claim is received to when the claim data are entered into the payer's system, there is a chance the claim could be lost. There are no tracking mechanisms with paper claims.

No Proof of Receipt

There is no proof of receipt indicating when the payer received the claim unless the claim is sent by registered or certified mail, which can be costly. When payment is not received for a claim, a provider representative will contact the payer to find out the status of the claim.

This inquiry may result in the payer indicating the claim was never received. Unless the provider can show proof that the payer received the claim, it must be resubmitted. Resubmission of claims will delay the reimbursement process. Reimbursement will be denied if the claim is not filed within the timely filing period specified by the payer.

Longer Processing Time

The time to process a manual claim will vary by payer. If the payer does not have the ability to scan the claim, manual input of claim data will delay reimbursement and increase the potential for error. If the payer does scan the claim it will be processed in a more timely fashion.

Delayed Reimbursement

Because of the processing time required for manual claims, reimbursement from payers for manual claims generally takes longer than reimbursement for electronic claims. The average turnaround time for processing a paper claim can be 4 to 8 weeks, as opposed to a turnaround time of 7 to 14 days for claims submitted electronically.

BOX 10-3 ■ KEY POINTS

Manual Claim Submission Disadvantages

- No tracking
- No proof of receipt
- Longer processing time
- Delayed reimbursement

Electronic Claim Submission

In an effort to improve the efficiency of processing claims and reduce associated costs, payers have been moving toward a "paperless" claim process. Electronic claim transmission greatly improves the time it takes for payers to process a claim. Many payers accept paper claims; however, many require claims to be submitted electronically. For example, the Centers for Medicare and Medicaid Services (CMS) requires covered entities to submit claims electronically.

The electronic claim process can be accomplished in two ways: direct transmission to the payer or transmission through a clearinghouse. Direct transmission is when a provider transmits a claim directly to various payers. Providers can also submit a claim through a clearinghouse that reformats the data to meet payer requirements and then forwards the claim to various payers.

Direct Transmission of Claims

Direct transmission requires software that can transmit claim data in the format required for receipt by the payer's computer system. This can pose a problem for providers because it requires software that is compatible with the software of various payers, such as Medicare, Medicaid, TRICARE, Blue Cross/Blue Shield, Aetna, Cigna, and a number of others. To eliminate this problem, many providers use a clearinghouse.

BOX 10-4 ■ KEY POINTS

Electronic Claim Process

The transmission of claims to payers through electronic data interchange (EDI)

Direct Transmission

Transmit to the payer directly, which requires software that can transmit claim data in the format required for receipt by the payer's computer system.

Clearinghouse

Transmit to a clearinghouse that reformats claim data received from various providers to meet compatibility specifications for submission to various payers.

Transmission of Claims Through a Clearinghouse

A **clearinghouse** is an organization that reformats claim data received from providers to meet compatibility specifications for submission to various payers. After the claim data are reformatted and edited, the claim is electronically transmitted by the clearinghouse to the appropriate payer.

The electronic claim submission process for a hospital is illustrated in Figure 10-2. The process begins with the hospital's Patient Accounts Department. Information about a claim is recorded on the patient's computerized account during the patient visit. Before submission of the claim information, the hospital's computer system performs edits on the claim. The edits identify problems with the claim data. Issues identified during the edit can be resolved before transmission. Claims are then prepared for transmission in batches. A **batch** is a group of claims that are prepared and submitted together. Transmission to the payer directly or through a clearinghouse is performed. The clearinghouse may also conduct edits. The clearinghouse and/or payer will provide a notice to the hospital indicating that the batch was received. After the claim has satisfied the payer's edit, payment determination is made. Remittance advice (RA) is forwarded to the hospital explaining payment determination. RA statements can also be transmitted electronically by various payers. The major disadvantage to electronic claim submission is the need for various versions of software or a clearinghouse. Another disadvantage is that claims requiring attachments cannot be submitted electronically. Despite these disadvantages, many providers elect to transmit claims

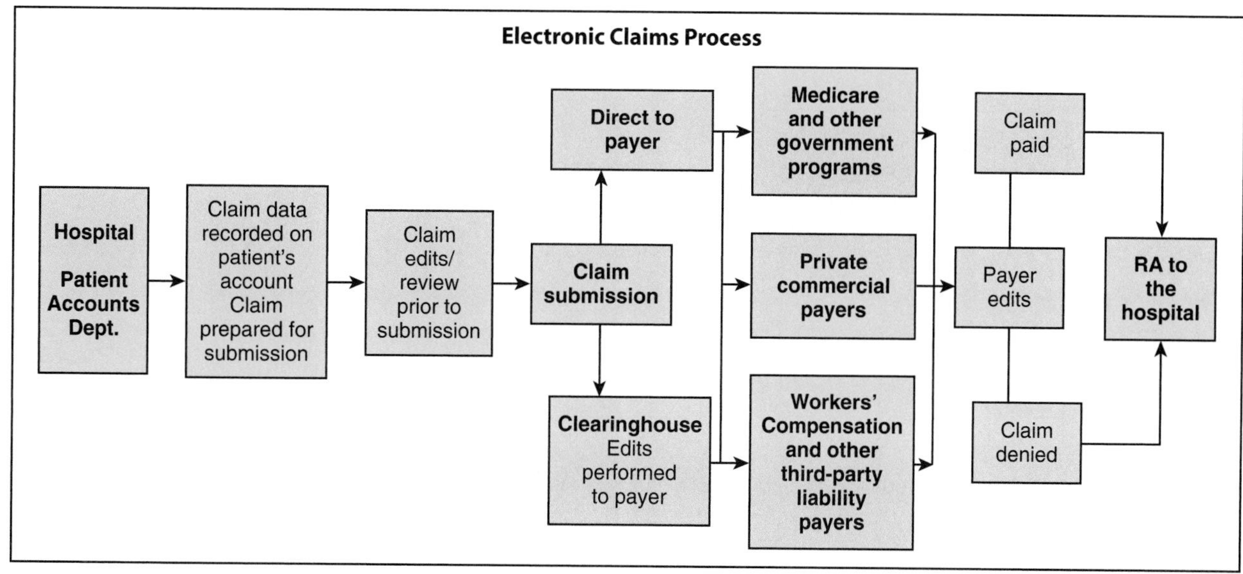

Figure 10-2 The hospital Patient Accounts Department prepares the claim, and it is submitted to the payer directly or through a clearinghouse. *(Modified from Fordney MT:* Insurance handbook for the medical office, *ed 11, St Louis, 2010, Elsevier.)*

electronically because the advantages are greater than the disadvantages.

Advantages of Electronic Claim Submission

Tracking

Electronic claim submission eliminates the potential for claims to be lost in the mail. The clearinghouse or payer confirms batches submitted electronically. This confirmation can be utilized for tracking when the payer received the claim.

Proof of Receipt

The clearinghouse and/or the payer provides a notification report indicating the date the batch was received. This report is referred to as a transmission report; it outlines the claims received in the batch. The transmission report is used as proof of receipt of the claim.

Processing Time

Electronic claim data are received in the payer's computer system. This eliminates any manual handling and data entry of claim information, which eliminates the potential for entry errors. The electronic claim process reduces the amount of time required to process the claim.

Reimbursement

The reduction in time required to process the claim improves the amount of time it takes for the payer to remit a payment determination. Reimbursement on claims transmitted electronically is generally about 7 to 14 days, as opposed to 4 to 8 weeks for a paper claim.

BOX 10-5 ■ KEY POINTS

Advantages of Electronic Claim Submission

Ability to track claims
Proof of receipt is provided
Shorter processing time
Faster reimbursement

CLAIM FORM VARIATIONS

Two claim forms are universally accepted by payers today: the CMS-1500 and the CMS-1450 (UB-04). It is necessary to complete these claim forms in accordance with payer guidelines and specifications. Claim form completion specifications vary by payer. Hospital billing professionals are required to gain knowledge regarding various payer specifications for claim form completion. The category of service dictates which claim form is utilized. Claim form variations for outpatient, inpatient, and nonpatient services are outlined in Table 10-1.

CMS-1500

The CMS-1500 is utilized by noninstitutional providers to submit professional charges for physician and outpatient services to payers for reimbursement.

CMS-1450 (UB-04)

The CMS-1450 (UB-04) is utilized by institutional providers to submit facility charges for services, procedures, and items to payers for reimbursement.

TEST YOUR *Knowledge* BOX 10-1

PURPOSE AND SUBMISSION OF A CLAIM

1. Explain the purpose of claim forms.
2. Define provider.
3. Define reimbursement.
4. Discuss the relationship between the claim form and reimbursement.
5. List two ways a claim form can be submitted.
6. Outline the difference between manual and electronic claim submission.
7. Name two claim forms that are used for submission of claims to payers.
8. Explain how and why computer templates are used.
9. Describe optical scanning.
10. Provide an explanation of how scanning has improved claim processing.
11. State four disadvantages of manual claim submission.
12. Outline two ways that the electronic claims process can be accomplished.
13. Discuss the purpose of a clearinghouse.
14. State four advantages of electronic claim submission.
15. Discuss the difference in the processing time for manual versus electronic claim submission and reimbursements.

TABLE 10-1 Claim Form Variations

Hospital Service Categories (Facility Charges)	CMS-1500	CMS-1450 (UB-04)	Variations
Outpatient			
Ambulatory surgery performed in a hospital outpatient surgery department		√	**Some payers require** ambulatory surgery charges to be submitted on the CMS-1500
Ambulatory surgery performed in a certified Ambulatory Surgery Center (ASC)		√	**Some payers require** outpatient department charges to be submitted on the CMS-1500
Emergency Department		√	**Some payers require** outpatient department charges to be submitted on the CMS-1500
Ancillary Departments: Radiology; Laboratory; Physical, Occupational and Speech Therapy		√	**Some payers require** outpatient department charges to be submitted on the CMS-1500
Other Outpatient Services: Infusion Therapy and Observation		√	**Some payers require** outpatient department charges to be submitted on the CMS-1500
Hospital Based Primary Care Office	√		Physician services may be included if employed by the hospital
Other Hospital Based Clinic	√		
Inpatient			
All services and items provided by the hospital during the inpatient stay		√	Emergency department charges are included on the inpatient claim when the patient is admitted from the emergency department.
Nonpatient			
A specimen received and processed; the patient is not present		√	**Some payers require** outpatient department charges to be submitted on the CMS-1500

Figure 10-3 illustrates which providers are required to utilize the CMS-1500 to report physician and outpatient services and which providers are required to utilize the CMS-1450 (UB-04) to submit facility charges.

BOX 10-6 ■ KEY POINTS

CMS-1450 (UB-04) Submission Requirements for Institutional Providers

Hospitals utilize the CMS-1450 (UB-04) to report facility charges for outpatient, nonpatient, and inpatient services.

Nursing Homes utilize the CMS-1450 (UB-04) to report facility charges for services provided for prolonged and short-term care.

Rehabilitation Centers submit facility charges for rehabilitation services utilizing the CMS-1450 (UB-04).

Ambulatory Surgery Services are reported on the CMS-1450 (UB-04). Independent ambulatory surgery centers may be required to submit charges on a CMS-1500.

CMS-1500 CLAIM FORM OVERVIEW

The CMS-1500 is the universal claim form accepted by most payers for submission of charges for physician and outpatient services. The Health Insurance Association of America (HIAA) and the American Medical Association (AMA) developed the CMS-1500, formerly known as the HCFA-1500, in 1958. The claim form was developed in an attempt to standardize the form used to submit charges to payers. In 1992, the claim form was printed in red ink and adopted by the CMS for use in submission of claims for Medicare patients. Other payers followed suit, and the claim form is now accepted by most payers. Completion requirements and specifications vary by payer to accommodate their computer systems and plans.

Claim Form Data

The form consists of 33 blocks utilized to record information about the patient, provider, and charges. The

CMS-1500 Used by noninstitutional providers to submit professional charges for services provided by physicians or outpatient services	CMS-1450 (UB-04) Used by noninstitutional providers to submit facility charges
Single or group practice physicians Physicians providing services in a primary care or walk-in clinic Hospitals billing for professional services provided by physicians who are employed by or under contract with the hospital Emergency room physicians Radiologists performing interpretation on radiology examinations Surgeons providing surgical services in hospitals and ambulatory surgery centers	Hospitals—technical portion of outpatient, non-patient, and inpatient services Nursing homes—technical portion of short-term and long-term care Rehabilitation centers—technical portion of rehabilitation services provided Ambulatory surgery centers (hospital based)–technical portion of surgeries performed on an outpatient basis
Claim Form Data	Claim Form Data
• Section I–Patient and insurance information (block 1-13) • Section II–Patient diagnosis information (block 14-23) • Section III–Charge information (block 24-24K) • Section IV–Provider information (block 25-33)	• Section I–Facility, patient, discharge, occurrence, and value information (form locator 1-41) • Section II–Charge information (form locator 42-49) • Section III–Payer, insured, employer, and authorization information (form locator 50-65) • Section IV–Procedure, diagnosis, and provider information (form locator 66-81)
Coding System Requirements	Coding System Requirements
• Procedures HCPCS Level I CPT HCPCS Level II Medicare National Codes • Diagnosis ICD-9-CM Volume I and II	• Procedures HCPCS Level I CPT HCPCS Level II Medicare National Codes ICD-9-CM Volume III Procedures • Diagnosis ICD-9-CM Volume I and II

Figure 10-3 Comparison of the CMS-1500 versus CMS-1450 (UB-04) claim forms.

CMS-1500 claim form can be viewed in four major sections, as illustrated in Figure 10-4.

Section I: Patient and Insurance Information (Blocks 1 to 13)

Information about the patient such as name, address, zip code, phone, sex, and employer is recorded in this area. The patient's insurance information, including the name of the plan, the insured's identification number, and other insurance information, is also recorded in this section so the payer can identify the patient and plan within their system.

Section II: Patient Diagnosis Information (Blocks 14 to 23)

This section is utilized to report information about the patient's condition, including the diagnosis code(s).

Section III: Charge Information (Blocks 24A to 24J)

Charge information for each service or item on the claim is required, including the date of service, place of service, procedure code, days or units, and the charge. The diagnosis code(s) that explains the medical necessity for services provided is referenced in Block 24E.

Section IV: Provider Information (Blocks 25 to 33)

This area is used to record information about the provider who rendered the services that are reported on the claim. The provider's name, address, identification number, and tax identification are listed. When services are provided at a location other than the provider's address, the name and address of that location is indicated in this section.

CMS-1500 Instructions

Most hospital facility charges are submitted utilizing the UB-04; therefore, this chapter will focus on completion requirements for the UB-04. This section will provide a brief review of charges submitted on a CMS-1500 and general claim form completion instructions. The completion instructions outlined in Table 10-2 follow guidelines provided by the CMS with some payer variations. Place of service codes are required for completion

1500

HEALTH INSURANCE CLAIM FORM

APPROVED BY NATIONAL UNIFORM CLAIM COMMITTEE 08/05

PICA | PICA

CARRIER

SECTION I PATIENT AND INSURANCE INFORMATION

1. MEDICARE (Medicare #) MEDICAID (Medicaid #) TRICARE CHAMPUS (Sponsor's SSN) CHAMPVA (Member ID#) GROUP HEALTH PLAN (SSN or ID) FECA BLK LUNG (SSN) OTHER (ID) | 1a. INSURED'S I.D. NUMBER (For Program in Item 1)

2. PATIENT'S NAME (Last Name, First Name, Middle Initial) | 3. PATIENT'S BIRTH DATE MM DD YY SEX M F | 4. INSURED'S NAME (Last Name, First Name, Middle Initial)

5. PATIENT'S ADDRESS (No., Street) | 6. PATIENT RELATIONSHIP TO INSURED Self Spouse Child Other | 7. INSURED'S ADDRESS (No., Street)

CITY STATE | 8. PATIENT STATUS | CITY STATE

ZIP CODE TELEPHONE (Include Area Code) ( ) | Employed Full-Time Student Part-Time Student | ZIP CODE TELEPHONE (Include Area Code) ( )

9. OTHER INSURED'S NAME (Last Name, First Name, Middle Initial) | 10. IS PATIENT'S CONDITION RELATED TO: | 11. INSURED'S POLICY GROUP OR FECA NUMBER

a. OTHER INSURED'S POLICY OR GROUP NUMBER | a. EMPLOYMENT? (Current or Previous) YES NO | a. INSURED'S DATE OF BIRTH MM DD YY SEX M F

b. OTHER INSURED'S DATE OF BIRTH MM DD YY SEX M F | b. AUTO ACCIDENT? YES NO PLACE (State) | b. EMPLOYER'S NAME OR SCHOOL NAME

c. EMPLOYER'S NAME OR SCHOOL NAME | c. OTHER ACCIDENT? YES NO | c. INSURANCE PLAN NAME OR PROGRAM NAME

d. INSURANCE PLAN NAME OR PROGRAM NAME | 10d. RESERVED FOR LOCAL USE | d. IS THERE ANOTHER HEALTH BENEFIT PLAN? YES NO *If yes,* return to and complete item 9 a-d.

READ BACK OF FORM BEFORE COMPLETING & SIGNING THIS FORM.

12. PATIENT'S OR AUTHORIZED PERSON'S SIGNATURE I authorize the release of any medical or other information necessary to process this claim. I also request payment of government benefits either to myself or to the party who accepts assignment below.

SIGNED DATE

13. INSURED'S OR AUTHORIZED PERSON'S SIGNATURE I authorize payment of medical benefits to the undersigned physician or supplier for services described below.

SIGNED

PATIENT AND INSURED INFORMATION

SECTION II PATIENT DIAGNOSIS INFORMATION

14. DATE OF CURRENT: MM DD YY ILLNESS (First symptom) OR INJURY (Accident) OR PREGNANCY(LMP) | 15. IF PATIENT HAS HAD SAME OR SIMILAR ILLNESS. GIVE FIRST DATE MM DD YY | 16. DATES PATIENT UNABLE TO WORK IN CURRENT OCCUPATION MM DD YY FROM TO

17. NAME OF REFERRING PROVIDER OR OTHER SOURCE | 17a. 17b. NPI | 18. HOSPITALIZATION DATES RELATED TO CURRENT SERVICES MM DD YY FROM TO

19. RESERVED FOR LOCAL USE | 20. OUTSIDE LAB? YES NO $ CHARGES

21. DIAGNOSIS OR NATURE OF ILLNESS OR INJURY (Relate Items 1, 2, 3 or 4 to Item 24E by Line) 1. 2. 3. 4. | 22. MEDICAID RESUBMISSION CODE ORIGINAL REF. NO.

23. PRIOR AUTHORIZATION NUMBER

SECTION III CHARGE INFORMATION

24. A. DATE(S) OF SERVICE From MM DD YY To MM DD YY	B. PLACE OF SERVICE	C. EMG	D. PROCEDURES, SERVICES, OR SUPPLIES (Explain Unusual Circumstances) CPT/HCPCS MODIFIER	E. DIAGNOSIS POINTER	F. $ CHARGES	G. DAYS OR UNITS	H. EPSDT Family Plan	I. ID. QUAL.	J. RENDERING PROVIDER ID. #
1								NPI	
2								NPI	
3								NPI	
4								NPI	
5								NPI	
6								NPI	

PHYSICIAN OR SUPPLIER INFORMATION

SECTION IV PROVIDER INFORMATION

25. FEDERAL TAX I.D. NUMBER SSN EIN | 26. PATIENT'S ACCOUNT NO. | 27. ACCEPT ASSIGNMENT? (For govt. claims, see back) YES NO | 28. TOTAL CHARGE $ | 29. AMOUNT PAID $ | 30. BALANCE DUE $

31. SIGNATURE OF PHYSICIAN OR SUPPLIER INCLUDING DEGREES OR CREDENTIALS (I certify that the statements on the reverse apply to this bill and are made a part thereof.) | 32. SERVICE FACILITY LOCATION INFORMATION | 33. BILLING PROVIDER INFO & PH # ( )

SIGNED DATE | a. NPI b. | a. NPI b.

NUCC Instruction Manual available at: www.nucc.org | APPROVED OMB-0938-0999 FORM CMS-1500 (08-05)

Figure 10-4 CMS-1500 claim form illustrating four sections of information.

of the form. Table 10-3 on page 363 highlights some common place of service codes.

Hospitals utilize the CMS-1500 claim form to submit charges that represent the professional component of patient care services provided by a physician or other nonphysician clinical provider such as a physician's assistant. As discussed previously, hospitals may submit charges for professional services when the provider is employed by or under contract with the hospital. For example, a hospital physician providing patient care services in a walk-in clinic or primary care office will have charges submitted through the hospital.

General claim form completion guidelines require claims to be completed in black ink. All data must be within the field and must be written in upper case lettering. No punctuation should be used on the form, and dates must be reported using eight digits (MMDDCCYY).

CMS-1450 (UB-04) CLAIM FORM OVERVIEW

The CMS-1450 is also referred to as the UB-04 because it is the universal bill accepted by most payers. UB-04 is used to submit facility charges for outpatient, inpatient, and nonpatient services. This claim form was developed and is maintained by the National Uniform Billing Committee (NUBC). The **National Uniform Billing Committee (NUBC)** was formed by the American Hospital Association in 1975 to develop a single billing form and a standard data set that could be used nationally by institutional providers. The original standard form was

TABLE 10-2 CMS-1500 (08/05) Completion Instructions

Block/Item	Description
Top right	***Carrier block***. Enter the carrier name and address in the upper right hand corner of the claim form in 4 lines as follows: (1) Name (2) Address 1 (3) Address 2 (4) City, State and Zip
1	***Type of insurance coverage***. Indicate the type of insurance coverage for the claim. Place an "X" in the appropriate box: Medicare, Medicaid, Champus, Champva, Group, FECA/Black Lung or Other. *(Other indicates an HMO, Commercial Insurance, Auto Insurance or Workers' Compensation.)*
1A	***Insured's identification number.*** Enter the insured's ID or the ID of the person who holds the policy. Medicare requires the Health Insurance Claim Number (HICN), regardless of whether Medicare is primary or secondary. *Do not use characters or spaces.*
2	***Patient's name.*** Enter the patient's last name, first name, and middle initial, separated by a space. This field is required by Medicare and most other payers. Hyphens may be used for hyphenated names. Do not use periods. For Worker's Compensation enter the Employee ID number.
3	***Patient birth date and sex.*** Enter the patient's date of birth (MMDDCCYY). Enter an X to indicate the patient's sex.
4	***Name of the primary insured.*** Enter the primary insured's name (last, first, middle initial), separated by a space. *If the patient is the insured, write SAME. If Medicare is primary, leave blank.*
5	***Patient's mailing address and telephone number*** on three lines: (1) street address (2) city, state (3) zip and telephone number. *Do not use commas, periods, or other punctuation.*
6	***Patient relationship to insured.*** Check the appropriate box to indicate the relationship to the insured when block 4 is completed.
7	***Insured's address and telephone number.*** Enter the insured's address and telephone number when Block 4 is completed. For Worker's Compensation claims enter the employer's address. *When the address is the same as the patient's, write SAME. If Medicare is primary, leave blank.*
8	***Patient status.*** Check the appropriate box to indicate the patient's marital and employment status.
9	***Other insured's last name, first name, middle initial***. When additional group health coverage exists and block 11D is completed, enter the other insured's name. Enter the name of the enrollee in a Medigap policy if different from the patient's name in Block 2. Otherwise enter SAME. *If there is no Medigap policy, leave blank.* This field may be used in the future for supplemental insurance plans.
9A	***Other insured's policy or group number.*** Leave blank if Block 9 is blank. Otherwise enter the policy and/or group number of the other insured or Medigap insured, preceded by MEDIGAP, MG, OR MGAP.
9B	***Other insured's date of birth and sex.*** Leave blank if Block 9 is blank. Otherwise, enter the other insured's or Medigap insured's birth date (MMDDCCYY) and sex.
9C	***Other insured's employer name or school name***. Leave blank if Block 9 is blank or if a Medigap Payer ID is entered in 9D. Otherwise enter the other insured's employer or school. If other coverage is Medigap, enter the claim processing address of the Medigap insurer and *use an abbreviated street address, two-letter postal code, and zip code.*
9D	***Other insurance plan name or program name.*** Leave blank if Block 9 is blank. Otherwise, enter the other insured's insurance plan or program name or the 9-digit PAYERID number of the Medigap insurer. If no PAYERID number exists, then enter the Medigap insurance program or plan name.
10A-C	***Patient's condition related to***. Place an "X" in the appropriate box to indicate whether the patient's condition was related to employment, auto accident, or other accident. *If an X is entered in the YES box for auto accident, enter the state postal code.* Any item checked "YES" indicates there may be other insurance that is primary. Identify the primary insurance information in Block 11.
10D	***Reserved for local use***. Use this item exclusively for Medicaid (MCD) information. If the patient is entitled to Medicaid, enter the patient's Medicaid number preceded by MCD.
11	***Insured's policy group or FECA number***. Enter the insured's policy or group number when block 4 is completed. *This field must be completed for Medicare claims. (When completed the provider acknowledges a good faith effort was made to determine Medicare primary or secondary payer status.)* If there is no insurance primary to Medicare enter the word "NONE" and proceed to Block 11B. Some payers may indicate this block should be left blank if there is no secondary insurance. If there is secondary insurance, complete Block 9-9D.
11A	***Insured's date of birth and sex***. Enter the insured's birth date (MM DD CCYY) and sex when different from Block 3.

TABLE 10-2 CMS-1500 (08/05) Completion Instructions—*cont'd*

Block/Item	Description
11B	***Employer's name or school name***. Enter employer's name or school, if applicable. If there is a change in the insured's insurance status (e.g., RETIRED), enter an eight-digit (MMDDCCYY) retirement date preceded by the word *retired*. Otherwise, leave blank.
11C	***Insurance plan name or program name***. Enter the 9-digit PAYERID number of the primary insurance. If no PAYERID number exists, enter the complete primary payer's program or plan name. If the primary payer's explanation of benefits (EOB) does not contain the claim processing address, record the primary payer's claims processing address directly on the EOB. This block is required if there is other primary insurance that is listed in Block 11.
11D	***Is there another health benefit plan***? Leave blank—not required by Medicare. Other payers require "yes" or "no" to indicate if there is another health plan. If "yes," Blocks 9A-D must be completed.
12	***Patient's or authorized person's signature and date.*** A signature in this block authorizes the release of medical information for claims processing. If the patient's signed consent form is on file, write "Signature on File".
13	***Insured's or authorized person's signature***. Signature or "signature on file" in this field authorizes payment of medical benefits to be sent to the participating physician or supplier. This block must be completed when "yes" is indicated in the Accept Assignment, Block 27.
14	***Date of current illness, injury, pregnancy***. Enter the date (MM DD CCYY) the patient's first symptoms occurred from the current illness if stated in the medical record; date of injury or accident; or for pregnancy, first day of last menstrual period. No information is required here if the visit is an annual or physical examination.
15	***If patient has had same or similar illness***. Enter the date of any prior, same or similar illness. If unknown, leave blank. This block is not required by Medicare.
16	***Date patient unable to work***. Enter the date (MMDDCCYY) that the patient is unable to work in their current occupation if documented in patient's records. An entry in this field may indicate employment-related insurance coverage. Otherwise, leave blank.
17	***Name of referring physician or other source***. Enter the name and credentials of the referring, ordering, or supervising physician. Format: first name, middle initial, last name, and credentials. When multiple providers are involved, use the following priority order to determine the physician to be listed: (1) Referring Provider (2) Ordering Provider (3) Supervising Provider. Medicare guidelines state "When a claim involves multiple referring and/or ordering physicians, a separate Form CMS-1500 shall be used for each ordering/referring physician."
17A	***Other ID number*** of the referring, ordering, or supervising provider. Medicare guidelines state, effective 5/23/08, that 17A is no longer used for reporting.
17B	***National provider identifier (NPI)***. Enter the NPI number of the referring, ordering, or supervising provider listed in block 17.
18	***Hospitalization dates related to current services***. Enter the eight-digit (MMDDCCYY) admitting and discharge dates when a medical service is furnished as a result of, or subsequent to, a related hospitalization. Leave discharge date blank if patient hasn't been discharged by the time the claim is completed.
19	***Reserved for local use.*** Leave blank.
20	***Outside lab?*** Enter "yes" or "no" when billing diagnostic laboratory tests subject to price purchase limitations. NO means the tests were performed by the billing physician or laboratory. YES means that the laboratory test was performed outside of the physician's office and that the physician is billing for the laboratory service.
21	***Diagnosis or nature of illness or injury***. Enter ICD-9-CM code(s) that represents the patient's diagnosis/condition. Enter one code on each of the four reference lines in priority order.
22	***Medicaid resubmission***. Leave blank for other payers.
23	***Prior authorization number***. Enter the Quality Improvement Organization (QIO) authorization number for those procedures requiring peer review organization approval. Do not use spaces or hyphens.
24A Line (1–6)	***Dates of service***. Enter the six-digit (MMDDYY) date of service for each service, procedure, or item in the "from" and "to" fields. When "from" and "to" dates are shown for a series of identical services, enter the number of consecutive days or units in column G. This is a required field for all payers.
24B (1–6)	***Place of service code (POS)***. Enter the two-digit place of service code to identify the location where the service was performed. This block is required by Medicare and other payers. Place of service codes are outlined in Table 10-3.

Continued

TABLE 10-2	CMS-1500 (08/05) Completion Instructions—*cont'd*
Block/Item	**Description**
24C (1–6)	***EMG.*** Enter Y (YES) or N (NO) in the bottom, unshaded area of the field when required by payer. This field is not required by Medicare.
24D (1–6)	***Procedures, services, or supplies***. Enter the appropriate HCPCS Level I CPT code or Level II Medicare National code and HCPCS modifier(s) as appropriate. You may use up to four modifiers per line item using one space between each one.
24E (1–6)	***Diagnosis pointer***. Enter the appropriate reference number from Block 21 to relate the service(s) with the primary diagnosis. Only one reference number may be used per line. Some payers may require more than one reference number per line. Medicare allows only one reference number.
24F (1–6)	***Charges.*** Enter the charge amount for each listed service.
24G (1–6)	***Days/units***. This field is most commonly used for multiple visits, unit of supplies, anesthesia minutes, or oxygen volume. If only one service is performed, the number 1 must be entered.
24H (1–6)	***ESPDT (Early, periodic, screening, diagnosis and treatment)***. This block is utilized for Medicaid preventive medical examinations. Medicare and other payers do not require completion of this field.
24I	***ID qualifier***. Enter the qualifier ID in the shaded area of 24I if the number is a non-NPI. The list of NUBC-defined qualifiers are outlined in block 17A.
24J	***Rendering provider ID number***. Enter the non-NPI ID No. of the rendering provider in the shaded area of the field. Enter the NPI No. in the unshaded area of the field. *Report the ID No. in blocks 24I and 24J only when different from data recorded in blocks 33A and 33B. Enter numbers left justified in the field.*
25	***Federal Tax ID Number***. Enter the provider's Federal Tax ID No., Employer Identification No., or Social Security No. of the provider billing the services (listed in block 33). Enter an "X" in the appropriate box to indicate the number reported. Only one box can be marked. *Do not enter hyphens with numbers. Enter numbers left justified in the field.*
26	***Patient's account number***. Enter the patient's account number assigned by the provider's accounting system. The number is printed on the payer's EOB. *Do not enter hyphens with numbers.*
27	***Accept assignment***. Check the appropriate box to indicate whether the provider of service accepts the assignment.
28	***Total charges***. Enter the total of all charges listed on the claim in Block 24F.
29	***Amount paid***. Enter the total amount the patient paid for charges listed on the claim. Medicare requires the total amount the patient paid on the covered services only.
30	***Balance due.*** Enter the difference between Total charges (Block 28) and amount paid (Block 29). Completion of this field is not required by Medicare.
31	***Signature of physician or supplier***. Enter the signature of the provider of service or their representative and the eight-digit date (MM DD CCYY) that the form was signed.
32	***Name and address of facility where services were rendered***. Enter the name, address, and zip code of the location where the services were rendered if other than the physician office (i.e., hospital). Line format: (1) Name (2) Address (3) City State Zip Code.
32A	***NPI number.*** Enter the NPI number of the billing provider in 32.
32B	***Other ID number***. Enter the two-digit qualifier identifying the non-NPI number followed by the ID number. The list of NUCC-defined qualifiers outlined in block 17A. *Medicare not reported; effective 5/23/08.*
33	***Billing provider information and phone number.*** Enter the provider's or supplier's billing name, address, and zip code on three lines. Enter the phone number in the area to the right of the title at the ( ). Medicare-required field.
33A	***NPI number.*** Enter the NPI number of the service facility location in 33.
33B	***Other ID number.*** Enter the two-digit qualifier identifying the non-NPI number followed by the ID number. The list of NUCC-defined qualifiers outlined in block 17A. *Medicare not reported; effective 5/23/08.*

Reference Medicare Claims Processing Manual, Chapter 26, and National Uniform Claim Committee, Page 1.

TABLE 10-3 CMS-1500 Block 24B Place of Service Codes

Code	Description
01	Pharmacy
02	Unassigned
03	School
04	Homeless shelter
05	Indian health service freestanding facility
06	Indian health service provider-based facility
07	Tribal 638 freestanding facility
08	Tribal 638 provider-based facility
09	Prison/correctional facility
9–10	Unassigned
11	Office
12	Home
13	Assisted living facility
14	Group home
15	Mobile unit
16	Temporary lodging
17–19	Unassigned
20	Urgent care facility
21	Inpatient hospital
22	Outpatient hospital
23	Emergency department–hospital
24	Ambulatory surgical center
25	Birthing center
26	Military treatment facility/uniformed service treatment facility
27–30	Unassigned
31	Skilled nursing facility (swing bed visits)
32	Nursing facility (intermediate/long-term care facilities)

the UB-82, which was adopted for use in 1982. The form underwent revisions again in 1992, and the UB-92 was adopted. Today, the role of the NUBC is to maintain the integrity of the UB-04 data set, adopted in 2004. The data set is the information required for each field on the claim form. **State Uniform Billing Committees (SUBCs)** have been created to oversee implementation of the UB-04 at the state level.

FOR IMMEDIATE RELEASE—UB-04 scheduled to replace CMS-1450 (UB-92)

NUBC Announces 45-day Public Comment Period, ending February 1, 2005, for the New UB-04 Data Set and Form

December 17, 2004

The National Uniform Billing Committee (NUBC) announced today the opening of a 45-day public comment period, ending February 1, 2005, for the new UB-04 data set and form to replace the UB-92. The UB-04 contains a number of improvements and enhancements that resulted from nearly four years of research. The NUBC is conducting this final survey to better understand the timelines and transition issues surrounding the implementation of the UB-04. Those wishing to comment on the UB-04 are encouraged to visit the NUBC website http://www.nubc.org/ for further information.

NUBC ANNOUNCES APPROVAL OF UB-04

Following the close of a public comment period and careful review of comments received, the National Uniform Billing Committee approved the UB-04 as the replacement for the UB-92 at its February 2005 meeting.

Receivers (health plans and clearinghouses) need to be ready to receive the new UB-04 by March 1, 2007.

Submitters (health care providers such as hospitals, skilled nursing facilities, hospice, and other institutional claim filers) can use the UB-04 **beginning March 1, 2007,** however, they will have a transitional period between March 1, 2007 and May 22, 2007 where they can use the UB-04 or the UB-92.

Starting May 23, 2007 all institutional paper claims must use the UB-04; the UB-92 will no longer be acceptable after this date.

The final image of the UB-04 form, a summary of the public comments/NUBC responses, and information on how to obtain the UB-04 Data Specifications Manual will be posted to the NUBC website.

Figure 10-5 NUBC announcement indicating the UB-04 is scheduled to replace the UB-92. *(Modified from National Uniform Billing Committee*: NUBC announces UB-04 schedule to replace UB-92, www.nubc.org*)*

The NUBC announced in December 2004 that the UB-04 was approved to replace the UB-92 (Figure 10-5). Receivers (health plans and clearinghouses) needed to be ready to receive the new UB-04 by March 1, 2007. Submitters (health care providers such as hospitals) were still able to use the UB-04 on March 1, 2007; however, they had a transitional period between March 1, 2007 and May 22, 2007. Starting May 23, 2007, all paper claims had to be submitted using the UB-04. The following section provides instructions for the UB-04.

Claim Form Data

The UB-04 consists of 81 data fields that are referred to as **form locators (FLs)**. The billing requirements for each field and the revenue codes are revised on an ongoing basis by the NUBC, SUBCs, and the CMS. The UB-04 can be viewed in four sections, in which information about the patient, facility, charges, and physicians involved in the patient's care is recorded, as illustrated in (Figure 10-6).

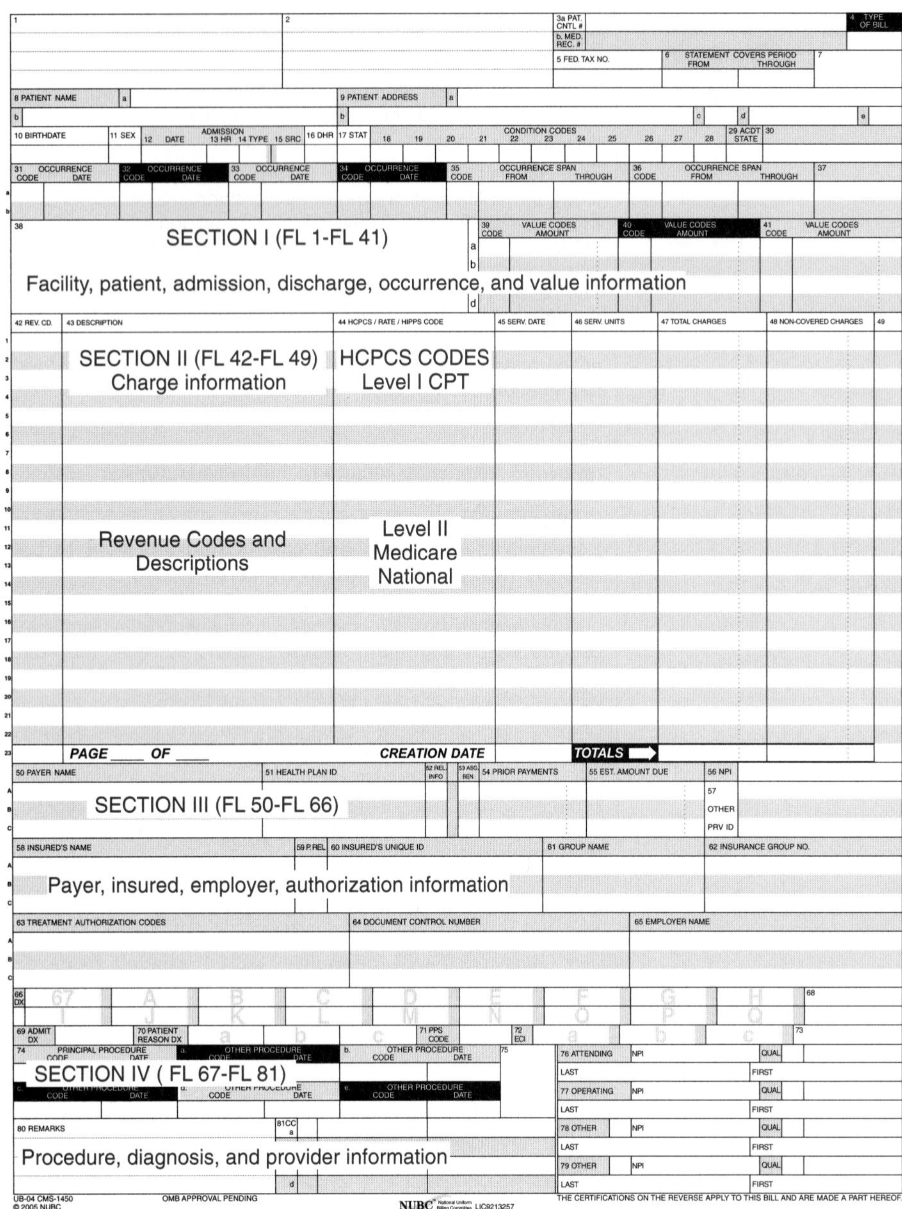
1
2
3a PAT. CNTL #
b. MED. REC. #
4 TYPE OF BILL
5 FED. TAX NO.
6 STATEMENT COVERS PERIOD FROM THROUGH
7
8 PATIENT NAME a b
9 PATIENT ADDRESS a b c d e
10 BIRTHDATE
11 SEX
ADMISSION 12 DATE 13 HR 14 TYPE 15 SRC
16 DHR
17 STAT
CONDITION CODES 18 19 20 21 22 23 24 25 26 27 28
29 ACDT STATE
30
31 OCCURRENCE CODE DATE
32 OCCURRENCE CODE DATE
33 OCCURRENCE CODE DATE
34 OCCURRENCE CODE DATE
35 OCCURRENCE SPAN CODE FROM THROUGH
36 OCCURRENCE SPAN CODE FROM THROUGH
37
38
39 VALUE CODES CODE AMOUNT
40 VALUE CODES CODE AMOUNT
41 VALUE CODES CODE AMOUNT
SECTION I (FL 1-FL 41)
Facility, patient, admission, discharge, occurrence, and value information
42 REV. CD.
43 DESCRIPTION
44 HCPCS / RATE / HIPPS CODE
45 SERV. DATE
46 SERV. UNITS
47 TOTAL CHARGES
48 NON-COVERED CHARGES
49
SECTION II (FL 42-FL 49)
Charge information
HCPCS CODES
Level I CPT
Revenue Codes and Descriptions
Level II Medicare National
PAGE ___ OF ___
CREATION DATE
TOTALS
50 PAYER NAME
51 HEALTH PLAN ID
52 REL. INFO
53 ASG. BEN.
54 PRIOR PAYMENTS
55 EST. AMOUNT DUE
56 NPI
57 OTHER PRV ID
SECTION III (FL 50-FL 66)
58 INSURED'S NAME
59 P. REL
60 INSURED'S UNIQUE ID
61 GROUP NAME
62 INSURANCE GROUP NO.
Payer, insured, employer, authorization information
63 TREATMENT AUTHORIZATION CODES
64 DOCUMENT CONTROL NUMBER
65 EMPLOYER NAME
66 DX
67 A B C D E F G H I J K L M N O P Q
68
69 ADMIT DX
70 PATIENT REASON DX
71 PPS CODE
72 ECI
73
74 PRINCIPAL PROCEDURE CODE DATE
a. OTHER PROCEDURE CODE DATE
b. OTHER PROCEDURE CODE DATE
75
76 ATTENDING NPI QUAL LAST FIRST
SECTION IV (FL 67-FL 81)
c. OTHER PROCEDURE CODE DATE
d. OTHER PROCEDURE CODE DATE
e. OTHER PROCEDURE CODE DATE
77 OPERATING NPI QUAL LAST FIRST
80 REMARKS
81CC a b c d
78 OTHER NPI QUAL LAST FIRST
Procedure, diagnosis, and provider information
79 OTHER NPI QUAL LAST FIRST
UB-04 CMS-1450 © 2005 NUBC
OMB APPROVAL PENDING
NUBC National Uniform Billing Committee LIC9213257
THE CERTIFICATIONS ON THE REVERSE APPLY TO THIS BILL AND ARE MADE A PART HEREOF.

Figure 10-6 CMS-1450 (UB-04) claim form is utilized to submit facility charges for outpatient, nonpatient, and inpatient services.

Section I: Facility, Patient, Admission, Discharge, Occurrence, and Value Information (FL 1 to 41)

Detailed information about the facility, patient admission, patient control number, medical record number, admission, and discharge is recorded in FL 1 to 17. Codes that provide information regarding the condition are recorded in FL 18 to 30. Occurrence and value codes are listed in FL 31 to 41 to provide information used by the payer to determine the need for medical services. The payer utilizes these codes in their benefit determination process.

Section II: Charge Information (FL 42 to 49)

This section requires detailed information about the charges submitted, including revenue code and description, Health Care Common Procedure Coding System (HCPCS) code and rates, service date, service units, total charges, and noncovered charges. Charge capture data gathered during the patient visit are utilized to print a detailed itemized statement and to complete FL 42 to 49. Charges are captured during the patient visit through the chargemaster. Each item in the chargemaster is associated with the appropriate revenue code category, HCPCS code, and other charge information. The detailed itemized statement lists each charge individually. Completion of FL 42 to 49 requires all charges captured during the patient stay to be grouped in revenue code categories. Each revenue code category is listed on one line in FL 42 to 49 along with other associated data, such as HCPCS code, charge, and units.

Section III: Payer, Insured, Employer, and Authorization Information (FL 50 to 66)

Information about the primary, secondary, and tertiary payers that are responsible for payment on the claim is submitted in these fields. **Tertiary payer** refers to the third insurance. Information in FL 50 to 66 includes the payer name, insured's name and identification number, group name and number, treatment authorization, and employer.

Section IV: Procedure, Diagnosis, and Provider Information (FL 67 to 81)

Diagnosis and procedure information related to the charges submitted is recorded in FL 66 to 75. Information regarding the attending and other physician, the payer's name and address, and provider signature is recorded in FL 76 to 81.

TEST YOUR *Knowledge* BOX 10-2

CLAIM FORM VARIATIONS; CMS-1500 AND CMS-1450 (UB-04) CLAIM FORM OVERVIEW AND DATA

1. Name two claim forms used to submit charges to payers.
2. What claim form is used for physician and outpatient services?
3. Name all the coding systems used on the CMS-1500.
4. State what claim form is used for inpatient services.
5. Name all the coding systems used on the CMS-1450 (UB-04).
6. State how many fields are on the CMS-1500 and the CMS-1450 (UB-04).
7. State what section of the CMS-1500 is used to report the patient's diagnosis.
8. Discuss the information recorded in Blocks 24A to 24J.
9. What organization developed and maintains the CMS-1450 (UB-04)?
10. What date was the UB-92 replaced and what form replaced it?
11. Explain what section and fields on the CMS-1500 and CMS-1450 (UB-04) are used to record patient information.
12. Describe what section and fields on the claim forms are used to record the provider information.
13. Discuss the relationship between charge capture and FL 42 to 49.
14. What blocks are used to record diagnosis and procedure codes on the CMS-1500?
15. State where diagnosis and procedure codes are recorded on the CMS-1450 (UB-04).

CMS-1450 (UB-04) Instructions

The UB-04 is a summary of the hospital stay and charges incurred. Information used to complete the claim form is entered into the patient's account on the computer. Required claim data for each field are pulled from the patient's account and the hospital data file. Information about charges for services provided is outlined on the detailed itemized statement, which may be attached to manual claims. Payers who receive electronic claims may request a detailed itemized statement after review of the UB-04 claim data. Completion requirements and specifications for the UB-04 vary by payer; therefore, it is critical to obtain payer specifications to ensure compliance with payer guidelines. Detailed instructions for completion of the claim form for Medicare claims can be viewed on the CMS Web site at www.cms.gov. General instructions for each FL are outlined below in four sections to provide a basic understanding of the data required.

Section I: Facility, Patient, Admission, Discharge, Occurrence, and Value Information (FL 1 to 41)

Section one consists of FL 1 to 41. This section is used to provide information about the facility, when the patient was admitted and discharged, the patient's name and address, and other information about the patient visit, as illustrated in Figure 10-7. An overview of data required for each FL is outlined below.

FL 1: Billing Provider Name, Address, Telephone Number

Record the name, complete service location, mailing address, and telephone number of the provider (hospital) that is submitting the claim. List each on a separate line, with a total of four lines. Abbreviation of the state is acceptable. The zip code may be five or nine digits.

When the address is outside the United States, a two-digit country code is also recorded to the right of the telephone number. The country code for the United States is US. This information is required by Medicare and other payers to forward payments and other communications to the hospital.

1. COMMUNITY GENERAL HOSPITAL
2. 8192 SOUTH STREET
3. MARS FLORIDA 37373-XXXX
4. 7477221800 US

FL 2: Billing Provider's Designated Pay-to Address

This field is completed when the provider requires payment to be sent to an address other than the address recorded in FL1. Record the pay-to name; street address; city, state, zip code, and country code on three lines. Line four is reserved for assignment by the NUBC. The country code is required when the address is outside the United States.

1. COMMUNITY HOSPITAL INC
2. 79632 18TH STREET
3. MARS FLORIDA 37373-XXXX US

FL 3A: Patient Control Number (PCN)

FL 3A is used to record the patient control number (PCN). The PCN is a unique number assigned by the hospital to identify the patient account for the claim. The PCN is used to identify the patient's account for posting payments and retrieving information. This field allows 20 alphanumeric characters with no spaces between digits. When the PCN is placed in this field, the payer records the number on the remittance advice. The PCN is generally different from the medical record number.

FL 3B: Medical/Health Record Number (MRN)

FL 3B is used to record the **medical or health record number (MRN or HRN)**. The MRN is a

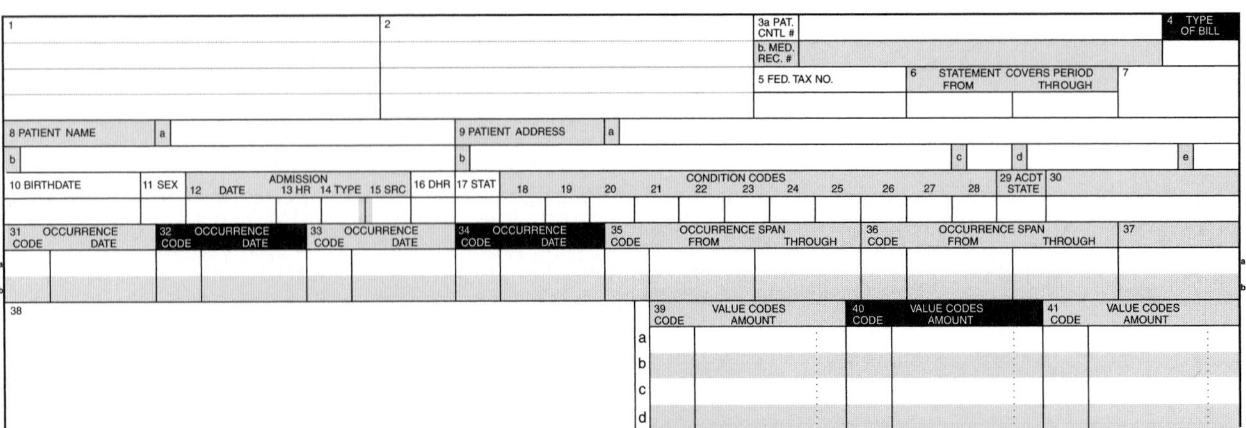
1
2
3a PAT. CNTL #
b. MED. REC. #
4 TYPE OF BILL
5 FED. TAX NO.
6 STATEMENT COVERS PERIOD FROM THROUGH
7
8 PATIENT NAME a
b
9 PATIENT ADDRESS a
b c d e
10 BIRTHDATE
11 SEX
ADMISSION 12 DATE 13 HR 14 TYPE 15 SRC
16 DHR
17 STAT
CONDITION CODES 18 19 20 21 22 23 24 25 26 27 28
29 ACDT STATE
30
31 OCCURRENCE CODE DATE
32 OCCURRENCE CODE DATE
33 OCCURRENCE CODE DATE
34 OCCURRENCE CODE DATE
35 OCCURRENCE SPAN CODE FROM THROUGH
36 OCCURRENCE SPAN CODE FROM THROUGH
37
a
b
38
39 VALUE CODES CODE AMOUNT
40 VALUE CODES CODE AMOUNT
41 VALUE CODES CODE AMOUNT
a
b
c
d

Figure 10-7 CMS-1450 (UB-04) FL 1 to 41 is used to record information about the facility, the patient, and the patient admission.

24-alphanumeric number assigned by the facility to a patient's medical record, and it is used to identify, track, and retrieve the medical record for a patient. The medical record number is not the same as the PCN, which is assigned by the facility to a specific claim. The MRN is also referred to as the health record number (HRN). This field is required by Medicare, and most other payers require completion of this field.

FL 4: Type of Bill

The four-digit type of bill (TOB) number is recorded in this field to provide information about the facility bill type. The first digit is zero. The second digit describes the facility type. The third digit indicates the type of care. The fourth digit is designed to let the payer know the expected frequency of the bills that will be submitted. TOB code options range from 000X to 0999. Three-digit TOB options and common fourth-digit frequency code options are outlined in Key Points Box 10-7.

FL 5: Federal Tax ID Number or Employer ID Number

Record the hospital's federal tax identification number in this field. The federal tax identification number (TIN) is a number assigned to the facility by the Internal Revenue Service for tax reporting purposes. The tax identification number is also referred to as the employer identification number (EIN). The tax identification number is recorded in the following format: XX-XXXXXXX including the dash. Most payers require completion of this field. Medicare does not require this field.

FL 6: Statement Covers Period

Dates indicating when services were provided are recorded in this field. The date service began is recorded in the field labeled "From." The date service ended is recorded in the field labeled "Through." When the Statement Covers period is one day, record the date in both the "From" and "Through" fields. The required format for dates to be displayed is as follows: month,

BOX 10-7 ■ KEY POINTS

CMS-1450 (UB-04) Type of Bill Options

010x Reserved for assignment by the National Uniform Billing Committee (NUBC)
011x Hospital Inpatient (Including Medicare Part A)
012x Hospital Inpatient (Medicare Part B only)
013x Hospital Outpatient
014x Hospital–Laboratory Services–Nonpatients
015x-017x Reserved for assignment by NUBC
018x Hospital–Swing Beds
019x-020x Reserved for assignment by NUBC
021x Skilled Nursing–Inpatient (Medicare Part A)
022x Skilled Nursing–Inpatient (Medicare Part B)
023x Skilled Nursing–Outpatient
024x-027x Reserved for assignment by NUBC
028x Skilled Nursing–Swing Beds
029x-031x Reserved for Assignment by NUBC
032x Home Health–Inpatient (Part B only)
033x Home Health–Outpatient (Part A, Durable Medical Equipment [DME] Part A)
034x Home Health–Other (for medical and surgical services not under a plan of treatment)
035x-040x Reserved for assignment by NUBC
041x Religious Nonmedical Health Care Institutions–Hospital Inpatient
042x Reserved for assignment by NUBC
043x Religious Nonmedical Health Care Institutions–Outpatient Services
044x-064x Reserved for assignment by NUBC
065x Intermediate Care–Level I
066x Intermediate Care–Level II
067x-070x Reserved for assignment by NUBC
071x Clinic–Rural Health
072x Clinic–Hospital Based or Independent Renal Dialysis Center
073x Clinic–Freestanding
074x Clinic–Outpatient Rehabilitation Facility (ORF)
075x Clinic–Comprehensive Outpatient Rehabilitation Facility (CORF)
076x Clinic–Community Mental Health Center
077x Clinic–Federally Qualified Health Center (FQHC)
078x Reserved for Assignment by NUBC
079x Clinic–Other
080x Reserved for assignment by NUBC
081x Special Facility–Hospice (nonhospital based)
082x Special Facility–Hospice (hospital based)
083x Special Facility–Ambulatory Surgery Center
084x Special Facility–Freestanding Birthing Center
085x Special Facility–Critical Access Hospital
086x Special Facility–Residential Facility
087x-088x Reserved for assignment by NUBC
089x Special Facility–Other
090x-9999 Reserved for assignment by NUBC

CMS-1450 (UB-04) Fourth-Digit Options

0-Nonpayment/Zero Claim
1-Admit Through Discharge Claim
2-Interim: First Claim
3-Interim: Continuing Claim
4-Interim: Last Claim
5-Late Charge (s) Only
6-Reserved for Assignment by the NUBC
7-Replacement of Prior Claim
8-Void/Cancel of Prior Claim
9-Final Claim for Home Health PPS Episode

day, and year (MMDDYY), with no dashes or slashes. The "From" date is used to determine whether the claim was filed within the required time frame, which is referred to as timely filing.

Timely filing refers to the period of time in which claims must be filed, such as 90 days. The time required to file claims varies by payer. Timely filing is generally calculated from the date of service. FL 6 is required by all payers. The dates in this field must coincide with the total number of days in the covered and noncovered FLs listed on the claim.

BOX 10-8 ■ KEY POINTS

Required Format for Dates

MMDDYY

Month, Day, Year

Example

Statement covers period from July 10, 2010 through July 20, 2010

Date in Required Format

071010 072010

FL 7: Reserved for Assignment by the National Uniform Billing Committee (NUBC)

FL 8 (A-B): Patient Name/Identifier

The patient identification number assigned by the payer is recorded in FL 8A when it is different from the insured's ID number in FL 60. The patient's name is recorded in 8B in the following format: last, first, and middle initial; each is separated by a space.

The name in this field should match the name listed on the patient's insurance or Medicare card, including hyphenated names or references such as Jr. or Sr., as illustrated below. Most payers require this field.

BOX 10-9 ■ KEY POINTS

Required Format for Name

Name on Insurance/ Medicare Card	Record in FL 8B
John M. James, Sr.	James Sr John M
Sara M. Jones-Smith	Jones Smith Sara M
Daniel J. D'Oreo	D'Oreo Daniel J

FL 9 (A-E): Patient Address

The patient's complete mailing address is recorded in this field. The address should be a permanent address, and it should include the street address, city, state, and zip code. The entire address is recorded as follows:

9A Street address
9B City
9C State
9D Zip code
9E Country code (when address is outside the United States)

Payers require this information to ensure that communication is forwarded to the correct patient address.

FL 10: Patient Birth Date

Report the patient's birth date in this field by month, day, and year. The required format for dates to be displayed is as follows: month, day, century, and year, (MMDDCCYY), with no dashes or slashes; for example, a birthday of April 26, 1968 is reported as 04261968. Enter 8 zeros in the field when the patient's full date of birth is not known. Medicare and other payers require this field. This field is compared with FL 11 (Patient sex), FL 67–72 (Diagnosis), and FL 74 (Procedure) to ensure that the procedure is age appropriate.

FL 11: Patient Sex

A single alphabetic character indicating the patient's sex and the date of admission, are recorded in this field. The standard options are:

M-Male
F-Female
U-Unknown

This field is compared with FL 67–70 (Diagnosis) and FL 74 (Procedure) to ensure that the procedure is gender appropriate. Medicare and other payers require this field.

FL 12: Admission/Start of Care Date

The date the patient was admitted or care was started as an inpatient or outpatient is recorded in this field. The required format for dates to be displayed is as follows: month, day, and year (MMDDYY), with no dashes or slashes. Medicare requires completion of this field. Other payers may require this field.

FL 13: Admission Hour

The hour the patient was admitted for inpatient or outpatient care is recorded in this field. A two-digit hour code representing the hour in military time is recorded, not the actual hour. The two-digit hour code options are outlined in Table 10-4. Completion of this field is required on inpatient claims.

FL 14: Priority (Type) of Visit

A single numeric digit is reported in this field to describe the priority (type) of the admission or visit. It is used to communicate the priority of an admission, such as an emergency admission.

TABLE 10-4 CMS-1450 (UB-04) Code Options for FL 13 and 16 Hour Codes

Code	AM (Midnight)	Code	PM (Noon)
00	12:00–12:59	12	12:00–12:59
01	01:00–01:59	13	01:00–01:59
02	02:00–02:59	14	02:00–02:59
03	03:00–03:59	15	03:00–03:59
04	04:00–04:59	16	04:00–04:59
05	05:00–05:59	17	05:00–05:59
06	06:00–06:59	18	06:00–06:59
07	07:00–07:59	19	07:00–07:59
08	08:00–08:59	20	08:00–08:59
09	09:00–09:59	21	09:00–09:59
10	10:00–10:59	22	10:00–10:59
11	11:00–11:59	23	11:00–11:59

Medicare requires completion of this field for inpatient claims. The field is not required for outpatient claims. Other payers may require completion of this field based on the admission type.

BOX 10-10 ■ KEY POINTS

CMS-1450 (UB-04) DATA CODE OPTIONS

FL 14: Priority (Type of Visit)

Code options for the type of admission

1—Emergency
2—Urgent
3—Elective
4—Newborn
5—Trauma
6–8—Reserved for assignment by the NUBC
9—Information Not Available

FL 15: Point of Origin for Admission or Visit

A single-digit code is entered here to explain the point of origin for the admission or visit. This field was previously used to indicate the referral for the admission or visit. Completion of this field is required for Medicare inpatient and outpatient claims. Other payers may require this field. Patient status code options are outlined in Key Points Box 10-11.

FL 16: Discharge Hour

Enter the appropriate two-digit hour code that represents the hour the patient was discharged from inpatient care. The two-digit hour code representing the hour in military time is recorded in this field, not the actual hour. The two-digit hour code options are outlined in Table 10-4. Completion of this field is required for inpatient claims.

BOX 10-11 ■ KEY POINTS

CMS-1450 (UB-04) DATA CODE OPTIONS

FL 15: Point of Origin for Admission or Visit

1. Non–Health Care Facility Point of Origin
2. Clinic
3. Reserved for assignment by the National Uniform Billing Committee (NUBC)
4. Transfer from Hospital (Different Facility)
5. Transfer from Skilled Nursing Facility (SNF) or Intermediate Care Facility (ICF)
6. Transfer from Another Health Care Facility
7. Emergency Room
8. Court/Law Enforcement
9. Information Not Available
   - A. Reserved for assignment by the NUBC
   - B. Transfer from Another Home Health Agency (HHA)
   - C. Readmission to Same HHA
   - D. Transfer from One Distinct Unit of the Hospital to Another Distinct Unit of the Same Hospital, Resulting in a Separate Claim to the Payer
   - E. Transfer from Ambulatory Surgery Center
   - F. Transfer from Hospice and Is Under a Hospice Plan of Care or Enrolled in a Hospice Program
   - G.-Z. Reserved for assignment by the NUBC

Code Structure for Newborn

1–4 Reserved for assignment by the NUBC
5 Born Inside This Hospital
6 Born Outside of This Hospital
7–9 Reserved for assignment by the NUBC

FL 17: Patient Discharge Status

A two-digit code is entered here to explain the patient status at the end of the hospital stay. Completion of this field is required for Medicare inpatient and outpatient claims. Other payers may require this field. Patient status code options are outlined in Table 10-5.

FL 18 to 28: Condition Codes

This field is used to communicate to the payer conditions or events that may affect the processing of the claim. A two-digit alphanumeric code indicating the condition is entered. More than one condition code may be required. Each FL accommodates one condition code. The payer uses these codes for determination of medical necessity, primary and secondary coverage, eligibility, and payment. Medicare and other payers may require completion of this field under certain circumstances. There are approximately 100 condition codes. Some of the most common condition codes are given in Key Points Box 10-12. A complete listing is located in Appendix B.

TABLE 10-5	CMS-1450 (UB-04) Code Options for FL 17 Patient Status Codes
01	Discharged to home or self care (routine discharge)
02	Discharged/transferred to another short-term general hospital for inpatient care
03	Discharged/transferred to skilled nursing facility (SNF) with Medicare certification in anticipation of skilled care
04	Discharged/transferred to an intermediate care facility (ICF)
05	Discharged/transferred to designated cancer center or children's hospital
06	Discharged/transferred to home under care of organized home health service organization in anticipation of covered, skilled care
07	Left against medical advice (AMA) or discontinued care
08	Reserved for assignment by the NUBC
09	Admitted as an inpatient to this hospital
10–19	Reserved for assignment by the NUBC
20	Expired
21–29	Reserved for assignment by the NUBC
30	Still patient
31–39	Reserved for assignment by the NUBC
40	Expired at home (Medicare and TRICARE hospice claims only)
41	Expired in a medical facility, such as hospital, SNF, ICF or freestanding hospice. (Medicare and TRICARE hospice claims only)
42	Expired—Place Unknown
43	Discharged/transferred to a federal health care facility
44–49	Reserved for assignment by the NUBC
50	Discharged to hospice–home
51	Discharged to hospice–medical facility (certified) providing hospice level of care
52–60	Reserved for assignment by the NUBC
61	Discharged/transferred to a hospital-based Medicare-approved swing bed
62	Discharged/transferred to an inpatient rehabilitation facility (IRF) including rehabilitation–distinct part unit of a hospital
63	Discharged/transferred to a Medicare-certified long-term care hospital (LTCH)
64	Discharged/transferred to a nursing facility certified under Medicaid but not certified under Medicare
65	Discharged/transferred to a psychiatric hospital or psychiatric–distinct part unit of a hospital
66	Discharged/transferred to a critical access hospital (CAH)
67–69	Reserved for assignment by the NUBC
70	Discharged/transferred to another type of health care institution not defined elsewhere in this code list
71–99	Reserved for assignment by the NUBC

FL 29: Accident State

When services reported are related to an auto accident, a two-digit abbreviation of the state where the accident occurred must be recorded in this field. The appropriate occurrence code and date should also be recorded in FL 31–34 when this field is completed.

FL 30: Reserved for Assignment by the National Uniform Billing Committee (NUBC)

FL 31 to 34 (A-B): Occurrence Codes and Dates

This field is used to explain an event associated with the claim that may affect the processing of the claim.

BOX 10-12 ■ KEY POINTS

CMS-1450 (UB-04) DATA CODE OPTIONS

FL 18–28: Condition Codes

Code	Description
01	Military Service Related
02	Condition Is Employment Related
03	Patient Covered by Insurance Not Reflected Here
04	Information-Only Bill
05	Lien Has Been Filed
06	End-Stage Renal Disease (ESRD) Patient in the First 30 Months of Coverage by Employer Group Health Plan (EGHP)
07	Treatment of Nonterminal Condition for Hospice Patient
08	Beneficiary Would Not Provide Information Concerning Other Insurance Coverage
09	Neither Patient Nor Spouse Is Employed
10	Patient and/or Spouse Is Employed But No EGHP Exists

A two-digit alphanumeric code indicating the occurrence is entered along with the date of that occurrence. A maximum of seven occurrence codes may be entered in FL 31 to 34. Enter codes in alphanumeric order on line A and continue on line B if required. The required format for dates to be displayed is as follows: month, day, and year (MMDDYY), with no dashes or slashes. The payer uses these codes to evaluate liability, coordinate benefits, and review coverage. There are approximately 70 occurrence codes. Some of the most common occurrence codes are outlined in Key Points Box 10-13. A complete listing of occurrence codes is located in Appendix B. This field is required for Medicare and other payers under certain conditions. For example, occurrence code 09 may be used to indicate that a claim relates to the start of an infertility treatment cycle on 9/24/07.

FL 35 to 36 (A-B): Occurrence Span Codes and Dates

This field is used to explain the span and dates of an occurrence(s) that may affect the claim processing. The span code and date further explain an event associated with the claim that happened over a span of time. A two-digit alphanumeric code indicating the occurrence span date is entered in the "From" and "Through" columns. Enter the codes and dates in alphanumeric order on line A, and continue on line B if more space is required. The required format for dates to be displayed is as follows: month, day, and year (MMDDYY), with no dashes or slashes. Medicare and other payers may require completion of this field in certain circumstances. Table 10-6 outlines occurrence span codes that may be utilized in FL 35 to 36 (A-B). A complete listing of occurrence span codes is also located in Appendix B.

BOX 10-13 ■ KEY POINTS

CMS-1450 (UB-04) DATA CODE OPTIONS

FL 31–34 (A-B) Occurrence Codes and Dates

Code	Description
01	Accident/Medical Coverage
02	No-Fault Insurance, Including Auto, Accident/Other
03	Accident/Tort Liability
04	Accident/Employment Related
05	Accident/No Medical or Liability Coverage
06	Crime Victim
07–08	Reserved for assignment by the National Uniform Billing Committee (NUBC)
09	Start of Infertility Treatment Cycle
10	Last Menstrual Period
A0	Reserved for assignment by the NUBC
Al	Birth Date–Insured A
A2	Effective Date–Insured A Policy
A3	Benefits Exhausted–Payer A
A4	Split Bill Date
A5–AZ	Reserved for assignment by the NUBC

TABLE 10-6 CMS 1450 (UB-04) Code Options for FL 35 to 36 (A-B) Occurrence Span Codes and Dates

Code	Description
70	Qualifying Stay Dates for Skilled Nursing Facility (SNF) Use Only
71	Prior Stay Dates
72	First/Last Visit Dates
73	Benefit Eligibility Period
74	Noncovered Level of Care/Leave of Absence Dates
75	SNF Level of Care Dates
76	Patient Liability
77	Provider Liability Period
78	SNF Prior Stay Dates
79	Payer Code
80	Prior Same-SNF Stay Dates
81–99	Reserved for assignment by the NUBC
M0	QIO/UR Approved Stay Dates
M1	Provider Liability–No Utilization
M2	Inpatient Respite Care Dates
M3	Intermediate Care Facility (ICF) Level of Care
M4	Residential Level of Care
M5–MQ	Reserved for assignment by the NUBC
MR–ZZ	Reserved for assignment by the NUBC

Using the example from the occurrence code and date section in FL 31 to 34, the following is an outline of how the occurrence code and span codes would be recorded. The period of the infertility treatment cycle is 092107 through 092507. To report to the payer that this will be the first and last visit, we would record 72 under Occurrence Span Code, and the dates 09/21/07 through 09/25/07 would be recorded to indicate the span of time as illustrated below.

CODE	FROM	THROUGH
72	092107	092507

FL 37: Reserved for Assignment by the National Uniform Billing Committee (NUBC)

FL 38 1–5: Responsible Party Name and Address

This field is used to report the name and address of the individual who is responsible for paying the claim. A responsible party can be the patient, a guardian, or an individual who has power of attorney and handles the patient's affairs. This field is required for Medicare and other payers under certain conditions. List the responsible party's complete name and address on three or four lines as follows:

John M James Sr.
3755 First Street
Miami Florida 35672 6795

FL 39 to 41 (A-D) Value Codes and Amounts

FL 39 to 41A to D are used to report two-digit alphanumeric value codes and the dollar amount associated with the code. Value codes describe information such as room rates, professional component charges, coinsurance, deductibles, cost share amount, and patient liability amount. The monetary value is reported with the value code. Payers utilize this information to determine benefits. There are four lines for each FL 39 to 41. Codes and values are entered in the fields in the following order: FL (39A to 49A) and then FL (39B to 49B). The NUBC lists more than 100 value codes that can be used to describe information required by the payer. A listing of some of the value code options is given in Key Points Box 10-14. A complete listing is located in Appendix B.

BOX 10-14 KEY POINTS

CMS-1450 (UB-04) DATA CODE OPTIONS

FL 39 to 41: Value Codes and Amount

Code	Description
01	Most Common Semiprivate Room Rate
02	Hospital Has No Semiprivate Rooms
05	Professional Component
A1	Deductible Payer A
A2	Coinsurance Payer A
A3	Estimated Patient Responsibility Payer A
A4	Covered Self-Administrable Drugs–Emergency
A5	Covered Self-Administrable Drugs—Not Self-Administrable in Form and Situation Furnished by Patient

Section II: Charge Information (FL 42 to 49)

FL 42 to 49 is used to provide information about charges submitted on the claim form. As illustrated in Figure 10-8, information recorded in FL 42 to 49 includes

	42 REV. CD.	43 DESCRIPTION	44 HCPCS / RATE / HIPPS CODE	45 SERV. DATE	46 SERV. UNITS	47 TOTAL CHARGES	48 NON-COVERED CHARGES	49	
1									1
2									2
3									3
4									4
5									5
6									6
7									7
8									8
9									9
10									10
11									11
12									12
13									13
14									14
15									15
16									16
17									17
18									18
19									19
20									20
21									21
22									22
23		PAGE ____ OF ____	CREATION DATE		TOTALS ➡				23

Figure 10-8 CMS-1450 (UB-04) FL 42 to 49 is used to record information about charges for services provided during the hospital visit.

TEST YOUR *Knowledge* BOX 10-3

CMS-1450 (UB-04) CLAIM FORM SECTION I (FL 1 TO 41)

1. Provide a brief explanation of what information is recorded in FL 1 to 41.
2. Explain what the patient control number is and which FL is used to record it on the CMS-1450 (UB-04).
3. State what each of the last three digits in FL 4 represents.
4. List the bill type that would be recorded in FL 4 for a hospital ambulatory surgery claim.
5. Describe the difference between tax identification number (TIN) and employer identification number (EIN) in FL 5.
6. List what information is recorded in FL 6, Statement Covers period.
7. Provide three options that can be recorded in FL 11, patient sex.
8. Explain if a patient is admitted through the ER, what will be recorded in FL 15, point of origin?
9. List the code that would be listed in FL 13 for an admission time of 7:42 PM.
10. Describe the data that are recorded in FL 39 to 41 and explain how payers use this information.

revenue code, description, HCPCS/rates, service date, service units, total charges, and noncovered charges.

Charges for services, procedures, and items provided during the hospital stay are posted to the patient's account through the chargemaster. Each item in the chargemaster is assigned a revenue code and an HCPCS code. The claim process is initiated after the patient is discharged. A detailed itemized statement listing all charges incurred during the patient stay is prepared. The length of the statement varies based on the number of charges incurred during the stay. An outpatient stay may be two pages, whereas a week-long inpatient stay may be 20 pages. Figure 10-9 illustrates one page of a detailed itemized statement. All charges incurred during the patient visit, reflected on the patient statement, are summarized and reported in FL 42 to 49 by revenue code category, as illustrated in Table 10-7.

Revenue codes are four-digit numeric codes developed and maintained by the NUBC to categorize like services and items. Revenue code categories represent various services, procedures, and items provided by facilities, such as anesthesia, emergency room, and laboratory services. A listing of revenue code categories is outlined in Table 10-8.

Within each revenue code category there are subcategories used to further specify services and items. Each revenue code contains an "X," which indicates that the last digit is variable. Each revenue code category has the standard first three numbers, such as "025" for pharmacy, with a listing of the last digit options (subcategories) to provide further specification. The last digit replaces the "X" when recording the code, and it is used to further specify the service or item.

For example, code range 025X provides various options to further describe pharmacy items. Table 10-9 illustrates revenue code last-digit specifications for the revenue code categories Pharmacy and Medical/Surgical Supplies. If the item is an experimental drug, revenue code 0256 would be recorded to describe the item as Pharmacy, Experimental Drugs. A more comprehensive listing of revenue code categories and subcategories is located in Appendix B.

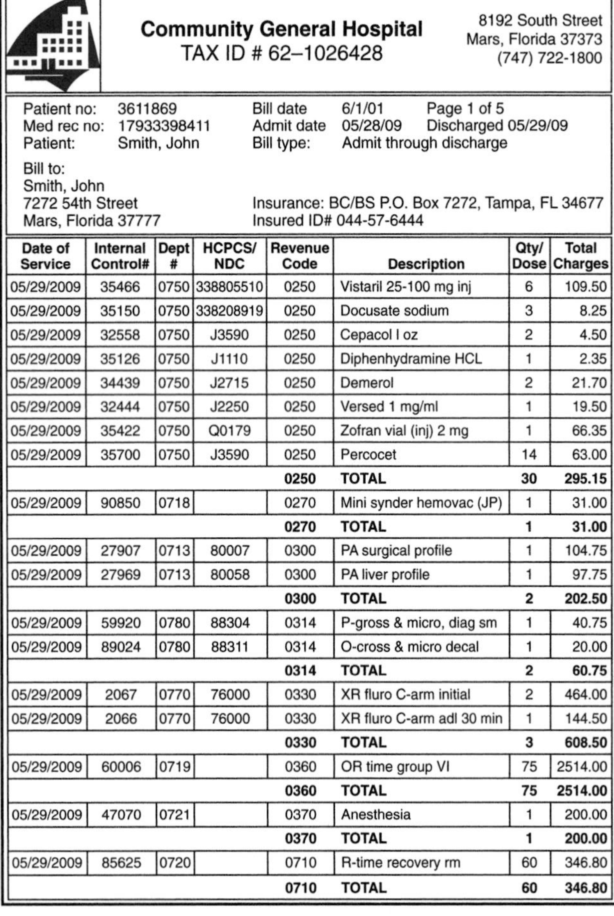

Community General Hospital
TAX ID # 62–1026428

8192 South Street
Mars, Florida 37373
(747) 722-1800

Patient no: 3611869 Bill date 6/1/01 Page 1 of 5
Med rec no: 17933398411 Admit date 05/28/09 Discharged 05/29/09
Patient: Smith, John Bill type: Admit through discharge

Bill to:
Smith, John
7272 54th Street
Mars, Florida 37777

Insurance: BC/BS P.O. Box 7272, Tampa, FL 34677
Insured ID# 044-57-6444

Date of Service	Internal Control#	Dept #	HCPCS/ NDC	Revenue Code	Description	Qty/ Dose	Total Charges
05/29/2009	35466	0750	338805510	0250	Vistaril 25-100 mg inj	6	109.50
05/29/2009	35150	0750	338208919	0250	Docusate sodium	3	8.25
05/29/2009	32558	0750	J3590	0250	Cepacol I oz	2	4.50
05/29/2009	35126	0750	J1110	0250	Diphenhydramine HCL	1	2.35
05/29/2009	34439	0750	J2715	0250	Demerol	2	21.70
05/29/2009	32444	0750	J2250	0250	Versed 1 mg/ml	1	19.50
05/29/2009	35422	0750	Q0179	0250	Zofran vial (inj) 2 mg	1	66.35
05/29/2009	35700	0750	J3590	0250	Percocet	14	63.00
				0250	**TOTAL**	**30**	**295.15**
05/29/2009	90850	0718		0270	Mini synder hemovac (JP)	1	31.00
				0270	**TOTAL**	**1**	**31.00**
05/29/2009	27907	0713	80007	0300	PA surgical profile	1	104.75
05/29/2009	27969	0713	80058	0300	PA liver profile	1	97.75
				0300	**TOTAL**	**2**	**202.50**
05/29/2009	59920	0780	88304	0314	P-gross & micro, diag sm	1	40.75
05/29/2009	89024	0780	88311	0314	O-cross & micro decal	1	20.00
				0314	**TOTAL**	**2**	**60.75**
05/29/2009	2067	0770	76000	0330	XR fluro C-arm initial	2	464.00
05/29/2009	2066	0770	76000	0330	XR fluro C-arm adl 30 min	1	144.50
				0330	**TOTAL**	**3**	**608.50**
05/29/2009	60006	0719		0360	OR time group VI	75	2514.00
				0360	**TOTAL**	**75**	**2514.00**
05/29/2009	47070	0721		0370	Anesthesia	1	200.00
				0370	**TOTAL**	**1**	**200.00**
05/29/2009	85625	0720		0710	R-time recovery rm	60	346.80
				0710	**TOTAL**	**60**	**346.80**

Figure 10-9 Detailed itemized statement.

FL 42: Revenue Code

FL 42 is used to record the four-digit revenue code number. Revenue code categories are based on the type of service or item. Remember, each item in the chargemaster is assigned a revenue code. Revenue codes are listed in numerical order in FL 42 on lines 1 through 23. The last line, on the last page of the claim, should indicate a revenue code of 0001 to indicate the Total Charge, the page numbers, the creation date of the claim, and the total charges in the covered and noncovered charge columns. Medicare requires completion of this field, as do most other payers. There are more than 90 revenue code categories, and more than one revenue code can be associated with a category. A complete listing of revenue code categories is outlined in Appendix B.

FL 43: Revenue Code Descriptions

This field is used to record a description of the revenue code used. Each revenue code has a general narrative description and a standard abbreviated description. The standard abbreviated description is required in this field. For example, revenue code 0624 describes "Medical/Surgical Supplies, FDA Investigational Device". The standard abbreviated description FDA INVEST DEVICE is recorded in FL 43. Completion of this field is not required by Medicare except when you are billing FDA investigational devices.

FL 42	FL 43
0624	FDA Invest Device

FL 44: HCPCS/Rates/HIPPS Code

FL 44 is utilized to record the Health Care Common Procedure Coding System (HCPCS) code, Health Insurance Prospective Payment System (HIPPS) rate code where applicable, or the daily accommodation rate

TABLE 10-7 Charge Detail CMS-1450 (UB-04) FL 42–49 Charge Information

42 Rev Code	43 Description	44 HCPCS/ Rates	45 Serv Date	46 Serv Units	47 Total Charges	48 Noncovered Charges	49
0250	PHARMACY		05 29 2001	29	295.15		
0300	LABORATORY		05 28 2001	2	202.50		
0314	PATHOL/BIOPSY		05 28 2001	2	60.75		
0330	RX X-RAY	76000	05 28 2001	3	608.50		
0360	OR TIME GROUP VI	43752	05 28 2001	75	2514.00		
0370	ANESTHESIA	43752	05 28 2001	1	200.00		
0710	RECOVERY ROOM		05 28 2001	60	346.80		
0001	TOTAL CHARGE			172	4227.70		

TABLE 10-8 **CMS-1450 (UB-04) FL 42 Revenue Code Categories**

Category Description Service/Item	Revenue Code Category(ies)
Accommodations (Room and Board)	011X, 012X, 013X, 014X, 015X, 016X
Anesthesia	037X
Audiology	047X
Blood	038X, 039X
Cardiology	048X
Coronary Care	021X
EKG/ECG	073X, 074X
Emergency Room	045X
Gastrointestinal Services	075X
Inpatient Renal Dialysis Services	080X
Intensive Care	020X
IV Therapy	026X
Laboratory, Clinical	030X
Laboratory, Pathological	031X
Labor/Delivery Room	072X
Lithotripsy	079X
Medical/Surgical Supplies	027X, 062X
Nursery	017X, 023X
Occupational Therapy	043X
Oncology	028X
Operating Room	036X
Organ Acquisition	081X
Patient Convenience Items	099X
Pharmacy	025X, 063X
Physical Therapy	042X
Professional Fees	096X, 097X, 098X
Radiological Services	032X, 033X, 034X, 035X, 040X, 061X
Recovery Room	071X
Respiratory Services	041X
Speech/Language Therapy	044X
Treatment or Observation	076X
Total Charges	0001

for inpatient claims. HCPCS Level I CPT and Level II National codes and two-digit modifiers are recorded in this field for services and items on outpatient claims. This field can accommodate up to four modifiers. For example, an entry for radiology, chest X-ray CPT code 71010 is recorded along with the rate $92.00, as illustrated below.

44 HCPCS/RATE/HIPPS CODE
71010 92.00

The HIPPS rate code is for skilled nursing facilities and home health. HIPPS codes will be discussed in Chapter 13. The daily rate for room and board is required when accommodation revenue codes are recorded for inpatient claims. Most payers require completion of this field; however, payer specifications regarding completion of the field will vary.

FL 45: Service Date

This field is utilized to report a date of service in the required format—month, day, and year (MMDDYY)—when an HCPCS code is listed in FL 43, as required by the payer. Most payers require this field for outpatient claims. Payer specifications for the service date for inpatient claims vary.

FL 46: Service Units

Information about the number of units for services and/or items within the revenue code category is recorded here. A unit can represent number of days, quantity of items, or dose of medication. For example, a unit might represent one day in the hospital, one chest X-ray or a 1-mL injection. The total units for all items in the revenue code category are recorded. For example, the detailed itemized statement in Figure 10-9 shows a total of 30 units under the Qty/Dose column for revenue code category 0250. The number 30 is recorded in FL 46. Medicare and most other payers require completion of this field.

FL 47: Total Charges

FL 47 is used to report the total charges of all items in the revenue code category for the claim on line 23 of the last page of the claim. The charges reported on the claim must be incurred during the Statement Covers period recorded in FL 6. FL 47 is a 10-position numeric field for the dollar amount. Additional space is available for a dollar sign, comma, and period. The format for dollars and cents is $2514.00.

Medicare requires this field to be completed with the total of all charges (covered and noncovered). Other payers may require the total of covered charges only.

FL 48: Noncovered Charges

This field is used to report the total of noncovered charges for the primary payer in a specific revenue code

TABLE 10-9 CMS-1450 (UB-04) FL 42 Sample Revenue Code Specifications

Code—General Description	Standard Description
025X PHARMACY	
Subcategory	*Standard Abbreviation*
0—General Classification	PHARMACY
1—Generic Drugs	DRUGS/GENERIC
2—Nongeneric Drugs	DRUGS/NONGENERIC
3—Take Home Drugs	DRUGS/TAKE HOME
4—Drugs Incident to Other Diagnostic Services	DRUGS/INCIDENT ODX
5—Drugs Incident to Radiology	DRUGS/INCIDENT RAD
6—Experimental Drugs	DRUGS/EXPERIMT
7—Nonprescription	DRUGS/NONPSCRPT
8—IV Solutions	IV SOLUTIONS
9—Other Pharmacy	DRUGS/OTHER
027X MEDICAL/SURGICAL SUPPLIES AND DEVICES (SEE ALSO 062X, AN EXTENSION OF 027X)	
Subcategory	*Standard Abbreviation*
0—General Classification	MED/SUR SUPPLIES
1—Nonsterile Supply	NONSTER SUPPLY
2—Sterile Supply	STERILE SUPPL
3—Take Home Supplies	TAKE HOME SUPPLY
4—Prosthetic/Orthotic Devices	PROSTH/ORTH DEV
5—Pacemaker	PACEMAKER
6—Intraocular Lens	INTRAOC LENS
7—Oxygen–Take Home	O2/TAKE HOME
8—Other Implants	SUPPLY/IMPL
9—Other Supplies/Devices	SUPPLY/OTHER

category. The noncovered charges reported on the claim must be incurred during the Statement Covers period. This field holds 10 digits for the dollar amount. Additional space is available for a dollar sign, comma, and period.

FL 49: Reserved for Assignment by the National Uniform Billing Committee (NUBC)

Section III: Payer, Insured, Employer, and Authorization Information (FL 50–65)

Information about the insured and payer is recorded in this field, as illustrated in Figure 10-10. The payer(s) that is responsible for payment on this claim is listed in FL 50. Information in FL 50 to 65 includes the payer's name, insured's name and identification number, group name and number, treatment authorization, and employer.

FL 50 A, B, and C: Payer Identification

FL 50 consists of three lines labeled A, B, and C to record the name and payer identification number for each payer that is responsible for payment on the claim. The primary payer is listed on line A along with the appropriate payer identification number, when required. The payer identification number may also be referred to as the carrier code. The second and third payers are listed on lines B and C with the payer identification, when required. The completion of FL 50 when there are primary, secondary, and tertiary payers is illustrated below. Medicare is the primary insurance listed on line A, Blue Cross/Blue Shield is the secondary insurance listed on line B, and Medicaid is the tertiary insurance listed on line C.

FL 50: Payer Identification

A	007	Medicare
B	816	Blue Cross/Blue Shield
C	700	Medicaid

The three lines A, B, and C in FL 50 correspond to information recorded for these payers in FL 51 to 66. Information for Medicare will be recorded on line A of each of the FLs. Information for Blue Cross/Blue Shield will be recorded on line B, and Medicaid information

50 PAYER NAME	51 HEALTH PLAN ID	52 REL INFO	53 ASG BEN.	54 PRIOR PAYMENTS	55 EST. AMOUNT DUE	56 NPI
A						57 A
B						OTHER B
C						PRV ID C

58 INSURED'S NAME	59 P. REL	60 INSURED'S UNIQUE ID	61 GROUP NAME	62 INSURANCE GROUP NO.
A				A
B				B
C				C

63 TREATMENT AUTHORIZATION CODES	64 DOCUMENT CONTROL NUMBER	65 EMPLOYER NAME
A		A
B		B
C		C

Figure 10-10 CMS-1450 (UB-04) FL 50 to 65 is used to record information about the insured and payer.

TEST YOUR *Knowledge* BOX 10-4

CMS-1450 (UB-04) CLAIM FORM SECTION II (FL 42 TO 49)

1. Provide an overview of the information recorded in FL 42 to 49.
2. List what information is outlined on a detailed itemized statement.
3. Explain what revenue codes are and their purpose.
4. Describe the meaning of the "X" in a revenue code such as 025X.
5. State how revenue codes are listed in FL 42.
6. Outline what description is used in FL 43.
7. Provide an explanation of what HCPCS means in FL 44.
8. List the levels in HCPCS that are used in FL 44.
9. State what information is recorded on line 23 in FL 42 to 49.
10. Describe what type of information is recorded in FL 46.

will be recorded on line C. Some payers may require the **North American Industry Classification System (NAIC) code**, which is the unique code assigned to each business within the United States. The NAIC code classifies the business and is used for statistical purposes by various agencies in the United States. Completion of this field is required by Medicare and other payers. NAIC numbers can be found on the NAIC Web site, http://www.claimsnet.com/public/solutions/payersearch.asp.

FL 51 A, B, and C: Health Plan Identification Number

FL 51 A, B, and C is used to record the health plan's identification number assigned by the payer. Under HIPAA the National Plan Identifier will be required when mandated. The proposed rule for implementation is pending.

FL 56 A, B, and C: National Provider Identifier (NPI)

FL 56 A, B, and C is used to record the national provider identifier number assigned to the provider.

FL 51 A, B, and C: Provider Number

The field consists of three lines labeled A, B, and C. The provider number for the primary payer is listed on line A. The provider numbers for the second and third payers are listed on lines B and C, as illustrated below. The example outlines the provider number for each of the payers listed in FL 50. Medicare is the primary insurance listed on line A, Blue Cross/Blue Shield is the secondary insurance listed on line B, and Medicaid is the tertiary insurance listed on line C. The provider numbers assigned by each of these payers are recorded in FL 51.

FL 51: Provider Number

A 236592
B 472755
C 895722

Historically, a provider number was assigned to the provider by each payer. Effective May 23, 2007, the National Provider Identifier (NPI) is required. All covered health care providers, health plans (except for small health plans), and health care clearinghouses must use the 10-digit NPI in standard transactions, as mandated under the Health Insurance Portability and Accountability Act (HIPAA). The NPI is the standard, unique health identifier for health care providers to use in filing and processing health care claims and other transactions. NPIs are being issued through the National Provider System (NPS), which is being developed by CMS. CMS began assigning NPIs in 2004. The NPI replaces all identifiers that are currently being used. CMS publishes an overview of NPIs along with a copy of the final rule on the Web site at http://www.cms.hhs.gov/nationalProvIdentstand/.

FL 52 A, B, and C: Release of Information Certification Indicator

FL 52 is used to record an alphabetic character that indicates whether there is a release of information, signed by the patient, on file. The options for this field are outlined in Key Points Box 10-15 below:

BOX 10-15 ■ KEY POINTS

CMS-1450 (UB-04) DATA CODE OPTIONS

FL 52: Release of Information Certification Indicator

I—Informed consent to release medical information for conditions or diagnoses regulated by Federal statutes
Y—Yes, provider has a signed statement permitting release of medical billing data related to a claim

The field consists of three lines labeled A, B, and C. An "I" or "Y" is recorded for the primary payer on line A. Information for the second and third payers is recorded on lines B and C. Medicare requires this field on all paper claims and adjustments. Other payers may also require this field.

FL 53: Assignment of Benefits

Assignment of benefits is written authorization from a patient for the payer to forward benefits to the provider. "Y" is recorded if permission is on file for the payer to send payment to the provider. "N" is recorded if there is no permission on file; the payer then will send payment to the patient. "W" indicates *not applicable.* Medicare and Medicaid do not require completion of this field. Other payers may require this field.

FL 54 A, B, and C: Prior Payments

Payments received from patients before claim submission are recorded in this field on lines A, B, and C, which correspond to the primary, secondary, and tertiary payers listed in FL 50 A, B, and C. Money collected from the patient that represents a deductible or coinsurance is recorded in the field labeled "DUE FROM PATIENT." This field is not required for inpatient and skilled nursing facility claims. Other payers may require completion of this field.

FL 55 A, B, and C: Estimated Amount Due

FL 55 is used to record an estimated amount due from the payer. The total in this field equals the hospital's estimated amount less any payments made previously by the payer. There are three lines in this field, labeled A, B, and C, which correspond to the primary, secondary, and tertiary payers listed in FL 50 A, B, and C. This field is not required for Medicare claims. Other payers may require completion of this field.

BOX 10-16 ■ KEY POINTS

Assignment of Benefits

The transfer of the patient's rights to receive benefits under an insurance plan to a designated provider.

When the patient signs a written authorization for the insurance company to send payment for services to the provider, the patient has assigned the benefits to the provider.

FL 56 National Provider Identifier (NPI)

Record the NPI for the provider who is submitting the claim. The NPI is entered on payer line A, B or C in FL 56 as follows: primary payer, line A; secondary payer, line B; and tertiary payer, line C. FL 56 is a required field.

FL 57: Other (Billing) Provider Identifier

This field is used to record the unique identification number that is assigned by the payer to the provider before the NPI implementation date or when the payer requires a secondary identifier.

FL 58 A, B, and C: Insured's Name

The insured's name for the payer(s) listed in FL 50 A, B, and C is recorded in this field on the corresponding line A, B, or C. Enter the insured's last name, first name, and middle initial as it is listed on the program or insurance card. For example, John James, Sr. is indicated on the Medicare card. Medicare is the primary payer. The insured's name is recorded in FL 58 A as follows: James, John Sr.

FL 59 Patient's Relationship to Insured

This field is used to indicate the patient's relationship to the insured. A two-digit code is used to report the relationship. Most payers require completion of this field. Medicare requires this field under specific circumstances. The Patient's Relationship to Insured code options are outlined in Table 10-10.

FL 60 (A-C): Insured Unique Identifier

This field is used to record the insured's identification number, which was assigned to the insured by the payer whose name is listed in FL 50 A, B, or C. This identification number can be referred to by the following names as determined by each payer: certificate number, social security number, health insurance claim number, or identification number. For example, Medicare refers to the identification number as the health insurance claim number. Medicare and other payers require completion of this field.

TABLE 10-10 CMS-1450 (UB-04) Code Options for FL 59 Patient's Relationship Codes

Code	Description
01	Spouse
04	Grandfather or Grandmother
05	Grandson or Granddaughter
07	Nephew or Niece
10	Foster Child
15	Ward
17	Stepson or Stepdaughter
18	Self
19	Child
20	Employee
23	Sponsored Dependent
24	Dependent of a Minor Dependent
29	Significant Other
32	Mother
33	Father
36	Emancipated Minor
39	Organ Donor
40	Cadaver Donor
41	Injured Plaintiff
43	Child Where Insured Has No Financial Responsibility

FL 61 (A-C): Insured Group Name

FL 61 is used to record the group name of the insured's plan. The group name is assigned to the insured group by the payer. There are three lines labeled A, B, and C that correspond to the payers listed in FL 50 A, B, and C. Medicare requires this field under certain circumstances. Other payers may require completion of this field.

FL 62 (A-C): Insurance Group Number

FL 62 is used to record the group number of the insured's plan. The group number is assigned to the insured's group plan by the insurance company. There are three lines labeled A, B, and C that corresponds with the payers listed in FL 50 A, B, and C. Medicare requires this field under certain circumstances. Other payers may require completion of this field.

FL 63 (A-C): Treatment Authorization Code

This field is used to record a treatment authorization code. The payer provides a treatment authorization code when treatment reported on the claim was authorized by the payer. There are three lines labeled A, B, and C that correspond to the payers listed in FL 50 A, B, and C. Medicare requires this field for home health services. Other payers may require completion of this field.

FL 64 (A-C): Document Control Number (DCN)

Enter the internal control number assigned to the original claim by the payer.

FL 65 (A-C): Employer Name (of the Insured)

The employer's name of the insured listed in FL 58 A, B, and C is recorded in this field. There are three lines labeled A, B, and C that correspond to the payers listed in FL 50 A, B, and C. Medicare requires this field when Medicare is the secondary or tertiary payer. Other payers, if applicable, require completion of this field.

FL 66: Diagnosis and Procedure Code Qualifier (International Classification of Diseases [ICD] Version Indicator)

This field is used to report the ICD version indicator. The indicator 9 is used for the ninth revision and the indicator 0 for the tenth revision.

Section IV: Diagnosis, Procedure, and Provider Information (FL 67 to 81)

This section is used to provide the payer with information about the patient's diagnosis, procedure(s), and the provider(s) involved with the patient's care, as illustrated in Figure 10-11.

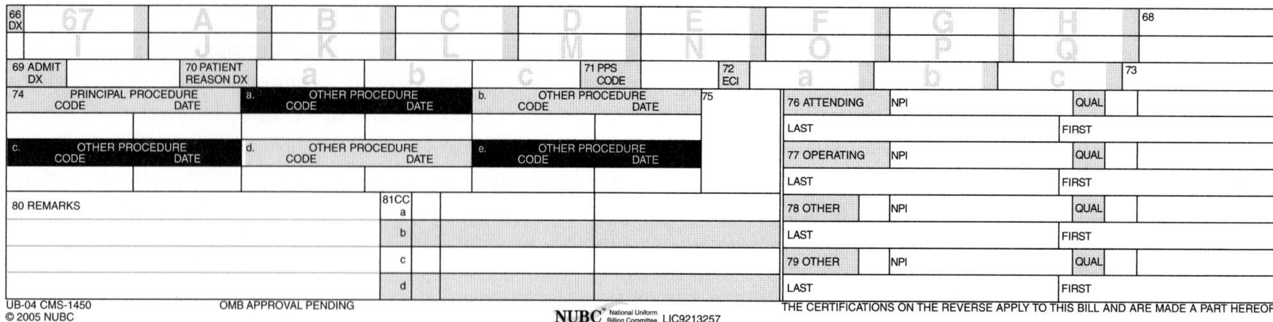

66 DX | 67 | A | B | C | D | E | F | G | H | 68
I | J | K | L | M | N | O | P | Q
69 ADMIT DX | 70 PATIENT REASON DX | a | b | c | 71 PPS CODE | 72 ECI | a | b | c | 73
74 PRINCIPAL PROCEDURE CODE DATE | a. OTHER PROCEDURE CODE DATE | b. OTHER PROCEDURE CODE DATE | 75 | 76 ATTENDING NPI QUAL
LAST FIRST
c. OTHER PROCEDURE CODE DATE | d. OTHER PROCEDURE CODE DATE | e. OTHER PROCEDURE CODE DATE | 77 OPERATING NPI QUAL
LAST FIRST
80 REMARKS | 81CC a | 78 OTHER NPI QUAL
b | LAST FIRST
c | 79 OTHER NPI QUAL
d | LAST FIRST
UB-04 CMS-1450 © 2005 NUBC | OMB APPROVAL PENDING | NUBC National Uniform Billing Committee LIC9213257 | THE CERTIFICATIONS ON THE REVERSE APPLY TO THIS BILL AND ARE MADE A PART HEREOF.

Figure 10-11 CMS-1450 (UB-04) FL 66 to 81 is used to record information about procedures, diagnoses, and the physicians involved in patient care.

TEST YOUR *Knowledge* BOX 10-5

CMS-1450 (UB-04) CLAIM FORM SECTION III (FL 50 TO 66)

1. Provide an overview of what information is recorded in FL 50 to 66.
2. State what information is recorded in FL 50 on Lines A, B, and C.
3. Where is the provider number recorded for the primary insurance on the UB-04?
4. Discuss what information is reported in FL 52.
5. Provide an explanation of what assignment of benefits means and where it is recorded.
6. List what information is recorded in FL 58A, B, and C.
7. Outline the meaning of certificate number, Social Security number, or health insurance claim number recorded in FL 60.
8. State what a group name and number is and where it is recorded.
9. Provide an explanation of a treatment authorization code.
10. Where is a treatment authorization code obtained and recorded for secondary insurance on the UB-04?

FL 67: Principal Diagnosis Code and Present on Admission (POA) Indicator

FL 67 is used to report an ICD-9-CM Volume I diagnosis code that represents the patient's principal diagnosis. The principal diagnosis is the condition determined after study, as discussed in earlier chapters. A three- to five-digit diagnosis code is entered in FL 67, without a decimal. Remember, it is critical to code to the highest level of specificity. Guidelines on selecting the principal diagnosis were reviewed in Chapter 9. Completion of this field is required by Medicare for outpatient and inpatient claims (except for religious nonmedical health care institutions). Most other payers require completion of this field.

All inpatient claims require a POA indicator. Reporting options include the following: "Y," the condition was present on admission; "N," condition not present on admission; "U," no information in the record; and "W," clinically undetermined.

FL 67 (A-Q): Other Diagnosis Codes and POA Indicators

FL 67 A-Q is used to report other ICD-9-CM Volume I diagnosis codes that represent all other conditions existing at the time of admission or developing after admission and those conditions affecting treatment, the length of stay, or both. The principal diagnosis is the condition determined after study, as discussed in earlier chapters. Each FL allows a three to five-digit diagnosis code that is recorded without a decimal point. A three- to five-digit diagnosis code is entered in FL 67 A-Q, without a decimal. Remember, it is critical to code to the highest level of specificity. Completion of this field is required by Medicare and other payers (except for religious nonmedical institutions). A POA indicator is also required for inpatient claims. POA indicator options are outlined under FL 67.

FL 68: Reserved for Assignment by the National Uniform Billing Committee (NUBC)

FL 69: Admitting Diagnosis Code

FL 69 is used to report the patient diagnosis or other reason the patient was admitted. A three- to five-digit ICD-9-CM Volume I diagnosis code that describes the condition, sign, symptom, illness, injury, disease, or other reason why the patient was admitted is entered in this field. Medicare and other payers require completion of this field.

FL 70 a-c: Patient's Reason for Visit

FL 70 is used to report the patient diagnosis that is the reason for the visit at the time of an outpatient registration. A three- to five-digit ICD-9-CM Volume I diagnosis code that describes the condition, sign, symptom, illness, injury, disease, or other reason why the patient was admitted is entered. One code is entered into each of the fields a-c, as required. Medicare and other payers require completion of this field.

FL 71: Prospective Payment System (PPS) Code

The Prospective Payment System (PPS) code is recorded in this field for the inpatient admission. A Medicare Severity Diagnosis-Related Group (MS-DRG) code is required for inpatient claims.

FL 72 (a-c): External Cause of Injury (E-Code) and POA Indicator

This field is used to provide a description of the external cause of the injury or illness for which the patient is being admitted. A four to five-digit ICD-9-CM external cause of injury code that begins with an "E," which describes the external cause, is entered in this field without a decimal. Completion of this field is not required for Medicare. Other payers may require the field. Although payers in many cases do not require this field, hospitals are encouraged to complete this field when an external cause of the injury or illness is reported.

FL 73: Reserved for Assignment by the National Uniform Billing Committee (NUBC)

FL 74: Principal Procedure Code and Date

FL 74 is used to record significant procedures utilizing ICD-9-CM Volume III procedure codes that represent the principal procedure performed during the stay and the date the procedure was performed. The Uniform Hospital Discharge Data Set (UHDDS), as published in the Federal Register, Volume 50, Number 147, July 31, 1985, includes data items for reporting procedures. The definitions included can be used to determine which codes should be reported. Item 12 of UHDDS states that all significant procedures are to be reported and defines a significant procedure as one that is

1. surgical in nature, or
2. carries a procedural risk, or
3. carries an anesthetic risk, or
4. requires specialized training.

Infusions, catheterization, and surgeries are examples of significant procedures. An electrocardiogram, complete blood count, and magnetic resonance imaging (MRI) are examples of services that are not significant procedures.

The principal procedure is the procedure performed for definitive treatment of the principal diagnosis or the procedure that is the most closely related to the principal diagnosis. The principal procedure must be a significant procedure, as discussed in previous chapters. A three- to four-digit code is entered without a decimal. The format required for dates is as follows: month, day, and year (MMDDYY), with no dashes or slashes. Effective January 1, 2005, this field is not required for Medicare outpatient claims. Completion of this field is required for Medicare inpatient claims. Other payers may require this field for inpatient and outpatient claims.

FL 74 a-e: Other Procedure Codes and Dates

FL 74 a-e is used to record up to five additional ICD-9-CM Volume III procedure codes that represent other significant procedures performed during the patient stay. The date each procedure was performed is also reported in this field. A three- to four-digit code is entered without a decimal. The format required for dates is as follows: month, day, and year (MMDDYY), with no dashes or slashes. The principal procedure is not listed in this field. Codes should be listed in order of complexity. This field is required for Medicare inpatient claims. Effective January 1, 2005, this is not a required field for Medicare outpatient claims. Other payers may require this field for outpatient and inpatient claims.

FL 75 Reserved for Assignment by the National Uniform Billing Committee (NUBC)

FL 76: Attending Physician Name and Identifier

The physician **National Provider Identifier (NPI)** number and name of the attending physician are recorded in this field. Enter the attending physician's last name, first name, and middle initial. The **attending physician** is the provider who is responsible for the patient's care during the inpatient hospital stay. Claims for outpatient services require the provider identification number and name of the physician who ordered or requested the outpatient services. The completion of this field is required by Medicare and other payers (except for religious nonmedical health care institutions).

The field has two lines. The first line is optional; it can be used to record the attending's NPI or the physician's state license number, which is required by some payers and is considered a secondary qualifier. Secondary qualifiers may include the following:

OB = State license number
1G = Unique Provider Identification Number (UPIN)
G2 = Provider commercial number

Record the attending physician's name (last, first) on line 2 as outlined below.

FL 82 A and B: Attending Physician ID

NPI	1234675423	QUAL	OB
LAST	Smith MD	FIRST	John J

FL 77: Operating Physician Name and Identifiers

The NPI number and name of the operating physician are recorded in this field. Enter the NPI and the secondary identifier qualifier required before the mandated HIPAA NPI implementation on Line 1. Enter the operating physician's last name and middle initial on Line 2. Secondary identifier qualifiers include the following:

OB = State license number
1G = UPIN
G2 = Provider commercial number

FL 78–79: Other Provider (Individual) Names and Identifiers

The physician identification and name of other providers are entered in this field. Enter the referring provider's information on outpatient claims when different from the attending physician. Enter other operating physician information when more than one surgeon performs a surgery.

Enter the provider type qualifier, the NPI, and the secondary identifier qualifier required before the mandated HIPAA NPI implementation on Line 1. Enter the name of other physicians (last name, first name, and middle initial) on Line 2.

Provider Type Qualifiers
DN = Referring Provider
ZZ = Other Operating Physician
82 = Rendering Provider
Secondary Identifier Qualifiers
OB = State License Number
1G = UPIN
G2 = Provider Commercial Number

The numbers and names of additional physicians involved in the patient's care are recorded in this field on lines A and B. This field is required under certain circumstances by Medicare and other payers. Payers define what other physicians they require in this field. Some payers may require that the number and name of the physician who performed the principal procedures be recorded. There are two lines in this field, so up to two other physicians can be listed.

FL 80: Remarks

This field is used to provide additional information required by the payer for the claim to be processed. There are four lines in the field, and it is recommended that payer-specific information that is not reported in any other field on the claim be recorded in this field. Completion requirements for this field vary by payer.

FL 81: Code-Code-Field

FL 81 is used to report additional condition or occurrence codes describing more information.

TEST YOUR *Knowledge* BOX 10-6

CMS-1450 (UB-04) CLAIM FORM SECTION IV (FL 67 TO 81)

1. Provide a brief explanation of the information recorded in FL 67 and 74.
2. Where are the principal diagnosis and other diagnosis codes recorded on the UB-04?
3. Explain the difference between principal diagnosis and other diagnosis(es).
4. Describe what information is listed in FL 69 and FL 72.
5. Explain what E codes are used to describe.
6. What information is recorded in FL 74?
7. Item 12 of Uniform Hospital Discharge Data Set (UHDDS) states that all significant procedures are to be reported and defines a significant procedure as one that is: ______________, ______________, ______________, and ______________.
8. Explain the difference between the principal procedure and other procedures.
9. Define attending physician and indicate where the name of the attending physician is recorded.
10. Provide an explanation of what information is recorded in FL 80.

CHAPTER SUMMARY

Claim forms are used to submit charges to payers for reimbursement. There are two claim forms hospital may use to submit charges, the CMS-1500 and the CMS-1450 (UB-04). The CMS-1500 is used to submit charges for physician and outpatient services. The UB-04 is used to submit "facility" charges for the technical portion of outpatient, inpatient, and nonpatient services. Claim forms can be submitted manually or electronically. Advantages to electronic claim submission include proof of receipt, faster processing time, and quicker receipt of reimbursement.

This chapter reviews both claim forms. A brief overview of the CMS-1500 is provided for a refresher. The UB-04 is the primary claim form used for submission of hospital facility charges; therefore, the chapter focuses on the UB-04 claim form instructions. The NUBC maintains the claim form and data requirements. Guidelines and instructions for completion of the UB-04 claim form vary by payer. The instructions for each field, which is referred to as an FL, are outlined within the chapter. This outline provides a basic overview of data required for each FL. Hospital billing professionals are required to have an understanding of payer specifications and guidelines for completion of the UB-04 to ensure that claim forms are completed in accordance with payer guidelines. Remember, the goal in claim submission is to submit a "clean claim" the first time the claim is sent. Submission of a clean claim means compliance with payer specifications and will ensure that appropriate reimbursement is obtained.

CHAPTER REVIEW 10-1

True/False

1. The purpose of a claim form is to submit charges to a patient. T F
2. Manual claim submission is more efficient than electronic claim submission. T F
3. The CMS-1500 is used to submit facility charges to a payer for reimbursement. T F
4. The CMS-1450 (UB-04) has 33 blocks. T F

Fill in the Blank

5. Codes recorded in FL 42 are used to ____________________ like services and items.
6. A patient's written permission for the payer to send payment to the provider is called ____________________.
7. The condition determined after study is the ____________________ diagnosis.
8. ____________________ procedures are recorded in FL 74a-e.
9. The procedure performed for definitive treatment of the principal diagnosis is called the ____________________.

Match the Form Locators in Which the Data Below Are Recorded

10. ___ Codes that represent the category of service or item that is submitted on the claim form
11. ___ Principal procedure
12. ___ Standard abbreviated description of revenue codes
13. ___ Principal and other diagnosis
14. ___ HCPCS Level II National codes

A. FL 44
B. FL 42
C. FL 67 to 72
D. FL 74
E. FL 43

CHAPTER REVIEW 10-2

Claim Form Completion

Review the patient face sheet/charge detail documents on the following pages and manually complete a claim form for each of the following cases. Utilize guidelines and instructions within the chapter and refer to the CMS-1450 (UB-04) form locator data in Appendix B when required to identify appropriate UB-04 code options and revenue code numbers.

Research Project

Research Medicare claim form completion requirements for the UB-04 on the CMS and National Uniform Billing Committee (NUBC) Web sites and make an outline of information required for each form locator.

CASE SCENARIO 10-1

Community General Hospital
Federal Tax ID# 62-1026428
NPI 1234567890

8192 South Street Mars, Florida 37373 (747)722-1800
Federal Tax ID# 62-1026428

PATIENT FACE SHEET AND CHARGE DETAIL

Admit/Discharge Date	Admit/Discharge Hour	Admission Source	Admission Type	Med Record/ Soc Sec #	Patient Control #	
07 19 2006 07 19 2006				L7463527	4370563	
Patient Name DEBRA P. LUPE	DOB 04 19 1974	Release Info Y	Assignment Ben N	Discharge Status SENT HOME	Sex F	Marital Status S

Patient Address	City, ST Zip	Phone
616 MONTESORI AVENUE	ALBANY, NY 12303	518-344-2345

INSURANCE INFORMATION

Primary Carrier AETNA HOME PLAN	Insured's Name DEBRA P. LUPE	Identification # 67 479273	
		Group Name and # 606B	
Secondary Carrier	Insured's Name	Identification #	
		Group Name and #	
Pt Relationship SELF	Employer Name WESTERN UNION	Employer Location CENTRAL AVE ALBANY 12303	Treatment Authorization # 502769 3C
Pt Relationship	Employer Name	Employer Location	Treatment Authorization #

PHYSICIANS/CLINICAL INFORMATION/DIAGNOSIS/PROCEDURE

Attending/Referring/Ordering Physician NPI	Other Physician NPI	Occurrence Date	Condition/Value Info
DR. SAMUAL BLACKSTONE NPI 14273492310			

Admitting Diagnosis	Principal Diagnosis		Other Diagnosis	Other Diagnosis
719.46 Knee Pain	836.1 Meniscus Tear			

Principal Procedure/Date | Other Procedure/Date | Other Procedure/Date

CHARGE DETAIL

Revenue Code	Service Description	HCPCS/Rates	Service Units	Total Charges	Non-covered Charges
	DIAGNOSTIC RADIOLOGY MRI JOINT LOWER EXTREMITY NO CONTRAST	73721	1	$1,240.00	
	TOTAL CHARGE				

CASE SCENARIO 10-2

Community General Hospital
NPI 1234567890

8192 South Street, Mars, Florida 37373
Federal Tax ID# 62-1026428

PATIENT FACE SHEET AND CHARGE DETAIL

Admit/Discharge Date	Admit/Discharge Hour	Admission Source	Admission Type	Med Record/Soc Sec #	Patient Control #	
08 15 2006 08 15 2006	ELECTIVE ADMISSION	1		A6748754	8973452	
Patient Name	**DOB**	**Release Info**	**Assignment Ben**	**Discharge Status**	**Sex**	**Marital Status**
APPLETON DAVID	02 26 1957	Y	N	SENT HOME	M	M

Patient Address	City, ST Zip	Phone
16736 ROUTE 19	CLEARWATER FL 33759	727 323 6794

INSURANCE INFORMATION

Primary Carrier	Insured's Name	Identification #	
CIGNA	APPLETON DAVID	432 77 6599	
		Group Name and # SOUTH STREET HOTEL	
Secondary Carrier	Insured's Name	Identification #	Provider #
		Group Name and #	
Pt Relationship SELF	Employer Name SOUTH STREET HOTEL	Employer Location 4752 SOUTH STREET ST PETERSBURG FL	Treatment Authorization # ZW43796232
Pt Relationship	Employer Name	Employer Location	Treatment Authorization

PHYSICIANS/CLINICAL INFORMATION/DIAGNOSIS/PROCEDURE

Attending/Referring/Ordering Physician NPI	Other Physician NPI / Occurrence Date	Condition/Value Info
DR. PETER HOUSERTON NPI 17769573210		Condition: Neither patient or spouse is employed

Admitting Diagnosis	Principal Diagnosis Other Diagnosis	Other Diagnosis
239.2 Squamous Cell Carcinoma	239.2 Squamous Cell Carcinoma	

Principal Procedure/Date Other Procedure/Date	Other Procedure/Date
14040 Adjacent Tissue	

CHARGE DETAIL

Revenue Code	Service Description	HCPCS/Rates	Service Units	Total Charges		Non-covered Charges
	ANESTHESIA		2	320.00		
	EKG/ECG	93000		166.00		
	IV SOLUTIONS		3	72.75		
	LAB-BLOOD WORK	85025		124.00		
	MEDICAL/SURGICAL		26	930.00		
	OPERATING ROOM	14040	2	2640.0		
	PATHOLOGY-BIOPSY	88305	1	383.00		
	PHARMACY		8	331.00		
	RECOVERY ROOM			99.00		
	STERILE SUPPLIES		1	120.50		
TOTAL CHARGE						

CASE SCENARIO 10-3

Community General Hospital
NPI 1234567890

8192 South Street Mars, Florida 37373 (747)722-1800
Federal Tax ID# 62-1026428

PATIENT FACE SHEET AND CHARGE DETAIL

Admit/Discharge Date	Admit/Discharge Hour	Admission Source	Admission Type	Med Record/Soc Sec#	Patient Control #	
08 03 2006 08 04 2006	6:00 AM 10:00 AM	PHYSICIAN REFERRAL	URGENT	J7253647	5630437	
Patient Name TINA JOHNSTORM	DOB 04 17 1962	Release Info Y	Assignment Ben Y	Discharge Status DISCHARGE TO HOME	Sex F	Marital Status M
Patient Address 7952 SW 10TH ST		City, ST, Zip OCALA FL 33429				Phone 352 799 1284

INSURANCE INFORMATION

Primary Carrier	Insured's Name	Identification #	
BLUE CROSS BLUE SHIELD	JOHNNY JOHNSTORM	236767411	
		Group Name and #	
Secondary Carrier	Insured's Name	Identification #	
		Group Name and #	
Pt Relationship SELF	Employer Name OCALA HOME CARE	Employer Location 24 CALHOON PLACE OCALA FLORIDA	Treatment Authorization # 509A64361
Pt Relationship	Employer Name	Employer Location	Treatment Authorization #

PHYSICIANS/CLINICAL INFORMATION/DIAGNOSIS/PROCEDURE

Attending/Referring/Ordering Physician NPI	Other Physician NPI	Occurrence Date	Condition/Value Info
DR. JENNY HALSTOMET NPI 14972676532	DR. CHARLES BURGESTER NPI 16765324792	INSURED DOB: 04 16 1992	MOST COMMON SEMIPRIVATE ROOM RATE COVERED DAYS 1

Admitting Diagnosis	Principal Diagnosis	Other Diagnosis	Other Diagnosis
530.81 Esophageal Reflux Disease	553.3 Hiatal Hernia		

Principal Procedure/Date	Other Procedure/Date	Other Procedure/Date
44.67 08 03 2006 Nissen Fundiplication		

CHARGE DETAIL

Revenue Code	Service Description	HCPCS/Rates	Service Units	Total Charges	Non-covered Charges
	RECOVERY ROOM		3	506.00	
	ANESTHESIA		6	1364.00	
	STERILE SUPPLY		2	120.50	
	RESPIRATORY		1	39.25	
	ROOM AND BOARD		1	430.00	
	OPERATING ROOM		6	4637.75	
	DRUGS OTHER		11	423.75	
	IV SOLUTIONS		4	309.25	
	MEDICAL/SURGICAL		56	10820.00	
	TOTAL CHARGE				

GLOSSARY

Assignment of benefits Written authorization from a patient for the payer to forward benefits to the provider.

Attending physician The provider who is responsible for the patient's care during the inpatient hospital stay.

Batch A group of claims that are prepared and submitted together.

Clearinghouse An organization that reformats claim data received from providers to meet compatibility specifications for submission to various payers.

Electronic data interchange (EDI) The process of sending data from one computer to another by telephone line or cable.

Electronic media claim (EMC) A claim that is transmitted through electronic data interchange (EDI).

Form locator (FL) A term used to describe each data field on the CMS-1450 (UB-04). The UB-04 consists of 81 fields, referred to as FL 1 through FL 81.

Insurance claim form A form completed by providers for the purpose of submitting charges for medical services and supplies to various third-party payers such as insurance companies and government programs.

Medical record number (MRN) A number assigned to a patient's medical record by the facility (hospital). The medical record number is also referred to as the health record number (HRN).

National Provider Identifier (NPI) The standard unique health identifier for health care providers to use in filing and processing health care claims and other transactions. NPIs are being issued through the National Provider System (NPS) that is being developed by CMS. Effective May 23, 2007, the NPI replaces all identifiers that are currently being used.

National Uniform Billing Committee (NUBC) Committee formed by the American Hospital Association in 1975 to develop a single billing form and standard data set that could be used nationally by institutional providers. Today, the role of the NUBC is to maintain the integrity of the UB-04 data set.

North American Industry Classification System (NAIC) code A unique code assigned to each business within the United States. The NAIC code classifies the business, and it is used for statistical purposes by various agencies in the United States.

Optical scanning A process whereby the claim form is scanned, and data on the claim are transferred into a computer system.

Paper claim A claim that is typed or computer generated on paper and sent by mail.

Provider An individual or entity such as a doctor or hospital that provides medical services and/or supplies to patients.

Reimbursement The payment received from a third-party payer for services rendered to patients by the provider.

Revenue codes Codes developed and maintained by the National Uniform Billing Committee (NUBC) to categorize like services and items. Revenue codes are four numeric digits.

State Uniform Billing Committees (SUBC) Committees created to oversee implementation of the CMS-1450 (UB-04) at the state level.

Tertiary payer Refers to the third insurance.

Timely filing Refers to the period of time that claims have to be filed within, such as 90 days. Timely filing is generally calculated from the date of service.

Unique Provider Identification Number (UPIN) A unique number assigned to the provider by the Medicare Fiscal Intermediary.

SECTION FIVE

Payers

Third-Party Payers

Government Payers

Prospective Payment Systems

Chapter 11

Third-Party Payers

The objective of this chapter is to provide an overview of third-party payers that provide coverage for health care services. Over the past decades the health insurance industry has evolved (Figure 11-1). Insurance began in 1929 when the first prepaid health plan was introduced by Blue Cross. Growth in the population, complexities of care, and the rising cost of health care has contributed to the evolution of the industry. Today the health insurance industry consists of a large number of companies offering a wide spectrum of coverage through many different plans.

Hospitals provide services to patients for treatment of conditions that are covered by various third-party payer plans. The processing of claims for hospital services is complex because of the variations among payers, plan types, coverage, and reimbursement and billing requirements. It is important for hospital personnel involved in billing and coding services to have an understanding of third-party payer plans and specifications. A discussion of all third-party payer plan variations and specifications is beyond the scope of this text. In fact, the insurance industry is so diverse that much of the required knowledge can be gained only through experience with the various payers. This chapter will provide a basic overview of third-party payers; plan types, terms, and specifications; reimbursement methods; and basic billing principles.

Chapter Objectives

- Define terms, phrases, abbreviations, and acronyms related to third-party payers.
- Discuss the relationship between third-party payers and private health insurance.
- Distinguish among different insurance plans.
- List other types of insurance that provide coverage for health care services.
- Demonstrate an understanding of basic terms and specifications found in insurance plans.
- Define managed care.
- Discuss the differences between traditional fee-for-service and managed care plans.

Outline

Key Terms

Accrued charges
Appeals process
Basic health insurance
Birthday rule
Capitation
Co-insurance
Co-payment
Coordination of benefits (COB)
Deductible
Exclusive Provider Organization (EPO)
Fee-for-service plan
Group health insurance
Health Maintenance Organization (HMO)
Individual health insurance
Major medical insurance
Managed care plan
Medicare Secondary Payer (MSP)
Participating provider
Patient Responsibility
Point of service (POS)
Preauthorization
Preexisting condition
Preferred Provider Organization (PPO)
Primary care physician (PCP)
Private health insurance
Provider network
Referral
Third-party payers
Timely filing
Utilization review

Acronyms and Abbreviations

APC—Ambulatory Payment Classification
CMS—Centers for Medicare and Medicaid Services
COB—Coordination of benefits
CPT—Current Procedural Terminology
EPO—Exclusive Provider Organization
FFS—fee-for-service
HCPCS—Healthcare Common Procedure Coding System
HMO—Health Maintenance Organization
ICD-9-CM—International Classification of Diseases, 9th Revision, Clinical Modification
MS-DRG—Medicare Severity Diagnosis Related Groups
MSP—Medicare Secondary Payer
PAR—participating provider
PCP—primary care physician
POS—Point of Service
PPO—Preferred Provider Organization
PPS—Prospective Payment System
RBRVS—resource-based relative value scale
RVU—relative value unit
UCR—Usual, customary, and reasonable
UM—utilization management
UR—utilization review

THIRD-PARTY PAYERS (TPP)

Payment for hospital services is received from patients and various third-party payers. **Third-party payers** are organizations or other entities that provide coverage for health care services. Third-party payers represent the largest portion of reimbursement for hospital services. They provide coverage for health care services through many different types of plans that represent variations in the billing and coding process for hospital services. Hospital services may be covered under private health insurance, other insurance, or government-sponsored health insurance, as illustrated in Table 11-1. It is important for hospital personnel involved in the billing and coding process to understand the differences in these plan types. As discussed previously, this chapter will focus on private and other third-party payers. Government payers will be discussed in the next chapter.

Private Health Insurance

Private health insurance is any type of health insurance plan that is paid for by someone other than the government. Private payers offer coverage for health care services to members of employer groups, organizations, or individuals who purchase health insurance. Private payers offer a wide range of health care benefits through a variety of different plans. The group or individual who purchases private health insurance can select the plan that provides coverage needed and is within specified budget parameters. Health insurance plan coverage and billing specifications vary by plan. Plan provisions include details regarding coverage, determination of primary or secondary payer status, patient responsibility, claim submission, and the appeals process. Private health insurance can be categorized as group health insurance or individual health insurance. Figure 11-2 illustrates some of the differences between group health insurance and individual health insurance.

Group Health Insurance

Group health insurance is insurance purchased by an employer or other organization for the purpose of providing coverage for medical services rendered to employees or members of the group. Groups offering health insurance coverage generally offer more than one type

BEFORE 1929

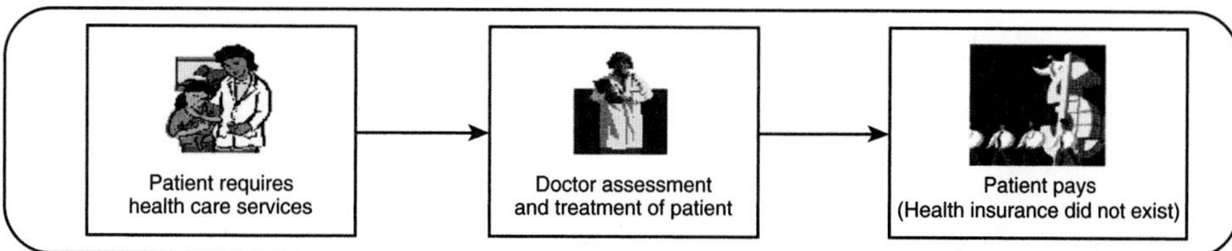

TODAY

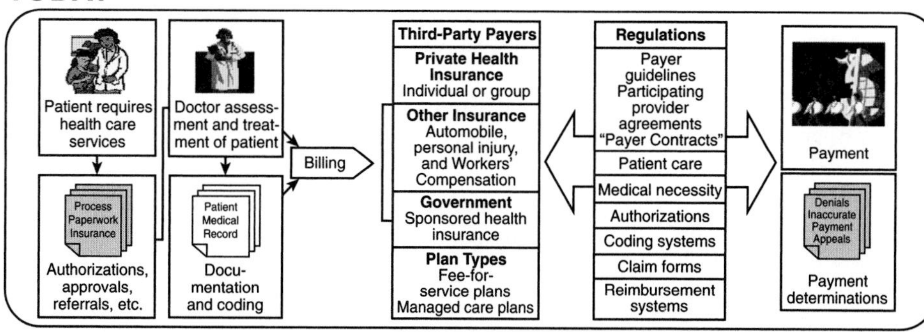

Figure 11-1 Evolution of the health insurance industry.

TABLE 11-1 Third-Party Payers

Private Health Insurance	Other insurance	Government-Sponsored Insurance
Group health insurance	Automobile insurance	Medicare
Individual health insurance	Personal injury protection insurance	Medicaid
	Workers' Compensation	TRICARE/TRICARE for Life

BOX 11-1 ■ KEY POINTS

Third-Party Payers

Private health insurance
Other insurance
Government-sponsored insurance

BOX 11-2 ■ KEY POINTS

Private Health Insurance

Private health insurance is a health insurance plan that is paid for by someone other than the government.

Private plans provide coverage for health care services provided to members of employer groups, organizations, or individuals who purchase health insurance.

of plan so that members can select the coverage that best meets their needs. Group health insurance plans can cover an individual member of the group and various family members, such as a child or spouse. Group plans provide coverage for a wide range of health care services. Plan premiums are generally lower than individual health insurance premiums because the cost of the plan is spread among all the members who are enrolled in the plan.

Group Health Insurance Coverage	Individual Health Insurance Coverage
• Purchased by a group such as employer, organization, or association to provide coverage for members. • Members may have the option of more than one plan. • Health insurance coverage is provided for all members of the group. • Coverage is provided for a wide range of health care services. • Premiums are less expensive as cost is spread among the group members.	• Purchased by an individual directly from the insurance company. • Health insurance coverage is provided for individual and family members as selected by the individual purchasing the plan. • Premiums are higher than group insurance premiums as the cost of the plan is placed on one individual. • Range of services may be limited. • Coverage for all medical conditions is not guaranteed and may be limited.

Figure 11-2 Comparison of group and individual health insurance.

> **BOX 11-3 ■ KEY POINTS**
>
> **Group Health Insurance**
>
> Group health insurance is health insurance purchased by an employer or other organization for the purpose of providing health insurance coverage for its employees or members.

Individual Health Insurance

Individual health insurance is insurance that is purchased by an individual directly from an insurance company. The individual's employer may not offer coverage, or the individual may be self-employed. Individual health insurance plans cover the individual and can also cover various family members, such as a child or spouse. Premiums for an individual plan are generally higher than premiums for a group plan because the cost is not spread among members of a group. Individual plans may not provide the wide range of benefits that a group plan might provide.

> **BOX 11-4 ■ KEY POINTS**
>
> **Individual Health Insurance**
>
> Individual health insurance is health insurance that is purchased by an individual directly from the insurance company.

Other Insurance

Hospitals provide diagnostic and therapeutic services to patients who are covered under other types of insurance such as liability insurance or Workers' Compensation insurance. An example of liability insurance is automobile or personal injury insurance. Liability insurance covers losses to a third party caused by the insured, by an object owned by the insured, or on premises owned by the insured. Liability policies also provide coverage for health care services required as a result of illness or injury related to liability. Hospitals may also provide health care services to diagnose and treat conditions that are work related and covered under Workers' Compensation insurance.

> **BOX 11-5 ■ KEY POINTS**
>
> **Other Insurance**
>
> Other types of insurance policies that provide coverage for medical care.
>
> - Automobile
> - Personal injury
> - Workers' Compensation

Automobile Insurance

Automobile insurance protects an individual against financial loss resulting from an automobile accident. It is a contract between the insured and the insurance company. The insured pays a premium and the insurance company agrees to cover losses incurred as defined in the policy. Automobile insurance provides coverage for damaged property, and many policies cover health care services.

Hospitals require patients in need of health care services related to an automobile accident to provide information regarding the automobile insurance such as the insurance company name, the policy number, and the name of the insured. The hospital will submit a claim to the automobile insurance company outlining charges for services rendered. The claim must be completed accurately with information required to tell the payer the claim is for services related to an automobile accident.

Automobile insurance provisions vary by state. In most states, insurance options include bodily injury and personal injury protection. Bodily injury is generally required by all states, as it covers injuries caused by the insured to someone else while the insured party is driving. Most states do not require personal injury protection.

Personal Injury Insurance

Personal injury insurance, commonly referred to as personal injury protection (PIP), provides coverage for losses incurred as a result of another individual or company's negligence. Personal injury losses can involve property damage and/or health care issues. A personal injury claim must be filed, and many times this begins a lengthy legal process. In the meantime, health care services are required. Hospitals have policies and procedures regarding payment for services involving personal injury liability. Some facilities require the patient to pay for services and seek reimbursement from the liability insurance company. If liability is not determined the medical insurance plan may be billed.

Workers' Compensation Insurance

Workers' Compensation insurance is generally paid for by employers to cover the cost of medical services for injuries that occur on the job. State laws require employers with a specified number of employees to provide insurance for work-related injuries. Workers' Compensation laws vary by state. Workers suffering from work-related injuries or diseases are entitled to benefits for lost wages and medical expenses arising as a result of the injury or disease.

Hospital procedures for Workers' Compensation cases vary according to the plan. All Workers' Compensation cases require a Notice of Injury report to be filed

TEST YOUR *Knowledge* BOX 11-1

THIRD-PARTY PAYERS

1. Provide a definition of a third-party payer.
2. Explain where the largest portion of reimbursement for hospital services comes from.
3. Name three types of insurance provided by private payers.
4. Describe private health insurance.
5. Name two types of private health insurance.
6. Provide an explanation of the difference between group and individual health insurance.
7. Discuss why premiums for group plans are generally less expensive than those for individual plans.
8. Provide three examples of other types of insurance that may provide health care benefits.
9. What insurance information is obtained when services related to an automobile accident are provided?
10. Provide an explanation of who may be covered under a Workers' Compensation insurance plan.

with the employer within a specified amount of time. Workers' Compensation insurance is regulated by the state and federal government.

The hospital will submit a claim that summarizes all charges for services required to treat the work-related injury. The payer may require a written report of the patient's medical condition and treatment. The information submitted by the hospital is used by the payer to determine whether the injury was work related.

Government-Sponsored Health Insurance

The government is one of the largest payers of health care services in the United States today. Government-sponsored health insurance is provided for the elderly, low-income individuals, government employees and dependents, and veterans and their families. Private payers contract with the government to provide health care coverage that meets the needs of these groups. Government-sponsored health insurance, including Medicare, Medicaid, and TRICARE, will be discussed in Chapter 12.

Third-party payers offer health insurance coverage through various plans. The plans may be individual or group plans. They may be health insurance, liability, or government-sponsored plans. Insurance plans today fall into two general categories: traditional fee-for-service plans and managed care plans.

PLAN CATEGORIES

Historically, third-party payers provided health insurance coverage for most health care services provided to patients. Payment for health care services was made on a fee-for-service (FFS) basis. These third-party health insurance plans are commonly referred to as traditional fee-for-service plans. Over the past decades, third-party payers have implemented plans to control the rising cost of health care by managing health care services provided to patients. These plans are referred to as managed care plans. There are distinct differences between traditional fee-for-service and managed care plans. The following sections provide a review of fee-for-service plans and managed care plans. It is critical for hospital personnel to understand the difference between these plans in order to obtain the appropriate insurance information and to understand billing requirements for services provided by the hospital.

BOX 11-6 ■ KEY POINTS

Health Insurance Plan Categories

Traditional fee-for-service plans
Managed care plans

BOX 11-7 ■ KEY POINTS

Traditional Fee-for-Service Plans

Traditional health insurance plans are known as fee-for-service plans. These plans provide health insurance coverage for services rendered by providers of the patient's choice, and reimbursement is determined for each service rendered based on a fee schedule. Traditional fee-for-service plans are also referred to as indemnity plans.

Traditional Fee-for-Service Plans

Traditional health insurance plans are fee-or-service plans, also referred to as indemnity plans. A **fee-for-service plan** provides health insurance coverage for services rendered by providers of the patient's choice, and reimbursement is determined for each service rendered based on a fee schedule. Fee-for-service plans do not require referrals or preauthorizations. A claim is submitted by the hospital summarizing the total accrued charges. **Accrued charges** represent the total amount of all charges incurred during the patient visit. Fee-for-service plans generally pay a percentage of accrued charges, such as 80%, as outlined in the plan. The patient is generally responsible for a deductible and co-insurance, which is a percentage of the charges. Figure 11-3 provides an example of FFS reimbursement.

In Figure 11-3 the hospital charged a separate fee for each service. The total of $388.00 represents the accrued charges. The fee-for-service plan calculated the reimbursement to the hospital at 80% of the accrued charges, or $310.40. The patient is responsible for $77.60, which represents 20% of the accrued charges.

Patient Name: John J. Smith
Date of Service: 10/25/05

COMMUNITY GENERAL HOSPITAL

PATIENT STATEMENT

HOSPITAL DIAGNOSTIC STUDIES

Complete blood count (CBC)	$ 72.00
EKG	139.00
Chest X-ray 2 views	177.00
Total accrued charges	$ 388.00
Payment received insurance (Fee-for-service reimbursement 80% of accrued charges)	−310.40
Patient responsibility (20% of accrued charges)	$ 77.60

PLEASE REMIT WITHIN 10 DAYS

Figure 11-3 Example of reimbursement under a fee-for-service plan.

Features of Fee-for-Service Plans

Traditional fee-for-service plans differ from other plans offered today. Features of these plans are illustrated in Figure 11-4.

- Coverage is provided for services required for diagnosis and treatment of patient conditions. Preventive services are generally not covered.
- Health care services may be obtained from providers of the patient's choice. The patient is not required to obtain care from providers within the plan.
- Authorizations or referrals are not required.
- The hospital charges a fee for each service and a claim is submitted by the hospital for accrued charges.
- Reimbursement is based on a percentage of the accrued charges.
- The patient is responsible for a co-insurance which is a percentage of accrued charges.

Coverage provided under a traditional fee-for-service plan can be categorized as basic health insurance coverage or major medical insurance coverage. The benefits under basic and major medical health insurance vary according to the plan.

Basic Health Insurance

Basic health insurance provides coverage for the cost of health care services required to diagnose and treat the patient's condition. Health care services required on a day-to-day basis, including physician services, diagnostic studies, surgeries, and hospitalizations, generally are covered by a basic health insurance plan.

Major Medical Insurance

Major medical insurance provides coverage for large medical expenses incurred as a result of a catastrophic

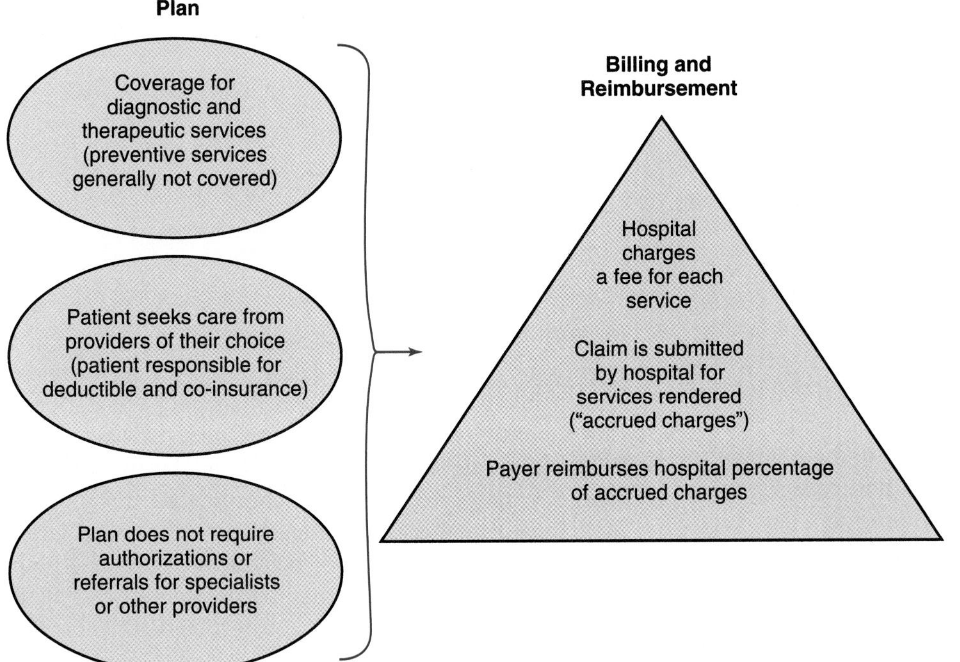

Figure 11-4 Features of traditional fee-for-service plans.

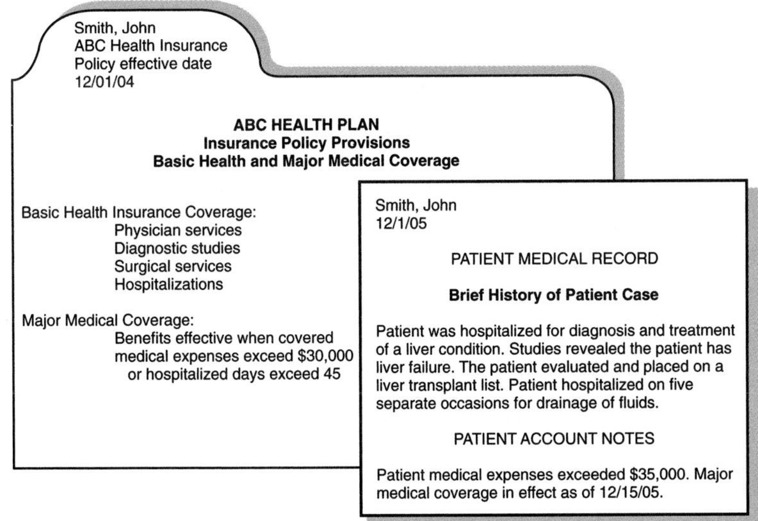
Smith, John
ABC Health Insurance
Policy effective date
12/01/04

ABC HEALTH PLAN
Insurance Policy Provisions
Basic Health and Major Medical Coverage

Basic Health Insurance Coverage:
Physician services
Diagnostic studies
Surgical services
Hospitalizations

Major Medical Coverage:
Benefits effective when covered medical expenses exceed $30,000 or hospitalized days exceed 45

Smith, John
12/1/05

PATIENT MEDICAL RECORD

Brief History of Patient Case

Patient was hospitalized for diagnosis and treatment of a liver condition. Studies revealed the patient has liver failure. The patient evaluated and placed on a liver transplant list. Patient hospitalized on five separate occasions for drainage of fluids.

PATIENT ACCOUNT NOTES

Patient medical expenses exceeded $35,000. Major medical coverage in effect as of 12/15/05.

Figure 11-5 Insurance policy provisions for basic and major medical insurance coverage.

or prolonged illness. Services required for treatment of a prolonged illness can result in the accumulation of large medical expenses. The key distinction between basic and major medical insurance coverage has to do with the expense of medical treatment or the number of hospital days required.

The major medical plan outlines a specific dollar amount or total number of hospitalization days that need to be exceeded before major medical coverage becomes effective as illustrated in Figure 11-5. A patient may initially require basic medical health care coverage and later require major medical benefits.

BOX 11-8 ■ KEY POINTS

Basic Health Insurance

Basic health insurance provides health insurance coverage for services required to diagnose and treat patient conditions on a day-to-day basis, including physician services, diagnostic studies, surgeries, and hospitalizations.

Major medical insurance provides health insurance coverage for large medical expenses incurred as a result of a catastrophic or prolonged illness.

For instance, John Smith received health care services required to diagnose and treat his liver failure (see Figure 11-5.) The expenses exceeded $35,000, as indicated on the patient's account. According to his plan, the major medical coverage becomes effective when medical expenses exceed $30,000 or hospitalization exceeds 45 days. Major medical benefits are generally paid on an FFS basis in accordance with the plan.

Managed Care Plans

Managed care plans are health insurance plans that incorporate the provision of coordinated health care services and cost-containment measures to monitor and manage health care services provided to members of the plan. Monitoring and managing patient care services is accomplished through the use of a primary care physician, who coordinates care for patients within a network of providers defined by the plan. Cost-containment measures include referrals, preauthorizations, and utilization review requirements. Utilization review is a formal review of services provided to evaluate the medical necessity and appropriateness of care Preauthorization requirements outline specific services that require prior authorization from the plan before services are provided. Managed care plans reimburse providers using various methods including fee-schedule, discounted FFS, and capitation. A majority of managed care plans provide reimbursement based on a **capitation** method by which payment is a predetermined, fixed amount paid per member, per month.

Managed care plans are designed to provide a wide range of preventive, diagnostic, and therapeutic services to plan members effectively and cost efficiently. Managed care plans are different from traditional fee-for-service plans, as they provide coverage for preventive services and incorporate key cost-containment measures.

BOX 11-9 ■ KEY POINTS

Managed Care Plans

Managed care plans are designed to provide comprehensive health care services effectively and cost efficiently.

Managed care plans are health insurance plans that incorporate the provision of coordinated health care services and cost-containment measures to monitor and manage health care services provided to members of the plan.

Cost-Containment Measures

Cost-containment measures utilized by managed care plans include the use of primary care physicians, provider networks, referrals, preauthorization, and utilization review.

BOX 11-10 ■ KEY POINTS

Managed Care Cost-Containment Measures

Primary care physician (PCP)
Provider network
Referral
Preauthorization
Utilization management review

Primary Care Physician (PCP)

A **primary care physician (PCP)** is the plan provider responsible for monitoring and managing the patient's care according to the managed care plan provisions. The PCP is referred to as the "gatekeeper" because all services for the patient must be coordinated through the PCP. Each member of a managed care plan must select a PCP from the network of providers within the plan. The following physicians may be designated as a PCP: family practitioner, internist, obstetrician/gynecologist, or pediatrician.

BOX 11-11 ■ KEY POINTS

The "Gatekeeper"

In managed care plans the primary care physician (PCP) is referred to as the "gatekeeper" because all services for the patient must be coordinated through the PCP.

Provider Networks

A **provider network** consists of providers who agree to offer health care services to plan members for a predetermined fixed payment. Managed care plans provide health care services to members through the network of providers. The provider network includes physicians, imaging centers, laboratories, and hospitals.

Referrals

A **referral** is the process of one physician transferring the care of a patient for a specific illness or injury to another physician. All health care services are coordinated through the PCP. When diagnostic, therapeutic, or specialty care is required that is beyond the scope of the PCP, a referral is made by the PCP to another provider. A referral form is prepared by the PCP and forwarded to the referred provider. The managed care plan will not pay for services rendered without the appropriate referral. Figure 11-6 illustrates a sample referral form.

Preauthorization

Preauthorization is a process required by a managed care plan to obtain approval for a service before the service is rendered. Information regarding the patient's

Dr. Alan Jones
(775) 643-2929

Referral Form

PATIENT NAME: John J. Smith

Physician referred to: Dr. Stephanie Tara

Referred for: Treatment of Cardiac Congenital condition
- ❑ Consult only
- ❑ Follow-up
- ❑ Lab
- ❑ X-ray
- ❑ Procedure
- ✓ ❑ Other

Reason for visit: consult confirmed congenital condition which requires treatment

Number of visits: as required

Appointment Scheduled: Please contact patient; phone: 776-447-8111

Referring Physician's Name: Alan Jones, M.D.

Referring Physician's Signature: Alan Jones, M.D.

Figure 11-6 Sample referral form.

ABC HEALTH PLAN
PREAUTHORIZATION REQUEST

AUTHORIZATION FOR:

❑ Hospitalization _____ Elective _________ Emergency
❑ Surgery _____ Elective _________ Emergency

Patient Name:	Date:
Address:	City, State, Zip:
__M __F DOB:	(H) Phone:
Insured Name:	Employer name:
Hospital Name:	Hospital Provider #:
Admit Date:	Estimated Length of Stay:
Admitting DX:	Other DX:
Treatment Plan:	

Treatment Authorization requested:
______ Diagnostic______ Therapeutic______ Surgical

Principal Procedure	Other Procedure

ABC HEALTH PLAN **Authorized Personnel**

Approved ________ Not approved ________

Signature______________________ Date ________

Authorization Number________________

Comments:

Figure 11-7 Sample preauthorization form.

condition and plan for treatment is presented to the managed care plan by the provider's representative. Preauthorization is granted if the plan approves the service. Services that require preauthorization are defined by the managed care plan. For example, most managed care plans require preauthorization for hospital admissions to be obtained prior to the patient admission. If an emergency admission is necessary, the plan requires authorization of the admission be obtained within a specified period of time after the admission. Payment for services will be denied if preauthorization is not obtained. Figure 11-7 illustrates a sample preauthorization request form.

Utilization Review

Utilization review is a function of the utilization management process that involves the review of patient cases to determine whether the care provided meets

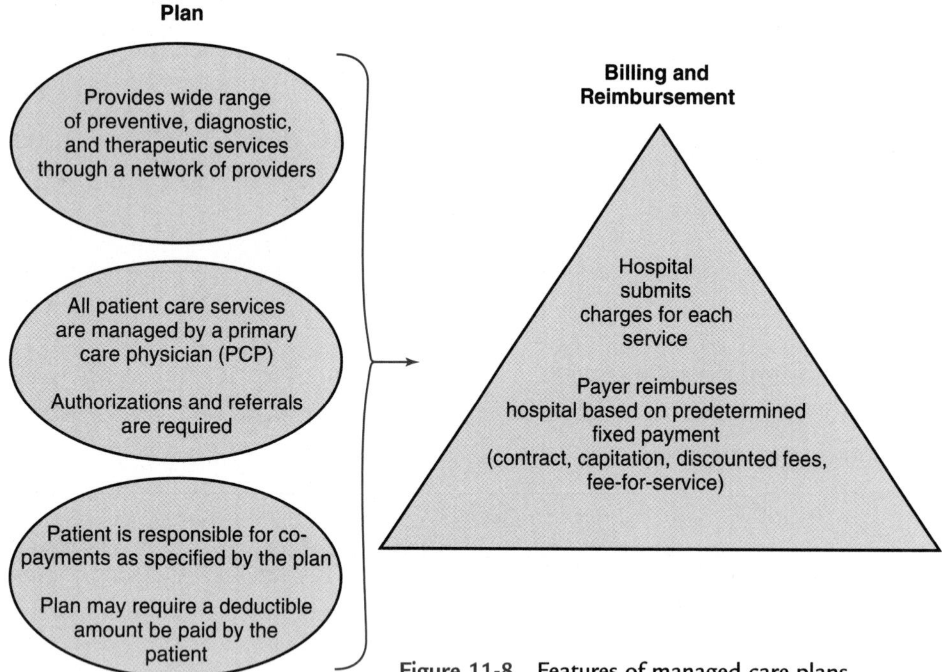

Figure 11-8 Features of managed care plans.

medical necessity requirements. Cases are also reviewed to determine if care was appropriate based on the patient's condition.

Features of Managed Care Plans

Managed care plans provide comprehensive health care coverage while incorporating cost-containment measures used by the plan. Figure 11-8 highlights the following features of managed care plans:

- A wide range of preventive, diagnostic, and therapeutic services are covered.
- Patient care services must be coordinated through the PCP.
- Health care services are provided within a network of providers as defined by the plan.
- A referral from the PCP is required for the patient to seek care from other providers.
- Preauthorization is required from the plan for specific services before the service can be provided.
- The plan requires the patient to pay a co-payment for specified services. Payment of a deductible may also be required by the plan.
- Reimbursement is determined on a capitation basis, which is a predetermined fixed periodic payment for services provided.

Types of Managed Care Plans

Managed care systems attempt to control health care costs by discouraging unnecessary hospitalization and over utilization of health care services. There are several types of managed care plans, including Health Maintenance Organization (HMO) and Preferred Provider Organization (PPO), Point of Service (POS), and Exclusive Provider Organization (EPO) plans. A comparison of these plans is outlined in Table 11-2.

BOX 11-12 ■ KEY POINTS

Managed Care Plans

Health Maintenance Organizations (HMO)
Preferred Provider Organization (PPO)
Point of Service Plan (POS)
Exclusive Provider Organization (EPO)

Health Maintenance Organization (HMO)

A **Health Maintenance Organization (HMO)** is a managed care organization that provides comprehensive health care services (preventive, diagnostic, and therapeutic) to members through a network of participating providers. Care is monitored and managed by a PCP. Members are required to obtain care from providers within the plan network. Utilization management techniques such as referrals, preauthorization, and utilization review are employed to optimize the use of health care services. Some providers are paid on a capitation basis, a predetermined fixed payment. HMO members are responsible for co-payments for specified services as outlined within the plan. The plan may require the patient to pay co-insurance or deductible amounts.

TABLE 11-2 Managed Care Plans

Type of Plan	Services	Monitored Care "Gatekeeper"	Care Providers		Utilization Management	Reimbursement	Patient Responsibility	
	Preventive, Diagnostic, and Therapeutic Services	Primary Care Physician (PCP)	Participating Network Providers	Non-participating Out-of-Network Providers	Referrals, Precertification, Second Opinion	Periodic Fixed Payment Predetermined	Co-Payment	Co-Insurance/ Deductible
Health Maintenance Organization (HMO)	Yes	Yes	Yes	No benefits	Yes	Contract capitation	Yes	Varies by plan
Preferred Provider Organization (PPO)	Preventive service coverage varies	No	Yes	Yes Higher out of pocket cost	Authorization required No referrals required	Contract discounted fees or capitation	Yes	Yes Varies by plan
Point of Service (POS)	Yes Reduced benefits	Yes	Yes	Yes Higher out of pocket cost	Yes Varies by plan	Contract capitation or fee-for-service	Yes	Yes Varies by plan
Exclusive Provider Organization (EPO)	Yes	Yes	Yes	No benefits	Yes	Contract discounted fees or capitation	Yes	Yes Varies by plan

Preferred Provider Organization (PPO)

A **Preferred Provider Organization (PPO)** is a managed care organization that provides diagnostic, therapeutic, and preventive services to its members. The PPO negotiates discounted fees with a group of providers such as hospitals, physicians, clinics, ambulatory surgical centers, diagnostic imaging centers, and laboratories. Members are encouraged to seek care from providers in the preferred network. Patient care services rendered by providers outside the network generally results in a higher out-of-pocket cost to the member. The plan may have higher co-insurance or deductible requirements for care obtained outside the network. Providers are reimbursed a discounted fee as negotiated or on a capitation basis.

Point of Service (POS)

Point of Service (POS) plans are HMOs or PPOs that provide diagnostic, therapeutic, and preventive services to members. POS plans generally have reduced benefits. Care is managed by a PCP. The plan allows members to obtain care from providers within or outside the provider network. Higher co-insurance and deductible payments may be required when care is obtained from an out-of-network provider. Utilization management requirements vary by plan however, a referral must be obtained for care beyond the scope of the PCP, whether seeking care from a network or an out-of-network provider.

Exclusive Provider Organization (EPO)

An **Exclusive Provider Organization (EPO)** is a managed care organization that provides diagnostic, therapeutic, and preventive services to members. EPO plans have many of the same features as PPO plans. Care is managed by a PCP. The EPO negotiates discounted fees with a group of providers such as hospitals, physicians, clinics, ambulatory surgical centers, diagnostic imaging centers, and laboratories. A major difference between PPOs and EPOs is that members are required to obtain care from the PPO network of providers. The plan includes referral and preauthorization requirements. Providers are reimbursed a discounted fee as negotiated or on a capitation basis. The patient may be responsible for co-payment, co-insurance and deductible amounts as outlined in the plan.

All health insurance plans contain different provisions regarding covered services, the appropriate process for obtaining care, patient responsibility, and submission of charges. Plan provisions are generally distributed to providers in a provider manual, through news bulletins, or on the plan's Web site. It is important for hospital billing and coding personnel to gain an understanding of various plan types and provisions. Having this knowledge will ensure compliance with payer specifications, which will help to prevent claim denials and to optimize reimbursement.

PLAN TERMS AND SPECIFICATIONS

A variety of health insurance plans are provided in today's health insurance industry. Private health insurance plans vary to accommodate the health care needs of the population served. The variations in health insurance plans relate to benefits, coverage limitations, how care is to be obtained, cost, the billing process and payment for health care services. Private payers require terms and specifications of the plan to be complied with as a condition for payment of health care services. Provider representatives negotiate with payers to arrive at mutually agreeable terms. Hospital personnel involved in the billing and coding process must have an understanding of the terms and specifications contained in insurance plans in order to obtain accurate information from the patient, code services provided, prepare claims, process payments, and follow-up on outstanding accounts.

A discussion of all payer specifications is beyond the scope of this text; however, there are basic terms and specifications that are written into most health care plans as discussed in previous chapters. This section discusses common terms and specifications related to covered services, coverage limitations, primary versus secondary payer responsibility, patient responsibility, and provider agreements.

BOX 11-13 ■ KEY POINTS

Plan Terms and Specifications

Covered services
Coverage limitations
Primary, secondary, tertiary payer status
Patient responsibility
Provider agreements

Covered Services

All health insurance plans define what services are covered under the patient's plan. Benefits are not provided for services that are not covered under the plan. The payer will not make payment for services when medical necessity requirements of the plan are not met. A health insurance plan may also outline limitations or exclusions for specific conditions. Common reasons for delay or denial of a claim related to coverage include the following:

- Service not covered under the patient's plan.
- Services provided do not meet medical necessity requirements of the plan.

TEST YOUR *Knowledge* BOX 11-2

PLAN TYPES

1. Discuss the historical transition from traditional fee-for-service plans to managed care plans.

2. Describe how fee-for-service plans reimburse providers.

3. Explain accrued charges.

4. State the patient responsibility amounts generally required in fee-for-service plans.

5. Provide an explanation of the difference between basic health insurance coverage and major medical coverage.

6. Define managed care.

7. Provide an explanation of how managed care plans reimburse providers.

8. List five cost-containment measures incorporated into managed care plans.

9. Explain the role of a primary care physician (PCP) in managed care plans.

10. Outline four different types of managed care plans.

- Benefits excluded for treatment related to the condition.

Non-covered Services

Services that are not covered under a patient's plan are generally billable to the patient. It is important to understand why the service is not covered: service is not a benefit under the plan, condition is excluded from coverage, or medical necessity requirements as defined by the plan are not met. Examples of non-covered services are elective or cosmetic surgeries and services that are not medically necessary.

BOX 11-14 ■ KEY POINTS

Common Reasons for Denial of Coverage

Services not covered under the patient's plan
Services do not meet medical necessity requirements of the plan
Benefits excluded for treatment related to the condition

Medical Necessity

All services provided must be considered medically necessary for the patient's condition before the plan will provide coverage. Medically necessary services are procedures or services performed that are considered reasonable and medically necessary to address the patient's condition based on standards of medical practice. Interpretations of medical necessity based on standards of medical practice may vary by payer.

BOX 11-15 ■ KEY POINTS

Medical Necessity

Medically necessary services are those that are considered reasonable and medically necessary to address the patient's condition based on standards of medical practice.

Coverage Limitations

Health insurance plans may contain exclusions or coverage limitations as defined in the plan. When a plan contains exclusions or limitations, language defining limitations of coverage for specific conditions is included in the plan. For example, two common exclusions defined in health insurance plans are preexisting conditions and self-inflicted injuries.

BOX 11-16 ■ KEY POINTS

Coverage Limitations

Coverage is not provided for the following in accordance with the plan:
Preexisting conditions
Self-inflicted injuries

Preexisting Conditions

A **preexisting condition** is a medical condition that was diagnosed or treated before coverage began under the current plan or insurance contract. An insurance plan may include a clause indicating that coverage is not provided for medical services related to a specific preexisting condition.

Self-Inflicted Injuries

Many health insurance plans will not provide benefits for treatment of conditions related to self-inflicted injuries. An example of a self-inflicted injury could be a drug overdose or an injury resulting from an attempted suicide.

Exclusions or limitations in coverage may be for a defined period of time, or coverage may be excluded indefinitely. Benefits will not be paid for conditions excluded from the patient's plan.

Figure 11-9 illustrates policy limitations included in John Smith's policy involving exclusion of conditions related to chondromalacia of the patella for 12 months and an indefinite exclusion period for conditions related to patent foramen ovale.

Primary, Secondary, and Tertiary Payer Responsibility

When a patient has coverage under more than one plan, there is often confusion about what plan is responsible to pay benefits as the primary payer. Coverage under multiple plans requires hospital personnel to determine which plan is primary, responsible to pay first on the claim. Determination of payer responsibility is a critical function that can have a negative impact on cash flow if the appropriate payer is not billed first. Patients are asked to provide all insurance information on the registration form (Figure 11-10). There are standards used to determine primary payer responsibility when the

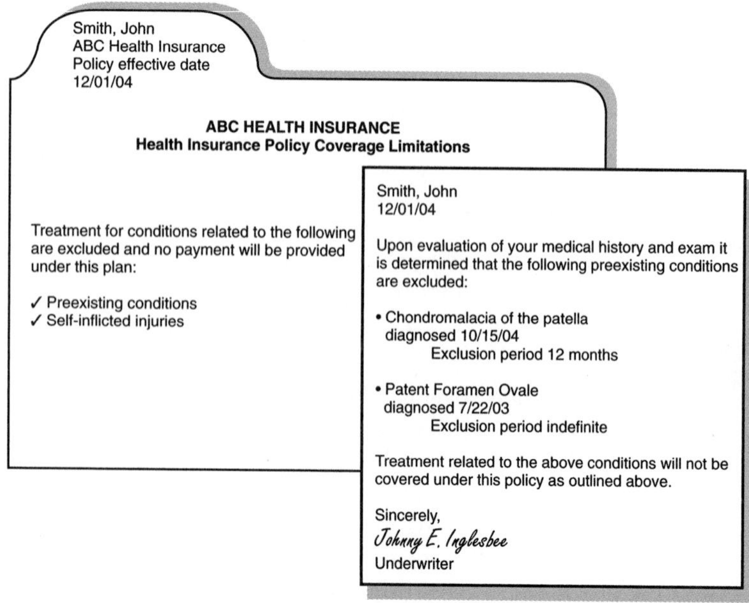
Smith, John
ABC Health Insurance
Policy effective date
12/01/04

ABC HEALTH INSURANCE
Health Insurance Policy Coverage Limitations

Treatment for conditions related to the following are excluded and no payment will be provided under this plan:

✓ Preexisting conditions
✓ Self-inflicted injuries

Smith, John
12/01/04

Upon evaluation of your medical history and exam it is determined that the following preexisting conditions are excluded:

• Chondromalacia of the patella
diagnosed 10/15/04
Exclusion period 12 months

• Patent Foramen Ovale
diagnosed 7/22/03
Exclusion period indefinite

Treatment related to the above conditions will not be covered under this policy as outlined above.

Sincerely,
Johnny E. Inglesbee
Underwriter

Figure 11-9 Health insurance policy coverage limitations.

patient is covered under two or more plans, as illustrated in Table 11-3.

Employer-Sponsored Plan: Insurance coverage provided by patient's employer is generally considered primary. For example, an individual may have employer-sponsored health insurance and may also be covered under the spouse's plan. The individual's employer-sponsored health insurance is primary.

Supplemental Plan: A supplemental plan is secondary to the plan it is meant to supplement. For example, an individual may purchase a cancer policy as a supplemental plan to an individual or group health insurance plan obtained through an employer. The individual or group health insurance coverage is primary.

Coverage under Two Employer Plans: A retired individual may have employer-sponsored coverage through a current employer in addition to the coverage from the employer from which he or she has retired. The plan through the active employer is primary.

Automobile Accident, Workers' Compensation, or Other Liability Coverage: Health insurance policies do not provide coverage for care that is required as a result of an automobile accident, work-related injury, or other liability-related incident, when there is coverage available under another insurance. The claim may be submitted under the patient's health insurance plan only if a determination is made that the condition is not the result of an automobile accident, work-related injury, or other liability-related incident or when benefits are exhausted under those plans.

Child Covered under Plans of Both Parents: When a child is covered under plans of both parents, generally the father's plan is considered primary. Exceptions to this include plans that have adopted the Birthday Rule or a court-ordered arrangement outlining the primary plan.

Coordination of Benefits

Coordination of benefits (COB) is the process of determining primary, secondary or tertiary responsibility when the patient is covered under multiple plans. A COB clause is written into an insurance policy to define how benefits will be paid when the member is covered under multiple plans. Insurance companies combine efforts to coordinate benefits paid by the plan through COB provisions. These provisions help to ensure the following:

- The plans pay as primary, secondary, or tertiary payer appropriately.
- Total payments for the claim do not exceed more than 100% of the charges.
- There is no duplication of payments for health care services.

Community General Hospital

PATIENT INFORMATION
Acct. No. | Admit Date | Time | PT | FC | Room | Bed | Svc | Med Rec No/Soc Sec No
Patient Name | DOB | Age | Race | Religion | Sex | Ma Stat
Patient Address | City, ST Zip | Phone
Employer | Employer Address | Occupation | Phone
Next of Kin | Address | Phone
NOK Employer | NOK Employer Address | Relat. | Phone

INSURANCE INFORMATION
Primary Insurance | Subscriber | Auth/Group/Plan Identification #
Secondary Insurance | Subscriber | Auth/Group/Plan Identification #
Tertiary Insurance | Subscriber | Auth/Group/Plan Identification #

GUARANTOR INFORMATION
Guarantor Name | Relation | Address | Phone
Guarantor Employer | Address | Phone | Guar Soc Sec No

DIAGNOSIS/PHYSICIANS
Referring/Admit/Attend/Ed Phys | Phys No | Diagnosis/Chief Complaint (ED)
Accident Date | Time | Previous Service | Adm By | Discharge Date | Time
Assem By | Analysis By | Advance Directive | On File | Arrive By
Comments

Figure 11-10 Patient registration form.

TABLE 11-3 Primary Payer Determination

Coverage Under	Primary Plan
Employer-sponsored plan and spouse's plan	Individual's employer-sponsored plan
Individual or group insurance and coverage under a supplemental plan	Individual or group insurance
Employer-sponsored plan through active employer and coverage through an employer from which the individual retired	Active employer plan
Health insurance plan and automobile, Workers' Compensation, or other liability plan	Automobile, Workers' Compensation, or other liability insurance
Child covered under plans of both parents	Father's plan unless Birthday Rule is adopted or by court-ordered agreement

First Health Insurance Company
Explanation of Benefits

ID#772-45-3727 DATE: 11/05/05 | Patient Name: Smith, John
Claim #4332765TB | Provider: Dr. Peters
Primary payer

Service Code	Type of Service	Place of Service	Service Dates From	To	Total Charges	Allowed Amount	Benefit %	Patient Deductible	Patient Resp	Provider Payment
55810	SURG	HOSP	102306	102306	$2,567.22	$1,925.00	70	$500.00	$927.50	$997.50

Second Supplemental Plan
Explanation of Benefits

ID#772-45-3727 DATE: 11/05/05 | Patient Name: Smith, John
Claim #4332765TB | Provider: Dr. Peters
Secondary payer total benefits payable at 100% of the plan's allowed amount less payment(s) made by primary payers.

Service Code	Type of Service	Place of Service	Service Dates From	To	Total Charges	Allowed Amount	COB Other Coverage	Benefit %	Patient Deductible	Patient Resp	Provider Payment
55810	SURG	HOSP	102306	102306	$2,567.22	$1,925.00	$997.50	100	$0.00	$0.00	$927.50

Figure 11-11 Illustration of claims processed by a primary and secondary payer in accordance with coordination of benefits provisions.

When a patient has multiple insurance plans, it is necessary to determine which plan is responsible to pay first. A patient may be required to fill out a COB form at the beginning of each plan year. Plans that include a COB clause will define when the plan is primary and how payment will be determined. Payer guidelines may require the provider to submit a copy of the remittance advice (RA) from the primary payer when submitting the claim to the secondary payer. The secondary payer disallows the portion of the charge paid by the primary payer, and the payment is calculated based on the balance. Figure 11-11 illustrates an Explanation of Benefits or RA for a primary and secondary plan that processed a claim submitted for John Smith's surgery. The payment calculations are outlined below.

John Smith has coverage under an employer-sponsored insurance called First Health Insurance Company. He also has coverage for cancer treatment under a Second Supplemental Plan. Dr. Peters participates with the first plan. The secondary plan does not have a deductible requirement.

Total charges submitted to primary plan $2,567.22
Primary plan
Allowed amount $1,925.00
The plan pays 70% of the allowed amount less $500.00
Total payment made by primary payer $997.50
Charges considered by the secondary plan
$2,567.22—642.22 (adjustment)—997.50 (primary plan payment) $927.50

Secondary plan
A claim is submitted to the Supplemental Plan. Payment is calculated as follows:
The allowed amount is $1925.00
The charges submitted are within the allowed amount and payment is calculated at 100% $927.50
Patient responsibility $0.00

Total payments for John Smith's surgery, $1925.00, do not exceed 100% of the total charges $2567.22.

The amount approved by each payer may vary. Many secondary payers will consider charges at the approved amount of the primary payer.

Coordination of benefits procedures are also required when a child is covered under the plans of both parents. The standard for determination of primary payer indicates the father's plan is primary. However, there may be some exceptions to this standard. When the parents are divorced, generally the custodial parent's plan is primary. A divorce agreement may also indicate which plan is primary. Many states have adopted a law that specifies primary coverage when a child is covered under plans of both parents. The law is called the Birthday Rule.

BOX 11-17 ■ KEY POINTS

Birthday Rule

- Plan of the parent whose birthday is first in the calendar year is the primary plan.
- When parents have the same birthday, the plan of the parent who has had the plan longer is primary plan.

Birthday Rule

The **Birthday Rule** is a law adopted by most states that defines which health insurance plan is considered "primary" when a child is listed as dependents on multiple health insurance plans. When adopted, this law supersedes the traditional standard that indicates the father's insurance is primary. The Birthday Rule determines which plan is primary based on the birthday, month and day, of each parent. The rule states that the primary plan is that of the parent whose birthday is first in the calendar year. For example:

John Smith, Jr., is covered under the insurance plans of both parents, John and Dora, and their birthdays are as follows:

John Smith, Sr.	Dora Smith
September 24	March 10

Dora's birthday occurs first in the calendar year, therefore, her plan will be billed as the primary payer. Under the Birthday Rule, when parents have the same birthday, the parent that had the plan longer pays first.

BOX 11-18 ■ KEY POINTS

Medicare as Secondary Payer (MSP)

Coverage primary to Medicare
Automobile insurance
Other liability insurance
Group health insurance
Black lung program
Veterans Benefits
Workers' Compensation
End-stage renal disease

Medicare as Secondary Payer (MSP)

A Medicare beneficiary may have coverage under another plan in addition to the Medicare coverage. Federal regulations prohibit Medicare from paying as the primary payer when other payers are responsible. To ensure that Medicare benefits are paid appropriately, legislation known as the **Medicare Secondary Payer (MSP)** Law was passed. The Medicare Secondary Payer (MSP) Law outlines coverage circumstances in which Medicare is considered the secondary payer. Providers are required by law to know when they may bill Medicare as the primary payer and when they are required to bill another insurer as the primary payer. In accordance with MSP laws, Medicare is considered the secondary payer when the beneficiary has coverage related to the following circumstances, as outlined in Table 11-4.

Automobile Insurance

Services provided to treat injury or illness that resulted from an automobile accident are generally covered under automobile liability insurance or no-fault insurance. Services are billed to the automobile insurance as the primary payer. Medicare may provide coverage as the secondary payer if benefits are exhausted.

TABLE 11-4 Medicare Secondary Payer Determination

Health Care Services	Other Insurance Coverage	Primary Coverage	Secondary Coverage
Automobile accident	Automobile liability insurance or no-fault insurance	Automobile insurance or No Fault	Medicare (MSP)
Accident on property belonging to someone else	Homeowners or business liability insurance	Liability insurance	Medicare (MSP)
Illness or injury; elderly employee or spouse; age 65 or older	Employee group health plan (EGHP)	EGHP	Medicare (MSP)
Illness related to black lung disease; coal miner or former coal miner	Federal Black Lung Act (FECA); Workers' Compensation provisions	FECA	Medicare does not apply
Injury or illness that is service related	Department of Veterans Affairs	Department of Veterans Affairs	Medicare (MSP)
Injury or illness; active duty military or dependent of active duty service person	TRICARE	TRICARE	Medicare (MSP)
Injury or illness; retired military	TRICARE for Life	TRICARE for Life	Medicare (MSP)
Injury or illness occurring on the job	Workers' Compensation	Workers' Compensation	Medicare does not apply
End-stage renal disease; current or former employees	Employer group coverage	Employer group coverage	Medicare (MSP)
Disability (except end-stage renal disease); employee or dependent younger than age 65	Employer group coverage	Employer group coverage	Medicare (MSP)

Other Liability Insurance

Services provided to treat injury or illness that occurred as a result of a fall or other accident involving an object or property owned by someone else may be covered under some other liability insurance such as homeowners or PIP insurance. Services are billed to the liability insurance as the primary payer. Medicare may provide coverage as the secondary payer if benefits are exhausted or if liability is not established.

Group Health Insurance Coverage

Medicare is the secondary payer when an individual is covered under a group health insurance plan and has Medicare. Services provided for treatment of an injury or illness are billed to the group health insurance plan as primary. Group health insurance may be acquired through an active employer, a former employer, or a family member such as a spouse. Medicare may be billed as a secondary payer for amounts not paid by the group plan.

Black Lung Program

The Federal Coal Mine Health and Safety Act of 1969 established the Black Lung Program, which provides coverage for coal miners for medical services resulting from black lung respiratory conditions. Services provided for treatment of black lung conditions are billed to the Federal Black Lung Program as the primary payer. Medicare may be billed as the secondary payer.

Veterans Benefits

Veterans who are also entitled to Medicare have a choice as to which program will be responsible for payment when both programs cover the services. When a veteran elects Medicare coverage, claims should be submitted to Medicare as the primary insurer. Claims should not be submitted to the Department of Veterans Affairs for the Medicare deductible and co-insurance amounts.

Military Benefits

Services provided to retired military personnel are billed under TRICARE for Life as the primary plan. Services provided to active military personnel or dependents are billed under TRICARE as the primary plan. Medicare may be billed as the secondary payer.

Workers' Compensation

Services provided to treat an injury or illness resulting from a work-related incident are billed to the Workers' Compensation plan as the primary payer. Medicare does not provide coverage for work-related injury unless it is determined the injury or illness is not work related.

End-Stage Renal Disease

An individual may require services related to end-stage renal disease (ESRD). The employer group health insurance is billed as primary payer during the first 30-month coordination period. Medicare may be billed as the secondary payer.

Patient Responsibility

All health insurance plans contain terms and specifications regarding the patient's responsibility. **Patient responsibility** refers to the amount the patient must pay to share in the cost of health care services as outlined in the plan. Patient's responsibility requirements may include a co-payment for specific services, co-insurance payments, or a deductible amount the patient pays before the plan will pay. Most fee-for-service plans require the patient to pay a co-insurance and deductible amount. Managed care plans usually require a co-payment for specific health care services, and they may include requirements for co-insurance or a deductible.

It is critical for hospital personnel involved in collecting monies from patients to understand the patient's responsibility as outlined in the plan to ensure that the appropriate amount is collected. Hospitals generally require payment of patient responsibility amounts at the time of visit for scheduled services. Each plan defines the patient's responsibility amounts outlined in the following sections, as illustrated in Figure 11-12.

Co-payment (Copay)

A **co-payment** is a set dollar amount the patient is required to pay for a specific service, as outlined in the patient's plan. Co-payment is also referred to as copay. Co-payment amounts can range from $10.00 to $250.00 based on the type of service. For example, the plan may require a co-payment of $15.00 for physician office visits and $25.00 for specialty physician office visits. Co-payment amounts can also be set for services such as Emergency Department or ambulatory surgery visits. Emergency Department copays can range from $50.00 to $75.00. Ambulatory surgery copays can range from $250.00 to $350.00.

BOX 11-19 ■ KEY POINTS

Patient Responsibility

Patient responsibility refers to the amount the patient is required to pay in accordance with his or her health care plan.

- Deductible—annual amount, determined by the payer, that the patient must pay before the plan pays benefits
- Co-insurance—a percentage of the approved amount that the patient is required to pay
- Co-payment—a fixed amount determined per service that the patient must pay

ABC HEALTH POS

Summary of Benefits for the ABC Health POS

Percentages shown are what the plan pays; dollar amounts shown are patient's responsibility (co-payment, co-insurance, and deductible)

BENEFIT	REFERRED CARE	SELF-REFERRED CARE
Annual Deductible	N/A DEDUCTIBLE →	$500 individual; $1,500 family
Annual Out of Pocket Maximum	N/A CO-PAYMENT	$2,500 individual; $7,500 family
Physician Office Visits, including	PCP: 100% after $15 per visit; 70%* after deductible Specialist: $25 per visit; then 100% routine well child care to age 16 only	
Allergy Shots	PCP: $15 if charged; Specialist: $25 if charged	70%* after deductible
Mammograms	100% after $25	100%, no deductible; age 35+ annually
Independent X-ray and Lab	100% after $25	70%* after deductible
Prescription Drugs When purchased at participating pharmacies		
Benefits for purchase out of network	60% Patient	
Brand	100% after $20	100% after $20
Non-formulary Formulary	100% after $35 100% after $50	100% after $35 100% after $35
Emergency Care		
Emergency	100% after $25 per visit	70%* after deductible
Emergency Room/ Urgent Care Facility	100% after $50 per visit, waived if admitted	100% after $50 per visit, waived if admitted
Hospital	100%	70%* after deductible
In Network – Hospital Inpatient Care including physician services, diagnostic, and therapeutic services.	100% after $300/day, 5-day maximum	70%* after deductible
Non-network – Hospital Inpatient Care including physician services, diagnostic, and therapeutic services. Patient is required to obtain pre-certification. Plan will not pay if pre-certification is not obtained. CO-INSURANCE →	80% after $300/day, 70%* after deductible Patient 20% 5-day maximum	
Preadmission Certification	Required (Performed by PCP)	No payment is provided if services are not pre-certified

Figure 11-12 Health insurance benefit plan illustrating a patient's responsibility (co-payment, co-insurance and deductible).

Co-insurance

Co-insurance is a percentage of the charges approved by the plan that the patient is required to pay. Co-insurance percentages vary according to the plan, and they can range from 20% to 50%. Some plans define a higher co-insurance amount when care is received from a provider who is not in the provider network. For example, a co-insurance amount of 30% may be required for services provided by a non-network hospital as opposed to a 20% co-insurance amount for an in-network hospital.

Deductible

A **deductible** is a specified dollar amount as defined in the plan that the patient is required to pay annually, before the plan will begin to pay benefits. Claims submitted by the provider are processed and the approved charges are applied to the deductible. An RA is sent to the provider indicating the approved amount has been applied to the patient's deductible. The patient also receives a notice from the payer regarding the amount applied to the deductible. Deductible amounts can range from $500.00 to $5,000.00 as outlined in the patient's plan. The plan may indicate an individual deductible amount and a family deductible amount.

Preauthorization

When care is obtained from a provider that does not contract with the patient's plan, the patient is generally responsible for obtaining the required preauthorization. Individuals are required to comply with the terms and specifications regarding obtaining care as outlined in their plan. The plan may require prior authorization for services rendered. In this instance, the patient would contact the insurance company to obtain necessary authorizations. The patient assumes financial responsibility for services when authorizations are not obtained.

The hospital will require the patient to pay the total amount of hospital charges. The hospital in most cases will submit a claim for the patient.

Participating providers (PAR) of managed care and other plans are generally responsible for obtaining preauthorization in accordance with the PAR agreement. In this case the hospital will make contact with the patient's plan to obtain required preauthorization.

Many providers require patients to pay amounts for which they are responsible at the time of service. Procedures must be followed to notify the patient when payment is required at the time of the visit. Many providers have a written financial policy posted. When monies are collected at the time of the visit, it is critical that hospital personnel understand the amount that should be collected from the patient as outlined in the plan. Many insurance cards indicate the co-payment amount for specific services. Insurance cards also indicate a phone number to use for verification of benefits and coverage and to obtain required preauthorization as illustrated in Figure 11-13. Many hospitals make contact with payers to verify insurance and obtain current information because information on insurance cards can be outdated.

TEST YOUR *Knowledge* BOX 11-3

PLAN TERMS AND SPECIFICATIONS

1. Discuss why it is important for hospital personnel to understand various plan terms and specifications.
2. Name three common reasons for delay or denial of a claim involving coverage.
3. Explain the relationship between insurance plan benefits and medical necessity.
4. Describe two common coverage limitations found in a health insurance policy.
5. Explain the standards utilized to determine primary and secondary payer when a patient is covered under multiple plans, and provide an example.
6. Provide an explanation of coordination of benefits.
7. State how the Birthday Rule is used to determine the primary plan for a child covered under multiple plans.
8. Briefly explain the Medicare Secondary Payer Law.
9. Provide an explanation of patient responsibility.
10. List three terms that describe the patient's responsibility amounts.

Front

ABC HEALTH INSURANCE **HMO BASIC** GRP#: X02604 **ID* MEMBER NAME** XXHB3TGA JOHN J. SMITH	VALID 01/01/2005 RX	
Member services 800-428-9999 Precertification 800-429-6060 Behavioral Health Vendor 800-428-9609	DR 20 SP 35 AS 300	ER 100 HO 700/A UC 50 35-20V

Back

ABC HEALTH INSURANCE P.O. Box 72256 Atlanta, GA 453221	
Direct access: benefits, referrals, hospitals	1-800-773-4949
Pre-Certification	1-800-773-6649
Emergency/Urgent Care Contact Primary Care Physician or Health Plan	1-800-773-7772

Figure 11-13 Health insurance card illustrating co-payment amounts and payer contact information.

PARTICIPATING PROVIDER AGREEMENT

Providers who elect to participate with an insurance plan or government program enter into a written agreement with each payer. The written contract is referred to as a participating provider agreement (PAR agreement, PAR contract, provider contract). The provider agreement outlines the terms and specifications for participation in the plan. Reimbursement for services provided to plan members is contingent on the provider's compliance with plan terms and specifications. It is critical for hospital personnel involved in the billing process to have an understanding of the terms in the provider agreement to ensure compliance with plan specifications and to optimize reimbursement. Participating provider agreements were discussed in previous chapters, however, this section provides a brief review of common provisions in the PAR agreement.

> **BOX 11-20 ■ KEY POINTS**
>
> **Participating Provider Agreement**
>
> A written contract between a provider and an insurance plan that outlines the terms of participation, including the following:
> - Provision of services
> - Utilization management
> - Billing requirements
> - Patient financial responsibility
> - Reimbursement

A **participating provider (PAR)** is a physician, hospital, or other entity that enters into a contract with an insurance company or government program to provide health care services to the plan's members. The provider agreement is between the payer and the provider. It outlines the terms of participation with the payer. Terms in the PAR agreement relate to provision of service, utilization management, medical necessity requirements, billing requirements, patient financial responsibility, and reimbursement (Figure 11-14).

Provision of Service

The PAR agreement outlines the services that will be provided to plan members. Details regarding how and where services are provided are also included. The provider is also required to meet all of the plan's medical necessity requirements. The payer agrees to list the provider in provider directories and other marketing material so that plan members know the facility is a PAR.

Utilization Management

PARs are required to follow all plan utilization management requirements. The provider must obtain required referrals and preauthorization as outlined in the plan.

Billing Requirements

Billing requirements vary according to the plan. The PAR agreement is a legal contract, and providers are legally obligated to comply with all provisions contained in the contract. Noncompliance can also affect reimbursement. Billing specifications are outlined in the provider manual that is given to the provider when the participating agreement is approved.

Patient Financial Responsibility

The PAR agreement outlines the patient responsibility for services rendered. As outlined in the PAR agreement, it is the provider's responsibility to make every attempt to collect amounts for which the patient is financially responsible.

Reimbursement

Reimbursement is the amount the plan pays the provider for services rendered. Payers use various

Participating Provider Agreement

This Agreement is entered into by and between **Community Hospital,** contracting on behalf of itself, **ABC Health Insurance, Inc.** and the other entities that are ABC Affiliates (collectively referred to as "ABC") and Community ("Hospital").

This Agreement is effective on the later of the following dates (the "Effective Date"):
i) December 31, 2006 or the first day of the first calendar month that begins at least thirty days after the date when this Agreement has been executed by all parties. Through contracts with physicians and other providers of health care services, ABC maintains one or more networks of providers that are available to Customers. Hospital is a provider of health care services. ABC wishes to arrange to make Hospital's services available to Customers. Hospital wishes to provide such services, under the terms and conditions set forth in this Agreement. The parties therefore enter into this Agreement.

Article I. Definitions

The following terms when used in this Agreement have the meanings set forth below:

1.1 "Benefit Plan" means a certificate of coverage or summary plan description, under which a Payer is obligated to provide coverage of Covered Services for a Customer.

1.2 "Covered Service" is a health care service or product for which a Customer is entitled to receive coverage from a Payer, pursuant to the terms of the Customer's Benefit Plan with that Payer.

1.3 "Customary Charge" is the fee for health care services charged by Hospital that does not exceed the fee Hospitals would ordinarily charge another person regardless of whether the person is a Customer.

1.4 "Customer" is a person eligible and enrolled to receive coverage from a Payer for Covered Services.

1.5 "Hospital" is duly licensed and qualified under the laws of the jurisdiction in which Covered Services are provided, who practices as a shareholder, partner, or employee of Hospital, or who practices as a subcontractor of Hospital.

Article II. Representations and Warranties

2.1 Representations and Warranties of Hospital. Hospital, by virtue of its execution and delivery of this Agreement, represents and warrants as follows:

(a) Hospital is a duly organized and validly existing legal entity in good standing under the laws of its jurisdiction of organization.

(b) Hospital has all requisite corporate power and authority to conduct its business as presently conducted, and to execute, deliver and perform its obligations under this Agreement.

(c) The execution, delivery and performance of this Agreement acknowledges the **Hospital does not and will not violate or conflict with** (i) the organizational documents of Hospital, (ii) any material agreement or instrument to which Hospital is a party or by which Hospital or any material part of its property is bound, or (iii) **applicable law.**

(d) Hospital has reviewed the Protocols and Payment Policies and acknowledges it is bound by the Protocols and that claims under this Agreement will be paid in accordance with the Payment Policies.

(f) **Each submission of a claim** by Hospital pursuant to this Agreement shall be deemed to constitute the representation and warranty by it to ABC that (i) the representations and warranties of it set forth in this section 2.1 and elsewhere in this Agreement are true and correct as of the date the claim is submitted, (ii) it has complied with the requirements of this Agreement with respect to the Covered Services involved and the submission of such claim, (iii) the charge amount set forth on the claim is the Customary Charge and (iv) the claim is a valid claim.

Article III. Applicability of this Agreement

3.1 Hospital's Services. This Agreement applies to services that are medically necessary and reasonable to diagnose and treat customer's condition.

3.2 Services not covered under a Benefit Plan. This Agreement does not apply to services not covered under the applicable Benefit Plan. Hospital may seek and collect payment from a Customer for such services, provided that the Hospital first obtains the Customer's written consent. This section does not authorize Hospital to bill or collect from Customers for Covered Services for which claims are denied or otherwise not paid. That issue is addressed in section 7 of this Agreement.

–1–

A

Figure 11-14 Common plan terms and specifications highlighted in A, Participating provider agreement, page 1.

reimbursement methods to determine payment. These methods were discussed in previous chapters. This section highlights reimbursement based on payer and service categories. The PAR agreement outlines the method of reimbursement for the provider. It also stipulates that the provider will accept the plan-approved amount as payment in full. This means the provider cannot bill the patient for more than the allowed amount or approved amount. This is referred to a balance billing and it is prohibited in accordance with most PAR agreements. Before entering into the agreement, the provider typically reviews the fee schedule outlining payment for services and determines the financial feasibility of participating in the plan. Payers also state in the agreement the time frame within which payment is to be made to the provider.

REIMBURSEMENT METHODS

Health insurance plans use various reimbursement methods to determine payment for services rendered to plan members. As outlined in previous chapters, reim-

Participating Provider Agreement

3.4 Health Care. Hospital acknowledges that this Agreement does not dictate the health care provided by Hospital or Hospital Professionals, or govern Hospital's or Hospital Professionals' determination of what care to provide their patients, even if those patients are Customers. The decision regarding what care is to be provided remains with Hospital and Hospital Professionals and with Customers, and not with ABC or any Payer. Hospital will not allow coverage decisions to determine or influence treatment decisions.

Article V. Duties of Hospital

5.1 Provide Covered Services. Hospital will provide Covered Services that are considered Medically Necessary to Customers at the location specified in section 3.1.

5.2 Cooperation with Protocols. Hospital will cooperate with and be bound by ABC's and Payers' Protocols. The Protocols include but are not limited to all of the following:

1. Hospital will use reasonable commercial efforts to direct Customers only to other providers that participate in ABC's network, except as otherwise authorized by ABC or Payer.
2. Hospital will follow Utilization Management protocols and provide notification for certain Covered Services as defined by ABC or Payer, including the following requirements:
   (a) Provide notification, as further described in the Protocols, prior to a scheduled inpatient admission of a Customer, by telephone, at least five (5) business days prior to the admission; in cases in which the admission is scheduled less than five business days in advance, Hospital will give notice at the time the admission is scheduled.
   (b) With regard to the inpatient admission of a Customer, provide notification, as further described in the Protocols, no later than the next business day, by telephone, if a Customer is admitted on an emergency basis or for observation.
   (c) Obtain required authorizations and certifications and authorizations as outlined in Appendix B.
3. Hospital will obtain customer consent to release Medical Record information.
4. Hospital will follow ABC protocols and fulfill responsibility for the collection of deductible, co-payment or co-insurance amounts outlined in Appendix C as the Customer's responsibility.

Article VII. Submission, Processing and Payment of Claims

7.1 Form and content of claims. Hospital must submit claims for Covered Services in a manner and format prescribed by ABC, as further described in the Protocols. Unless otherwise directed by ABC, Hospital shall submit claims using current CMS-1500 or CMS-1450 (UB-04) forms, whichever is appropriate, with applicable coding including, but not limited to, ICD, CPT, Revenue and HCPCS coding. Hospital shall comply with all claim form completion guidelines as outlined in Appendix C.

7.2 Electronic filing of claims. Within six months after the Effective Date of this Agreement, Hospital will use electronic submission for all of its claims under this Agreement that ABC is able to accept electronically.

7.3 Time to file claims. All information necessary to process a claim must be received by ABC no more than 90 days from the date that Covered Services are rendered. Payment to the hospital may be denied if the Hospital does not comply with Timely Filing Protocols in Appendix D and does not file a timely claim.

7.4 Denial of Claims. Hospitals may appeal claim denials in accordance with Protocols outlined in Appendix E.

7.5 Reimbursement - Payment of claims. ABC will pay claims for Covered Services according to the lesser of, the Hospital's Customary Charge or the applicable fee schedule, as provided in Appendix F. Payment determinations are subject to the Payment Policies, and minus any co-payment, deductible, or coinsurance as applicable under the Customer's Benefit Plan. The obligation for payment under this Agreement is solely that of ABC.

7.6 Timely payment. In accordance with provisions in this Agreement and legal statutes, ABC is obligated to process claims and remit payment or explanation of non-payment within 30 days of the date the claim is received.

–2–

B

Figure 11-14, ***cont'd*** **B,** Participating provider agreement, page 2.

bursement methods can be categorized as traditional, fixed-payment, and Prospective Payment System (PPS) methods, as outlined in Table 11-5. Reimbursement methods vary by payer. Traditional fee-for-service plans use methods that base payment on each service provided. Managed care plan reimbursements are generally predetermined, fixed payments. Government programs use reimbursement methods implemented under the PPS. Some private and managed care plans have begun to adopt PPS-type reimbursement methods.

TABLE 11-5 Reimbursement Methods

Methods	Outpatient, Professional, and Non-Patient Services	Ambulatory Surgery Services	Inpatient Services
Traditional Methods: Traditional plans, Blue Cross/Blue Shield, Aetna, and Humana	Fee-for-service (FFS); fee schedule; usual, customary, and reasonable (USR); relative value scale (RVU)	Fee-for-service (FFS), case rate, contract rate, percentage of accrued charges	Fee-for-service (FFS), percentage of accrued charges, per diem, flat rate, case rate, contract rate
Fixed-Payment Methods: Managed care plans	Capitation, fee schedule, contract, discounted fee	Case rate, contract rate, capitation, discounted fee	Case rate, contract rate
Prospective Payment Methods Government plans and other third-party payers. Implemented under Prospective Payment System (PPS)	Resource-based relative value scale (RBRVS)	Ambulatory Payment Classification (APC)	Medicare Severity Diagnosis Related Groups (MS-DRG)

BOX 11-21 ■ KEY POINTS

Reimbursement

Charges for services rendered are submitted to payers for reimbursement using a claim form.

Reimbursement is payment from a third-party payer to a provider for services rendered.

Reimbursement is provided when services are covered in accordance with the patient's plan and when the services are considered medically necessary.

BOX 11-22 ■ KEY POINTS

Reimbursement Methods

Payers use various reimbursement methods to calculate payment for services provided. Three categories of reimbursement methods are:

- Traditional methods
- Fixed-payment methods
- Prospective Payment System (PPS) methods

Traditional Methods

Traditional reimbursement methods typically used by traditional fee-for-service plans include percentage of accrued charges; fee schedules; usual, customary, and reasonable (UCR) fees; relative value scale (RVU); and FFS methods.

Fixed-Payment Methods

Fixed-payment methods include fee schedules, contract rates, capitation, and case rates. Managed care plans typically have fee schedules that indicate reimbursement fees for services determined by one of these methods.

Prospective Payment System (PPS) Methods

Government programs use PPS methods. In recent years, traditional and managed care plans have begun to adopt PPS reimbursement methods. PPS reimbursement methods include resource-based relative value scales (RBRVS), Ambulatory Payment Classifications (APC) and Medicare Severity Diagnosis Related Groups (MS-DRG).

A review of payment method definitions is provided in Table 11-6.

BILLING REQUIREMENTS

The purpose of the billing process is to obtain reimbursement for services rendered. The billing process involves collection of pertinent billing information, documentation of services and patient conditions, preparation of claims, and collection of outstanding accounts (Figure 11-15). Charges for services are submitted to payers by means of claim forms. The CMS-1500 and CMS-1450 (UB-04) claim forms are used according to payer requirements. The information collected and prepared during the patient visit is recorded on the claim form for submission to payers. Reimbursement is determined based on the information submitted on the claim. Payer requirements for completion and submission of claims vary. A review of the various payer specifications for billing is beyond the scope of this text. Basic principles of billing can be reviewed and applied for all payers. Some of the basic principles involve documentation, coding, claim forms, timely filing, and the appeals process.

TABLE 11-6 Reimbursement Methods Defined

Reimbursement Method	Definition
Traditional Reimbursement Methods	
Fee-for-service	A reimbursement method in which hospitals are paid for each service provided, based on an established fee schedule.
Fee schedule	A listing of established allowed amounts for specific medical services and procedures.
Percentage of accrued charges	A reimbursement method used to calculate payment based on charges accrued during a hospital stay. Payment is based on a percentage of approved charges.
Usual, customary, and reasonable (UCR)	Reimbursement is based on review of three fees: 1) Usual fee—the fee usually submitted by the provider of a service or item; 2) Customary fees—fees that providers of the same specialty in the same geographic area charge for a service or item; 3) Reasonable fee—the fee that is considered reasonable
Fixed-Payment Reimbursement Methods	
Capitation	Reimbursement method used to determine payment based on a fixed amount, paid per member, per month. Capitation methods are generally used to provide reimbursement for primary care physician (PCP) other specified services.
Case rate	A set rate is paid to the hospital for the case. The payment rate is based on the type of case and resources used to treat the patient.
Contract rate	Reimbursement to the hospital is at a set rate as agreed to in the contract between the hospital and the payer.
Flat rate	Reimbursement is at a set rate for a hospital admission regardless of charges accrued.
Per diem	The hospital is paid a set rate per day rather than payment based on total accrued charges.
Relative value scale (RVS)	A relative value that represents work, practice expense, and cost of malpractice insurance is assigned to professional services.
Prospective Payment System (PPS) Reimbursement Methods	
Ambulatory Payment Classifications (APC)	An Outpatient Prospective Payment System (OPPS) that is used by Medicare and other government programs to provide reimbursement for hospital outpatient services including ambulatory surgery performed in a hospital outpatient department. The hospital is paid a fixed fee based on the procedure(s) performed.
Medicare Severity Diagnosis Related Groups (MS-DRG)	An Inpatient Prospective Payment System (IPPS) that is used by Medicare and other government programs to provide reimbursement for hospital inpatient cases. The hospital is paid a fixed fee based on the patient's condition and relative treatment.
Resource-based relative value scale (RBRVS)	A reimbursement method implemented under PPS for Medicare and other government programs to provide reimbursement for physician and outpatient services. A unit value is assigned to each procedure. The unit value represents physician time, skill, practice expense and cost of malpractice insurance.

Documentation

Documentation of all patient conditions and services is required during a patient visit. The documentation of the patient visit supports and explains to the payer the services provided and the reasons. Documentation is not submitted with every claim; however, the payer may request documentation after initial review of the claim. It is critical for hospital billing and coding personnel to understand that services and conditions that are not documented should not be coded. Reimbursement is not provided for services, procedures, and items that are not documented (Figure 11-16).

TEST YOUR *Knowledge* BOX 11-4

PARTICIPATING PROVIDER AGREEMENT AND REIMBURSEMENT METHODS

1. Outline why it is important for hospital personnel to understand the terms of the participating provider agreement.
2. Define participating provider.
3. Discuss utilization requirements that may be outlined in a participating provider agreement.
4. Briefly describe why compliance with payer billing specifications is important.
5. Provide an explanation of the provider's responsibility regarding collection of the amount the patient is financially responsible for.
6. Discuss the relationship between provider contracts and reimbursement.
7. What is balance billing?
8. List three categories of reimbursement methods used to reimburse providers for services rendered.
9. Discuss the difference between traditional reimbursement methods and fixed-payment methods.
10. List payer types that utilize reimbursement methods implemented under the Prospective Payment System (PPS).

BOX 11-23 ■ KEY POINTS

Coding Systems

It is important to remember that coding system utilization is determined based on the type of provider and service.

Procedure Coding Systems

HCPCS Level I—CPT codes
HCPCS Level II—Medicare National codes
ICD-9-CM Volume III Procedure codes

Diagnosis Coding System

ICD-9-CM Volumes I and II Diagnosis codes

Coding

Coding is the process of translating written descriptions of conditions and services in the patient's record into codes. Submission of claims requires codes to describe the services provided and the patient conditions that were treated. There are variations in the coding systems utilized that are determined by the type of provider and service. Each payer defines the coding systems required for describing patient conditions and services. The coding system used for reporting patient conditions is the International Classification of Diseases, 9th

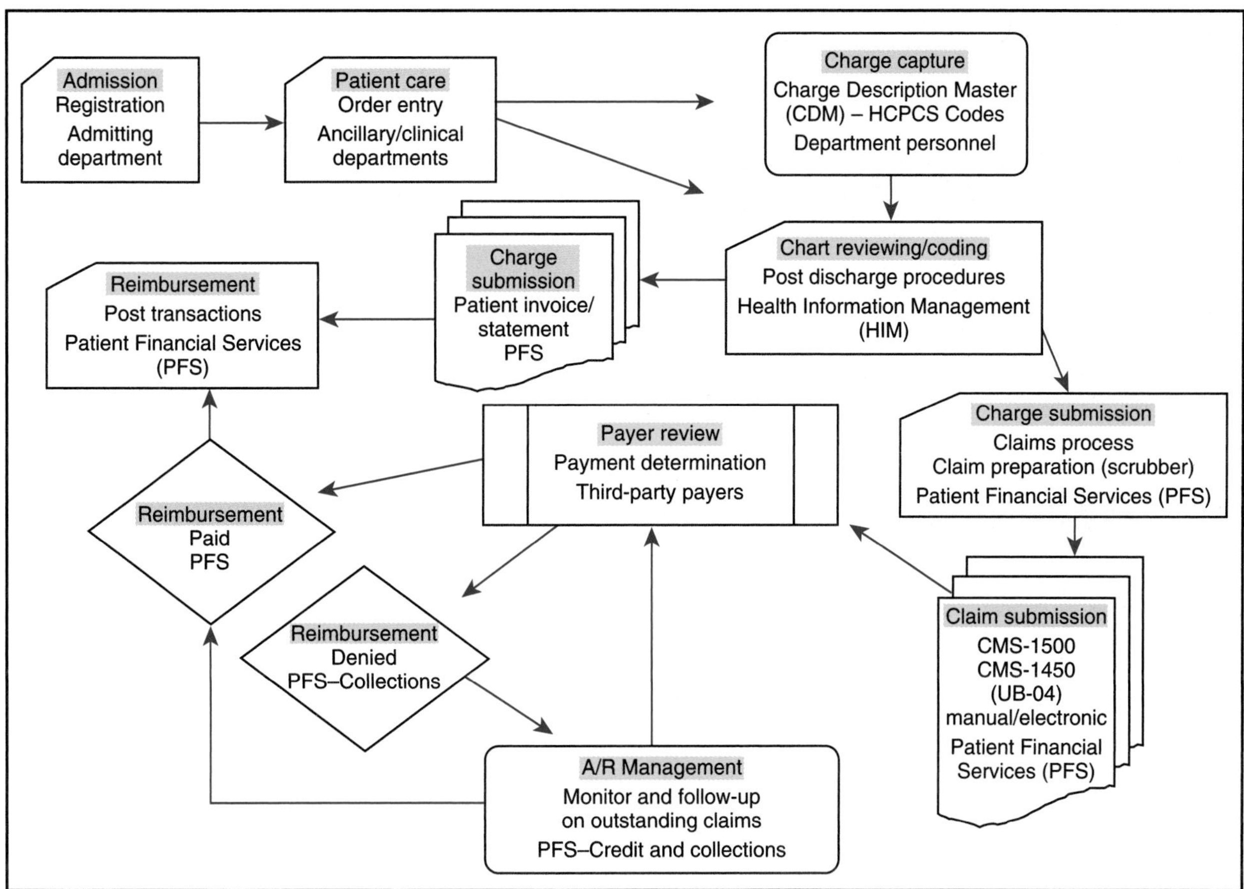

Figure 11-15 The hospital billing process: key functions and the primary departments involved in performing those functions. *(Revision of illustration courtesy Sandra Giangreco.)*

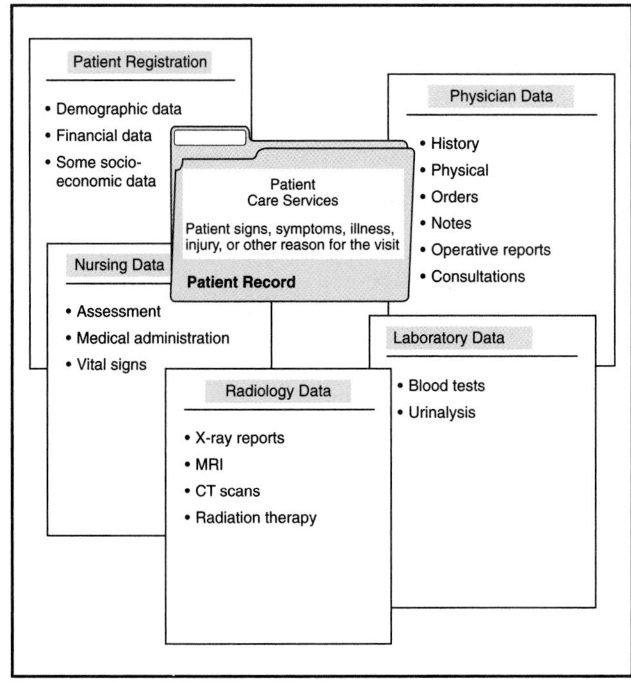

Figure 11-16 Medical record. *(Modified from Davis N, LaCour M:* Introduction to health information technology, *ed 1, St Louis, 2002, Saunders.)*

Revision, Clinical Modification (ICD-9-CM). Coding services can be performed utilizing HCPC Level I CPT, Level II Medicare National or ICD-9-CM Volume III procedure codes. Coding system requirements also vary by category of service for outpatient, inpatient, and non-patient services. Figure 11-17 provides an overview of coding system requirements for various payers and services.

Claim Forms

Claim forms are used to submit charges to payers for reimbursement. The claim form required is defined by the payer: either the CMS-1500 or the CMS-1450 (UB-04) (Figure 11-18). Almost all payers require the CMS-1500 for physician and outpatient services. Payer's requirements regarding claim forms for ambulatory surgery services vary. Some require the CMS-1500, whereas others may require the UB-04. The UB-04 is required by most payers for outpatient, inpatient, and non-patient services provided by hospitals, skilled nursing facilities, and rehabilitation centers.

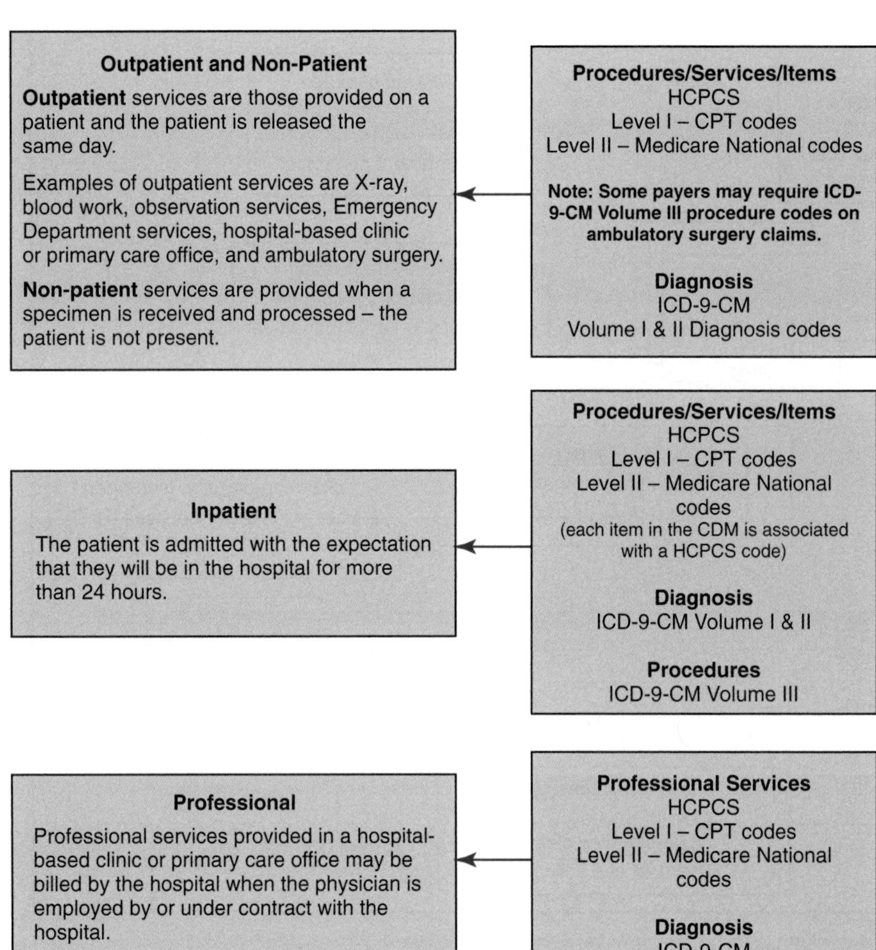

Outpatient and Non-Patient
Outpatient services are those provided on a patient and the patient is released the same day.
Examples of outpatient services are X-ray, blood work, observation services, Emergency Department services, hospital-based clinic or primary care office, and ambulatory surgery.
Non-patient services are provided when a specimen is received and processed – the patient is not present.
Procedures/Services/Items
HCPCS
Level I – CPT codes
Level II – Medicare National codes
Note: Some payers may require ICD-9-CM Volume III procedure codes on ambulatory surgery claims.
Diagnosis
ICD-9-CM
Volume I & II Diagnosis codes
Inpatient
The patient is admitted with the expectation that they will be in the hospital for more than 24 hours.
Procedures/Services/Items
HCPCS
Level I – CPT codes
Level II – Medicare National codes
(each item in the CDM is associated with a HCPCS code)
Diagnosis
ICD-9-CM Volume I & II
Procedures
ICD-9-CM Volume III
Professional
Professional services provided in a hospital-based clinic or primary care office may be billed by the hospital when the physician is employed by or under contract with the hospital.
Professional Services
HCPCS
Level I – CPT codes
Level II – Medicare National codes
Diagnosis
ICD-9-CM

Figure 11-17 Coding system variations for outpatient, non-patient, inpatient, and professional services.

BOX 11-24 ■ KEY POINTS

CMS Claim Forms

CMS-1500

Physician and outpatient services

CMS-1450 (UB-04)

Facility charges for services provided on an outpatient, non-patient, and inpatient basis

Instructions for completion of the claim form vary by payers. Payer requirements outline what claim form and data are required. Payers define the method of claim submission. Some payers require claims be submitted electronically, and some allow submission of paper claims. It is important for hospital personnel to understand variations in claim form instructions and submission requirements as outlined in Chapter 10. An understanding of payer requirements helps to ensure compliance with payer specifications and to optimize reimbursement.

Timely Filing

All payers require claims be submitted within a specific period after services are provided. **Timely filing** requirements outline the time frame during which claims must be submitted to the payer for reimbursement. If a claim is not submitted within the timely filing period defined by the payer, reimbursement will not be made for those services.

Appeals Process

The purpose of the appeals process is for payers to provide a formal way for providers to ask for reconsideration of a claim determination. The **appeals process** involves standard procedures required by the payer, for submission of a request for reconsideration of a claim determination. All payers have a formal appeals process for providers to follow when they do not agree with how the claim was paid or a claim denial. The payer guidelines will outline a specific time frame for which appeals can be submitted, how appeals should

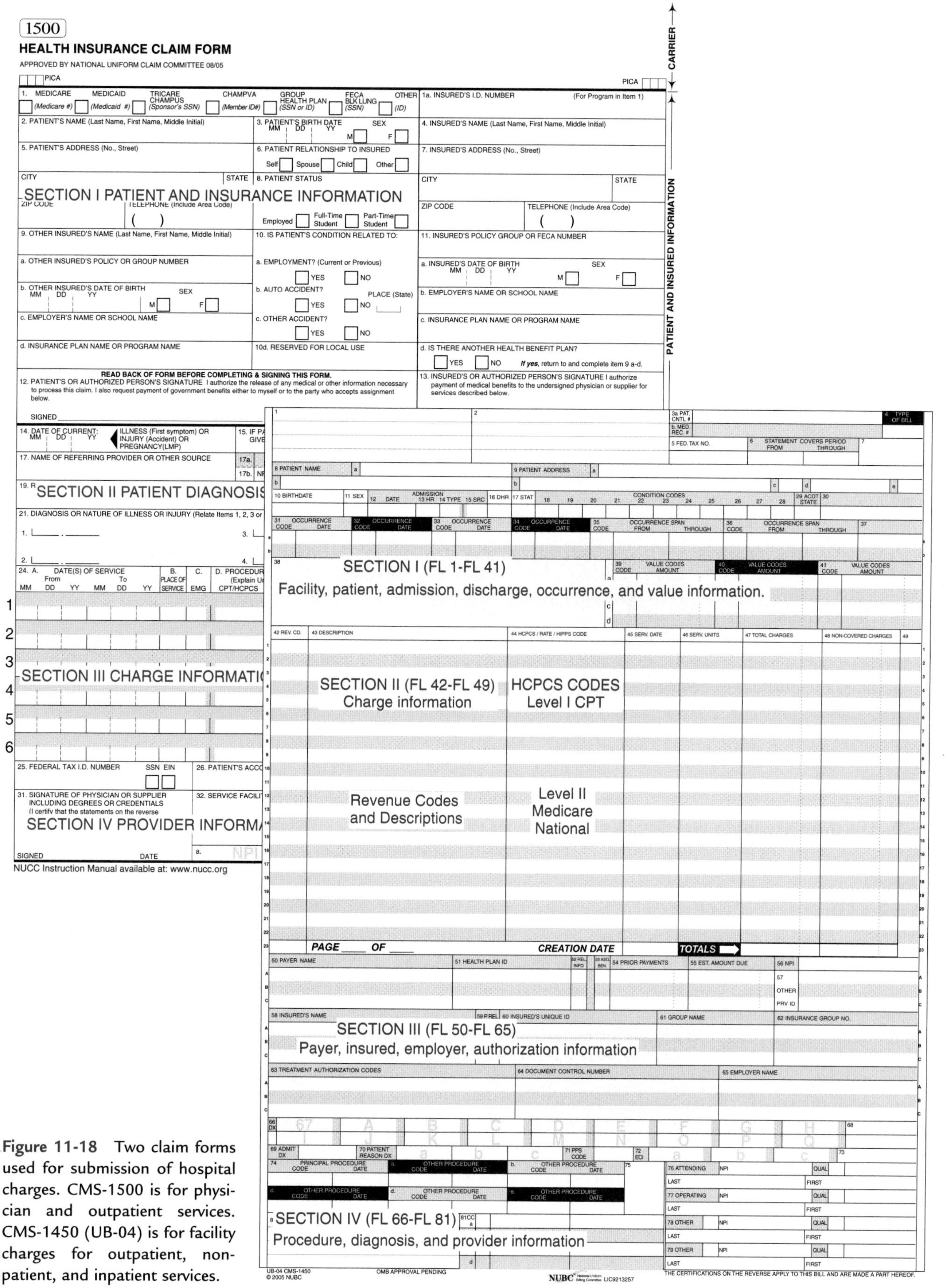

1500

HEALTH INSURANCE CLAIM FORM

APPROVED BY NATIONAL UNIFORM CLAIM COMMITTEE 08/05

PICA

CARRIER

SECTION I PATIENT AND INSURANCE INFORMATION

PATIENT AND INSURED INFORMATION

SECTION II PATIENT DIAGNOSIS

SECTION III CHARGE INFORMATION

SECTION IV PROVIDER INFORMATION

NUCC Instruction Manual available at: www.nucc.org

SECTION I (FL 1-FL 41)
Facility, patient, admission, discharge, occurrence, and value information.

SECTION II (FL 42-FL 49)
Charge information

HCPCS CODES
Level I CPT

Revenue Codes
and Descriptions

Level II
Medicare
National

PAGE ___ OF ___ CREATION DATE TOTALS

SECTION III (FL 50-FL 65)
Payer, insured, employer, authorization information

SECTION IV (FL 66-FL 81)
Procedure, diagnosis, and provider information

UB-04 CMS-1450 © 2005 NUBC OMB APPROVAL PENDING NUBC LIC9213257

THE CERTIFICATIONS ON THE REVERSE APPLY TO THIS BILL AND ARE MADE A PART HEREOF.

Figure 11-18 Two claim forms used for submission of hospital charges. CMS-1500 is for physician and outpatient services. CMS-1450 (UB-04) is for facility charges for outpatient, nonpatient, and inpatient services.

be submitted and what type of claim issues can be appealed. Guidelines for appeals will explain what type of denials can be appealed. Most payers require that appeal requests be submitted in writing. The payer also defines the time frame during which an appeal may be submitted. For example, a payer may require appeals to be submitted within 60 days of the denial.

It is essential for hospital personnel involved in the billing process to understand how compliance with payer guidelines can affect payment. Claims can be delayed or denied if they are not completed accurately. Services may not be paid if guidelines are not followed. The opportunity to appeal a denial can be lost if the appeal is not submitted within the appropriate time frame.

BOX 11-25 ■ KEY POINTS

Timely Filing

After services are rendered, each payer requires the claim for the service to be submitted within a specific period of time.

Timely filing requirements must be met or payment will not be made.

TEST YOUR *Knowledge* BOX 11-5

BILLING REQUIREMENTS

1. Explain the relationship between documentation and payment for services from payers.
2. Define coding.
3. State the purpose of coding systems in the billing process.
4. Provide an outline of various coding systems used for inpatient services.
5. List two claim forms that may be used to submit charges to payers.
6. Provide a brief explanation of what services can be reported on each of the claim forms.
7. Discuss how completion of a claim form may vary by payer.
8. Define timely filing, and explain its importance in the billing process.
9. State the purpose of the appeals process.
10. Provide a brief explanation of payer variations related to the appeals process.

CHAPTER SUMMARY

Hospitals provide services to patients who are covered under various health insurance plans offered by third-party payers. Hospital services may be covered under private health insurance, other insurance such as liability insurance, or government programs. The plans may be group or individual plans. Traditional plans are referred to as fee-for-service plans, in which the provider is paid based on the total accrued charges. Today, managed care plans are dominant. They provide coordinated care and incorporate cost-containment measures. Fees paid to providers are fixed, predetermined fees.

All health insurance plans have terms and specifications that define how services are obtained, what services are covered, how providers are to bill for services and how reimbursement will be determined. Hospitals may elect to participate with various health insurance plans. Participation requirements vary by plan. Payments for health care services are contingent on compliance with plan requirements by both the provider and patient. These variations require hospital personnel to have an understanding of plan terms and specifications in order to ensure compliance with the plan requirements and to optimize reimbursement. While this chapter provides an overview of the terms and specifications found in insurance plans, hospital professionals must extend their knowledge base through experience with the various plans. To accomplish this, hospital personnel may attend payer specific seminars, join associations, subscribe to industry newsletters, and communicate with various payers regarding the terms and specifications found in the plan contracts.

CHAPTER REVIEW 11-1

True/False

1. Third-party payers represent the largest portion of reimbursement for hospital services. T F
2. Private health insurance is insurance that is paid for by someone other than the government. T F
3. Fee-for-service plans reimburse providers on a capitation basis. T F
4. Major medical insurance provides coverage for large medical expenses incurred as a result of a catastrophic or prolonged illness. T F
5. Managed care organizations do not incorporate cost-containment measures in their plans. T F

Fill in the Blank

6. The provider responsible for monitoring and managing patient care is the ________________.
7. Managed care plans require provider to obtain a ________________ for specific services before the services are rendered.
8. ________________ conditions are those that were diagnosed and/or treated before coverage under an insurance policy began.
9. A fixed amount for specific services that a patient is required to pay is a ________________.
10. The time period set by a plan during which a claim must be filed is ________________.

Match the Following Definitions with the Terms at Right

11. ___ The process of reviewing patient cases to determine whether care provided met medical necessity requirements and was appropriate based on the patient's condition.
12. ___ A managed care plan that allows members to obtain care from providers within or outside the provider network.
13. ___ Refers to the amount the patient must pay to share in the cost of health care services.
14. ___ A managed care organization that provides health care services managed by a primary care physician (PCP) through a network of providers. This plan does not allow members to obtain care from providers outside the plan network.
15. ___ A physician, hospital, or other entity that enters into a contract with an insurance company or government program to provide health care services to the plan members.

A. Patient responsibility
B. Participating provider
C. Utilization review
D. Health Maintenance Organization (HMO)
E. Point of Service (POS)

CHAPTER REVIEW 11-1—*cont'd*

Research Project

The purpose of this project is to further research variations in insurance plans to apply basic concepts reviewed in this chapter.

Conduct research through the Internet or contact with payers or hospitals to outline the following.

1. Identify two different companies that offer a:
   a. Fee-for-service plan
   b. Managed care plan

2. Research and identify the following elements for each plan:
   a. Does the plan incorporate cost-containment measures? If so, provide a brief explanation of at least two measures.
   b. Outline covered services.
   c. State the medical necessity requirements.
   d. Discuss coverage limitations listed in each plan.
   e. Explain how you would determine whether the plan is a primary or secondary plan.
   f. List patient responsibility requirements for the plan.

3. Research what a provider is required to do to participate with the plan, and discuss the following:
   a. Briefly describe two or three of the terms for participation for each plan.
   b. Is the provider required to obtain a referral to provide care to a patient?
   c. How does the plan reimburse the provider?
   d. Discuss what claim form is required.
   e. State the timely filing requirements for the plan.
   f. Provide an overview of the appeals process for the plan.

Provide a separate report for each plan and outline all the above.

GLOSSARY

Accrued charges The total amount of all charges incurred during the patient visit.

Appeals process Standard procedures required by the payer, for submission of a request for reconsideration of a claim determination.

Basic health insurance Provides coverage for the cost of health care services required on a day-to-day basis, to diagnose and treat the patient's condition.

Birthday Rule A "law" adopted by most states that defines which health insurance plan is considered "primary" when children are listed as dependents on multiple health insurance plans.

Capitation Reimbursement method by which payment is determined based on a predetermined fixed amount paid per member per month.

Co-insurance A percentage of the charges approved by the plan that the patient is required to pay

Co-payment A set dollar amount the patient is required to pay for a specific service as outlined in the patient's plan.

Coordination of Benefits (COB) The process of determining primary, secondary, or tertiary responsibility when the patient is covered under multiple plans.

Deductible A specified dollar amount as defined in the plan that the patient is required to pay annually before the plan will begin to pay benefits.

Exclusive Provider Organization (EPO) A managed care organization that provides health care service to members. Care is managed by a primary care physician (PCP); members must obtain care through the network of providers.

Fee-for-service plan A plan that provides health insurance coverage for services rendered and reimbursement determined for each service rendered based on a fee schedule. Traditional health insurance plans were fee-for-service plans.

Group health insurance Health insurance purchased by an employer or other organization for the purpose of providing coverage for medical services rendered to employees or members of the group.

Health Maintenance Organization (HMO) A managed care organization that provides comprehensive health care services to members, managed by a primary care physician (PCP), through a network of participating providers. Providers are paid a predetermined fixed payment, capitation.

Individual health insurance Health insurance coverage that is purchased by an individual directly from the insurance company.

Major medical insurance Provides coverage for large medical expenses incurred as a result of a catastrophic or prolonged illness.

Managed care plan A health insurance plan that incorporates the provision of coordinated health care services and cost-containment measures to monitor and manage health care services provided to members of the plan.

Medicare Secondary Payer (MSP) Legislation that outlines coverage circumstances in which Medicare is considered the secondary payer. The legislation is referred to as Medicare Secondary Payer (MSP) laws.

Participating provider A physician, hospital, or other entity that enters into a contract with an insurance company or government program to provide health care services to its members in accordance with the contract. Commonly referred to as a PAR provider.

Patient responsibility Refers to the amount the patient must pay to share in the cost of health care services as outlined in the patient's plan.

Point of Service (POS) A health maintenance or preferred provider organizations that provide health care services to members. Care is managed by a primary care physician (PCP). Members are allowed to obtain care outside the provider network from nonparticipating providers.

Preauthorization A process required by a managed care plan to obtain approval for a service before the service is rendered.

Preexisting condition A medical condition that was diagnosed or treated before coverage began under the current plan or insurance contract.

Preferred Provider Organization (PPO) A managed care organization that provides health care services to members. Members may obtain care from a non-network provider. PPOs negotiate discounted fees with providers.

Primary care physician (PCP) The plan provider responsible for monitoring and managing the patient's care according to the managed care plan provisions. The PCP is also referred to as the "gatekeeper."

Private health insurance Any type of health insurance plan that is paid for by someone other than the government.

Provider network Consists of providers who agree to provide health care services to plan members for a predetermined fixed payment. The provider network includes physicians, imaging centers, laboratories, and hospitals.

Referral The process of one physician transferring the care of a patient, for a specific illness or injury, to another physician.

Third-party payers Organizations or other entities that provide coverage for health care services.

Timely filing The submission of a claim within a required period of time after services are rendered.

Utilization review Part of the utilization management process whereby patient cases are reviewed to determine whether the care provided met medical necessity requirements and to determine if care was appropriate based on the patient's condition.

Chapter 12

Government Payers

The objective of this chapter is to provide an overview of government-sponsored health insurance. Hospitals provide services to patients for treatment of conditions that are covered under various government-sponsored health insurance plans. The processing of claims for hospital services is complex because of the variations in the government plan types, coverage, reimbursement, and billing requirements. It is important for hospital personnel involved in billing and coding services to have an understanding of these variations in order to ensure compliance with program requirements and to obtain accurate reimbursement. A discussion of all government payer plan variations is beyond the scope of this text. In fact, the insurance industry is so diverse that much of the required knowledge can be gained only through experience with the various government programs. This chapter provides an overview of key elements of various government-sponsored health insurance plans.

Chapter Objectives

- Define terms, phrases, abbreviations, and acronyms related to government-sponsored health insurance.
- Provide an overview of coverage for each government program.
- Discuss the relationship between third-party payers and government programs.
- Distinguish between traditional government plans and managed care plans.
- State primary versus secondary responsibility for Medicare, Medicaid, and TRICARE.
- Demonstrate an understanding of basic terms and specifications.
- Explain why government programs implemented managed care plans.
- Describe the role of the Centers for Medicare and Medicaid Services (CMS) in government plans.
- Provide a brief overview of eligibility requirements for each government program.

Outline

Key Terms

Benefit period
Categorically needy
Centers for Medicare and Medicaid Services (CMS)
Civilian Health and Medical Program of the Veterans Administration (CHAMPVA)
Defense Enrollment Eligibility Reporting System (DEERS)
Field activities
Fiscal agents (FA)
Lifetime Reserve Days
Local coverage determination (LCD)
Medicaid
Medically needy
Medicare
Medicare Administrative Contractor (MAC)
Medicare Part A
Medicare Part B
Medicare Part C
Medicare Part D
Medicare Summary Notice (MSN)
Medigap plan
Military Treatment Facility (MTF)
National coverage determination (NCD)
Non-Availability Statement (NAS)
Participating provider (PAR)
Quality Improvement Organization (QIO)
Regional contractors
State Children's Health Insurance Program (SCHIP)
TRICARE
TRICARE Extra
TRICARE for Life (TFL)
TRICARE Management Activity (TMA)
TRICARE Prime
TRICARE Remote
TRICARE Standard

Acronyms and Abbreviations

AFDC—Aid to Families with Dependent Children
APC—Ambulatory Payment Classification
BBA—Balanced Budget Act
CHAMPUS—Civilian Health and Medical Program of the Uniformed Services
CHAMPVA—Civilian Health and Medical Program of the Veterans Administration
CHIP—Children's Health Insurance Program
CMS—Centers for Medicare and Medicaid Services
COB—Coordination of benefits
CPT—Current Procedural Terminology
DEERS—Defense Enrollment Eligibility Reporting System
ESPDT—Early and Periodic Screening, Diagnostic, and Treatment
ESRD—end-stage renal disease
FA—fiscal agent
FFS—fee-for-service
FI—Fiscal Intermediary
FQHC—federally qualified health center
HCFA—Health Care Financing Administration
HCPCS—Health Care Common Procedure Coding System
HMO—Health Maintenance Organization
ICD-9-CM—International Classification of Disease, 9th Revision, Clinical Modification
LCD—local coverage determination
MAC—Medicare Administrative Contractor
MMA—Medicare Prescription Drug Improvement Modernization Act
MSN—Medicare Summary Notice
MS-DRG—Medicare Severity Diagnosis Related Groups
MSP—Medicare Secondary Payer
MTF—Military Treatment Facility
NAS—Non-Availability Statement
NCD—national coverage determination
PAR—participating provider
PCM—primary care manager
PCP—primary care physician
PIP—Personal injury protection
PPO—Preferred Provider Organization
QIO—Quality Improvement Organization
QMB—Qualified Medicare Beneficiary
SCHIP—State Children's Health Insurance Program
SSI—Supplemental Security Income
TFL—TRICARE for Life
TMA—TRICARE Management Activity

GOVERNMENT-SPONSORED PROGRAMS OVERVIEW

Over the past decade, the health insurance industry has evolved and the government has become the largest payer of health care services. In the 1960s a growing concern over the rising cost of health care and limited access to care for the poor and elderly resulted in the implementation of several federally sponsored government health insurance programs. In 1965, through an amendment of the Social Security Act of 1935, health insurance for the aged, called Medicare, was implemented. Another program, Medicaid, was implemented to provide coverage for health expenses to low-income individuals. In 1966 the U.S. Congress created the Civilian Health and Medical Program of the Uniformed Services (CHAMPUS), now known as TRICARE, to provide coverage for medical care provided to individuals in the military.

Government health care expenditures for Medicare, Medicaid, and military beneficiaries equaled $713 billion in 2002, as illustrated in Figure 12-1. Government-sponsored health care represented 45.5% of the total national health care expenditure of $1.55 billion in 2002, whereas private health insurance represented 54.5% of the total national health care expenditure. Figure 12-2 illustrates the percentage of health care expenditures according to payer: Medicaid, Medicare, military, and private third-party payers. The high percentage of government health care expenditures provides an explanation of why the government sets the pace in the health care industry regarding provision of care, processing claims, and payment for services.

Government-sponsored health care is provided under many programs such as Medicare, Medicaid, and TRICARE. Health care coverage provided under each program varies according to plan types, eligibility, coverage, and other key factors involving billing for services covered under each program. The following discussion of three major programs—Medicare, Medicaid, and TRICARE—provides hospital billing and coding professionals with an overview of key factors in billing for services covered under these programs, including administration, plan options, eligibility, coverage, and coordination of benefits. The chapter closes with a review of participating provider agreements, reimbursement methods, and billing requirements.

Box 12-1 ■ KEY POINTS

Medicare

Medicare is a federally funded program implemented under Title XVIII of the Social Security Act in 1965. The purpose of the program is to provide coverage for health care services provided to the following:

- Individuals 65 years of age or older
- Individuals who are eligible for social security disability
- Individuals with end-stage renal disease (ESRD)

MEDICARE

Medicare is a federally funded program implemented under Title XVIII of the Social Security Act in 1965. The purpose of the program is to provide coverage for health care services provided to the following:

- Individuals 65 years of age or older
- Individuals who are eligible for social security disability.
- Individuals with end-stage renal disease (ESRD)

Box 12-2 ■ KEY POINTS

Centers for Medicare and Medicaid Services

The Centers for Medicare and Medicaid Services (CMS) is a federal agency within the Department of Health and Human Services that is responsible for three national health care programs that benefit over 80 million Americans:

- Medicare
- Medicaid
- State Children's Health Insurance Program (SCHIP)

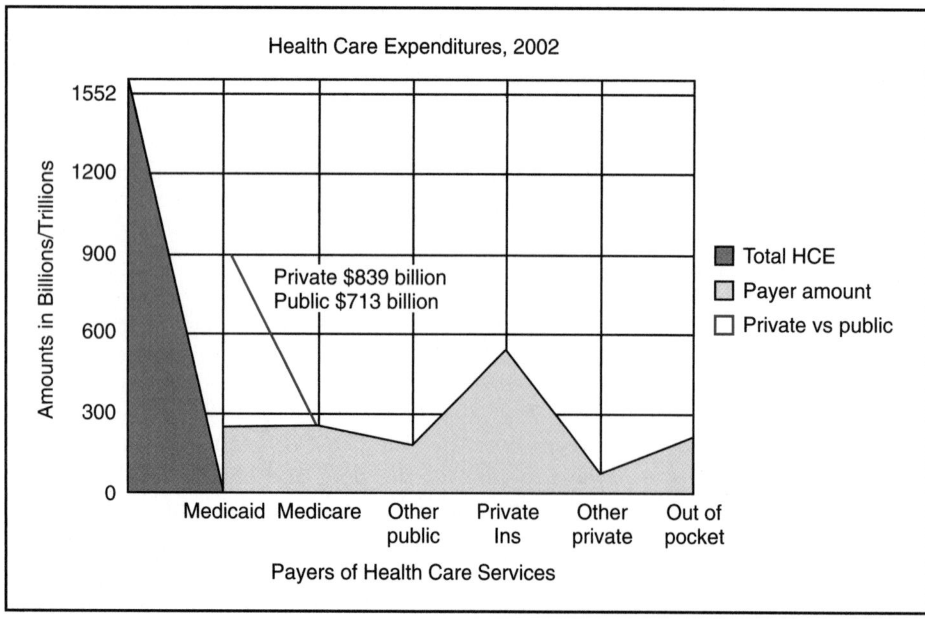

Figure 12-1 Health care expenditures chart illustrates total health care expenditures for 2002 of $1.55 trillion dollars. Private payer health care dollars amounted to $839 billion. Health care dollars by public payers totalled $713 billion. *(Data from Centers for Medicare & Medicaid Services:* Health Care Expenditures 2002, *www.cms.hhs.gov)*

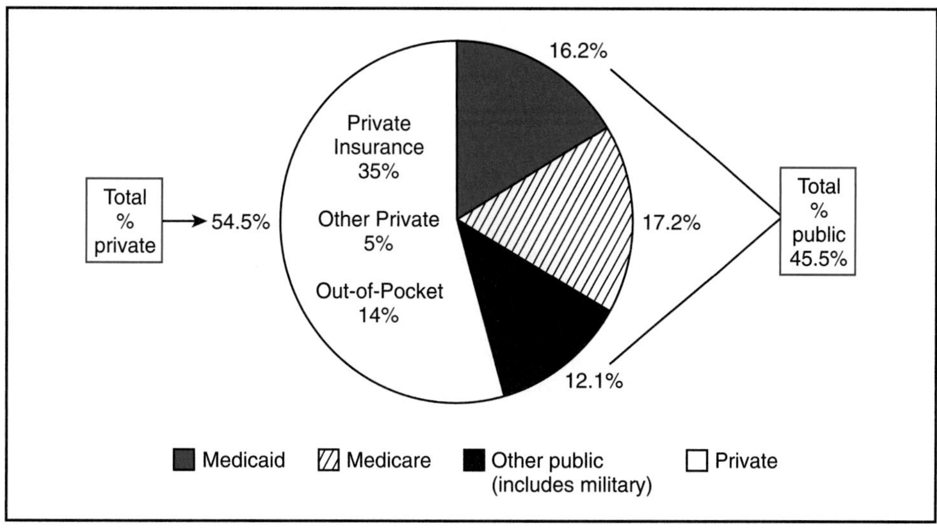

Figure 12-2 Health care expenditures chart illustrates the percentage of total health care dollars spent in 2002 by private payers and public payers. *(Data from Centers for Medicare & Medicaid Services:* Health Care Expenditures, *www.cms.hhs.gov)*

Administration

Medicare is administered by the **Centers for Medicare and Medicaid Services (CMS)**, a federal agency within the Department of Health and Human Services, as illustrated in Figure 12-3. CMS was formerly known as the Health Care Financing Administration (HCFA). CMS is responsible for three national health care programs that benefit over 81 million Americans:

- Medicare
- Medicaid.
- State Children's Health Insurance Program (SCHIP)

Two divisions within CMS that are chiefly responsible for the Medicare program are the Center for Medicare Management and the Center for Beneficiary Choices. Figure 12-4 illustrates the two divisions.

The Center for Medicare Management

The Center for Medicare Management is responsible for the oversight of traditional fee-for-service Medicare. It serves as the focal point for all interactions with health care providers, intermediaries, and carriers for issues relating to CMS policies and operations. Responsibilities of the Center for Medicare Management include the management of fee-for-service contractors and the development of policies regarding coding and payments.

The Center for Beneficiary Choices

The Center for Beneficiary Choices manages Medicare Advantage Plans, consumer research, and grievance and appeal functions for the Medicare program. The division serves as the focal point for all interactions with beneficiaries, their families, care givers, health care providers, and others operating on their behalf concerning improving beneficiaries' ability to make informed decisions about their health and about program benefits administered by CMS.

Fiscal Intermediary (FI)—Medicare Administrative Contractor (MAC)

A **Medicare Administrative Contractor (MAC)** is an insurance company or other entity that contracts with the federal government to handle functions related to

Box 12-3 ■ KEY POINTS

Centers for Medicare and Medicaid Services—Medicare Oversight Divisions

The Center for Medicare Management

Responsible for the oversight of traditional fee-for-service Medicare

The Center for Beneficiary Choices

Responsible for the management of the Medicare Advantage Plans, consumer research, and grievance and appeals functions for the Medicare program

Box 12-4 ■ KEY POINTS

Medicare Administrative Contractor (MAC)

A Medicare Administrative Contractor (MAC) is an insurance company or other entity contracted by the federal government to handle the functions related to enrollment and processing of claims for the Medicare program.

Medicare contractors were previously known as Fiscal Intermediaries (for Medicare Part A) or Medicare Carriers (for Medicare Part B). The Centers for Medicare and Medicaid Services (CMS) published a notice of change that states that, effective October 1, 2005, Medicare contractors will be referred to as Medicare Administrative Contractors.

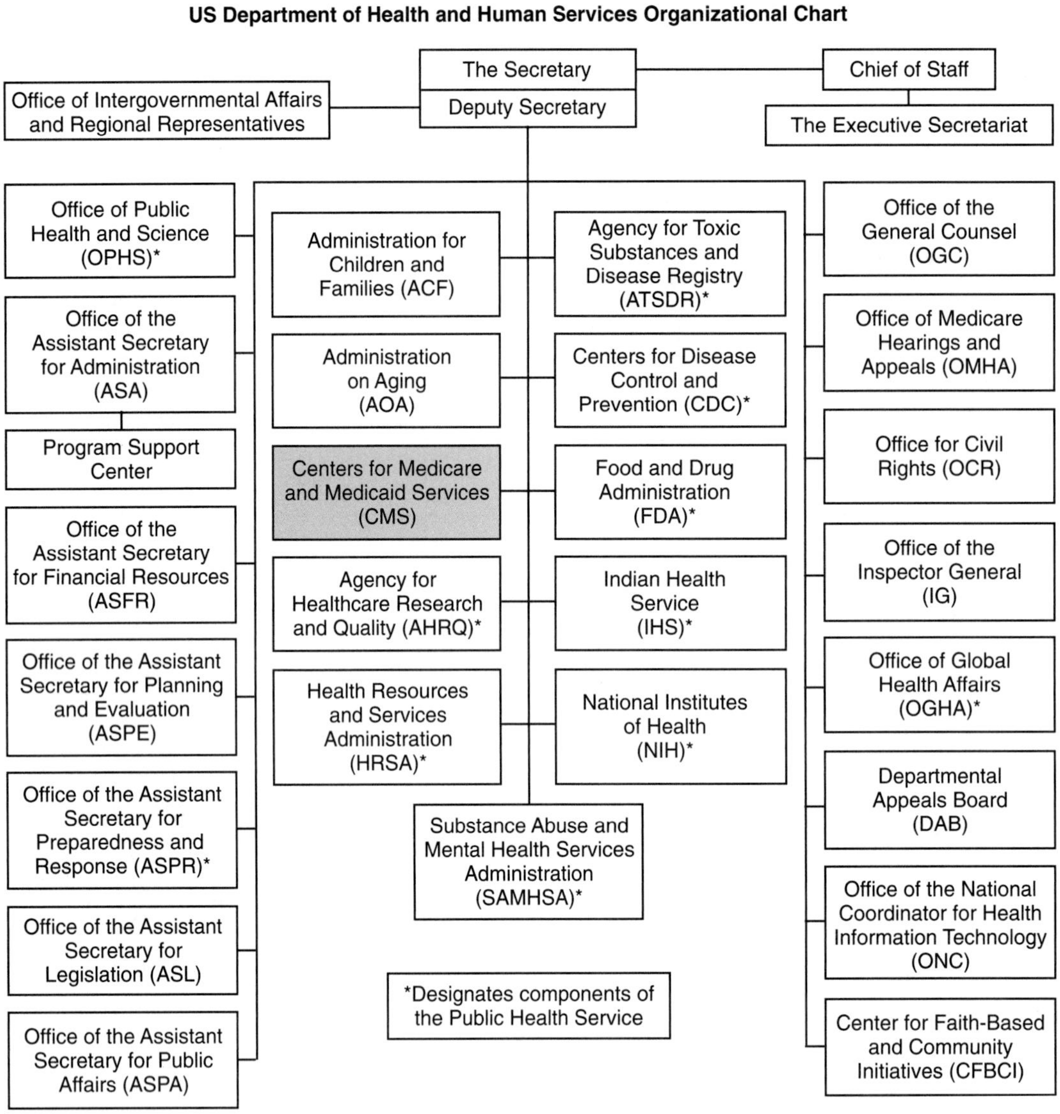

US Department of Health and Human Services Organizational Chart

The Secretary
Deputy Secretary
Chief of Staff
The Executive Secretariat
Office of Intergovernmental Affairs and Regional Representatives
Office of Public Health and Science (OPHS)*
Office of the Assistant Secretary for Administration (ASA)
Program Support Center
Office of the Assistant Secretary for Financial Resources (ASFR)
Office of the Assistant Secretary for Planning and Evaluation (ASPE)
Office of the Assistant Secretary for Preparedness and Response (ASPR)*
Office of the Assistant Secretary for Legislation (ASL)
Office of the Assistant Secretary for Public Affairs (ASPA)
Administration for Children and Families (ACF)
Administration on Aging (AOA)
Centers for Medicare and Medicaid Services (CMS)
Agency for Healthcare Research and Quality (AHRQ)*
Health Resources and Services Administration (HRSA)*
Agency for Toxic Substances and Disease Registry (ATSDR)*
Centers for Disease Control and Prevention (CDC)*
Food and Drug Administration (FDA)*
Indian Health Service (IHS)*
National Institutes of Health (NIH)*
Substance Abuse and Mental Health Services Administration (SAMHSA)*
Office of the General Counsel (OGC)
Office of Medicare Hearings and Appeals (OMHA)
Office for Civil Rights (OCR)
Office of the Inspector General (IG)
Office of Global Health Affairs (OGHA)*
Departmental Appeals Board (DAB)
Office of the National Coordinator for Health Information Technology (ONC)
Center for Faith-Based and Community Initiatives (CFBCI)
*Designates components of the Public Health Service

Figure 12-3 Department of Health and Human Services organizational chart illustrating agencies under the DHHS, such as the Centers for Medicare and Medicaid Services (CMS). *(Modified from U.S. Department of Health & Human Services:* Organizational Chart, *www.hhs.gov/about/orgchart/2010.)*

enrollment and processing of claims for the Medicare program. Medicare contractors were previously known as Fiscal Intermediaries (FIs) or Medicare Carriers. CMS published a notice of change that states that, effective on October 1, 2005, Medicare contractors will be referred to as Medicare Administrative Contractors (MAC) instead of FIs or Medicare Carriers. MAC vary by state or region. For example, First Coast Service Options, a division of Blue Cross and Blue Shield, is the MAC for Florida.

Eligibility

In accordance with Medicare eligibility requirements, individuals eligible for Medicare are those who meet the following criteria:

Box 12-5 ■ KEY POINTS

Medicare Eligibility

In accordance with Medicare eligibility requirements, individuals eligible for Medicare are those who meeting following the criteria:

- Have worked for at least 10 years as Medicare-covered employees
- Are age 65 years or older
- Are citizens or permanent residents of the United States
- Are eligible for social security disability benefits *or*
- Have end-stage renal disease (permanent kidney failure requiring dialysis or transplant)

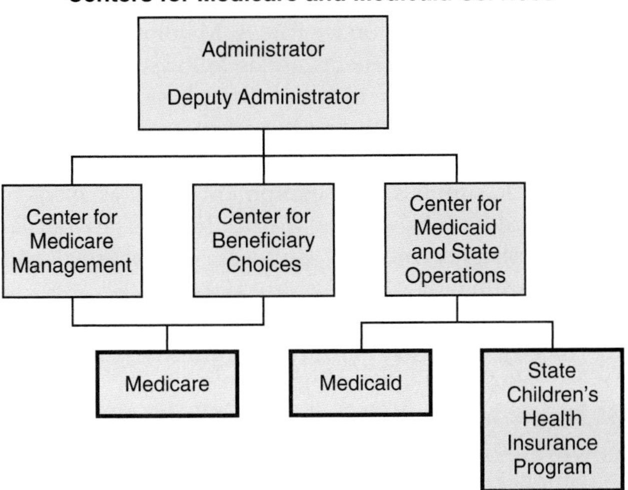

Figure 12-4 Centers for Medicare and Medicaid Services (CMS)—divisions chiefly responsible for oversight of the Medicare program. *(Modified from U.S. Department of Health & Human Services:* Organizational Chart, *www.hhs.gov)*

Medicare Health Care Coverage

PART A
Hospital Insurance

Hospital, skilled nursing, home health, hospital, hospice, and blood.

PART B
Medical Insurance

Medical expenses for physician and hospital outpatient diagnostic and therapeutic services including: laboratory, x-ray, physical therapy, emergency room and ambulatory surgical services.

PART C
Medicare Advantage Plans
Formerly known as Medicare + Choice

Beneficiaries may select from various managed care, preferred provider organization, fee-for-service, or Medicare specialty plans that provide Part A and B coverage.

PART D
Medicare Prescription Drug Plan

Beneficiaries may select from various prescription drug plan options to obtain coverage for prescription drugs. Medicare Part D was created under MMA, passed in 2003. Drug coverage under the prescription drug plans became available effective January 1, 2006.

Figure 12-5 Medicare Parts A, B, C, and D. Highlights coverage provided by Medicare.

- Worked for at least 10 years as Medicare-covered employees (contributions were made for social security)
- Are age 65 years or older
- Are citizens or permanent residents of the United States
- Are eligible for social security disability benefits *or*
- Have end-stage renal disease (ESRD) (permanent kidney failure requiring dialysis or transplant).

Coverage

Coverage provided under the Medicare program is defined in four parts: Medicare Part A, Part B, Part C, and Part D, as illustrated in Figure 12-5.

Medicare Part A

Medicare Part A is referred to as "hospital insurance," as it provides coverage for medically necessary inpatient care provided in a hospital, skilled nursing facility, or a psychiatric facility. Coverage for hospice, home health care, and blood is also provided under Medicare Part A.

Medicare Part A coverage is automatically assigned to individuals who are retired and receiving social security, railroad retirement beneficiaries, and individuals who are receiving social security disability benefits. Medicare Part A does not require the beneficiary to pay a premium unless they do not meet the Medicare 10-year covered employment requirement.

Medicare Part A Benefits

Medicare Part A benefits are paid based on a benefit period. A **benefit period** begins on the first day a patient is admitted to the hospital. The period ends when the patient has not been in the hospital for 60 consecutive days. This period is also referred to as an episode of care. Major categories of coverage under Medicare Part A are:

1. Inpatient hospitalization, which includes room and board (semi-private), medications, supplies, nursing care, and other hospital services.
2. Skilled nursing facility care provided by a Medicare-approved nursing facility. Nursing facility services are covered when the patient is admitted to a nursing facility from a hospital after a minimum stay of 3 days in the facility.
3. Home health care provided on a part-time or intermittent skilled care basis, including home health aide services, durable medical equipment, supplies, and other services.
4. Hospice care services provided to a patient who is terminally ill for the purpose of relieving pain and symptoms.
5. Blood required during a patient stay.

Medicare beneficiaries are required to pay a Medicare Part A deductible. The deductible for 2010 is $1100.00. The Part A co-insurance requirement is $275.00 a day for each day for inpatient hospital stays over 60 days and $550.00 per day for hospital stay of 91 to 150 days. Medicare beneficiaries are entitled to Lifetime Reserve Days. **Lifetime Reserve Days** are 60 days of hospitalization, per lifetime, that the beneficiary may use at his or her discretion. Lifetime Reserve Days may be used to cover patient stays beyond 150 days. The patient is responsible for all hospital charges for stays over 150 days, unless the patient elects to use the Lifetime Reserve Days. Table 12-1 illustrates Medicare Part A covered services, amounts paid by Medicare, and the patient's responsibility for the major classifications of coverage.

Medicare Part B

Medicare Part B is generally referred to as "medical insurance," that provides coverage for most care that is not covered under Medicare Part A. Coverage for medically necessary physician and outpatient services, including laboratory tests, X-ray examinations, physical therapy, emergency room services, and ambulatory surgery services, is provided under Medicare Part B. Unlike Medicare Part A, where coverage is assigned automatically, there is an enrollment process for Medicare Part B benefits. Individuals who are turning 65 may elect to enroll in Medicare Part B.

Medicare Part B Benefits

Medicare Part B benefits cover most services and items typically not covered under Part A. Major classifications of Medicare Part B benefits are as follows:

1. Medical expenses incurred for physician services, outpatient diagnostic and therapeutic services including diagnostic procedures, and ambulatory surgery; medical supplies and equipment such as oxygen, hospital beds or walkers; medically necessary outpatient therapy includes physical, occupational and speech therapy.
2. Clinical laboratory services includes hematology (blood), chemistry (specimens from any source), and microbiology (cultures).
3. Home health care includes skilled nursing care, therapy, home health aide, medical social services, supplies, and durable medical equipment, when there is no Part A coverage available.
4. Outpatient hospital treatment includes diagnostic and therapeutic services.
5. Blood required is covered if medically necessary.

TABLE 12-1 Medicare (Part A): Hospital Insurance-Covered Services for 2010*

Services	Benefit	Medicare Pays	Patient Pays
Inpatient Hospitalization Semi-private room and board, general nursing, and miscellaneous hospital services and supplies. (Medicare payments based on benefit periods.) Includes hospitalization in a hospital, psychiatric, rehabilitation facility, or long-term care facility.	First 60 days	All but $1100	$1100 deductible
	61st to 90th day 91st to 150th day	All but $275 a day	$275 a day
	60-reserve-days benefit†	All but $550 a day	$550 a day
	Beyond 150 days	Nothing	All costs†
Skilled Nursing Facility Care Patient must have been in a hospital for at least 3 days and enter a Medicare-approved facility generally within 30 days after hospital discharge.‡ (Medicare payments based on benefit periods.)	First 20 days	100% of approved amount	Nothing
	21st to 100th day	All but $137.50 a day	Up to $137.50 a day
	Beyond 100 days	Nothing	All costs
Home Health Care Part-time or intermittent skilled care, home health aide services, durable medical equipment and supplies, and other services.	Unlimited as long as Medicare conditions are met and services are declared "medically necessary"	100% of approved amount; 80% of approved amount for durable medical equipment	Nothing for services; 20% of approved amount for durable medical equipment
Hospice Care Pain relief, symptom management, and support services for the terminally ill.	If patient elects the hospice option and as long as doctor certifies need	All but limited costs for outpatient drugs and inpatient respite care	Limited cost sharing for outpatient drugs and inpatient respite care
Blood	Unlimited if medically necessary	All but first 3 pints per calendar year	For first 3 pints

Data from Medicare and you, 2010, U.S. Government Printing Office.
*Managed care and Preferred Provider Organization benefits and patient responsibility amounts vary by plan.
†This 60-Reserve-Days benefit may be used only once in a lifetime.
‡Neither Medicare nor private Medigap insurance will pay for most long-term nursing home care.
§To the extent that the blood deductible is met under Part B of Medicare during the calendar year, it does not have to be met under Part A.

Medicare beneficiaries are required to pay a monthly premium, an annual deductible, and a co-payment or co-insurance amount as outlined in the Medicare Plan selected. The monthly premium for 2010 is $110.50. The annual deductible for 2010 is $155.00. Table 12-2 illustrates Medicare Part B covered services, amounts paid by Medicare, and the patient's responsibility for the major classifications of coverage.

Medicare Part C

Medicare Part C provides various health insurance plan options for Medicare beneficiaries to select from to meet their specific health care needs. The Medicare Advantage Plan option, formerly known as Medicare + Choice, was created under the Balanced Budget Act (BBA) of 1997. Plan options under Medicare Part C vary according to geographic area. Under the Medicare Advantage Plan a beneficiary selects one plan that provides Part A and B coverage. Beneficiaries may choose one of the following plan types: Medicare Managed Plan, Preferred Provider Organization (PPO) Plan, a Private Fee-For-Service Plan, or a Medicare Specialty Plan. Medicare Advantage Plans are offered by private health insurance companies. Medicare pays a set amount to the private insurance company on a monthly basis for care provided to the beneficiary. Medicare Advantage Plan options available may not be the same in all areas. Premiums, co-payment, and co-insurance amounts will vary according to the plan.

Medicare Part D

Medicare Part D provides various plan options for beneficiaries to obtain prescription drug coverage. Medicare Part D was created under the Medicare Prescription Drug Improvement Modernization Act (MMA), passed in 2003. Drug coverage under the prescription drug plans became available effective January 1, 2006.

TABLE 12-2 Medicare (Part B): Medical Insurance-Covered Services for 2010*

Services	Benefit	Medicare Pays	Patient Pays
Medical Expenses Doctor's services (not routine physical examinations), outpatient medical and surgical services and supplies, diagnostic tests, ambulatory surgery center facility fees for approved procedures, and durable medical equipment (such as wheelchairs, hospital beds, oxygen, and walkers). Also covers second surgical opinions, outpatient mental health care, and outpatient physical and occupationaltherapy, including speech-language therapy.	Unlimited if medically necessary	80% of approved amount (after $124 deductible); reduced to 50% for most outpatient mental health services	$155 deductible plus 20% of approved amount or limited charges
Clinical Laboratory Services Blood tests, urinalyses, and others.	Unlimited if medically necessary	100% of approved amount	Nothing for services
Home Health Care Part-time skilled nursing care, physical therapy, occupational therapy, speech-language therapy, home health aide services, medical social services, durable medical equipment (such as wheelchairs, hospital beds, oxygen, and walkers), medical supplies, and other services.	Unlimited as long as patient meets conditions and benefits are declared medically necessary	100% of approved amount; 80% of approved amount for durable medical equipment	Nothing for services; 20% of approved amount for durable medical equipment
Outpatient Hospital Treatment Services for the diagnosis or treatment of illness or injury.	Unlimited if medically necessary	Medicare payment to hospital based on hospital cost	$100 deductible, plus 20% of whatever the hospital charges
Blood	Unlimited if medically necessary	80% of approved amount	First 3 pints plus 20% of approved amounts for additional pints (after the deductible)

Data from Medicare and you, 2010, *U.S. Government Printing Office.*
*Managed care and Preferred Provider Organization benefits and patient responsibility amounts vary by plan.
Note: Medicare Part B monthly premium is $110.50

Medicare Part D
Prescription Drug Plans

The 2006 Medicare and You Handbook outlines the following information regarding Medicare Prescription Drug Coverage

When a beneficiary obtains Medicare prescription drug coverage, they pay part of the cost, and Medicare pays part of the cost. The beneficiary pays a premium each month to join the drug plan. If the beneficiary has Medicare Part B, the monthly Part B premium must also be paid by the beneficiary. If the beneficiary belongs to a Medicare Advantage Plan or Medicare Cost Plan, the monthly premium for that plan may increase if you add prescription drug coverage.

Costs

The cost of prescription drug plan coverage will vary depending on the plan selected. The plan must, at a minimum, provide the beneficiary with a standard level of coverage. Some plans offer more coverage or lower premiums. Drug plans generally require the beneficiary to pay a monthly premium, an annual deductible and a copayment or co-insurance amount.

- Monthly premiums vary depending on the plan selected. Premiums can range from $25.00 to $105.00.
- Yearly deductible is an amount that must be paid before the drug plan will pay. Deductibles can range from $0 to $300.00 per year.
- A copayment or co-insurance amount will be defined by the drug plan. The copayment amount can range from $1.00 to $100.00. The co-insurance percentage can range from 11% to 75% of the approved amount.

Figure 12-6 Medicare Part D prescription drug plan. *(Modified from Centers for Medicare & Medicaid Services:* Medicare & you, *Baltimore, 2010.)*

Medicare contracted with private insurance companies to provide drug coverage to Medicare beneficiaries. Coverage under prescription drug plans became available January 1, 2006. Enrollment in Medicare Part D is voluntary; however, a Medicare beneficiary can enroll in Medicare Part D only if he or she has Parts A and B. Figure 12-6 highlights information provided by Medicare regarding prescription Part D prescription drug coverage and cost. It is important to remember that benefits and cost will vary by plan.

Plan Options

Medicare Parts A, B, C, and D coverage is provided through various plan options from which beneficiaries may select. The plan options include traditional plans, managed care plans, specialty plans, and prescription drug plans. Plans offered are not the same in all areas. Medicare provides a listing of plans available within the area in the *Medicare & You* publications provided to beneficiaries. Plan options can also be found on the Medicare Web site: www.medicare.gov. State-specific *Medicare & You* handbooks are available at www.cms.hhs.gov/partnerships/ tools/materials/publications/state/default.asp.

Traditional Medicare

The traditional Medicare plan is a fee-for-service plan. The providers charge a fee for each service or item provided. The plan reimburses the provider based on a fee schedule amount set for each service or item or the appropriate Ambulatory Payment Classification (APC) or Medicare Severity Diagnosis Related Groups (MS-DRG) rate. Traditional Medicare plan members may seek health care from Medicare-approved providers of their choice. A **Medicare Summary Notice (MSN)** is a notice sent to the beneficiary that outlines the amount the beneficiary is responsible to pay. Beneficiaries under the traditional fee-for-service plan are responsible to pay a deductible and co-insurance. Traditional Medicare plans require the patient to pay a co-insurance amount of 20% of approved charges, and Medicare pays 80% of approved charges. Out-of-pocket costs are typically higher in the fee-for-service plan. Traditional Medicare is available to beneficiaries nationwide.

Box 12-6 ■ KEY POINTS

Medicare Plan Options

Medicare provides plan choices for the beneficiaries covered under the program. Plan choices include the following:

- Traditional Medicare
- Medicare Managed Care Plans
- Medicare Preferred Provider Organizations (PPO)
- Medicare private fee-for-service organizations
- Medicare specialty plans

Medicare Managed Care Plans

Managed care plans require the patient's care to be managed by a primary care physician (PCP). Care must be obtained from providers within the plan network. Specialty care requires a referral from the PCP. Figure 12-7 illustrates a sample referral form. Managed care plan provisions also contain preauthorization requirements for specified services. Figure 12-8 illustrates a sample preauthorization form. Managed care plans generally require the beneficiary to pay a co-payment, which is a specific dollar amount, for each service received, and some have deductible requirements. Medicare managed care plans offered vary by area. Managed care plan guidelines and rules vary according to plan.

Medicare Preferred Provider Organizations (PPO)

PPOs allow the beneficiary to obtain care from providers who are out-of-network. Referrals for specialty care are not required. Out-of-pocket costs are higher when

Dr. Alan Jones
(775) 643-2929

Referral Form

PATIENT NAME: John J. Smith

Physician referred to: Dr. Stephanie Tara

Referred for: Treatment of Cardiac Congenital condition
- ❑ Consult only
- ❑ Follow-up
- ❑ Lab
- ❑ X-ray
- ❑ Procedure
- ☑ Other

Reason for visit: consult confirmed congenital condition which requires treatment

Number of visits: as required

Appointment Scheduled: Please contact patient; phone: 776-447-8111

Referring Physician's Name: Alan Jones, M.D.

Referring Physician's Signature: Alan Jones, M.D.

Figure 12-7 Sample referral form.

ABC HEALTH PLAN
PREAUTHORIZATION REQUEST

AUTHORIZATION FOR:

❑ Hospitalization	______ Elective	__________ Emergency
❑ Surgery	______ Elective	__________ Emergency

Patient Name:	Date:
Address:	City, State, Zip:
___M ___F DOB:	(H) Phone:
Insured Name:	Employer name:
Hospital Name:	Hospital Provider #:
Admit Date:	Estimated Length of Stay:
Admitting DX:	Other DX:
Treatment Plan:	
Treatment Authorization requested: ______ Diagnostic _______Therapeutic ______ Surgical	
Principal Procedure	Other Procedure

ABC HEALTH PLAN **Authorized Personnel**

Approved_________ Not approved _________

Signature______________________________ Date _________

Authorization Number______________________

Comments:

Figure 12-8 Sample preauthorization form.

care is obtained from providers who are not in the plan network. The patient's responsibility generally consists of a deductible and a co-insurance amount. PPO plans generally pay a lower percentage for services provided by an out-of-network provider.

Medicare Private Fee-for-Service Plans

Private fee-for-service plans are offered by private companies. Under the private plan a beneficiary may seek care from any Medicare-approved provider. The provider must accept the fee-for-service plan terms regarding payment for services. The beneficiary is required to pay a premium to join the plan. The plan may also require a deductible and a co-insurance amount (20% of the approved charges) to be paid by the beneficiary.

Medicare Specialty Plans

Medicare specialty plans are offered under Medicare Part C. They were created by Medicare to provide more focused health care to specific people. Medicare beneficiaries can select one plan to cover all health care needs including special needs such as long-term health care.

Medigap Plans

Medicare beneficiaries who have traditional Medicare are required to pay annual deductible and co-insurance amounts. Additionally, the beneficiary may be responsible for services or items that are not covered under the Medicare plan. This causes a "gap" between what Medicare pays and amounts required by the beneficiary. Many individuals purchase a private insurance plan designed to cover the "gap" which pay amounts not paid by Medicare. These plans are known as Medigap plans or policies. A **Medigap plan** is a supplemental insurance plan purchased by a Medicare beneficiary to provide coverage for amounts not paid by Medicare such as non-covered services or items, the annual deductible and co-insurance amounts. The government regulates Medigap plans. Standards are set by the government regarding basic benefits required under Medigap policies. Ten standardized plans have been approved by the government, and they are designated plans A through J. The basic benefits required by the government are included in all of the plans as illustrated in Table 12-3. Additional optional benefits vary according to the plan.

Basic Benefits

- Hospital inpatient benefits
  Coverage of Part A co-insurance
  Coverage for the cost of 365 extra days of hospital care during a lifetime
- Medical benefits
  Coverage of Part B co-insurance
- Blood
  Coverage for the first 3 pints of blood each year

Additional Optional Benefits

- Skilled nursing facility co-insurance
- Part A deductible
- Part B deductible
- Part B excess charges
- Drug benefits
- Preventive medicine visits

Coordination of Benefits (COB)

A Medicare beneficiary may have coverage under another plan in addition to Medicare coverage. Federal regulations prohibit Medicare from paying as the primary payer when other payers are responsible. To ensure Medicare benefits are paid appropriately, legislation known as the Medicare Secondary Payer (MSP) Law was passed in 1980. MSP legislation outlines coverage circumstances in which Medicare is considered the secondary payer. Providers are required by law to know when it is appropriate to bill Medicare as the primary payer and when it is necessary to bill another insurer as the primary payer. Under MSP laws Medicare is considered secondary when care provided is the responsibility of another plan as outlined in Table 12-4.

Box 12-7 ■ KEY POINTS

Medigap Plans

A Medigap policy is a supplemental insurance plan purchased by a Medicare beneficiary to provide coverage for amounts not paid by Medicare, such as for non-covered services or items, annual deductibles, and co-insurance amounts.

Box 12-8 ■ KEY POINTS

Medicare Secondary Payer

To ensure Medicare benefits are paid appropriately, legislation known as the Medicare Secondary Payer (MSP) Law was passed in 1980. MSP legislation outlines coverage circumstances in which Medicare is considered the secondary payer. Providers are required by law to know when it is appropriate to bill Medicare as the primary payer.

- Automobile liability or no-fault insurance
- Other liability insurance such as personal injury protection (PIP), homeowners or business liability insurance
- Group health insurance
- Black lung program coverage
- Department of Veterans Affairs benefits
- TRICARE benefits
- Workers' compensation
- End-stage renal disease.

MEDICAID

Medicaid is a program designed to provide health care coverage for specified eligible needy individuals. Medicaid was implemented in 1965 under Title XIX of the Social Security Act. Medicaid is a jointly funded cooperative venture between the federal and state

TABLE 12-3 Ten Standardized Medigap Plans A-J: Basic and Additional Benefits Provided under Each Plan

A	B	C	D	E	F	G	H	I	J
Basic	Basic	Basic	Basic	Basic	Basic	Basic	Basic	Basic	Basic
Basic Benefits Inpatient hospital benefits: Part A co-insurance and the cost of 365 extra hospital days during lifetime. Medical benefits: Part B co-insurance Blood: first 3 pints of blood each year									
A	**B**	**C**	**D**	**E**	**F**	**G**	**H**	**I**	**J**
		Skilled nursing co-insurance	Skilled nursing co-insurance	Skilled nursing co-insurance	Skilled nursing co-insurance	Skilled nursing co-insurance	Skilled nursing co-insurance	Skilled nursing co-insurance	Skilled nursing co-insurance
	Part A deductible	Part A deductible	Part A deductible	Part A deductible	Part A deductible	Part A deductible	Part A deductible	Part A deductible	Part A deductible
		Part B deductible			Part B deductible				
					Part B excess (100%)	Part B excess (100%)		Part B excess (100%)	
		Foreign travel emergency	Foreign travel emergency	Foreign travel emergency	Foreign travel emergency	Foreign travel emergency	Foreign travel emergency	Foreign travel emergency	Foreign travel emergency
			At home recovery			At home recovery		At home recovery	
							Basic drug benefit ($1,250 limit)	Basic drug benefit ($1,250 limit)	
				Preventive care					

Data from Medicare and you, 2010, *U.S. Government Printing Office.*
Note: Additional benefits vary by plan.

TABLE 12-4 Medicare Secondary Payer Determination

Health Care Services	Other Insurance Coverage	Primary Coverage	Secondary Coverage
Automobile accident	Automobile liability insurance or no-fault insurance	Automobile insurance or no fault	Medicare (MSP)
Accident on property belonging to someone else	Homeowners or business liability insurance	Liability insurance	Medicare (MSP)
Illness or injury; elderly employee or spouse; age 65 or older	Employee group health plan (EGHP)	EGHP	Medicare (MSP)
Illness related to black lung disease; coal miner or former coal miner	Federal Black Lung Act (FECA); Workers' Compensation provisions	FECA	Medicare does not apply
Injury or illness that is service related	Department of Veterans Affairs	Department of Veterans Affairs	Medicare (MSP)
Injury or illness; active duty military or dependent of active duty service person	TRICARE	TRICARE	Medicare (MSP)
Injury or illness; retired military	TRICARE for Life	TRICARE for Life	Medicare (MSP)
Injury or illness occurring on the job	Workers' Compensation	Workers' Compensation	Medicare does not apply
End-stage renal disease; current or former employees	Employer group coverage	Employer group coverage	Medicare (MSP)
Disability (except end-stage renal disease); employee or dependent younger than age 65	Employer group coverage	Employer group coverage	Medicare (MSP)

governments to assist states in the provision of adequate medical care to eligible needy individuals. The federal government sets broad national guidelines followed by the states to administer the program. Medicaid programs vary by state because each state designs its own program and has the flexibility to do the following:

- Establish eligibility standards
- Determine the type, amount, duration, and scope of services
- Set the rate of payment for services provided within the program
- Administer its own program.

Box 12-9 ■ KEY POINTS

Medicaid

- Medicaid is a program designed to provide health care coverage for specified eligible needy individuals.
- Medicaid was implemented in 1965 under Title XIX of the Social Security Act. Medicaid is a jointly funded cooperative venture between the federal and state governments to assist states in the provision of adequate medical care to eligible needy individuals.

Administration

The Medicaid program is administered at the state level, under federal guidelines. CMS oversees the Medicaid program. The division within CMS that is chiefly responsible for oversight of the Medicaid program is the Center for Medicaid and State Operations.

The Center for Medicaid and State Operations

The focus of this division is federal-state programs such as Medicaid and the State Children's Health Insurance Program (SCHIP). This division serves as the focal point for all Agency interactions with states and local governments regarding these programs. The responsibilities of the Center for Medicaid and State Operations include the following:

- Development of national Medicaid policies and procedures
- Evaluation of state agencies
- Support for states relative to the use of standardized measures for provider feedback and quality improvement activities.

TEST YOUR *Knowledge* BOX 12-1

MEDICARE

1. Discuss when and why the Medicare program was created.

2. ______________ is a federally funded program implemented under Title XVIII of the SSA of 1965 to provide coverage for health care services to individuals who are ______________, are ______________, or have ______________.

3. Explain what agency is responsible for the administration of Medicare.

4. List two divisions within CMS, which administers Medicare, that are chiefly responsible for the Medicare program.

5. Discuss the role of Medicare Administrative Contractors (MAC) in the Medicare program.

6. Outline the eligibility requirements for the Medicare program.

7. List four parts of Medicare coverage.

8. Medicare Part A is designed to provide coverage for ______________.

9. Medicare Part B is designed to provide coverage for what type of care?

10. State the purpose of Medicare Advantage Plans.

11. What type of coverage is provided under Medicare Part D?

12. List six different plans types a Medicare beneficiary may have.

13. Provide an explanation of the difference in patient responsibility under traditional Medicare and Medicare managed care plans.

14. What is a Medigap plan?

15. Provide an explanation of how coordination of benefits (COB) relates to Medicare Secondary Payer Law.

Box 12-10 ■ KEY POINTS

CMS Division Medicaid Oversight

The Center for Medicaid and State Operations

The division under CMS that is chiefly responsible for oversight of the Medicaid program is the Center for Medicaid and State Operations. The focus of this division is on federal-state programs such as Medicaid and the State Children's Health Insurance Program (SCHIP). The division serves as the focal point for all Agency interactions with state and local governments regarding these programs.

Fiscal Agent (FA)

A **fiscal agent (FA)** is an insurance company or other entity that contracts with the government to handle functions related to enrollment and the processing of claims for the Medicaid program. FAs are commonly referred to as Medicaid contractors. The government contracts with various FAs throughout the United States. For example, the FA for Florida Medicaid is ACS State Healthcare, formerly known as Consultec, Inc.

Box 12-11 ■ KEY POINTS

Medicaid Fiscal Agents

- A fiscal agent (FA) is an insurance company or other entity contracted by the government to handle functions related to enrollment and the processing of claims for the Medicaid program
- Medicaid contractors are commonly referred to as fiscal agents (FA)

Box 12-12 ■ KEY POINTS

Medicaid Eligibility Categories

- **Categorically Needy**—Groups of individuals who are in need of Medicaid benefits, such as the aged, blind, or disabled or children and families who meet specific eligibility requirements
- **Medically Needy**—Individuals with high medical expenses and low income

Eligibility

Medicaid eligibility requirements vary by state. Federal statutes identify over 25 different eligibility categories for which federal funds are available. These groups are referred to as "categorically needy." **Categorically needy** is a term used to identify groups of individuals who are in need of Medicaid benefits, such as the aged, blind, or disabled or children and families who meet specific eligibility requirements. States have an option to extend the Medicaid program to include additional medically needy persons. **Medically needy** is a term used to describe individuals with high medical expenses and low income who meet specific eligibility requirement. The following is a list of mandatory Medicaid categorically needy or medically needy eligibility groups as illustrated in Figure 12-9.

- Families, pregnant women, and children; individuals who meet the requirements for the Aid to Families with Dependent Children (AFDC) program
- Non-AFDC pregnant women and children whose family income is below the poverty level
- Recipients of adoption or foster care assistance under Title IV of the Social Security Act
- Aged or disabled persons who qualify under the Supplemental Security Income (SSI) or Qualified Medicare Beneficiary (QMB) program
- Specially protected groups (medically needy low-income individuals)
- Low-income persons losing employer health insurance coverage (Medicaid purchase of COBRA coverage).

Medicaid Eligibility Groups

Categorically Needy

Families, pregnant women, and children
- Aid to Families with Dependent Children (AFDC)-related groups
- Non-ADFC pregnant women and children
- Recipients of adoption or foster care assistance under Title IV of the Social Security Act

Aged and disabled persons
- Supplemental Security Income (SSI-related groups)
- Qualified Medicare Beneficiaries (QMB)

Persons receiving institutional or other long-term care in nursing facilities (NFs) and intermediate care facilities (ICF)
- Medicaid beneficiaries
- Medi/Medi beneficiaries

Medically Needy

Medically needy low-income individuals and families
Low-income persons losing employer health insurance coverage

Figure 12-9 Categorically needy and medically needy groups eligible for Medicaid. *(Modified from Centers for Medicare & Medicaid Services: Medicaid Eligibility Groups, www.cms.hhs.gov)*

Coverage

Medicaid programs have flexibility in determining services covered under the program. The federal government mandates the basic services that must be provided in order to receive federal matching funds.

Medicaid Services	
Mandatory Basic Service	Optional Services

• Hospital services (inpatient and outpatient)
• Prenatal care
• Physician services
• Nursing facility services for persons aged 21 or older
• Family planning services and supplies
• Rural health clinic services
• Home health care for persons eligible for skilled-nursing services
• Laboratory and X-ray services
• Pediatric and family nurse practitioner services including
  • Nurse-midwife services
  • Federally qualified health-center (FQHC) services and ambulatory services of an FQHC that would be available in other settings
  • Early and periodic screening, diagnostic, and treatment (EPSDT) services for children under age 21 and vaccines for children
	• Diagnostic services
	• Clinic services
	• Intermediate care facilities for the mentally retarded (ICFs/MR)
	• Prescribed drugs and prosthetic devices
	• Optometrist services and eyeglasses
	• Nursing facility services for children under age 21
	• Transportation services
	• Rehabilitation and physical therapy services
	• Home and community-based care to certain persons with chronic impairments

Figure 12-10 Services that Medicaid programs are mandated to provide and those that are optional. *(Modified from Centers for Medicare & Medicaid Services: Medicaid Services, www.cms.hhs.gov)*

Mandatory Basic Services

As outlined in Figure 12-10 the following are mandatory services that must be provided by Medicaid programs:

- Hospital services (inpatient and outpatient)
- Prenatal care
- Physician services
- Nursing facility services for persons aged 21 or older
- Family planning services and supplies
- Rural health clinic services
- Home health care for persons eligible for skilled nursing services
- Laboratory and x-ray services
- Pediatric and family nurse practitioner services
- Nurse-midwife services
- Federally qualified health center (FQHC) services, and ambulatory services of an FQHC that would be available in other settings
- Early and periodic screening, diagnostic, and treatment (EPSDT) services for children under age 21, and vaccines for children.

Optional Services

States may also receive federal matching funds if they provide certain optional services. The following list includes some of the most common optional Medicaid services:

- Diagnostic services
- Clinic services
- Intermediate care facilities for the mentally retarded
- Prescribed drugs and prosthetic devices
- Optometrist services and eyeglasses
- Nursing facility services for children under age 21
- Transportation services
- Rehabilitation and physical therapy services
- Home and community-based care to certain persons with chronic impairments.

Box 12-13 ■ KEY POINTS

Medicaid Coverage and Plan Options

Mandatory Basic Services

The federal government mandates the basic services such as hospital, physician, and laboratory services that must be provided in order for federal matching funds to be received.

Optional Services

States may also receive matching funds for the provision of certain optional services.

Medicaid Plan Options

- Plans offered by Medicaid vary by state. Many states maintain the traditional fee-for-service Medicaid.
- Most states encourage Medicaid beneficiaries to enroll in a managed care plan. Managed care plan options for Medicaid beneficiaries also vary by state.

Plan Options

Plan options offered under Medicaid programs vary by state. Many states maintain the traditional fee-for-service Medicaid. Most states encourage Medicaid beneficiaries to enroll in a managed care plan. Managed care plan options for Medicaid beneficiaries also vary by state.

Coordination of Benefits (COB)

Medicaid is considered the payer of last resort. When a Medicaid beneficiary has coverage under another plan such as Medicare, Medicaid is the secondary payer.

STATE CHILDREN'S HEALTH INSURANCE PROGRAM (SCHIP)

The **State Children's Health Insurance Program (SCHIP)** is a program designed to provide health care coverage for uninsured children up to the age of 19. The program is also referred to as the Children's Health

Insurance Program (CHIP). SCHIP was implemented as part of the BBA of 1997. Under this program, states can receive grants to implement a program or expand their existing Medicaid program to provide coverage to eligible uninsured children for health care costs. The federal government sets broad national guidelines followed by the states to design and administer the program. The government offers states three options when designing a program. The states can do one of the following:

- Use SCHIP funds to expand Medicaid eligibility to children who previously did not qualify for the program
- Design a separate children's health insurance program entirely separate from Medicaid
- Combine both the Medicaid and separate program options.

Administration

The SCHIP program is administered at the state level, under federal guidelines. CMS oversees the program in cooperation with the Health Resources Services Administration. The division within CMS that is chiefly responsible for oversight of the Medicaid and the SCHIP program is the Center for Medicaid and State Operations. Information on SCHIP by state can be located on the CMS Web site: http://www.cms.hhs.gov.

Eligibility

SCHIP programs are administered at the state level, and therefore they have flexibility in setting eligibility requirements within guidelines set by the federal government. Figure 12-11 outlines federal eligibility and coverage requirements for SCHIP programs. In accordance with federal guidelines, SCHIP programs are required to provide health insurance coverage to uninsured children who meet the following basic eligibility requirements:

- Not eligible for Medicaid
- Under the age of 19
- Family income level not exceeding 200% of the federal poverty level

In addition to the basic eligibility requirements, the following requirements also must be met:

- Not covered under another insurance plan or program
- Has not had group insurance coverage in the past 3 months
- Other requirements applied by the State.

Coverage

Because the SCHIP program is administered at the state level, each state has the flexibility to set coverage guidelines; however, in accordance with federal law, SCHIP programs must provide coverage for basic services such as the following:

- Doctor's visits
- Immunizations
- Emergency room visits
- Hospitalizations

State Children's Health Insurance Program (SCHIP)

Eligibility Requirements

Federal eligibility requirements

- Children not eligible for Medicaid
- Children under the age of 19
- Children whose family income level cannot be greater than 200% of the federal poverty level

In addition to the basic eligibility requirements outlined above the following requirements must also be met

- Not covered under another insurance plan or program
- Has not had group insurance coverage in the past three months
- Other requirements may apply according to the state

Basic Coverage

SCHIP programs are required to provide coverage for the following basic services as mandated by federal law

- Doctor's visits
- Immunizations
- Emergency room visits
- Hospitalizations

Figure 12-11 Eligibility requirements and basic services that SCHIP programs are required to provide. *(Modified from Centers for Medicare & Medicaid Services:* SCHIP Eligibility, *www.cms.hhs.gov)*

TRICARE

TRICARE is a federally funded health insurance program designed to provide coverage for health care services provided to military personnel and their families. TRICARE was formerly known as the Civilian Health and Medical Program of the Uniformed Services (CHAMPUS). In 1994 the Department of Defense changed the program name and introduced a three-tier program called TRICARE. TRICARE is a regionally managed health care program that brings together the health care resources of the armed services and supplements them with networks of civilian health care professionals to provide better access to high-quality service while maintaining the capability to support the military operation.

Administration

Tasks and responsibilities required for the administration of the TRICARE program are defined by the Department of Defense as **field activities.** The Department of Defense creates agencies to conduct field activities, various tasks and responsibilities required for the

TEST YOUR *Knowledge* BOX 12-2

MEDICAID AND THE STATE CHILDREN'S HEALTH INSURANCE PROGRAM (SCHIP)

1. Discuss why the Medicaid program was created and its purpose.
2. Provide an explanation of the relationship between the state and federal government as it relates to Medicaid.
3. Explain what federal agency is responsible for the oversight of the Medicaid program.
4. State the division within the federal oversight agency that is chiefly responsible for the Medicaid program.
5. Discuss the role of fiscal agents within the Medicaid program.
6. Outline two eligibility categories defined in Medicaid eligibility requirements.
7. Medicaid eligibility requirements define ____________ ____________ as groups of individuals in need of Medicaid benefits, such as aged, blind, or disabled individuals or children and families who meet specific eligibility requirements.
8. Individuals with high medical expenses and low income who meet specific Medicaid eligibility requirements fall into the ____________ ____________ eligibility category.
9. Explain the flexibility that states have in determining what services to cover under their Medicaid programs.
10. Discuss the type of plans offered under the Medicaid program.
11. Discuss the purpose of the SCHIP program.
12. Provide an explanation of the relationship between the state and federal government as it relates to the SCHIP program.
13. Explain what federal agency is responsible for the oversight of the SCHIP program.
14. Outline the federal basic eligibility requirements for the SCHIP program.
15. List examples of services covered under the SCHIP program.

operation of the Department of Defense. The Department of Defense created a field activity agency called **TRICARE Management Activity (TMA)** to oversee the TRICARE program. The organizational structure of the Department of Defense field activity agencies, including TMA, is outlined in Figure 12-12. The Department of Defense TMA is responsible for the management of all financial aspects of the Department's medical and dental programs and the execution of policy issued by the Assistant Secretary of Defense in the administration of the Department's medical and dental programs.

Regional Contractors

Regional contractors are insurance companies or other entities that contract with TRICARE to handle the functions related to enrollment and filing claims for TRICARE. Regional contractors are also known as TRICARE contractors. TMA awarded contracts to the following companies in three regions referred to as TRICARE North, South, and West:

- TRICARE South—Regional contractor is Humana Military Healthcare Services
- TRICARE North—Regional contractor is Health Net Federal Services
- TRICARE West—Regional contractor is TriWest Healthcare Alliance Corp.

Box 12-14 ■ KEY POINTS

TRICARE

Formerly known as CHAMPUS, TRICARE is a federally funded health insurance program designed to provide coverage for health care services provided to military personnel and their families.

- TRICARE Management Activity (TMA) is responsible for oversight of TRICARE.
- TMA awards contracts to TRICARE contractors for three regions: TRICARE South, North, and West.
- Eligibility is determined using the Defense Enrollment Eligibility Reporting System.

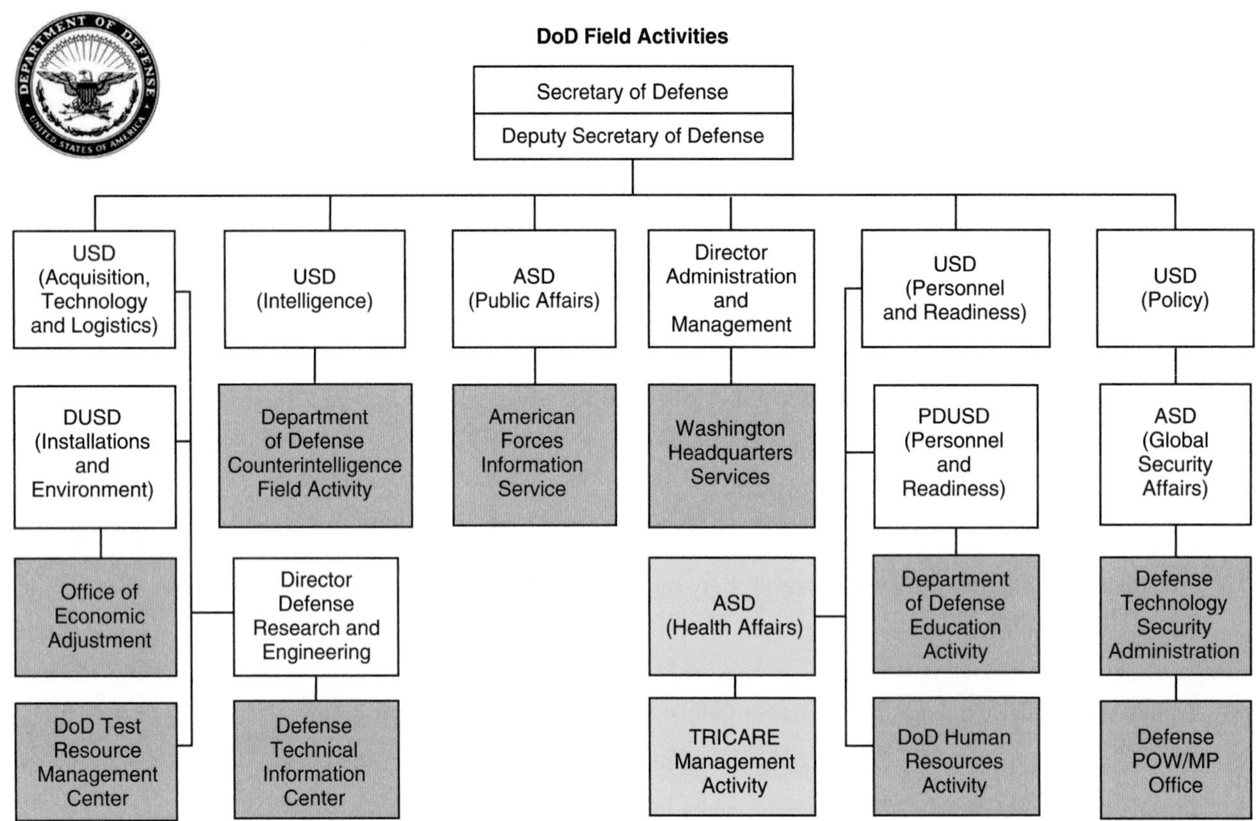

Figure 12-12 TRICARE Department of Defense organizational chart. *(Modified from U.S. Department of Defense:* Defense Agencies, *http://odam.defense.gov/omp/pubs/GuideBook/pdf/FldAct.pdf, 2010.)*

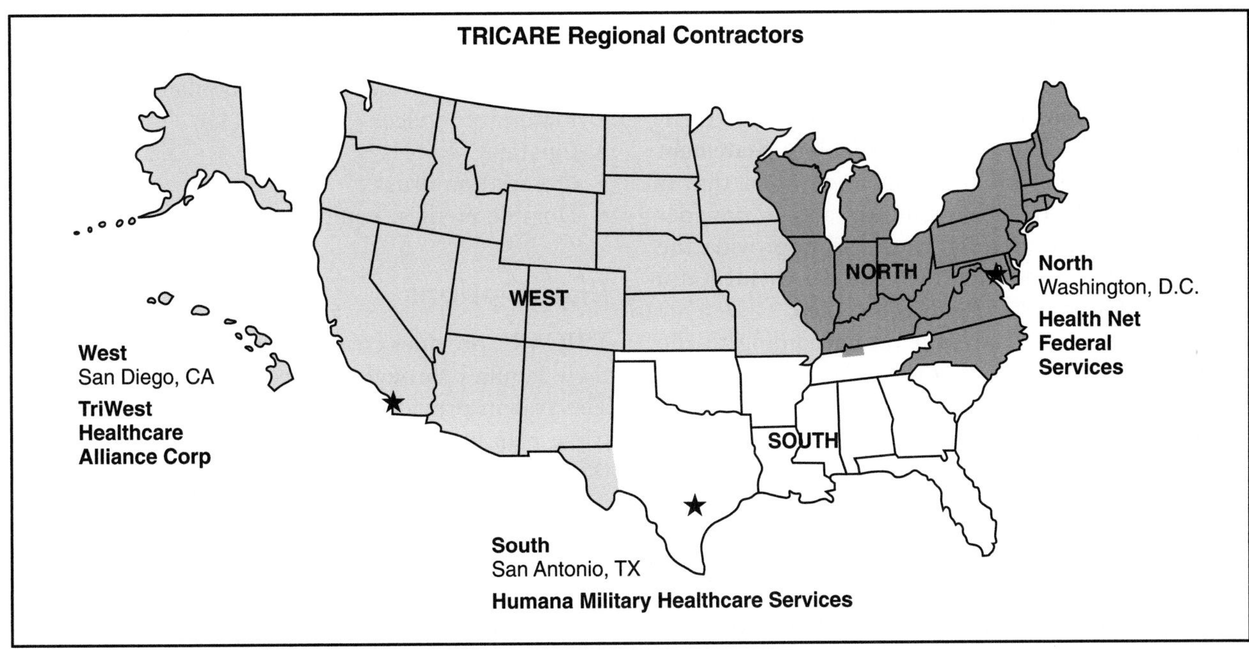

Figure 12-13 TMA awarded contracts to the companies illustrated in three regions referred to a TRICARE North, South, and West. *(Data from TRICARE, www.tricare.osd.mil, 2005.)*

The three TRICARE regions and the company awarded the contract by TMA for each region are illustrated in Figure 12-13. Regional contractors perform functions related to enrollment and claims processing, including the provision of information to beneficiaries regarding enrollment, network providers, and the claims process.

Eligibility

The **Defense Enrollment Eligibility Reporting System (DEERS)** is the system utilized by TRICARE to determine eligibility and maintain enrollment records. An individual's record on the DEERS system outlines the date of eligibility. Enrollment is conducted through personnel offices of the uniformed services. Updates to enrollment are also processed through personnel offices. The member of the military that obtains individual or family coverage is referred to as a "sponsor." Sponsors are required to ensure that information on the DEERS system regarding spouses, dependents, and address is current. Individuals eligible for TRICARE fall into one of several beneficiary categories:

- Active and retired members of the military, including Army, Navy, Marine Corps, Coast Guard, Reserve, and National Guard personnel
- Active and retired members' spouses and unmarried children (to age 21 or to age 23 if child is a full-time student)
- Reserve members when on active duty
- Reserve members' spouse and children (to age 21 or to age 23 if child is a full-time student)
- Retired members of the reserve and their spouses and children
- Deceased members' widows and children (to age 21 or to age 23 if child is a full-time student)
- Members of the military who have received a Medal of Honor and their family members
- Active or retired members' former spouses when eligible.

Box 12-15 ■ KEY POINTS

TRICARE Eligibility Categories

- Active and retired members of the military
- Active and retired members' spouses and unmarried children
- Reserve members when on active duty
- Reserve members' spouses and children
- Retired members of the reserves and their spouses and children
- Deceased members' widows and children
- Members of the military who have received a Medal of Honor and their family members
- Active or retired members' former spouses when eligible

Coverage

The TRICARE health care system provides coverage for health care services based on the plan selected by the member. Services are obtained at a Military Treatment Facility (MTF) or at other TRICARE-approved provider locations. Most of the care provided to TRICARE beneficiaries is provided at a **Military Treatment Facility (MTF)**. If the MTF is unable to provide inpatient care that is required, the member may obtain care at a civilian hospital by obtaining a Non-Availability Statement (NAS) (Figure 12-14). A **Non-Availability Statement** (NAS) is obtained from the military hospital that is unable to provide the care required and it provides certification that the hospital is unable to provide the care. TRICARE will not pay for services provided at a civilian hospital unless an NAS is obtained.

Health care services covered vary according to the plan and may include the following:

- Physician services
- Preventive services, including annual examinations, immunizations, and screening examinations
- Diagnostic and therapeutic services, including radiology, pathology, and laboratory services
- Outpatient services such as ambulatory surgery
- Maternity services
- Inpatient services
- Prescription drugs
- Durable medical equipment.

Plan Options

TRICARE provides coverage for military personnel and their families through a three-tier health care system. The system provides three plan options, referred to as triple plan options. Under this system, members select the plan that meets their needs. The plan options are

NONAVAILABILITY STATEMENT DEPENDENTS MEDICAL CARE PROGRAM

(AR 40-121, SECNAV INST 6320.8A, AFR 160-41, PHS GEN CIR NO 6)

(This Statement is issued for your immediate use)

THE ISSUANCE OF THIS STATEMENT MEANS:

1. The medical care requested is not available to you at a Uniformed Services facility in this area.
2. If you receive medical care from civilian sources and such care is determined to be authorized care under the Medicare Program, it will be paid for by the Government to the extent that the program permits.
3. If you receive medical care from civilian sources and it is determined that all or part of the care is not authorized under the Medicare Program, THE GOVERNMENT WILL NOT PAY for the unauthorized care.

The determination of whether medical care you may receive from civilian sources is authorized for payment cannot be made at this time because this determination depends, among other things, upon the care you actually receive. Further, no statement regarding your condition or diagnosis made hereon will be considered in any way determinative as to whether care rendered for such condition is payable under the Medicare Program.

The use of this statement is subject to the conditions and limitations set forth in the regulation issued under the Dependents' Medical Care Act as codified in 10 U.S.C. 1071–1085.

This form must be presented with your Uniformed Services Identification and Privilege Card (DD Form 1173), identified below, when you obtain civilian medical care.

DEPENDENT, SPOUSE OR CHILD, RESIDING WITH SPONSOR

DEPENDENT'S LAST NAME-FIRST NAME-MIDDLE INITIAL	UNIFORMED SERVICES IDENTIFICATION AND PRIVILEGE CARD (DD FORM 1173) CARD NUMBER: PREFIX	NUMERICAL	SUFFIX	EXPIRATION DATE
DOE, MARY B.	EU	18352	A	20XX JUNE 15

DEPENDENT'S ADDRESS (Complete mailing address)

503 CORN DRIVE, WOODLAND HILLS, XY 12345-0002

SPONSOR MEMBER OF UNIFORMED SERVICES ON ACTIVE DUTY

SPONSOR'S LAST NAME-FIRST NAME-MIDDLE INITIAL: DOE, JOHN B.

SERVICE NUMBER: 000-00-0001 GRADE OR RANK: LT/03

BRANCH OF SERVICE: ☐ ARMY ☒ NAVY ☐ AIR FORCE ☐ MARINE CORPS ☐ PUBLIC HEALTH ☐ COAST GUARD ☐ COAST & GEODETIC SURVEY

ORGANIZATION AND OFFICIAL DUTY STATION: POINT MUGU NAVAL STATION, POINT MUGU, CALIFORNIA

REMARKS

STATION AT WHICH PERMIT ISSUED: POINT MUGU NAVAL STATION, POINT MUGU, CALIFORNIA DATE ISSUED: 20XX MAY 12

GRADE OR RANK AND POSITION OF ISSUING OFFICER: COMMANDING OFFICER LT CMDR SIGNATURE OF ISSUING OFFICER: George M. Plates

DISTRIBUTION *(Three signed copies of this statement will be furnished the dependent for distribution as follows):* DEPENDENT *(Original Copy)* ATTENDING PHYSICIAN *(Duplicate copy)* CIVILIAN MEDICAL FACILITY *(Triplicate copy)*

Figure 12-14 TRICARE Non-Availability Statement. *(From Fordney MT:* Insurance handbook for the medical office, *ed 9, St Louis, 2005, Elsevier.)*

TRICARE Prime, TRICARE Extra, and TRICARE Standard.

TRICARE Prime

TRICARE Prime is a Health Maintenance Organization (HMO) type of plan that provides health care services that are managed by a Primary Care Manager (PCM). A PCM is assigned to each plan member for the purpose of managing and coordinating all health care services required by the member. TRICARE Prime members are not required to pay annual enrollment fees. TRICARE Prime requires co-payment amounts to be paid by the beneficiary for specified services. Table 12-5 outlines TRICARE Prime benefits and beneficiary costs for the outpatient and inpatient services and prescription drugs as follows:

Outpatient Services

Covered services obtained on an outpatient basis include physician services, ancillary (radiology, laboratory, and cardiac) services, immunizations, ambulatory surgery, eye examinations, emergency department services, outpatient behavioral health services, ambulance services, home health care, family health care, and durable medical equipment.

Inpatient Services

Hospitalization is covered, including maternity care, skilled nursing care, mental illness hospitalization, substance abuse treatment, partial hospitalization, and hospice care.

Prescription Drugs

Coverage and cost for prescriptions is determined by where the prescription is obtained: from a military facility, by mail order, or from a non-network pharmacy.

TRICARE Extra

TRICARE Extra is a Preferred Provider Organization (PPO) type of plan that has provisions for members to

TABLE 12-5 TRICARE Prime

TRICARE PRIME		
BENEFIT AND COVERAGE CHART		
ADFM = active duty family members	*RFMS = retirees, family members and survivors*	
ENROLLMENT OR DEDUCTIBLE	**ADFM**	**RFMS**
Annual Enrollment Fee* (per fiscal year)	$0	$230 *individual*/$460 *family*
Annual Deductible	$0 (except when using Point-of-Service option)	
OUTPATIENT BENEFITS AND BENEFICIARY COST		
Outpatient benefits include: Physician Services, Ancillary Services (certain radiology, laboratory, & cardiac services), Immunizations (for required overseas travel), Ambulatory Surgery (same day) and Eye Examinations. Costs outlined below are for care provided in civilian facilities.		
Outpatient Visits	$0	$12
Clinical Preventive Services	$0	$0
Durable Medical Equipment, Prosthetics, Orthotics and Supplies	$0	20% of negotiated fee
Emergency Services	$0	$30 co-pay per visit
Outpatient Behavioral Health	$0	$25 *(individual visit)*, $17 *(group visit)*
INPATIENT BENEFITS AND BENEFICIARY COST		
	ADFM	**RFMS**
Inpatient Hospitalization *(one or two days)* Inpatient Hospitalization *(more than two days)*	$0 $0	$25 *for the stay* $11 *per day*
Inpatient Hospitalization *at a Military Treatment Facility*	$0	$16.30 *per day for retiree family members*
Inpatient Skilled Nursing Care	$0	$11 *per day ($25 minimum charge)*
Inpatient Behavioral Health	$0	$40 *per day*

Data from US Department of Defense, http://www.tricare.mil/mybenefits/download/forms/bene_cost_br_unliked.pdf

obtain health care services from providers within the TRICARE network of approved civilian providers. Members of TRICARE Extra are required to pay an annual deductible ranging from $150 to $300 for family coverage, determined based on the member's military status. Co-insurance and co-payment amounts are required for specified services. Table 12-6 outlines TRICARE Extra benefits and beneficiary costs for the outpatient and inpatient services.

Outpatient Services

Covered services obtained on an outpatient basis include emergency services, physician services, ancillary (radiology, laboratory, and cardiac) services, outpatient behavioral health care, ambulance services, home health care, family health care, limited eye examinations, and ambulatory surgery services. TRICARE Extra also provides coverage for durable medical equipment.

Inpatient Services

Coverage includes hospitalization, including maternity care, skilled nursing care, mental illness hospitalization, substance abuse treatment, partial hospitalization, and hospice care.

Prescription Drugs

Coverage and cost for prescriptions is determined by where the prescription is obtained: from a military

TABLE 12-6 TRICARE Extra

TRICARE EXTRA		
BENEFIT AND COVERAGE CHART		
ADFM = active duty family members	*RFMS = retirees, family members and survivors*	
ENROLLMENT/DEDUCTIBLE	**ADFM**	**RFMS**
Annual Enrollment Fee *(per fiscal year)*	$0	$230 *individual*/$460 *family*
Annual Outpatient Deductible	Rank E4 *and below* $50 *individual*/$100 *family* Rank E5 *and above* $150 *individual*/$300 *family*	$150 *individual*/$300 *family*
OUTPATIENT BENEFITS AND BENEFICIARY COST		
Outpatient benefits include: Physician Services, Ancillary Services (certain radiology, laboratory, & cardiac services), Immunizations (for required overseas travel), Ambulatory Surgery (same day) and Eye Examinations. Costs outlined below are for care provided in civilian facilities.		
Outpatient Visits	15% *after annual deductible is met*	20% *after annual deductible is met*
Clinical Preventive Services	15% *after annual deductible is met*	20% *after annual deductible is met*
Durable Medical Equipment, Prosthetics, Orthotics and Supplies	15% *after annual deductible is met*	20% *after annual deductible is met*
Emergency Services	15% *after annual deductible is met*	20% *after annual deductible is met*
Outpatient Behavioral Health	15% *after annual deductible is met*	20% *after annual deductible is met*
INPATIENT BENEFITS AND BENEFICIARY COST		
	ADFM	**RFMS**
Inpatient Hospitalization	$16.30 per day *($25 minimum charge)*	$250 *per day or 25% of billed charges for institutional services, whichever is less,* **plus** 20% cost-share for separately billed services
Inpatient Behavioral Health	$20 per day *($25 minimum charge)*	20% of the total charge, **plus** 20% cost-share for separately billed services
Inpatient Skilled Nursing Care	$16.30 per day *($25 minimum charge)*	$250 *per day or 20% of billed charges for institutional services, whichever is less,* **plus** 20% cost-share for separately billed services

Data from US Department of Defense, Tricare Management Activity, http://www.tricare.mil/mybenefits/download/form/bene_cost_br_unliked.pdf

facility, by mail order, or from a non-network pharmacy.

TRICARE Standard

TRICARE Standard is the traditional fee-for-service CHAMPUS plan. Members under the TRICARE Standard plan may elect to obtain care from civilian doctors or at a MTF. Members are required to pay an annual deductible ranging from $50 to $300 for family coverage. TRICARE Standard members are required to pay co-payment and co-insurance amounts for specified services. Table 12-7 outlines TRICARE Standard benefits and beneficiary costs for the outpatient and inpatient services and prescription drugs as outlined below:

Outpatient Services

Covered services obtained on an outpatient basis include emergency services, physician services, ancillary (radiology, laboratory, and cardiac) services, outpatient behavioral health care, ambulance services, home health care, family health care, limited eye examinations, and ambulatory surgery services. TRICARE Standard also provides coverage for durable medical equipment.

Inpatient Services

Coverage includes hospitalization, maternity care, skilled nursing care, mental illness hospitalization, substance abuse treatment, partial hospitalization, and hospice care.

TABLE 12-7 **TRICARE Standard**

TRICARE STANDARD		
BENEFIT AND COVERAGE CHART		
ADFM = active duty family members	*RFMS = retirees, family members and survivors*	
ENROLLMENT/DEDUCTIBLE	**ADFM**	**RFMS**
Annual Enrollment Fee *(per fiscal year)*	$0	$230 *individual*/$460 *family*
Annual Outpatient Deductible	Rank E4 *and below* $50 *individual*/$100 *family* Rank E5 *and above* $150 *individual*/$300 *family*	$150 *individual*/$300 *family*
OUTPATIENT BENEFITS AND BENEFICIARY COST		
Outpatient benefits include: Physician Services, Ancillary Services (certain radiology, laboratory, & cardiac services), Immunizations (for required overseas travel), Ambulatory Surgery (same day) and Eye Examinations. Costs outlined below are for care provided in civilian facilities.		
Outpatient Visits	20% *after annual deductible is met*	25% *after annual deductible is met*
Clinical Preventive Services	20% *after annual deductible is met*	25% *after annual deductible is met*
Durable Medical Equipment, Prosthetics, Orthotics and Supplies	20% *after annual deductible is met*	25% *after annual deductible is met*
Emergency Services	20% *after annual deductible is met*	25% *after annual deductible is met*
Outpatient Behavioral Health	20% *after annual deductible is met*	25% *after annual deductible is met*
INPATIENT BENEFITS AND BENEFICIARY COST		
	ADFM	**RFMS**
Inpatient Hospitalization	$16.30 per day *($25 minimum charge)*	$535 *per day or 25% of billed charges for institutional services, whichever is less,* **plus** 25% cost-share for separately billed services
Inpatient Behavioral Health	$20 per day *($25 minimum charge)*	25% *of hospital-specific per diem (high-volume hospital) or* $197 *per day or 25% of billed charges for institutional services, whichever is less*
Inpatient Skilled Nursing Care	$16.30 per day *($25 minimum charge)*	25% of the allowed charges for institutional services, **plus** 25% cost-share for separately billed services

Data from US Department of Defense, Tricare Management Activity, http://www.tricare.mil/mybenefits/download/form/bene_cost_br_unliked.pdf

Prescription Drugs

Coverage and cost for prescriptions is determined by where the prescription is obtained: from a military facility, by mail order, or from a non-network pharmacy.

Box 12-16 ■ KEY POINTS

TRICARE Plan Options

TRICARE Prime

TRICARE Prime is a Health Maintenance Organization (HMO) type of plan that provides health care services that are managed by a Primary Care Manager (PCM).

TRICARE Extra

TRICARE Extra is a Preferred Provider Organization (PPO) type of plan that has provisions for members to obtain health care services from providers within the TRICARE network of approved civilian providers.

TRICARE Standard

The traditional fee-for-service CHAMPUS plan. Members under the TRICARE Standard plan may elect to obtain care from civilian doctors or at a Military Treatment Facility.

Coordination of Benefits (COB)

Coordination of benefits provisions outline circumstances in which TRICARE is secondary to other health care programs as follows:

Other Third-Party Liability

Injury or illness treated is the result of an automobile accident or personal injury where another third-party payer is liable, such as an auto insurance or personal injury policy.

Workers' Compensation

Injury or illness treated is work related. The Workers' Compensation carrier is required to pay benefits to cover health care services required.

Medicare Beneficiary

Medicare is considered primary to TRICARE for Life (TFL).

Other TRICARE Programs

In addition to the triple option plans, TRICARE offers additional programs designed to provide coverage under specific circumstances. Additional programs include: TRICARE Remote, TRICARE for Life (TFL) and CHAMPVA.

TRICARE Remote Program

The **TRICARE Remote** Program is designed to provide health care services to active duty members who work and live more than a specified distance from an MTF. The required distance for this program is more than 50 miles or 1 hour away. The program allows members to obtain care from civilian providers.

TRICARE for Life (TFL)

TRICARE for Life (TFL) offers expanded medical coverage for military retirees and veterans who have attained the age of 65, are Medicare eligible, and have purchased Medicare Part B. TFL is a permanent health care benefit, and it provides coverage that is secondary to Medicare.

CHAMPVA Program

The **Civilian Health and Medical Program of the Veterans Administration (CHAMPVA)** is designed to provide benefits for health care services provided to the spouse and children of a veteran with a permanent, total disability that is service connected or a veteran who is deceased as a result of a disability that is service connected.

Box 12-17 ■ KEY POINTS

Other TRICARE Programs

- TRICARE Remote Program
- TRICARE for Life (TFL)
- Civilian Health and Medical Program of the Veterans Administration (CHAMPVA)

PARTICIPATING PROVIDER AGREEMENT

Providers who elect to participate with various government programs enter into a written agreement with each program. The provider agreement outlines the terms and specifications for participation in the plan. Reimbursement for services provided to program members is contingent on the provider's compliance with plan terms and specifications. It is critical for hospital personnel involved in the billing process to have an understanding of the terms in the provider agreement to ensure compliance with program specifications and to optimize reimbursement.

A **participating provider** is a physician, hospital, or other entity that enters into a contract with an insurance company or a government program to provide health care services to the plans members. The provider agreement is a legal contract between the plan and the provider. It outlines the terms of participating with the payer. Terms in the participating provider agreement relate to provision of service, medical necessity, utilization management and billing requirements, patient financial responsibility, and reimbursement. Figure 12-15 illustrates provisions in a participating provider agreement.

Box 12-18 ■ KEY POINTS

Participating Provider Agreement Provisions

- Provision of service
- Medical necessity
- Utilization management
- Patient financial responsibility
- Reimbursement
- Billing requirements

Provision of Service

The participating provider agreement outlines the services that will be provided to program members. Details regarding how and where services are provided are also included. The provider is required to meet all the plan specifications. The program agrees to list the provider in provider directories and other marketing material so program members know the facility is a participating provider.

Medical Necessity

Providers are statutorily obligated to provide services to patients that are medically necessary. All payers have

Participating Provider Agreement

This Agreement is entered into by and between **Community Hospital,** contracting on behalf of itself, **ABC Health Insurance, Inc.** and the other entities that are ABC Affiliates (collectively referred to as "ABC") and Community ("Hospital").

This Agreement is effective on the later of the following dates (the "Effective Date"):
i) December 31, 2006 or the first day of the first calendar month that begins at least thirty days after the date when this Agreement has been executed by all parties. Through contracts with physicians and other providers of health care services, ABC maintains one or more networks of providers that are available to Customers. Hospital is a provider of health care services. ABC wishes to arrange to make Hospital's services available to Customers. Hospital wishes to provide such services, under the terms and conditions set forth in this Agreement. The parties therefore enter into this Agreement.

Article I. Definitions

The following terms when used in this Agreement have the meanings set forth below:

1.1 "Benefit Plan" means a certificate of coverage or summary plan description, under which a Payer is obligated to provide coverage of Covered Services for a Customer.

1.2 "Covered Service" is a health care service or product for which a Customer is entitled to receive coverage from a Payer, pursuant to the terms of the Customer's Benefit Plan with that Payer.

1.3 "Customary Charge" is the fee for health care services charged by Hospital that does not exceed the fee Hospitals would ordinarily charge another person regardless of whether the person is a Customer.

1.4 "Customer" is a person eligible and enrolled to receive coverage from a Payer for Covered Services.

1.5 "Hospital" is duly licensed and qualified under the laws of the jurisdiction in which Covered Services are provided, who practices as a shareholder, partner, or employee of Hospital, or who practices as a subcontractor of Hospital.

Article II. Representations and Warranties

2.1 Representations and Warranties of Hospital. Hospital, by virtue of its execution and delivery of this Agreement, represents and warrants as follows:

(a) Hospital is a duly organized and validly existing legal entity in good standing under the laws of its jurisdiction of organization.

(b) Hospital has all requisite corporate power and authority to conduct its business as presently conducted, and to execute, deliver and perform its obligations under this Agreement.

(c) The execution, delivery and performance of this Agreement acknowledges the **Hospital does not and will not violate or conflict with** (i) the organizational documents of Hospital, (ii) any material agreement or instrument to which Hospital is a party or by which Hospital or any material part of its property is bound, or (iii) **applicable law.**

(d) Hospital has reviewed the Protocols and Payment Policies and acknowledges it is bound by the Protocols and that claims under this Agreement will be paid in accordance with the Payment Policies.

(f) **Each submission of a claim** by Hospital pursuant to this Agreement shall be deemed to constitute the representation and warranty by it to ABC that (i) the representations and warranties of it set forth in this section 2.1 and elsewhere in this Agreement are true and correct as of the date the claim is submitted, (ii) it has complied with the requirements of this Agreement with respect to the Covered Services involved and the submission of such claim, (iii) the charge amount set forth on the claim is the Customary Charge and (iv) the claim is a valid claim.

Article III. Applicability of this Agreement

3.1 Hospital's Services. This Agreement applies to services that are medically necessary and reasonable to diagnose and treat customer's condition.

3.2 Services not covered under a Benefit Plan. This Agreement does not apply to services not covered under the applicable Benefit Plan. Hospital may seek and collect payment from a Customer for such services, provided that the Hospital first obtains the Customer's written consent. This section does not authorize Hospital to bill or collect from Customers for Covered Services for which claims are denied or otherwise not paid. That issue is addressed in section 7 of this Agreement.

–1–

A

Figure 12-15 A, Sample Participating Provider Agreement. Page 1, illustrating terms and specifications for participating in the plan.

Participating Provider Agreement

3.4 Health Care. Hospital acknowledges that this Agreement does not dictate the health care provided by Hospital or Hospital Professionals, or govern Hospital's or Hospital Professionals' determination of what care to provide their patients, even if those patients are Customers. The decision regarding what care is to be provided remains with Hospital and Hospital Professionals and with Customers, and not with ABC or any Payer. Hospital will not allow coverage decisions to determine or influence treatment decisions.

Article V. Duties of Hospital

5.1 Provide Covered Services. Hospital will provide Covered Services that are considered Medically Necessary to Customers at the location specified in section 3.1.

5.2 Cooperation with Protocols. Hospital will cooperate with and be bound by ABC's and Payers' Protocols. The Protocols include but are not limited to all of the following:

1. Hospital will use reasonable commercial efforts to direct Customers only to other providers that participate in ABC's network, except as otherwise authorized by ABC or Payer.
2. Hospital will follow Utilization Management protocols and provide notification for certain Covered Services as defined by ABC or Payer, including the following requirements:
   (a) Provide notification, as further described in the Protocols, prior to a scheduled inpatient admission of a Customer, by telephone, at least five (5) business days prior to the admission; in cases in which the admission is scheduled less than five business days in advance, Hospital will give notice at the time the admission is scheduled.
   (b) With regard to the inpatient admission of a Customer, provide notification, as further described in the Protocols, no later than the next business day, by telephone, if a Customer is admitted on an emergency basis or for observation.
   (c) Obtain required authorizations and certifications and authorizations as outlined in Appendix B.
3. Hospital will obtain customer consent to release Medical Record information.
4. Hospital will follow ABC protocols and fulfill responsibility for the collection of deductible, co-payment or co-insurance amounts outlined in Appendix C as the Customer's responsibility

Article VII. Submission, Processing and Payment of Claims

7.1 Form and content of claims. Hospital must submit claims for Covered Services in a manner and format prescribed by ABC, as further described in the Protocols. Unless otherwise directed by ABC, Hospital shall submit claims using current CMS-1500 or CMS-1450 (UB-04) forms, whichever is appropriate, with applicable coding including, but not limited to, ICD, CPT, Revenue and HCPCS coding. Hospital shall comply with all claim form completion guidelines as outlined in Appendix C.

7.2 Electronic filing of claims. Within six months after the Effective Date of this Agreement, Hospital will use electronic submission for all of its claims under this Agreement that ABC is able to accept electronically.

7.3 Time to file claims. All information necessary to process a claim must be received by ABC no more than 90 days from the date that Covered Services are rendered. Payment to the hospital may be denied if the Hospital does not comply with Timely Filing Protocols in Appendix D and does not file a timely claim.

7.4 Denial of Claims. Hospitals may appeal claim denials in accordance with Protocols outlined in Appendix E.

7.5 Reimbursement - Payment of claims. ABC will pay claims for Covered Services according to the lesser of, the Hospital's Customary Charge or the applicable fee schedule, as provided in Appendix F. Payment determinations are subject to the Payment Policies, and minus any co-payment, deductible, or coinsurance as applicable under the Customer's Benefit Plan. The obligation for payment under this Agreement is solely that of ABC.

7.6 Timely payment. In accordance with provisions in this Agreement and legal statutes, ABC is obligated to process claims and remit payment or explanation of non-payment within 30 days of the date the claim is received.

–2–

B

Figure 12-15, *cont'd* **B,** Sample Participating Provider Agreement. Page 2, illustrating terms and specifications for participating in the plan.

TEST YOUR *Knowledge* BOX 12-3

TRICARE

1. State the purpose of the government-sponsored health insurance program TRICARE.

2. Explain what organization was created by the Department of Defense to oversee the TRICARE program.

3. Discuss the role of Regional Contractors within the TRICARE program, and list the regions.

4. Explain the purpose of the Defense Enrollment Eligibility Reporting System (DEERS).

5. Provide a brief outline of TRICARE beneficiary categories for eligibility.

6. State the purpose and role of Military Treatment Facilities (MTF).

7. What is a Non-Availability Statement, and when is it used?

8. List three triple option plans offered under the TRICARE program.

9. ______________ ______________ is an HMO type of plan that provides health care services that are managed by a ______________.

10. ______________ ______________ is a PPO type of plan that has provisions for members to obtain health care services within the network of TRICARE-approved civilian providers.

11. What triple option plan is the traditional fee-for-service CHAMPUS Plan?

12. In accordance with coordination-of-benefits provisions, TRICARE is secondary to ______________, ______________, and ______________.

13. Provide a brief explanation of TRICARE Remote.

14. Provide a brief explanation of TRICARE for Life.

15. CHAMPVA is designed to provide benefits for ______________.

medical necessity guidelines that must be met as a condition for receiving payment for those services. Medically necessary services are those that are considered reasonable and medically necessary to address the patient's condition based on standards of medical practice. Interpretations of medical necessity based on standards of medical practice vary by payer.

National Coverage Determination (NCD)

Payers develop coverage policies that outline conditions that will meet medical necessity guidelines to ensure payment is made only for services that are medically necessary. Medicare coverage policies developed by CMS are referred to as national coverage determinations. A **national coverage determination (NCD)** describes coverage policies and outlines condition(s) that meet medical necessity standards for specified service(s) reported. National coverage policies are found in the *Medicare National Coverage Determinations Manual.* CMS also provides access to the national coverage database, which can be searched for coverage decisions on specific services. The Internet address for the national coverage database is http://cms.hhs.gov/coverage/. Figure 12-16 illustrates the NCD for ambulatory EEG monitoring.

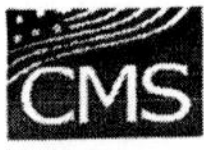

Centers for Medicare & Medicaid Services

Medicare Coverage Database

NCD for Ambulatory EEG Monitoring (160.22)

Publication Number
100-3

Manual Section Number
160.22

Version Number
1

Effective Date of this Version
6/12/1984

Benefit Category
Diagnostic Tests (other)

Note: This may not be an exhaustive list of all applicable Medicare benefit categories for this item or service.

Coverage Topic
Diagnostic Tests, X-rays, and Lab Services

Item/Service Description
Ambulatory, or 24-hour electroencephalographic (EEG) monitoring is accomplished by a cassette recorder that continuously records brain wave patterns during 24 hours of a patient's routine daily activities and sleep. The monitoring equipment consists of an electrode set, preamplifiers, and a cassette recorder. The electrodes attach to the scalp, and their leads are connected to a recorder, usually worn on a belt.

Indications and Limitations of Coverage
Ambulatory EEG monitoring is a diagnostic procedure for patients in whom a seizure diathesis is suspected but not defined by history, physical or resting EEG. Ambulatory EEG can be utilized in the differential diagnosis of syncope and transient ischemic attacks if not elucidated by conventional studies. Ambulatory EEG should always be preceded by a resting EEG.

Ambulatory EEG monitoring is considered an established technique and covered under Medicare for the above purposes.

Figure 12-16 National coverage determinations (NCDs). Illustrates coverage criteria from the Medicare NCD database for ambulatory EEG monitoring. *(Modified from Centers for Medicare & Medicaid Services:* Medicare Coverage Databases, *www.cms.gov)*

Local Coverage Determination (LCD)

MACs are required to incorporate and use national coverage policies when processing claims. **Local coverage determinations (LCD)**, formerly referred to as Local Medical Review Policies (LMRP), are developed by MAC to provide guidance and enhance understanding of coverage guidelines. LCD outline criteria for coverage of services along with information regarding coding and billing for services. Figure 12-17 illustrates an LCD for nail debridement, CPT code 11720.

Box 12-19 ■ KEY POINTS

Coverage Determinations

Coverage determinations describe coverage policies relating to medical necessity and billing and coding for services.

- **National coverage determination (NCD)**—developed by the Centers for Medicare and Medicaid Services (CMS)
- **Local coverage determination (LCD)**—developed by Local Medicare Administrative Contractors to provide guidelines and further define NCDs

Utilization Management

Utilization management involves monitoring and managing health care resources for the purpose of controlling costs and ensuring that high-quality care is provided. Utilization management may also be referred to as utilization review or quality improvement. The Utilization Management or Quality Improvement department within each facility performs utilization management functions internally. Government programs such as Medicare, Medicaid, and TRICARE also have implemented utilization management plans that include reviews of services rendered to determine appropriateness and necessity of those services. In accordance with the participating provider agreement, providers are required to follow all program utilization management requirements outlined by each payer. Government programs hire various organizations to conduct utilization reviews to ensure that guidelines are met and also to ensure that payment is made for services that are considered medically necessary. Reviews conducted by these organizations can be conducted prospectively, concurrently, or retrospectively.

- Prospective reviews are those conducted before services are rendered.
- Concurrent reviews are those conducted during the rendering of service.
- Retrospective reviews are those that are conducted after services are rendered.

Local Coverage Determination Implementation

11720: Nail Debridement

This local coverage determination is being developed to define coverage for nail debridement of all symptomatic mycotic nails.

Medicare will consider the treatment of fungal (mycotic) infection of the nails a covered service when the medical record substantiates:

- Clinical evidence of mycosis of the nail, by generally accepted clinical findings such as discoloration, onycholysis, subungual debris, thickening, or secondary skin infection;

One of the following must be documented for mycotic toenails:

- The ambulatory patient has marked limitation of ambulation, pain, or secondary infection resulting from the thickening and dystrophy of the infected nail plate(s) or;
- The non-ambulatory patient suffers from pain, or secondary infection resulting from the thickening and dystrophy of the infected nail plate(s).

In addition to the above, use of appropriate anti-fungal treatment or the contraindication of such treatment, must also be documented, to qualify nail debridement as a medically necessary and reimbursable service.

The following CPT codes are included in this policy:

- 11720 Debridement of nail(s) by any method(s); one to five
- 11721 Debridement of nail(s) by any method(s); six or more

The following ICD-9 codes that support medical necessity are listed in this policy:

- 110.1 Dermatophytosis of nail (Onychomycosis)
- 112.3 Candidiasis of skin and nails
- 117.0–117.9 Other mycoses

Patients need not have an underlying systemic condition to be covered for mycotic nail care. For treatment of non-symptomatic mycotic nails, refer to the Routine Foot Care policy.

The full-text of this LCD is available on our provider education website at *http://www.statemedicare.com.* This policy is effective for services rendered on or after January 1, 2005.

Figure 12-17 Local coverage determinations (LCD) coverage detail for nail debridement. *(Example from U.S. Department of Health and Human Services, Centers for Medicare and Medicaid Services.)*

Utilization management activities vary according to the third-party payer. Medicare, Medicaid, and TRICARE utilization management activities are outlined in the following sections.

Box 12-20 ■ KEY POINTS

Utilization Review

Three types of utilization reviews are:

- Prospective reviews—conducted before services are rendered.
- Concurrent reviews—conducted during the rendering of service.
- Retrospective reviews—that are conducted after services are rendered.

Utilization Management—Medicare and Medicaid

CMS contracts with an organization referred to as a **Quality Improvement Organization (QIO)** that conducts utilization and quality control reviews of health care services provided to Medicare and Medicaid members. QIO was formerly referred to as a Peer Review Organization (PRO). Some of the duties and responsibilities of the QIO are as follows:

- Identify violations of the provider agreement involving the provision of health care services and items
- Make recommendations to the Office of the Inspector General (OIG) if it is found that a provider is not meeting its obligations under the participating agreement
- Monitor claim activity in relation to hospital-issued notices of non-covered services
- Review suspicious or questionable procedures that are not covered
- Notify providers of violations to the provider's statutory obligations.

Utilization Management—TRICARE

The Department of Defense's Utilization Management Policy for services provided to TRICARE members is developed and maintained at the Regional Contractor level. The director of the Regional Contractor office has flexibility to develop utilization management processes. Goals of the Department of Defense's Utilization Management Policy are to:

- Maximize appropriate care
- Minimize and eliminate inappropriate care, which includes underutilization and overutilization
- Limit annual medical inflation

The objectives of the plans are to minimize and eliminate:

- Inappropriate level of care
- Inappropriate admissions
- Inappropriate stays
- Inappropriate procedures
- Inappropriate discharges.

Utilization review criteria incorporate program requirements regarding referrals and authorizations required for specific services. As outlined in the participating provider agreement, providers are required to obtain necessary referrals, authorizations, or precertifications as specified by the plan.

Patient Financial Responsibility

Participating provider agreements include information regarding the patient's financial responsibility under the plan. All health care plans require the patient to pay some portion of the charges for services rendered. Based on the plan the patient's responsibility amount may represent a deductible, co-insurance, or co-payment amount. The agreement further specifies the participating provider's contractual obligation to collect the deductible, co-insurance, and co-payment amount from the patient and the consequences if the provider does not make every attempt to collect the patient's share.

Reimbursement

Reimbursement for covered services will vary according to the plan. The participating provider agreement includes information about the reimbursement methods that will be used to calculate payment for covered services.

Billing Requirements

Billing requirements are outlined in each participating provider agreement. Billing requirements vary according to plan. Most plans outline provisions in the participating provider agreement regarding documentation, coding, claim forms, timely filing, and the appeals process, as discussed in the next section of this chapter.

REIMBURSEMENT METHODS

Health insurance plans use various reimbursement methods to determine payment for services rendered to plan members. As outlined in previous chapters, reimbursement methods can be categorized as traditional, fixed payment, and Prospective Payment System (PPS) methods, as outlined in Table 12-8. Reimbursement methods used vary by payer. Traditional fee-for-service plans use methods that base payment on a percentage of charges submitted for each service. Managed care plan reimbursements are generally predetermined, fixed payments. Government programs use reimbursement methods implemented under the PPS. PPS will be discussed in the next chapter.

Box 12-21 ■ KEY POINTS

Prospective Payment Systems (PPS)

- Resource Based Relative Value Scales (RBRVS)
- Ambulatory Payment Classifications (APC)
- Medicare Severity Diagnosis Related Groups (MS-DRG)

BILLING REQUIREMENTS

Basic Principles

Billing requirements vary according to program and plan. The participating provider agreement requires provider compliance with all billing specifications. Billing specifications are outlined in a provider manual that is given to the provider when the participating agreement is approved. The purpose of the billing process is to obtain reimbursement for services ren-

TABLE 12-8 Reimbursement Methods

Methods	Outpatient, Professional, and Non-Patient Services	Ambulatory Surgery Services	Inpatient Services
Traditional Methods Traditional plans, Blue Cross/Blue Shield, Aetna, and Humana	Fee-for-service (FFS); fee schedule; usual, customary, and reasonable (USR); relative value scale (RVU)	Fee-for-service (FFS), case rate, contract rate, percentage of accrued charges	Fee-for-service (FFS), percentage of accrued charges, per diem, flat rate, case rate, contract rate
Fixed-Payment Methods: Managed care plans	Capitation, fee schedule, contract, discounted fee	Case rate, contract rate, capitation, discounted fee	Case rate, contract rate
Prospective Payment Methods: Government plans and other third-party payers.	Resource-based relative value scale (RBRVS)	Ambulatory Payment Classification (APC)	Medicare Severity Diagnosis Related Groups (MS-DRG)
Implemented under Prospective Payment System (PPS)			

Data from U.S. Department of Defense, TRICARE Management Activity.

TEST YOUR *Knowledge* BOX 12-4

PARTICIPATING PROVIDER AGREEMENT

1. Outline why it is important for hospital personnel to understand the terms of the participating provider agreement.
2. Define participating provider.
3. A provider agreement is a ______________ ______________ between the provider and the plan.
4. Providers are ______________ ______________ to provide services to patients that are ______________ ______________.
5. What are national coverage determinations (NCD) and what payer develops them?
6. Explain the difference between national coverage determination and local coverage determination.
7. Discuss the purpose of utilization management and what it involves.
8. CMS contracts with an organization referred to as a ______________ ______________ ______________ to perform utilization management activities.
9. TRICARE utilization management policies are developed and maintained at the ______________ ______________ level.
10. The participating provider agreement includes information about the ______________ ______________ that will be used to ______________ ______________ for covered services.

dered. The billing process involves collection of pertinent billing information, documentation of services and patient conditions, preparation of claims, and collection of outstanding accounts (Figure 12-18). A patient registration form is used to collect patient demographic, financial, and insurance information (Figure 12-19). Collection of information includes obtaining insurance information for all plans of which the patient is a member. A copy of the patient's insurance card (front and back) is obtained for each plan. Figure 12-20 illustrates sample cards for Medicare, Medicaid, and TRICARE. Charges for services are submitted to payers via claim forms. The CMS-1500 and CMS-1450 (UB-04) claim forms are used according to payer requirements. The data collected and prepared during the patient visit are recorded on the claim form for submission to payers. Reimbursement is determined based on the information submitted on the claim. Payer requirements for completion and submission of claims vary by payer. It is critical for hospital billing and coding professionals to understand billing requirements to ensure compliance with those requirements and obtain accurate reimbursement. A review of the various payer specifications for billing is beyond the scope of this text. As discussed in previous chapters, basic principles of billing can be reviewed and applied for all payers. Some of the basic principles are documentation, coding, claim forms, timely filing, and the appeals process.

Hospital Billing Process

Admission
Registration
Admitting department

Patient care
Order entry
Ancillary/clinical departments

Charge capture
Charge Description Master (CDM) – HCPCS Codes
Department personnel

Chart reviewing/coding
Post discharge procedures
Health Information Management (HIM)

Charge submission
Patient invoice/ statement
PFS

Reimbursement
Post transactions
Patient Financial Services (PFS)

Payer review
Payment determination
Third-party payers

Charge submission
Claims process
Claim preparation (scrubber)
Patient Financial Services (PFS)

Reimbursement
Paid
PFS

Reimbursement
Denied
PFS–Collections

Claim submission
CMS-1500
CMS-1450 (UB-04)
manual/electronic
Patient Financial Services (PFS)

A/R Management
Monitor and follow-up on outstanding claims
PFS–Credit and collections

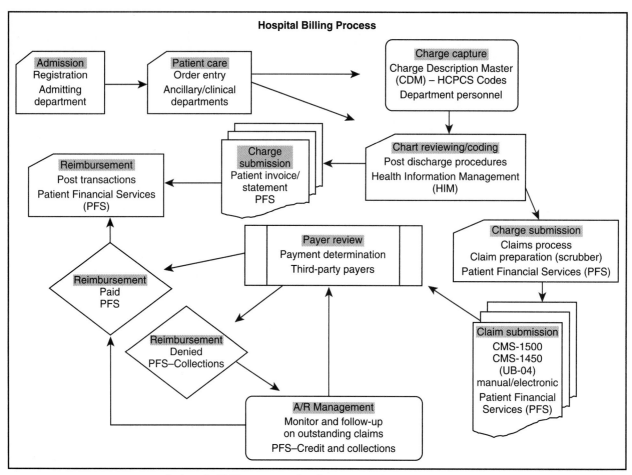

Figure 12-18 The hospital billing process: key functions and the primary departments involved in performing those functions. *(Revision of illustration courtesy Sandra Giangreco.)*

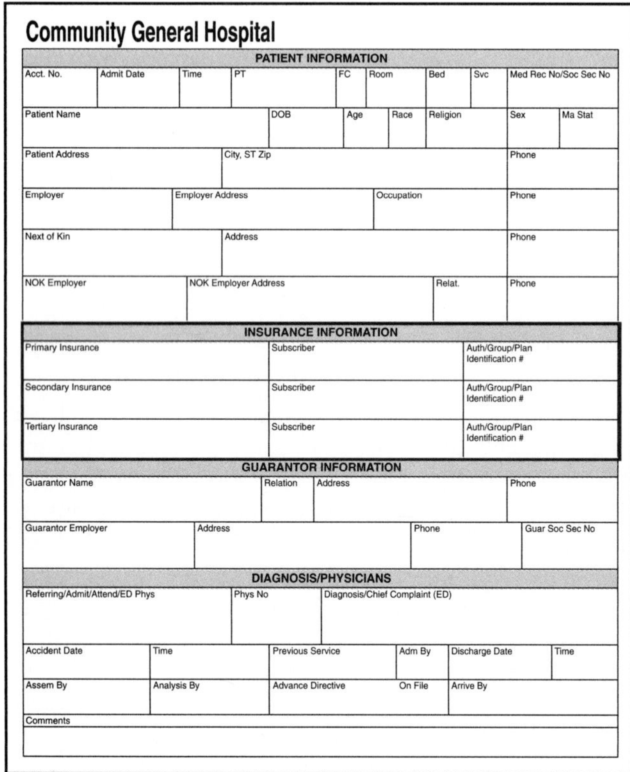

Community General Hospital

PATIENT INFORMATION								
Acct. No.	Admit Date	Time	PT	FC	Room	Bed	Svc	Med Rec No/Soc Sec No
Patient Name	DOB	Age	Race	Religion	Sex	Ma Stat		
Patient Address	City, ST Zip	Phone						
Employer	Employer Address	Occupation	Phone					
Next of Kin	Address	Phone						
NOK Employer	NOK Employer Address	Relat.	Phone					
INSURANCE INFORMATION								
Primary Insurance	Subscriber	Auth/Group/Plan Identification #						
Secondary Insurance	Subscriber	Auth/Group/Plan Identification #						
Tertiary Insurance	Subscriber	Auth/Group/Plan Identification #						
GUARANTOR INFORMATION								
Guarantor Name	Relation	Address	Phone					
Guarantor Employer	Address	Phone	Guar Soc Sec No					
DIAGNOSIS/PHYSICIANS								
Referring/Admit/Attend/ED Phys	Phys No	Diagnosis/Chief Complaint (ED)						
Accident Date	Time	Previous Service	Adm By	Discharge Date	Time			
Assem By	Analysis By	Advance Directive	On File	Arrive By				
Comments								

Figure 12-19 Sample patient registration form.

Medicare

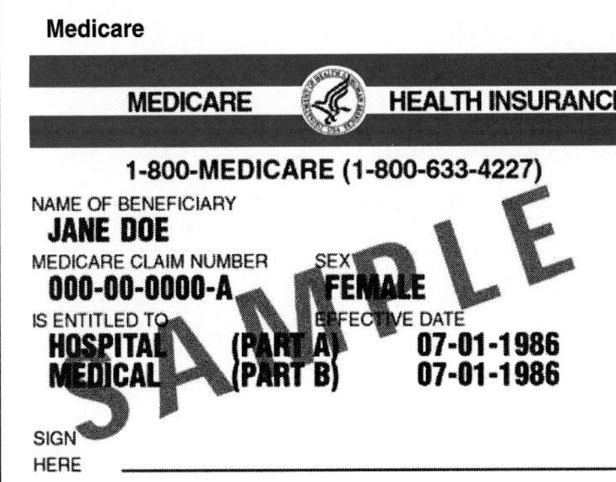

MEDICARE HEALTH INSURANCE

1-800-MEDICARE (1-800-633-4227)

NAME OF BENEFICIARY
JANE DOE

MEDICARE CLAIM NUMBER SEX
000-00-0000-A FEMALE

IS ENTITLED TO EFFECTIVE DATE
HOSPITAL (PART A) 07-01-1986
MEDICAL (PART B) 07-01-1986

SIGN HERE

SAMPLE

1. Carry your card with you when you are away from home.
2. Let your hospital or doctor see your card when you require hospital, medical, or health services under Medicare.
3. Your card is good wherever you live in the United States.

WARNING: Issued only for the use of the named beneficiary. Intentional misuse of this card is unlawful and will make the offender liable to penalty.

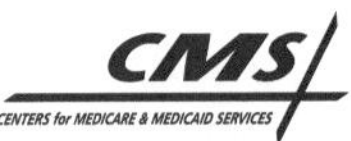

Centers for Medicare and Medicaid Services
Baltimore, MD 21244

If you have questions about Medicare, call 1-800-MEDICARE (1-800-633-4227) TTY/TDD: 1-877-486-2048 or visit us at www.medicare.gov.

Tricare

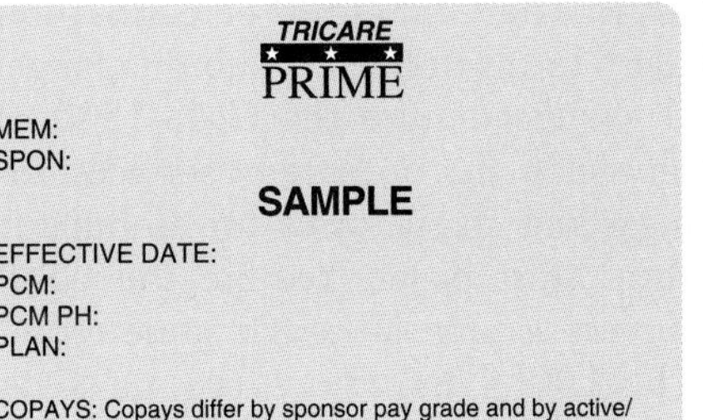

TRICARE PRIME

MEM:
SPON:

SAMPLE

EFFECTIVE DATE:
PCM:
PCM PH:
PLAN:

COPAYS: Copays differ by sponsor pay grade and by active/retired status. See Member Handbook or Provider Manual.

TRICARE PRIME PROVIDERS: This care is for identification only. Call the local Health Care Finder for Prime eligibility verification and certification of care. To determine applicable copayments see your Provider Manual.

COPAYMENTS: Copayments are required for most covered services. Refer to the TRICARE Prime Member Handbook for specific copayment information.

OUT-OF-AREA/EMERGENCY PROVIDERS: Call 1-800-242-6788

TRICARE PRIME MEMBERS: The Primary Care Manager (PCM) shown on the front of this card is responsible for all health care services. Referral by the Primary Care Manager and authorization by the Health Care Finder is required for all specialty care and hospitalization before services are rendered.

SAMPLE

If you have an emergency at any time which is life threatening, go directly to the nearest hospital. If emergency hospitalization is required, contact your Primary Care Manager or your Health Care Finder by the first working day after admission.

IF YOU MOVE: Please notify the Beneficiary Services Representative at or near your local Military Hospital or Clinic.

Medicaid

Expiration Date	Start Date	MISSOURI MEDICAID CARD	Pay Co.	Caseload No.
04-04-92	03-01-92		050	001

Recipient's Name	Birthdate S/R	Medicaid Number	Program Restriction	MEDI-CARE	Pharmacy Limit
	06-91 FW	2222222	A B	EPSDT MEDICAL	12345

B

COVERAGE	EXPLANATION
A	All available benefits (co-payment not required)
B	All available benefits (co-payment is required) for specified services
C	Client is eligible for outpatient care only, must reach spenddown for inpatient care
X	Client is eligible only for inpatient care, emergency room, and clinic services
Z	Limited benefits as explained in the shaded area on the face of this card

Figure 12-20 Sample insurance identification cards (Medicare, Medicaid, and TRICARE). *(Modified from Fordney MT:* Insurance handbook for the medical office, *ed 9, St Louis, 2005, Elsevier, and Adams WL:* Adams' coding and reimbursement: a simplified approach, *ed 2, St Louis, 2005, Elsevier.)*

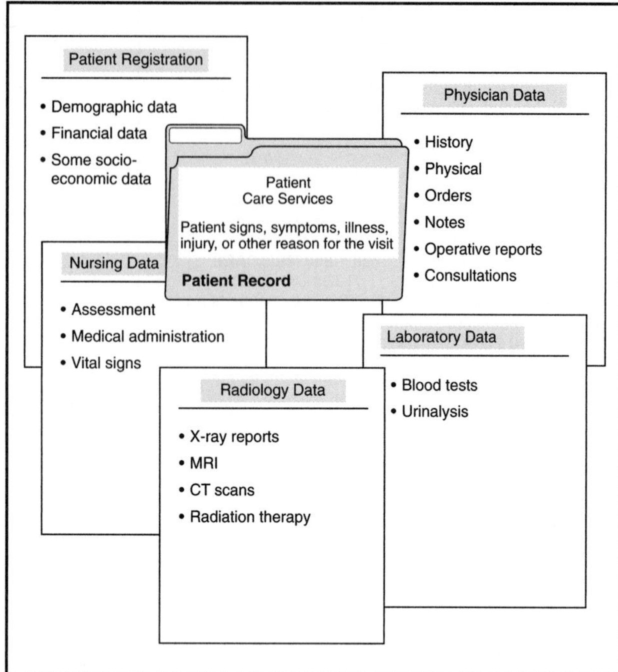

Figure 12-21 Patient medical record. *(Modified from Davis N, LaCour M:* Introduction to health information technology, *ed 1, St Louis, 2002, Saunders.)*

Documentation

Documentation of all patient conditions and services is required during a patient visit. The documentation of the patient visit supports and explains to the payer the services provided and the reasons for them. Documentation is not submitted with every claim; however, the payer may request documentation after initial review of the claim. It is critical for hospital billing and coding personnel to understand that services and conditions that are not documented should not be coded (Figure 12-21).

Coding

Coding is the process of translating written descriptions of conditions and services in the patient's record into codes. Submission of claims requires codes to describe the services provided and the patient conditions that were treated. There are variations in the coding systems used by payers. Each payer defines the coding systems required for describing patient conditions and services. The coding system used for reporting patient conditions is the International Classification of Diseases, 9th Revision, Clinical Modification (ICD-9-CM). Coding services can be performed using HCPCS Level I CPT, Level II Medicare National, or ICD-9-CM Volume III procedure codes. Coding systems requirements also vary for outpatient and inpatient services. Figure 12-22 provides an overview of coding system requirements for professional, outpatient and inpatient services.

Box 12-22 ■ KEY POINTS

Coding Systems

Patient Conditions

ICD-9-CM Volume I and II

Procedures

HCPCS Level I CPT and Level II Medicare National codes

ICD-9-CM Volume III

Claim Forms

Claim forms are used to submit charges to payers for reimbursement. Claim form requirements vary by payer. The CMS-1500 or CMS-1450 (UB-04) are two claim forms utilized to submit charges to payers. Almost all payers require the CMS-1500, (Figure 12-23), for physician and outpatient services. Payer's requirements regarding claim forms for ambulatory surgery services vary. Most payers require the UB-04 for ambulatory surgery claims, although some require the CMS-1500. The UB-04 is required by most payers for inpatient services provided by hospitals, skilled nursing facilities, and rehabilitation centers (Figure 12-24).

Claim form completion requirements and instructions vary by payer. Payer requirements outline what information should be required in certain fields. They also outline what fields are required. Payers define the method of claim submission. Some payers require that claims be submitted electronically, and some allow submission of paper claims. It is important for hospital personnel to understand variations in claim form instructions and submission requirements as outlined in Chapter 10. An understanding of payer requirements helps to ensure compliance with payer specifications and to optimize reimbursement.

Box 12-23 ■ KEY POINTS

Claim Forms

CMS-1500

Used to submit charges for physician and outpatient services

CMS-1450 (UB-04)

Used to submit facility charges for hospital services provided on outpatient, non-patient, and inpatient bases

Timely Filing

All payers require claims to be submitted within a specific period after services are provided. Timely filing requirements outline the time frame for submission of claims (Table 12-9). If a claim is not submitted within the timely filing period defined by the payer, reimbursement will not be made for those services.

Coding System Variations		
Professional Services	**Outpatient Services**	**Inpatient Services**
Report physician and outpatient services, procedures, and items using HCPCS Level I CPT and Level II National codes	Report facility charges for outpatient services, procedures, and items using HCPCS Level I CPT and Level II National codes	Report facility charges for inpatient services, procedures, and items using HCPCS Level I CPT and II National codes
Report procedure codes on CMS-1500 in block 24A-K	Report procedure codes on CMS-1450 (UB-04) in FL 44	Report procedure codes on CMS-1450 (UB-04) in FL 44 and FL 74a-e
Report diagnosis using ICD-9-CM Volume I and II codes	Report diagnosis using ICD-9-CM Volume I and II codes	Report diagnosis using ICD-9-CM Volume I and II codes
Report diagnosis codes on CMS-1500 in 21 and reference in 24E	Report diagnosis codes on CMS-1450 (UB-04) in FL 67, 69, 70, 72	Report diagnosis codes on CMS-1450 (UB-04) in FL 67, 69, 70, 72
Hospital may bill professional services when the provider is employed by or under contract with the hospital. Some payers may require ICD-9-CM Volume III procedure codes on ambulatory surgery claims.		

Current Procedural Terminology (CPT)	**HCPCS National Level II**	**ICD-9-CM Volume I and II**	**ICD-9-CM Volume III**
HCPCS LEVEL I Services and Procedures	HCPCS LEVEL II Services, Procedures, and Items	Diagnosis	Procedures

Figure 12-22 Coding systems used for submission of charges are determined based on the type of service: professional, outpatient, or inpatient.

TABLE 12-9 Timely Filing Requirements*

Medicare		Medicaid	TRICARE	
Claims must be submitted no later than the end of the calendar year following the fiscal year in which services were furnished. The fiscal year for claims begins October 1 and ends September 30th.		Timely filing requirements vary in accordance with individual state guidelines for claim submission. Some states may have a 30-day timely filing limit, and others may require claims to be submitted within 1 year.	TRICARE Prime, Extra, and Standard require claims to be submitted within 1 year of the date of service or date of discharge for inpatient services.	
Example			**Example**	
Date of Service	**Time Limit**		**Date of Service**	**Time Limit**
October 1, 2009	December 31, 2010		October 1, 2009	October 1, 2010
October 1, 2008	December 31, 2009		**Date of Discharge**	**Time Limit**
			October 1, 2008	October 1, 2009

From U. S. Department of Health and Human Services, Centers for Medicare & Medicaid Services, and U.S. Department of Defense, TRICARE Management Activity.

*Payers require claim submission within a specified period of time after services are provided.

Appeals Process

All payers have a formal appeals process for providers to follow when there is disagreement about the way the claim has been paid or denied. The payer guidelines will outline a specific time frame for the submission of appeals, the process by which appeals should be submitted, and what type of claim issues can be appealed. Guidelines for appeals will explain what type of denials can be appealed. Most payers require appeal requests be submitted in writing. The participating provider agreement also defines the time period during which an appeal may be submitted. For example, a payer may require appeals to be submitted within 60 days of the denial.

It is essential for hospital personnel involved in the billing process to understand how compliance with

1500

HEALTH INSURANCE CLAIM FORM

APPROVED BY NATIONAL UNIFORM CLAIM COMMITTEE 08/05

PICA PICA

CARRIER

1. MEDICARE (Medicare #) MEDICAID (Medicaid #) TRICARE CHAMPUS (Sponsor's SSN) CHAMPVA (Member ID#) GROUP HEALTH PLAN (SSN or ID) FECA BLK LUNG (SSN) OTHER (ID)

1a. INSURED'S I.D. NUMBER (For Program in Item 1)

2. PATIENT'S NAME (Last Name, First Name, Middle Initial)

3. PATIENT'S BIRTH DATE MM DD YY SEX M F

4. INSURED'S NAME (Last Name, First Name, Middle Initial)

5. PATIENT'S ADDRESS (No., Street)

6. PATIENT RELATIONSHIP TO INSURED Self Spouse Child Other

7. INSURED'S ADDRESS (No., Street)

CITY STATE

8. PATIENT STATUS

CITY STATE

SECTION I PATIENT AND INSURANCE INFORMATION

ZIP CODE TELEPHONE (Include Area Code) ( )

Employed Full-Time Student Part-Time Student

ZIP CODE TELEPHONE (Include Area Code) ( )

9. OTHER INSURED'S NAME (Last Name, First Name, Middle Initial)

10. IS PATIENT'S CONDITION RELATED TO:

11. INSURED'S POLICY GROUP OR FECA NUMBER

a. OTHER INSURED'S POLICY OR GROUP NUMBER

a. EMPLOYMENT? (Current or Previous) YES NO

a. INSURED'S DATE OF BIRTH MM DD YY SEX M F

b. OTHER INSURED'S DATE OF BIRTH MM DD YY SEX M F

b. AUTO ACCIDENT? PLACE (State) YES NO

b. EMPLOYER'S NAME OR SCHOOL NAME

c. EMPLOYER'S NAME OR SCHOOL NAME

c. OTHER ACCIDENT? YES NO

c. INSURANCE PLAN NAME OR PROGRAM NAME

d. INSURANCE PLAN NAME OR PROGRAM NAME

10d. RESERVED FOR LOCAL USE

d. IS THERE ANOTHER HEALTH BENEFIT PLAN? YES NO *If yes,* return to and complete item 9 a-d.

PATIENT AND INSURED INFORMATION

READ BACK OF FORM BEFORE COMPLETING & SIGNING THIS FORM.

12. PATIENT'S OR AUTHORIZED PERSON'S SIGNATURE I authorize the release of any medical or other information necessary to process this claim. I also request payment of government benefits either to myself or to the party who accepts assignment below.

SIGNED

13. INSURED'S OR AUTHORIZED PERSON'S SIGNATURE I authorize payment of medical benefits to the undersigned physician or supplier for services described below.

14. DATE OF CURRENT: MM DD YY ILLNESS (First symptom) OR INJURY (Accident) OR PREGNANCY(LMP)

15. IF PA... GIVE...

17. NAME OF REFERRING PROVIDER OR OTHER SOURCE 17a. 17b. NPI

19. R...

SECTION II PATIENT DIAGNOSIS

21. DIAGNOSIS OR NATURE OF ILLNESS OR INJURY (Relate Items 1, 2, 3 or...

1. 3.

2. 4.

24. A. DATE(S) OF SERVICE From MM DD YY To MM DD YY B. PLACE OF SERVICE C. EMG D. PROCEDURES (Explain U... CPT/HCPCS

1

2

3

SECTION III CHARGE INFORMATION

4

5

6

25. FEDERAL TAX I.D. NUMBER SSN EIN

26. PATIENT'S ACC...

31. SIGNATURE OF PHYSICIAN OR SUPPLIER INCLUDING DEGREES OR CREDENTIALS (I certify that the statements on the reverse

32. SERVICE FACILI...

SECTION IV PROVIDER INFORMATION

SIGNED DATE a. NPI

NUCC Instruction Manual available at: www.nucc.org

1 2 3a PAT. CNTL # b. MED. REC. # 4 TYPE OF BILL

5 FED. TAX NO. 6 STATEMENT COVERS PERIOD FROM THROUGH 7

8 PATIENT NAME SECTION I (FL 1-FL 41) 9 PATIENT ADDRESS

10 BIRTHDATE 11 SEX ADMISSION 12 DATE 13 HR 14 TYPE 15 SRC 16 DHR 17 STAT CONDITION CODES 18 19 20 21 22 23 24 25 26 27 28 29 ACDT STATE 30

31 OCCURRENCE CODE DATE 32 OCCURRENCE CODE DATE 33 OCCURRENCE CODE DATE 34 OCCURRENCE CODE DATE 35 OCCURRENCE SPAN CODE FROM THROUGH 36 OCCURRENCE SPAN CODE FROM THROUGH 37

38 39 VALUE CODES CODE AMOUNT 40 VALUE CODES CODE AMOUNT 41 VALUE CODES CODE AMOUNT

Facility, patient, admission, discharge, occurrence, and value information.

42 REV. CD. 43 DESCRIPTION 44 HCPCS / RATE / HIPPS CODE 45 SERV. DATE 46 SERV. UNITS 47 TOTAL CHARGES 48 NON-COVERED CHARGES 49

Revenue Codes and Descriptions

SECTION II (FL 42-FL49) Charge information

HCPCS CODES Level I CPT

Level II Medicare National

PAGE OF CREATION DATE TOTALS

50 PAYER Payer, insured, employer, authorization information PAYMENTS 55 EST. AMOUNT DUE 56 NPI 57 OTHER PRV ID

SECTION III (FL 50-FL 65)

58 INSURED'S NAME 59 P.REL 60 INSURED'S UNIQUE ID 61 GROUP NAME 62 INSURANCE GROUP NO.

63 TREATMENT AUTHORIZATION CODES 64 DOCUMENT CONTROL NUMBER 65 EMPLOYER NAME

66 DX 67 A B C D E F G H 68

Procedure, diagnosis, and provider information 72 ECI 73

74 PRINCIPAL PROCEDURE CODE DATE a. OTHER PROCEDURE CODE DATE b. OTHER PROCEDURE CODE DATE 75

SECTION IV (FL 66-FL 81)

c. OTHER PROCEDURE CODE DATE d. OTHER PROCEDURE CODE DATE e. OTHER PROCEDURE CODE DATE

76 ATTENDING NPI QUAL LAST FIRST

77 OPERATING NPI QUAL LAST FIRST

80 REMARKS 81CC a b c d

78 OTHER NPI QUAL LAST FIRST

79 OTHER NPI QUAL LAST FIRST

UB-04 CMS-1450 © 2005 NUBC OMB APPROVAL PENDING NUBC National Uniform Billing Committee LIC9213257 THE CERTIFICATIONS ON THE REVERSE APPLY TO THIS BILL AND ARE MADE A PART HEREOF.

Figure 12-23 Two claim forms used for submission of hospital charges. CMS-1500 is for physician and outpatient services. CMS-1450 (UB-04) is for facility charges for outpatient, nonpatient, and inpatient services.

payer guidelines can affect payment. Claims can be delayed or denied if they are not completed accurately. Services may not be paid if guidelines are not followed. The opportunity to appeal a denial can be lost if the appeal is not submitted within the appropriate time frame.

Box 12-24 ■ KEY POINTS

Timely Filing Requirements

Timely filing requirements are written into payer contracts to outline the time frame for submission of claims.

CHAPTER SUMMARY

Hospitals provide services to patients who are covered under various health insurance plans offered by various government programs. The plans may be traditional fee-for-service plans or managed care plans. Medicare, Medicaid, and TRICARE offer managed care plans, and therefore they provide coordinated care and incorporate cost containment measures. Fees paid to providers are fixed, predetermined fees.

All health insurance plans have terms and specifications that define how services are obtained, what services are covered, payment for services, and how

TEST YOUR *Knowledge* BOX 12-5

REIMBURSEMENT METHODS AND BILLING REQUIREMENTS

1. List three categories of reimbursement methods that are utilized by payers to determine payment.
2. Describe the methods USED by the following plan types:
   a. Traditional fee-for-service
   b. Managed care
   c. Government programs
3. List three reimbursement methods implemented under the Prospective Payment System (PPS).
4. Discuss briefly why it is important for hospital personnel involved in billing and coding to understand payer billing requirements.
5. Explain the relationship between documentation and payment for services from payers.
6. State the purpose of coding systems in the billing process.
7. Provide an outline of various coding systems used to submit claims.
8. List two claim forms that may be used to submit charges to payers.
9. Provide a brief explanation of what services can be reported on each of the claim forms.
10. Define timely filing, and explain its importance in the billing process.

FOR IMMEDIATE RELEASE—UB-04 scheduled to replace CMS-1450 (UB-92)

NUBC Announces 45-day Public Comment Period, ending February 1, 2005, for the New UB-04 Data Set and Form

December 17, 2004

The National Uniform Billing Committee (NUBC) announced today the opening of a 45-day public comment period, ending February 1, 2005, for the new UB-04 data set and form to replace the UB-92. The UB-04 contains a number of improvements and enhancements that resulted from nearly four years of research. The NUBC is conducting this final survey to better understand the timelines and transition issues surrounding the implementation of the UB-04. Those wishing to comment on the UB-04 are encouraged to visit the NUBC website http://www.nubc.org/ for further information.

NUBC ANNOUNCES APPROVAL OF UB-04

Following the close of a public comment period and careful review of comments received, the National Uniform Billing Committee approved the UB-04 as the replacement for the UB-92 at its February 2005 meeting.

Receivers (health plans and clearinghouses) need to be ready to receive the new UB-04 by March 1, 2007.

Submitters (health care providers such as hospitals, skilled nursing facilities, hospice, and other institutional claim filers) can use the UB-04 **beginning March 1, 2007,** however, they will have a transitional period between March 1, 2007 and May 22, 2007 where they can use the UB-04 or the UB-92.

Starting May 23, 2007 all institutional paper claims must use the UB-04; the UB-92 will no longer be acceptable after this date.

The final image of the UB-04 form, a summary of the public comments/NUBC responses, and information on how to obtain the UB-04 Data Specifications Manual can be found on the NUBC website.

Figure 12-24 NUBC announcement, the UB-04 is scheduled to replace the CMS-1450 (UB-92) effective May 23, 2007. *(Modified from National Uniform Billing Committee:* NUBC Announces UB-04 Scheduled to Replace UB-92, *www.nubc.org)*

providers are to bill for services. Hospitals may elect to participate with various health insurance plans. Participation requirements vary by plan. Payment for health care services is contingent on compliance with plan requirements. These variations require hospital personnel to have an understanding of various plan terms and specifications in order to ensure compliance with the plan requirements and to optimize reimbursement. Although this chapter provides an overview of the terms and specifications found in insurance plans, the hospital professional must extend his or her knowledge base through experience with the various plans. To accomplish this, hospital personnel are required to understand the basic terms and specifications found in plans and build on the basic knowledge through experience.

CHAPTER REVIEW 12-1

True/False

1. Government programs were created because third-party payers represent the largest portion of reimbursement for hospital services. T F
2. Medicare is a government program designed to provide health care coverage for the elderly and other selected groups. T F
3. Medicaid is a state program designed to provide health care coverage only for children. T F
4. TRICARE is a government program designed to provide health care coverage for military personnel and their families. T F
5. Most government programs offer managed care plans to their members. T F

Fill in the Blank

6. The provider responsible for monitoring and managing patient care in managed care plans is the ____________________.
7. Name four parts of the Medicare program: ____________________, ____________________, ____________________, and ____________________.
8. ________________ is a program developed to provide health care coverage for children to age 19.
9. ____________________ ____________________ enter into a contract with a private payer or government plan to provide health care services to the plan's members.
10. Medicare coverage determinations made at the national level are referred to as ________________, and coverage determinations made at the local level are referred to as ________________.

Match the Following Definitions With the Terms at Right

11. ___ An insurance company or other entity that contracts with a government program to perform functions related to enrollment and processing of Medicare claims.
12. ___ A statement needed to obtain coverage for services provided by a civilian provider. It is obtained from a Military Treatment Facility to certify the facility was not able to provide the care required.
13. ___ A government program designed to provide health care coverage for the elderly and other selected groups.
14. ___ A program funded by the federal and state governments that provides health care coverage to eligible needy individuals.
15. ___ An organization that conducts utilization and quality control reviews of health care services.

A. Medicare
B. Medicaid
C. Medicare Administrative Contractor and TRICARE Management Activity
D. Quality Improvement Organization
E. Non-Availability Statement

CHAPTER REVIEW 12-1—*cont'd*

Research Project

The purpose of this project is to further research variations in government plan options and to apply basic knowledge reviewed in this chapter.

Research government payers and discuss the following:

1. Identify one specific plan type offered by each of the following programs:
   - Medicare
   - Medicaid
   - TRICARE

   The plan types selected for each of the three programs should be different.

2. Research the plan type within the program and discuss the following for each of the three plans selected:
   a. Does the plan incorporate cost containment measures? If so, provide a brief explanation of at least two measures.
   b. Outline covered services.
   c. State the medical necessity requirements.
   d. Discuss coverage limitations listed in each plan.
   e. Explain how you would determine if the plan is a primary or secondary plan.
   f. List patient responsibility requirements for the plan.

3. Research what a provider is required to do to participate with the plan and discuss the following:
   a. Briefly describe two or three of the terms for participation for each plan.
   b. Is the provider required to obtain a referral to provide care to a patient?
   c. How does the plan reimburse the provider?
   d. Discuss what claim form is required.
   e. State the timely filing requirements for the plan.
   f. Provide an overview of the appeals process for the plan.

   Provide a separate report for each plan outlining all the above.

GLOSSARY

Benefit period (episode of care) A benefit period under Medicare is an episode of care that begins on the first day a patient is admitted to the hospital and ends when the patient has not been in the hospital for 60 consecutive days.

Categorically needy A term used to identify groups of individuals who are in need of Medicaid benefits, such as the aged, blind, or disabled or children and families who meet specific eligibility requirements.

Centers for Medicare and Medicaid Services (CMS) A federal agency within the Department of Health and Human Services, formerly known as the Health Care Financing Administration (HCFA), that oversees the Medicare and Medicaid programs.

Civilian Health and Medical Program of the Veterans Administration (CHAMPVA) A program designed to provide benefits for health care services provided to the spouse and children of a veteran with a permanent, total disability that is service connected or a veteran who is deceased as a result of a disability that is service connected.

Defense Enrollment Eligibility Reporting System (DEERS) The system used by TRICARE to determine eligibility and maintain enrollment records.

Field activities A term used by the Department of Defense to describe the tasks and responsibilities required for the administration of the TRICARE program.

Fiscal agents (FA) An insurance company or other entity that the federal government contracts with to handle functions related to enrollment and the processing of claims for the Medicaid program. Fiscal agents are Medicaid contractors.

Lifetime Reserve Days A benefit under Medicare Part A that provides coverage for 60 days of hospitalization, per lifetime, that the beneficiary may use at any time.

Local coverage determination (LCD) Developed by Medicare Administrative Contractors (MAC) to provide guidance and enhance understanding of coverage guidelines. LCDs outline criteria for coverage of services and they provide coding and billing information for the services. LCDs were formerly referred to as Local Medical Review Policies (LMRPs).

Medicaid A government program designed to provide health care coverage for specified eligible needy individuals. Medicaid is funded by a cooperative venture between the federal and state governments to assist states in the provision of adequate medical care to eligible needy individuals.

Medically needy A term used to describe individuals with high medical expenses and low income who meet specific eligibility requirements.

Medicare A federally funded program implemented under Title XVIII of the Social Security Act in 1965 to provide coverage for health care services to the elderly and other specified groups.

Medicare Administrative Contractor (MAC) Insurance company or other entity that the Federal government contracts with to handle functions related to enrollment and processing claims for the Medicare program. Medicare contractors were previously known as Fiscal Intermediaries (FI) or Medicare Carriers.

Medicare Part A Medicare benefits referred to as "hospital insurance" that provide coverage for medically necessary inpatient care provided in a hospital, skilled nursing facility, or psychiatric facility.

Medicare Part B Medicare benefit referred to as "medical insurance" that provides coverage for care that is not covered under Medicare Part A. Coverage for medically necessary physician and outpatient services is provided under Medicare Part B, including laboratory tests, X-ray examinations, physical therapy, emergency room services, and ambulatory surgery services.

Medicare Part C Medicare benefits also known as "Medicare Advantage Plans", that provides various health insurance plan options for Medicare beneficiaries to select from to meet their specific health care needs. Formerly known as "Medicare + Choice."

Medicare Part D Medicare benefit that provides various plan options for beneficiaries to obtain prescription drug coverage. Medicare Part D was created under the Medicare Prescription Drug Improvement Modernization Act (MMA), passed in 2003. Drug coverage under the prescription drug plans became available effective January 1, 2006.

Medicare Summary Notice (MSN) A notice sent to the beneficiary that provides detailed information about the charges and the amount the beneficiary is responsible to pay.

Medigap plan A supplemental insurance plan purchased by a Medicare beneficiary for the purpose of providing coverage for amounts not paid by Medicare, such as non-covered services or items, the annual deductible, and co-insurance amounts.

Military Treatment Facility (MTF) A military facility in which most of the care is provided to TRICARE beneficiaries.

National coverage determination (NCD) Describes coverage policies developed by the Center for Medicare and Medicaid Service (CMS) that outline condition(s) that meet medical necessity standards for specified service(s) reported.

Non-Availability Statement (NAS) A statement obtained from the military hospital that is not able to provide the care required. TRICARE will not pay for services provided at a civilian hospital unless an NAS is obtained.

Participating provider (PAR) A provider—physician, hospital, or other entity—that enters into a contract with an insurance company or government program to provide health care services to the plan's members.

Quality Improvement Organization (QIO) An organization that conducts utilization and quality control reviews of health care services provided to Medicare and Medicaid members. QIO was formerly known as the Peer Review Organization (PRO).

Regional contractor An insurance company or other entity that TRICARE administration contracts with to handle functions related to enrollment and filing claims. Regional contractors are also referred to as TRICARE contractors.

State Children's Health Insurance Program (SCHIP) A government program designed to provide health care coverage for uninsured children to the age of 19. The program is also referred to as the Children's Health Insurance Program (CHIP).

TRICARE A federally funded health insurance program designed to provide coverage for health care services provided to military personnel and their families.

TRICARE Extra A PPO type of plan that has provisions for members to obtain health care services from providers within the TRICARE network of approved civilian providers.

TRICARE for Life (TFL) A program that offers expanded medical coverage for military retirees and veterans who have attained the age of 65, are Medicare eligible, and have purchased Medicare Part B.

TRICARE Management Activity (TMA) A field activity agency created by the Department of Defense to oversee the TRICARE program.

TRICARE Prime An HMO type of plan that provides health care services that are managed by a Primary Care Manager (PCM).

TRICARE Remote A program designed to provide health care services to active duty members who work and live more than a specified distance from a Military Treatment Facility (MTF).

TRICARE Standard The traditional fee-for-service CHAMPUS plan. Members under the TRICARE Standard plan may elect to obtain care from civilian doctors or at a Military Treatment Facility (MTF).

Chapter 13

Prospective Payment Systems

The objective of this chapter is to provide an overview of Prospective Payment Systems (PPS). Hospitals provide services to patients for treatment of conditions that are covered under various government-sponsored health insurance plans. Since 1965, when Medicare and Medicaid were created, reimbursement for hospital services has shifted from the traditional cost-based reimbursement to PPS methods that use predetermined fixed payments for hospital services. An overview of the evolution of reimbursement to PPS provides an understanding of events leading to the implementation of PPS. Today, hospital services provided to beneficiaries of government-sponsored plans are paid based on various PPS methods. A discussion of each PPS used for hospital reimbursement will provide hospital professionals with an understanding of how the system is designed, and the basis for payment under each system. It is critical for hospital billing and coding professionals to understand these systems to ensure compliance and to obtain appropriate reimbursement.

Chapter Objectives

- Define terms, phrases, abbreviations, and acronyms related to Prospective Payment Systems.
- Demonstrate an understanding of the evolution of health care reimbursement from cost-based systems to Prospective Payment Systems.
- Describe the relationship between government programs and Prospective Payment Systems.
- Discuss various payment systems implemented under the Prospective Payment System.
- Demonstrate an understanding of Inpatient Prospective Payment System (IPPS) development, payment calculations, structure and assignment.
- Provide an overview of the Prospective Payment Systems used to reimburse hospitals for inpatient and outpatient services.
- Demonstrate an understanding of Outpatient Prospective Payment System (OPPS) development, payment calculations, structure, and assignment.
- Explain what coding systems are used to submit charges under Prospective Payment Systems, and how they affect reimbursement.

Outline

Key Terms

Ambulatory Payment Classification (APC)
Ambulatory Payment Classification (APC) outlier
Ambulatory surgery
Ambulatory surgery center (ASC)
Arithmetic mean length of stay (AMLOS)
Co-morbidity
Complications
Conversion factor (CF)
Geometric mean length of stay (GMLOS)
Inpatient Prospective Payment System (IPPS)
Major diagnostic category (MDC)
Medicare Severity Diagnosis Related Groups (MS-DRG)
Medicare Severity Diagnosis Related Groups (MS-DRG) grouper program
Medicare Severity Diagnosis Related Groups (MS-DRG) outlier modifiers
Outpatient Prospective Payment System (OPPS)
Outpatient Prospective Payment System (OPPS) grouper
Outpatient services
Relative weight (RW)
Transitional Pass-Through Payments

Acronyms and Abbreviations

AMLOS—arithmetic mean length of stay
APC—Ambulatory Payment Classification
ASC—ambulatory surgery center
BBA—Balanced Budget Act
CF—conversion factor
CMS—Centers for Medicare and Medicaid Services
CMS-DRG—Centers for Medicare and Medicaid Services Diagnosis Related Groups (1983–2007)
CORF—comprehensive outpatient rehabilitation facility
CPT—Current Procedural Terminology
DRG—Diagnosis Related Group
EIN—Employer Identification Number
E/M—evaluation and management
GMLOS—Geometric mean length of stay
HCPCS—Health Care Common Procedure Coding System
HH—home health
HIM—Health Information Management
ICD-9-CM—International Classification of Diseases, 9th Revision, Clinical Modification
IPPS—Inpatient Prospective Payment System
IRF—Inpatient rehabilitation facility
IRS—Internal Revenue Service
LCTH—long-term care hospital
MDC—major diagnostic category
MS-DRG—Medicare Severity Diagnosis Related Groups (implemented 2007–2009)
OBRA—Omnibus Budget Reconciliation Act
OPPS—Outpatient Prospective Payment System
PPS—Prospective Payment System
RW—relative weight
SI—status indicator
SNF—skilled nursing facility
TEFRA—Tax Equity and Fiscal Responsibility Act
TIN—Tax Identification Number
UB-04—CMS-1450 Universal Bill implemented in 2007.

PROSPECTIVE PAYMENT SYSTEM (PPS) DEFINED

A **Prospective Payment System (PPS)** is a method of determining reimbursement to health care providers based on predetermined factors, not on individual services. There are a number of insurance companies and government agencies that use PPS for reimbursement. Prospective Payment System is the term used to describe Medicare's reimbursement system for services provided by hospitals. Prospective payment is a statistically developed method that identifies the amount of resources that are directed toward a group of diagnoses or procedures, on average, and reimburses on that basis. For example, after a review of 10,000 inpatient pneumonia cases, it may be determined that patients tend to be hospitalized for 3 to 5 days in the absence of any significant co-morbidities (additional diagnoses) or complications (additional diagnoses or procedures that result from the original diagnosis or treatment of the diagnosis). Based on the amount of resources that a pneumonia patient would consume under these circumstances, a fixed amount is assigned to that case. Prospective payment may be based on diagnosis, procedure, or a combination of both.

BOX 13-1 ■ KEY POINTS

Prospective Payment System (PPS)

- A method of determining reimbursement to health care providers based on predetermined factors, not on individual services
- Basis for reimbursement is the amount of resources required for a group of diagnoses or procedures

PROSPECTIVE PAYMENT SYSTEM (PPS) EVOLUTION

Historically, payments for health care services were largely based on the provider's charge for the service or on a per diem basis for hospital inpatient services. Insurance companies and government programs processed payments for services by using fee-for-service (FFS); fee schedule; usual, customary, and reasonable; percentage of accrued charges; or per diem reimbursement methods, as discussed in previous chapters. These systems are commonly referred to as cost-based systems, because they determine reimbursement based on the reasonable cost of providing services.

Establishment of Government Programs

From 1965 to 1982 the government became one of the largest payers of health care services with the establishment of the Medicare, Medicaid, and TRICARE programs. Reimbursement to hospitals during this period was made based on accrued charges submitted for a hospital case. Medicare and other payers determined payments based on reasonable costs of the care provided, and paid a percentage of those costs. Again, hospital inpatient services were reimbursed on a per diem basis. Later, significant changes in reimbursement for health care services were seen as a result of the rising cost of health care and the growing aged and uninsured population.

BOX 13-2 ■ KEY POINTS

Prospective Payment System (PPS) Evolution, 1965–1982

The government became one of the largest payers of health care with the establishment of Medicare, Medicaid, and TRICARE.

Hospitals submitted accrued charges. Reimbursement was made based on the reasonable cost of care provided, and payment was a percentage of that cost or was calculated on a per diem basis.

Rising Cost of Health Care

From 1960 to 1980 the public sector's (Medicare, Medicaid, and TRICARE) share of health care expenditures increased from 21.4% to 40.3%, as illustrated in Figure 13-1. The government found it necessary to devise reimbursement methods that provided fixed payment amounts for health care services. One of the more significant changes was the implementation of the Medicare Inpatient PPS (IPPS).

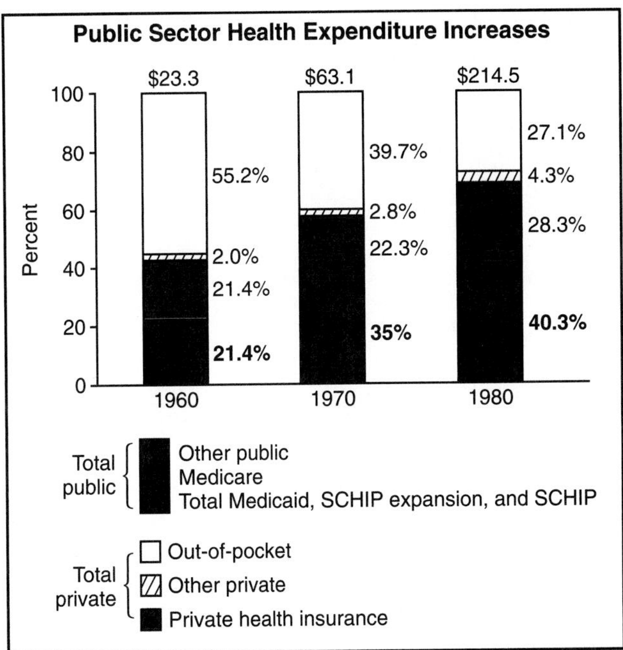

Figure 13-1 Figure illustrates the rising cost of health care between 1960 and 1980. Public sector's (Medicare, Medicaid, and TRICARE) share of health care expenditures increased from 21.4% to 40.3%. *(Data from Centers for Medicare & Medicaid Services, Office of the Actuary, National Health Statistics.)*

Inpatient Prospective Payment System (IPPS)

The **Inpatient Prospective Payment System (IPPS)** was established as mandated by the Tax Equity and Fiscal Responsibility Act (TEFRA) in 1983 to provide reimbursement for acute hospital inpatient services. The purpose of the PPS system was to control health care costs through provider incentives to manage the care provided. The system implemented under IPPS is known as the Diagnosis Related Group (DRG) system. Under this system, hospitals are reimbursed a predetermined fixed rate for services provided based on the patient's condition and the resources required to treat the condition. The implementation of the DRG system ended hospital reimbursement by government programs based on the amount of charges accrued during the inpatient stay. The DRG system provides incentives for hospitals to ensure cost-efficient care. The original DRG system, now known as CMS-DRG, was replaced with MS-DRG effective October 1, 2009.

During the remainder of the 1980s payment for hospital outpatient services remained on a cost-based system. Advancements in medical technology increased the number of surgeries performed on an outpatient basis. Congress began to focus on controlling costs for outpatient care through across-the-board reductions of payable amounts for hospital operating costs and capital costs. Different payment methods for specific outpatient services were created, including fee schedules for

BOX 13-3 ■ KEY POINTS

Inpatient Prospective Payment System (IPPS) Evolution, 1983

The establishment of a Prospective Payment System (PPS) for inpatient services was mandated by the Tax Equity and Fiscal Responsibility Act in 1983.

The Inpatient Prospective Payment System (IPPS) implemented to provide reimbursement for hospital inpatient acute care provided to Medicare beneficiaries is the Diagnosis Related Group (DRG) system. The DRG system was replaced with Medicare Severity Diagnosis Related Groups (MS-DRG) effective 10/1/2009.

diagnostic laboratory tests, orthotics, and durable medical equipment.

Outpatient Prospective Payment System (OPPS)

During the 1990s legislation was passed that mandated the implementation of a PPS for hospital outpatient services for members of government-sponsored health plans. The Omnibus Budget Reconciliation Act (OBRA) of 1986 paved the way for development of a PPS for hospital outpatient services. OBRA legislation included a mandate for hospitals to report services provided on an outpatient basis, using the Health Care Common Procedure Coding System (HCPCS). This information was used by the Centers for Medicare and Medicaid Services (CMS) for the development of a PPS. Revisions to OBRA in 1990 mandated CMS to develop a proposal to replace the existing hospital outpatient payment system with a PPS. The Balanced Budget Act (BBA) of 1997 required CMS to implement the OPPS effective January 1, 1999. The final rule outlining the establishment of an outpatient PPS was published by CMS in the *Federal Register* in April 2000. CMS implemented the OPPS, effective August 2000. The OPPS provides reimbursement for hospital outpatient services based on predetermined fixed rates. Table 13-1 outlines legislation that contributed to the development and implementation of PPSs.

BOX 13-4 ■ KEY POINTS

Outpatient Prospective Payment System (OPPS) Evolution, 2000

The Omnibus Budget Reconciliation Act (OBRA) of 1986 and the Balanced Budget Act (BBA) of 1997 led to the mandated implementation of a Prospective Payment System (PPS) to replace the traditional reimbursement systems for hospital outpatient services.

As mandated under the BBA, CMS implemented the Outpatient Prospective Payment System (OPPS), effective August 2000. OPPS provides reimbursement for hospital outpatient services provided to Medicare beneficiaries. The Outpatient Prospective Payment System (OPPS) used to provide reimbursement for hospital outpatient services is called Ambulatory Payment Classifications (APC).

Other Prospective Payment Systems (PPS)

In an effort to control the rising cost of health care, CMS implemented PPS for services provided by other facilities and providers. The BBA of 1997 required the creation of the following PPSs:

- Skilled nursing facility (SNF PPS)
- Home health (HH PPS)
- Inpatient rehabilitation facility (IRF PPS).

The Balanced Budget Refinement Act (BBRA) of 1999 and the Benefits Improvement Act (BIPA) of 2000 established the following PPS for long-term care:

- Long-term care hospital (LTCH PPS).

It is important for hospital personnel involved in billing and coding to understand the PPS that will be used to determine reimbursement for hospital services. The guidelines for coding and PPS assignment vary for each system. This chapter provides an overview of Medicare's IPPS for hospital inpatient services and OPPS for hospital outpatient services.

BOX 13-5 ■ KEY POINTS

Other Prospective Payment Systems (OPPS) Implemented by the Centers for Medicare and Medicaid Services (CMS)

- Skilled nursing facility (SNF PPS)—1997
- Home health (HH PPS)—1997
- Inpatient rehabilitation facility (IRF PPS)—1997
- Long-term care hospital (LTCH PPS)—2000

INPATIENT PROSPECTIVE PAYMENT SYSTEM (IPPS)

Medicare's Inpatient Prospective Payment System (IPPS) is a reimbursement system for hospital acute inpatient care under which the facility is paid a fixed amount for the stay, based on the patient's diagnosis and procedure. Medicare's IPPS was implemented in 1983 as a measure to control rising health care costs. Under this system hospitals are no longer paid based on charges accrued. Payment for the patient's stay is fixed, regardless of charges accrued. When hospital care provided during the stay costs less than the PPS payment, the hospital saves money. However, if the cost of care is greater than the PPS payment, the hospital will experience a loss of revenue. Under this system, hospitals are required to manage care to ensure that resources used during the stay are efficient.

TABLE 13-1 Legislation Affecting Reimbursement

Date	Legislation	Effect on Reimbursement
1965	Creation of Medicare and Medicaid	Original reimbursement methods: • Fee-for-service • Usual, customary, and reasonable (UCR) • Percentage of accrued charges
1967	Creation of TRICARE	Government share of health care costs increased
1970–1980s	Implementation of managed care plans	Fixed payment reimbursement methods. • Contract rates • Capitation • Per diem • Case rates
1982	Tax Equity and Fiscal Responsibility Act (TEFRA)	Established methods of controlling the cost of the Medicare program, set a limit on reimbursement, and required development of a Prospective Payment System (PPS)
1983	The Social Security Amendments of 1983	Mandated 3-year phase-in of Prospective Payment System (PPS) for hospital inpatient services
	Implementation of the Inpatient Prospective Payment System (DRG)	Reimbursement for hospital acute inpatient care reimbursed based on predetermined fixed payment assigned to DRG groups
1986	Omnibus Budget Reconciliation Act (OBRA)	Requires hospitals to report claims for services using the Health Care Common Procedure Coding System (HCPCS); data will be used to create a Prospective Payment System (PPS) for hospital outpatient services
1990	Revision of Omnibus Budget Reconciliation Act (OBRA)	Required CMS to develop and replace cost-based reimbursement for hospital outpatient services with a Prospective Payment System (PPS)
1997	Balanced Budget Act (BBA) Section 443	Authorizes CMS to implement a Prospective Payment System (PPS) for hospital outpatient services.
2000	Implementation of the Outpatient Prospective Payment System (OPPS)	Reimbursement for hospital-based outpatient services including ambulatory surgery
2007–2009	Implementation of MS-DRG	MS-DRG system replaced the CMS-DRG system

Diagnosis Related Group (DRG) Overview

The IPPS implemented in 1983 by CMS and other payers for reimbursement to hospitals for acute inpatient care is known as the CMS-Diagnosis Related Group (DRG) system. CMS-DRG is a payment classification system that defines patient categories based on diagnosis, procedure, and other clinical factors. Each CMS-DRG is a grouping that groups patient cases that are clinically similar and that require a similar level of resources during the stay. Under CMS-DRG, the facility is paid a fixed fee based on the patient's condition and relative treatments.

BOX 13-6 ■ KEY POINTS

Diagnosis Related Group (DRG)

- The Inpatient Prospective Payment System (IPPS) used by Medicare to provide reimbursement for hospital inpatient services is called Diagnosis Related Group (DRG).
- The DRG system was replaced by the MS-DRG system, October 1, 2009.
- The MS-DRG system provides a predetermined fixed payment based on the patient's condition and resources required to treat the patient's condition.
- A MS-DRG is assigned based on the principal and other diagnoses and relative treatment.

Diagnosis Related Group (DRG) Development

CMS-DRG classifications were developed by a group of researchers at Yale University in the late 1960s. The classification system was used as a tool to help clinicians and hospitals monitor quality of care and utilization of services. They proved to be so useful that Medicare adopted the system for use as the basis of the IPPS in 1983. The development of this system required analysis of a large number of actual inpatient cases from hospitals throughout the United States. A database was developed with information regarding inpatient cases including diagnoses, length of stay, procedure(s) performed, and cost. The database was analyzed and used to develop CMS-DRG groups that represented average resources required by hospitals to treat conditions included within that group. This system is the basis of the new Medicare Severity Diagnosis Related Group (MS-DRG) system. Significant changes were made to the CMS-DRG system to "better account for severity of illness and resource consumption for Medicare Beneficiaries." As published in the CMS Acute Care Hospital Inpatient Payment System Fact Sheet the CMS-DRG system was replaced by the MS-DRG system. "For discharges occurring on or after October 1, 2007 a new DRG system called Medicare Severity Diagnosis Related Group (MS-DRG) was adopted. The MS-DRG system was implemented and transitioned in during a two-year period." Final implementation of the MS-DRG System occurred as of October 1, 2009. The fact sheet can be viewed at http://www.cms.hhs.gov/MLNProducts/downloads/AcutePaymtSysfctsht.pdf.

TEST YOUR *Knowledge* BOX 13-1

PROSPECTIVE PAYMENT SYSTEMS DEFINED; PROSPECTIVE PAYMENT SYSTEM EVOLUTION

1. Provide a definition for Prospective Payment System (PPS).

2. Discuss the difference between PPSs and traditional methods of reimbursement.

3. State why PPS systems were developed and implemented.

4. Discuss the impact of the BBA of 1997 on outpatient reimbursement.

Match the acronyms listed below with the appropriate description of the reimbursement method.

5. IPPS

6. HH PPS

7. LTCH PPS

8. OPPS

9. IRF PPS

10. SNF PPS

A. Implemented to provide reimbursement for hospital outpatient services. The system is referred to as Ambulatory Payment Classifications (APC).
B. Implemented to provide reimbursement for services provided in a skilled nursing facility.
C. Implemented to provide reimbursement for hospital inpatient services.
D. Implemented to provide reimbursement for services provided in an inpatient rehabilitation facility.
E. Implemented to provide reimbursement for home health services.
F. Implemented to provide reimbursement for services provided in a long-term care hospital.

Medicare Severity Diagnosis Related Groups (MS-DRG) Payment Calculations

MS-DRG payments are based on the relative weight assigned to the MS-DRG group. The formula used by CMS and other payers is complex, as it takes into account the hospital's case mix, the geographic area, a wage index, and operating costs. These factors are used to determine the hospital's base rate. Hospital base rates are defined in accordance with federal regulations, and they are updated annually to include technical adjustments and to ensure that payments accurately reflect inflation. Hospital base rates are also determined largely based on budgetary constraints. The estimated payment for a MS-DRG can be calculated by multiplying relative weight for the MS-DRG by the hospital base rate (HBR) assigned, as illustrated in Figure 13-2. A **relative weight (RW)** is a value assigned to a MS-DRG or APC group or to a procedure code to reflect the relative resource consumption. The RW is used to calculate the total payment for the case. The higher the relative weight (RW), the higher the payment. The MS-DRG payment is intended to cover the necessary costs of the average patient assigned to that MS-DRG. Necessary costs included are pharmaceuticals, medical devices, imaging guidance, diagnostic tests, therapeutic services, and overhead items such as staff, supplies, meals, and linens.

BOX 13-7 ■ KEY POINTS

Medicare Severity Diagnosis Related Groups (MS-DRG) Payment

MS-DRG payments are based on the relative weight (RW) assigned to each MS-DRG.

The formula used by CMS and other payers to calculate payment takes into account the following:

- Hospital's case mix
- Geographic area
- Wage index
- Operating costs

The MS-DRG payment is intended to cover the necessary cost for the average patient assigned to the MS-DRG.

MS-DRG # 93	Relative Weight 1.4378
RW × HBR = MS-DRG Payment	
1.4378 × $2,877.759 = $4,137.64	
Relative weight (×) hospital base rate = MS-DRG Payment	
Hospital base rate for ABZ hospital	$2,877.759

Figure 13-2 MS-DRG payment calculations.

BOX 13-8 ■ KEY POINTS

Medicare Severity Diagnosis Related Groups Outliers and Inliers

Outliers are circumstances that result in a patient case that requires a much longer length of stay or an unusually high cost for treatment compared with most cases represented by the MS-DRG group.

Inliers are circumstances that result in a hospital case that falls below the mean average of expected length of stay.

BOX 13-9 ■ KEY POINTS

Medicare Severity Diagnosis Related Groups (MS-DRG) Elements

The following elements are assigned to each MS-DRG payment group:

- Geometric mean length of stay (GMLOS)
- Arithmetic mean length of stay (AMLOS)
- Relative weight (RW)

These elements are used to calculate the DRG payment rate.

CMS has made available a PRICER program that hospitals can use to obtain a more accurate estimate of a Medicare payment for the hospital inpatient case. The PRICER program for the IPPS can be downloaded from the CMS Web site: http://www.cms.hhs.gov/providers/ pricer/pricdnld.asp. Figure 13-3 illustrates the elements involved in the MS-DRG payment calculation as shown on a screen from the IPPS PRICER program, including outliers, pass-through amounts, operating cost, capital, MS-DRG weight, wage index, and national labor rates.

Medicare Severity Diagnosis Related Groups (MS-DRG) Outliers

MS-DRG outliers are inpatient cases that involve circumstances that result in a patient case that requires a much longer length of stay or an unusually high cost for treatment compared with most cases represented by the MS-DRG group. Hospitals may obtain higher reimbursement for these outlier circumstances. Typical outlier situations include the following:

- The patient has a unique combination of conditions that require more complex treatments, such as multiple surgeries that result in higher cost for the hospital
- The patient has a very rare condition
- The patient's length of stay is longer than usual, referred to as day outliers
- Low-volume MS-DRG

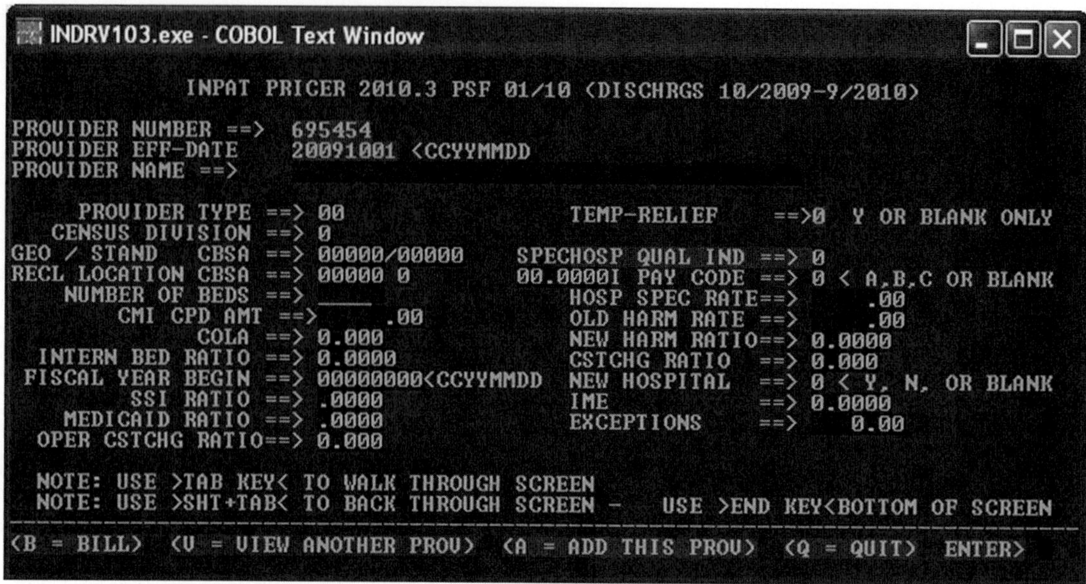

Figure 13-3 Illustration of the CMS IPPS MS-DRG PRICER program 2010 screen shows the elements involved in the MS-DRG payment calculations. *(Modified from Centers for Medicare & Medicaid Services, Pricer [Prospective Payment System], http://www.cms.hhs.gov/PcPricer/03_inpatient.asp#TopOfPage)*

Inliers are circumstances that result in a hospital case that falls below the mean average of expected length of stay. Typical inlier situations include the following:

- The patient passed away (Death)
- The patient left the hospital against medical advice (AMA)
- The patient was admitted and discharged on the same day.

Reimbursement for outliers under the MS-DRG system is calculated based on the full MS-DRG rate, plus payment for additional services required.

Medicare Severity Diagnosis Related Groups (MS-DRG) Structure

The MS-DRG system classifies hospital inpatient cases based on the patient's diagnosis and the procedures required to treat the patient's condition. There are 999 MS-DRG groups classified into categories based on the patient's diagnosis, referred to as a major diagnostic category (MDC), as discussed in the following section. There are two types of MS-DRG payment groups: surgical and medical. Each MS-DRG group contains related principal diagnoses and procedures where appropriate. MS-DRG assignment is determined based on the principal diagnosis and up to eight secondary diagnoses that describe comorbidities and complications. Figure 13-4 illustrates a sample MS-DRG #340, showing the MS-DRG number, type and description, MDC, principal diagnoses, and procedures for the group. The following elements are assigned to each MS-DRG payment group: geometric mean length of stay (GMLOS), arith-

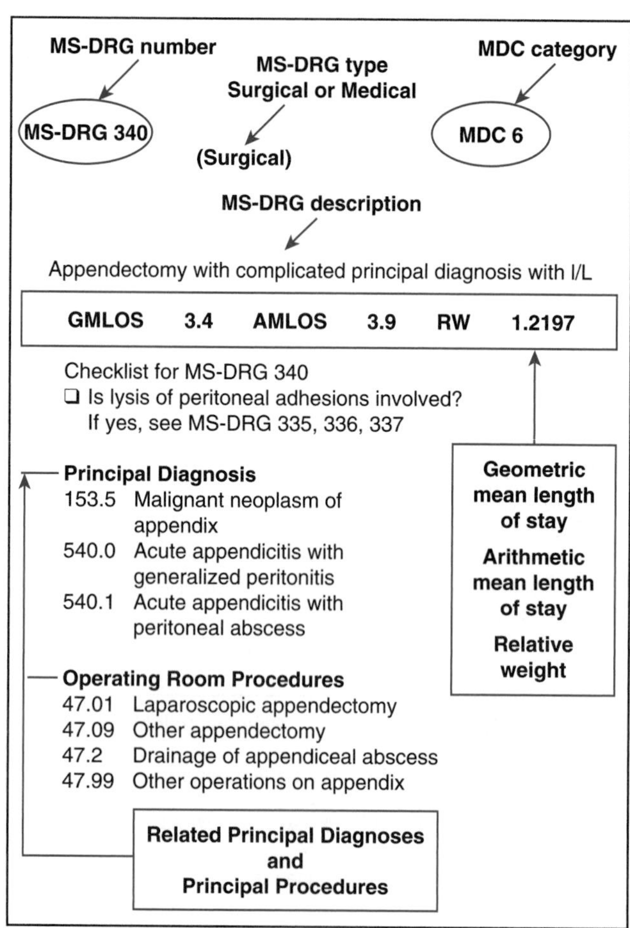

Figure 13-4 MS-DRG 164, illustrating MS-DRG elements. *(Data from Ingenix:* Medicode MS-DRG guide, *Eden Prairie, Minn., 2003, Ingenix.)*

TEST YOUR *Knowledge* BOX 13-2

INPATIENT PROSPECTIVE PAYMENT SYSTEMS (IPPS) AND DIAGNOSIS RELATED GROUP (DRG) OVERVIEW, DEVELOPMENT, AND PAYMENT CALCULATIONS

1. Provide a definition of Inpatient Prospective Payment System (IPPS).
2. Explain why IPPS was implemented.
3. What services are reimbursed under IPPS?
4. State when the IPPS was implemented and for what payer.
5. List the name of the IPPS system implemented.
6. Briefly describe MS-DRG.
7. Explain the relationship between relative weights and MS-DRG.
8. List factors considered in the MS-DRG payment formula.
9. Provide an explanation of the PRICER program and why it was made available by CMS.
10. Explain what outliers are and how they affect reimbursement.

metic mean length of stay (AMLOS), and relative weight (RW).

- **Geometric mean length of stay (GMLOS)** is a value assigned to each MS-DRG to represent an adjusted value for all cases, making allowances for outliers, transfer cases, and negative outlier cases that normally skew data. The GMLOS is used to calculate reimbursement for the MS-DRG.
- **Arithmetic mean length of stay (AMLOS)** is a value assigned to each MS-DRG to represent the average number of approved inpatient days for the MS-DRG.
- **Relative weight (RW)** is a value assigned to each MS-DRG to reflect relative resource consumption for the group. The relative weight is used to calculate the total payment for the case. The higher the RW, the higher the MS-DRG payment.

Information for these values was compiled from data from all U.S. hospital inpatient stays for Medicare patients. These values are used to calculate the DRG payment for the hospital inpatient case. CMS updates the RW, length of stay, and national average charge for each MS-DRG on an annual basis.

MS-DRG groups are organized into categories based on the patient's condition, referred to as major diagnostic categories (MDC).

Major Diagnostic Category (MDC)

A **major diagnostic category (MDC)** is a grouping of hospital inpatient cases based on body system, used to further categorize MS-DRG. MDCs were developed to further categorize 999 MS-DRG groups into smaller groups. Each MDC is based on conditions related to specific organ systems. All principal diagnoses within the MS-DRG system are grouped into 25 MDCs. For example, MDC 1 contains MS-DRG payment groups involving diseases or disorders of the nervous system.

Some MS-DRG groups may relate to any of the MDCs, such as MS-DRG 981, "Extensive Operative Room Procedure Unrelated to Principal Diagnosis." Table 13-2 illustrates the 25 MDCs and related MS-DRG ranges associated with all MDCs.

BOX 13-10 ■ KEY POINTS

Major Diagnostic Categories

MDC Defined

A major diagnostic category (MDC) is a grouping of hospital inpatient cases based on body system used to further categorize MS-DRG. MDCs were developed to further categorize over 999 MS-DRG groups into smaller groups. Each MDC is based on conditions related to specific organ systems.

Surgical versus Medical MS-DRG

MS-DRG are further categorized, with each major diagnostic category (MDC) as being either a surgical MS-DRG or a medical MS-DRG.

- Surgical–Principal diagnoses requiring surgical procedures are assigned to a surgical MS-DRG
- Medical–Principal diagnoses that do not require surgery are assigned to a medical MS-DRG

There are many MS-DRG groups associated with each MDC. For example, the MS-DRG groups assigned to MDC 1 and MDC 4 are as illustrated in Figure 13-5. MS-DRG groups 20 to 69 are assigned to MDC 1, because they involve diseases or disorders of the nervous system. MS-DRG groups 163 to 208 are assigned to MDC 4, because they involve diseases or disorders of the respiratory system.

Within each MDC the groups are further categorized as surgical or medical. Surgical MS-DRG include conditions that require surgical intervention. Medical MS-DRG include conditions that do not require surgical intervention.

Surgical MS-DRG

Principal diagnoses requiring one or more surgical procedures are assigned to a surgical MS-DRG. Surgical MS-DRGs are further classified based on the type of procedure, anatomic area, and whether complications or co-morbidities exist. Within these definitions, procedures are categorized as either major or minor operating room (OR) procedures, as illustrated in Figure 13-6. MS-DRG 116 is a surgical MS-DRG within MDC 2.

Medical MS-DRG

Principal diagnoses that do not require surgery are assigned to a medical MS-DRG. Medical MS-DRG are further divided based on the patient's specific diagnosis. Other factors such as age and whether complications or co-morbidities exist are considerations in the MS-DRG assignment. Figure 13-6 illustrates the medical MS-DRG 121.

Major Diagnostic Category (MDC) Decision-Making Tree

A decision-making tree was developed for each MDC. The decision tree follows the logic of MS-DRG assignment. Figure 13-7 outlines the decision-making tree for MDC 2 Diseases and Disorders of the Eye. Decision trees illustrate the surgical and medical partition. The surgical partition is followed if a surgical "OR procedure" is involved. The tree branches off to various MS-DRG according to body area and age in some areas. The RW for each MS-DRG is listed on the tree. The medical partition is followed when surgery is not required. The medical partition branches off to various MS-DRG based on the patient's diagnosis, age, and the presence of complications or co-morbidities.

Medicare Severity Diagnosis Related Groups (MS-DRG) Variables

Hospital inpatient cases are classified into MS-DRG based on the following variable information:

Principal and Secondary Diagnoses

The principal diagnosis assigned to a hospital case determines what MDC is used in assigning the MS-DRG. To obtain accurate reimbursement, it is essential that the correct principal diagnosis be assigned. Figure 13-7 illustrates the decision-making tree for MDC 2 and the weighted values for each MS-DRG. The incorrect principal diagnosis could lead to a MS-DRG that reimburses the hospital at a lower level. For example, a patient under age 17 with a principal diagnosis of "Other Disorders of the Eye" with no major co-morbidities or complications leads to the assignment of MS-DRG 125, with RW 0.6627. If the disorder of the eye is a neurologic disorder, a principal diagnosis of "Neurological Disorders" in the same MDC leads to a MS-DRG assignment of 123, which carries an RW of 0.7153. In addition to the principal diagnosis, up to eight secondary diagnoses may be assigned, including complications or co-morbidities, which generally contribute to a higher MS-DRG assignment.

Principal Procedure

The principal procedure is assigned to the case to describe the significant procedure performed for definitive treatment of the principal diagnosis, or the procedure that most closely relates to the principal diagnosis. Principal procedures are illustrated on the decision tree based on body areas. If the wrong principal procedure is selected, it could lead to incorrect MS-DRG assignment.

TABLE 13-2 **MDC Categories**

MDC	Category	MS-DRG Range
1	Diseases/Disorders Nervous System	020–103
2	Diseases/Disorders Eye	113–125
3	Diseases/Disorders Ears, Nose, Mouth, Throat	129–159
4	Diseases/Disorders Respiratory System	163–208
5	Diseases/Disorders Circulatory System	215–316
6	Diseases/Disorders Digestive System	326–395
7	Diseases/Disorders Hepatobiliary System/Pancreas	405–446
8	Diseases/Disorders Musculoskeletal System/Connective Tissue	453–566
9	Diseases/Disorders Skin, Subcutaneous Tissue, Breast	573–607
10	Endocrine, Nutritional, Metabolic Diseases/Disorders	614–645
11	Diseases/Disorders of the Kidney/Urinary Tract	652–700
12	Diseases/Disorders Male Reproductive System	707–730
13	Diseases/Disorders Female Reproductive System	734–761
14	Pregnancy, Childbirth, Puerperium	765–782
15	Newborns, Neonates with Conditions Originating in Perinatal Period	789–795
16	Diseases/Disorders Blood, Blood–Forming Organs/Immunological	799–816
17	Myeloproliferative Diseases/Disorders and Poorly Differentiated Neoplasms	820–849
18	Infectious/Parasitic Diseases	853–872
19	Mental Diseases/Disorders	876–887
20	Alcohol/Drug Use/Drug-Induced Organic Mental Disorders	894–897
21	Injuries, Poisonings, Toxic Effect Drugs	901–923
22	Burns	927–934
23	Factors Influencing Health Status, Other Contact Health Services	939–951
24	Multiple Significant Trauma	955–965
25	Human Immunodeficiency Virus Infections	969–977

MS-DRG Categories associated with all MDCs:
981–983—Extensive Operative Room Procedure Unrelated to Principal Diagnosis
984–986—Prostatic Operating Room Procedure Unrelated to Principal Diagnosis
987–989—Non-extensive Operative Room Procedure Unrelated to Principal Diagnosis
005–006—Liver Transplant
009—Bone Marrow Transplant
011–013—Tracheostomy
From www.cms.hhs.gov.

Complications and Co-morbidities (CC)

Complications are conditions that arise during the admission that may require additional treatment and increase the length of stay. Co-morbidities are preexisting conditions that have an impact on the principal condition being treated. Co-morbidities may increase the length of stay for the admission. Complications and co-morbidities affect the level of care required and therefore may increase resources used for the admission. CCs are factored into MS-DRG assignment and may contribute to a higher reimbursement. As published in the CMS Acute Care Hospital Inpatient Payment System Fact Sheet "there are three levels of severity in the MS-DRG based on secondary diagnosis codes:

1) MCC—Major Complication/Comorbidity, which reflects the highest level of severity;
2) CC—Complication/Co-morbidity, which is the next level of severity; and

MS-DRG Listing by MDC			
MDC 1 – Diseases/Disorders of the Nervous System		**MDC 4 – Respiratory System**	
MS-DRG		**MS-DRG**	
020	Intracranial Vascular Procedures W Pdx Hemorrhage W MCC	163	Major Chest Procedures W MCC
021	Intracranial Vascular Procedures W Pdx Hemorrhage W CC	164	Major Chest Procedures W CC
022	Intracranial Vascular Procedures W Pdx Hemorrhage W/O CC/MCC	165	Major Chest Procedures W/O CC/MCC
023	Cranio W Major Dev Impl/Acute Complex Cns Pdx W MCC Or Chemo Implant	166	Other Resp System O.R. Procedures W MCC
024	Cranio W Major Dev Impl/Acute Complex Cns Pdx W/O MCC	167	Other Resp System O.R. Procedures W CC
025	Craniotomy & Endovascular Intracranial Procedures W MCC	168	Other Resp System O.R. Procedures W/O CC/MCC
026	Craniotomy & Endovascular Intracranial Procedures W CC	175	Pulmonary Embolism W MCC
027	Craniotomy & Endovascular Intracranial Procedures W/O CC/MCC	176	Pulmonary Embolism W/O MCC
028	Spinal Procedures W MCC	177	Respiratory Infections & Inflammations W MCC
029	Spinal Procedures W CC Or Spinal Neurostimulators	178	Respiratory Infections & Inflammations W CC
030	Spinal Procedures W/O CC/MCC	179	Respiratory Infections & Inflammations W/O CC/MCC
031	Ventricular Shunt Procedures W MCC	180	Respiratory Neoplasms W MCC
032	Ventricular Shunt Procedures W CC	181	Respiratory Neoplasms W CC
033	Ventricular Shunt Procedures W/O CC/MCC	182	Respiratory Neoplasms W/O CC/MCC
034	Carotid Artery Stent Procedure W MCC	183	Major Chest Trauma W MCC
035	Carotid Artery Stent Procedure W CC	184	Major Chest Trauma W CC
036	Carotid Artery Stent Procedure W/O CC/MCC	185	Major Chest Trauma W/O CC/MCC
037	Extracranial Procedures W MCC	186	Pleural Effusion W MCC
038	Extracranial Procedures W CC	187	Pleural Effusion W CC
039	Extracranial Procedures W/O CC/MCC	188	Pleural Effusion W/O CC/MCC
040	Periph/Cranial Nerve & Other Nerv Syst Proc W MCC	189	Pulmonary Edema & Respiratory Failure
041	Periph/Cranial Nerve & Other Nerv Syst Proc W CC Or Periph Neurostim	190	Chronic Obstructive Pulmonary Disease W MCC
042	Periph/Cranial Nerve & Other Nerv Syst Proc W/O CC/MCC	191	Chronic Obstructive Pulmonary Disease W CC
052	Spinal Disorders & Injuries W CC/MCC	192	Chronic Obstructive Pulmonary Disease W/O CC/MCC
053	Spinal Disorders & Injuries W/O CC/MCC	194	Simple Pneumonia & Pleurisy W CC
054	Nervous System Neoplasms W MCC	194	Simple Pneumonia & Pleurisy W CC
055	Nervous System Neoplasms W/O MCC	195	Simple Pneumonia & Pleurisy W/O CC/MCC
056	Degenerative Nervous System Disorders W MCC	196	Interstitial Lung Disease W MCC
057	Degenerative Nervous System Disorders W/O MCC	197	Interstitial Lung Disease W CC
058	Multiple Sclerosis & Cerebellar Ataxia W MCC	198	Interstitial Lung Disease W/O CC/MCC
059	Multiple Sclerosis & Cerebellar Ataxia W CC	199	Pneumothorax W MCC
060	Multiple Sclerosis & Cerebellar Ataxia W/O CC/MCC	200	Pneumothorax W CC
061	Acute Ischemic Stroke W Use Of Thrombolytic Agent W MCC	201	Pneumothorax W/O CC/MCC
062	Acute Ischemic Stroke W Use Of Thrombolytic Agent W CC	202	Bronchitis & Asthma W CC/MCC
063	Acute Ischemic Stroke W Use Of Thrombolytic Agent W/O CC/MCC	203	Bronchitis & Asthma W/O CC/MCC
064	Intracranial Hemorrhage Or Cerebral Infarction W MCC	204	Respiratory Signs & Symptoms
065	Intracranial Hemorrhage Or Cerebral Infarction W CC	205	Other Respiratory System Diagnoses W MCC
066	Intracranial Hemorrhage Or Cerebral Infarction W/O CC/MCC	206	Other Respiratory System Diagnoses W/O MCC
067	Nonspecific Cva & Precerebral Occlusion W/O Infarct W MCC	207	Respiratory System Diagnosis W Ventilator Support 96+ Hours
068	Nonspecific Cva & Precerebral Occlusion W/O Infarct W/O MCC	208	Respiratory System Diagnosis W Ventilator Support <96 Hours
069	Transient Ischemia		

Figure 13-5 Illustration of MS-DRG categories associated with MDC 1 and MDC 4. *(Modified from www.cms.hhs.gov.)*

Medical and Surgical DRG

MS-DRG 116 (Surgical) MDC 2

Retinal procedures

GMLOS 2.7 AMLOS 4.0 RW 1.1418

Checklist for MS-DRG 116

- ❑ Is the procedure performed for an injury, with CCs? Yes, see MS-DRG 907
- ❑ Is the procedure performed for an injury, without CCs? Yes, see MS-DRG 908, 909
- ❑ Is there significant trauma to a minimum of two body sites? Yes, see MS-DRG 957, 958, 959

Operating Room Procedures

14.21	Destruction of chorioretinal lesion by diathermy
14.22	Destruction of chorioretinal lesion by cryotherapy
14.26	Destruction of chorioretinal lesion by radiation therapy
14.27	Destruction of chorioretinal lesion by implantation of radiation source
14.29	Other destruction of chorioretinal lesion
14.31	Repair of retinal tear by diathermy
14.32	Repair of retinal tear by cryotherapy
14.39	Other repair of retinal tear
14.41	Scleral buckling with implant
14.49	Other scleral buckling
14.51	Repair of retinal detachment with diathermy
14.52	Repair of retinal detachment with cryotherapy
14.53	Repair of retinal detachment with xenon arc photocoagulation

MS-DRG 121 (Medical) MDC 2

Acute major eye infections

GMLOS 4.4 AMLOS 5.6 RW 1.0006

Checklist for MS-DRG 121

- ❑ Is an eye disorder or another complication or comorbidity present in the patient? Yes, see MS-DRG 122

Principal Diagnosis

360.00	Unspecified purulent endophthalmitis
360.01	Acute endophthalmitis
360.02	Panophthalmitis
360.04	Vitreous abscess
360.13	Parasitic endophthalmitis NOS
360.19	Other endophthalmitis
370.00	Unspecified corneal ulcer
370.03	Central corneal ulcer
370.04	Hypopyon ulcer
370.05	Mycotic corneal ulcer
370.06	Perforated corneal ulcer
370.55	Corneal abscess
375.01	Acute dacryoadenitis
375.31	Acute canaliculitis, lacrimal
375.32	Acute dacryocystitis
376.01	Orbital cellulitis
376.02	Orbital periostitis
376.03	Orbital osteomyelitis
376.04	Orbital tenonitis

Figure 13-6 Illustration of surgical and medical DRG within MDC 2. *(Data from www.cms.hhs.gov., 2010.)*

3) Non-CC—Non-Complication/Co-morbidity, which does not significantly affect severity of illness and and resources used."

The major restructuring of the CMS-DRG system involved incorporating these severity levels into each of the 999 MS-DRG categories.

Present on Admission

Present on Admission diagnoses are also an important factor in the MS-DRG system. When completing the CMS-1450 (UB-04) for inpatient cases, present on admission indicators must be recorded. These indicators are utilised in determining the level of severity for the inpatient cases. When the condition is present on admission the level of severity is higher.

BOX 13-11 ■ KEY POINTS

Medicare Severity Diagnosis Related Group (MS-DRG) Variables

Hospital inpatient cases are classified into MS-DRG based on the following variable information:

- Principal and secondary diagnoses
- Principal procedure
- Complications and co-morbidities (CC)
- Age of patient
- Discharge status

Medicare Severity Diagnosis Related Groups (MS-DRG) Assignment

The following basic steps are followed to assign a MS-DRG to a hospital inpatient case.

- Step 1—Determine the correct MDC based on the principal diagnosis.
- Step 2—Determine whether the surgical or medical partition should be followed within the MDC.
- Step 3—Follow the logic through the partition, using information from the patient record to assign the correct MS-DRG. Be sure to identify other MS-DRG variables that affect MS-DRG assignment, such as complications and co-morbidities.

Coding for Medicare Severity Diagnosis Related Groups (MS-DRG) Assignment

MS-DRG were developed based on the patient's condition and resources required to treat the condition. Accurate diagnosis and procedure coding is critical to ensure the correct MS-DRG is assigned. The principal diagnosis is the condition determined after study to be the major, most significant reason for the hospital admission. The principal diagnosis code assigned to the patient case essentially drives the MS-DRG assignment. Inaccurate selection and coding of the principal diagnosis can lead to a MS-DRG assignment that is incorrect, resulting in lost revenue. Figure 13-8 illustrates correct and incorrect MS-DRG assignments for Patient Case 1. Patient Case 1 illustrates the effect of coding the wrong principal diagnosis on the MS-DRG assignment and the dramatic effect on reimbursement. The coder selected COPD as the principal diagnosis and pneumonia for the

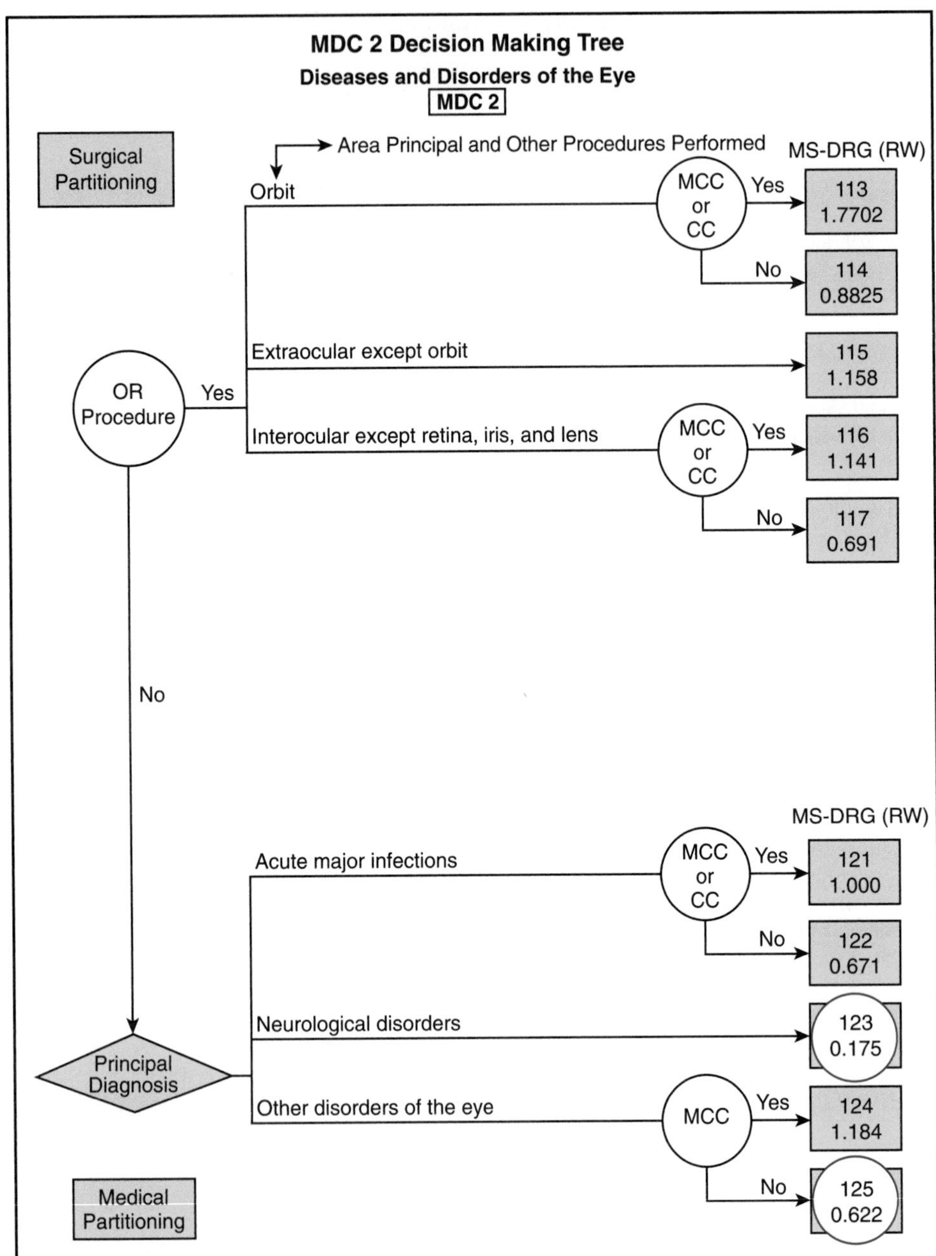

Figure 13-7 Illustration of the decision-making tree for MDC 2 highlights the partitioning, principal, and other diagnoses, complications, co-morbidities, and relative weights assigned to each. The principal diagnosis is used to determine what MDC is associated with the case. *(Modified from Ingenix:* MS-DRG Grouper Version 27.0, *Salt Lake City, UT, 2010.)*

secondary diagnosis. Bronchitis and emphysema were not coded. Based on this coding, MS-DRG 192 is assigned, which reimburses the hospital $2,064.79. Coding pneumonia as the principal diagnosis and emphysema and chronic bronchitis as secondary diagnoses would lead to the correct MS-DRG, 193, which provides reimbursement in the amount of $5,575.44.

Health information management (HIM) coding personnel abstract information from the patient's medical record for the purpose of coding and MS-DRG assignment. HIM coders must follow Inpatient Coding Guidelines as outlined in the ICD-9-CM. Some facilities use a coding worksheet or other form to abstract and code

BOX 13-12 ■ KEY POINTS

Basic Steps to Coding for MS-DRG Assignment

1. Identify and code diagnosis recorded in the patient record.
2. Identify and code significant procedures recorded in the record.
3. Identify the principal diagnosis and procedures.
4. List additional diagnoses and sequence in order of severity, including complications and co-morbidities.
5. Abstract other information required: length of stay, age, sex, discharge status, and birth weight if the patient is a neonate.

MS-DRG Patient Case 1			
Correct MS-DRG Assignment		**Incorrect MS-DRG Assignment**	
MDC 4: Respiratory System		MDC 4: Respiratory System	
Principal Diagnosis	Pneumonia (ICD-9-CM-486)	Principal Diagnosis	COPD (ICD-9-CM-496)
Secondary Diagnosis	Emphysema (ICD-9-CM-492.8)	Secondary Diagnosis	Pneumonia (ICD-9-CM-486)
Secondary Diagnosis	Chronic Bronchitis (ICD-9-CM-491.20)	Secondary Diagnosis	None
Principal Operative	None	Principal Operative	None
Procedure	None	Procedure	None
Secondary Operative	None	Secondary Operative	None
Procedure	None	Procedure	None
Age	69 Years	Age	69 Years
Discharge Status	Routine	Discharge Status	Routine
Sex	Male	Sex	Male
Length of Stay	15 Days	Length of Stay	15 Days
MS-DRG	**193**	MS-DRG	192
Average Length of Stay	4-22 Days	Average Length of Stay	3-19 Days
Rate	**$5,575.44**	Rate	**$2,064.79**

Figure 13-8 How inaccurate coding can lead to an incorrect MS-DRG assignment and incorrect reimbursement. *(Modified from Fordney MT:* Insurance handbook for the medical office, *ed 10, St Louis, 2008, Elsevier.)*

information in the patient's record. Figure 13-9 illustrates a sample coding worksheet. Coding worksheets may include the patient's name, medical record number, race, sex, address, admission date, discharge date, admitting physician, and operating physician name. Most facilities use a computer program called an encoder or grouper for coding and MS-DRG assignment. The following steps are followed in coding for MS-DRG assignment:

- **Step 1**—List diagnoses. Abstract from the patient's medical record all conditions that were treated and those that affect treatment, including complications and co-morbidities. Code conditions abstracted using ICD-9-CM Volumes I and II.
- **Step 2**—List procedures. Abstract from the patient's medical record all significant procedures that were performed during the admission. Code all significant procedures using ICD-9-CM Volume III procedure codes.
- **Step 3**—Identify the principal diagnosis and procedure. The principal diagnosis is the condition determined after study. The principal procedure is the procedure that addresses the principal diagnosis or the one that most closely relates to the principal diagnosis.
- **Step 4**—List additional diagnoses in order of severity. Include complications and co-morbidities.

HEALTH INFORMATION MANAGEMENT
CODING WORKSHEET

DEMOGRAPHICS		
Medical Record Number:	**Bill Type#:**	
Patient Name: Last, First, Middle Init:	Admit Hour Code: Admit Type Code: Admit Source Code:	Discharge Hour Code: Discharge Status Code:
Condition Code (s)	Occurrence Span Code and Date	Value Code and Amount

ADMISSION INFORMATION

Type of Admission: ER Facility Physician Referral Other Unknown

Admitting Diagnosis	**HIM Code(s)**
Principal Diagnosis (Including complications and co-morbidities if applicable)	**HIM Code**
Other Secondary Diagnoses (Including complications and co-morbidities if applicable)	**HIM Code(s)**
Principal Procedure (Significant procedure performed for definitive treatment or that most closely relates to the principal diagnosis) **Date:**	**HIM Code**
Other Significant Procedure(s) **Date:**	**HIM Code(s)**
Medications, supplies, equipment or other item (s) **Date:**	**HIM Code(s)**

DISCHARGE INFORMATION

Home Facility AMA Deceased Other

DRG ASSIGNMENT		APC ASSIGNMENT		
MDC:	Surgical/Medical:			

CONTRIBUTING FACTORS:				
Age	Sex	Discharge Status	Complications/Comorbidities	Birthweight

Questions/Need Clarification:

Figure 13-9 Sample coding worksheet used by Health Information Management (HIM) coding personnel to abstract and code the patient conditions and procedures recorded in the patient record. *(Modified from Davis N, LaCour M:* Introduction to health information technology, *ed 1, St Louis, 2002, Saunders.)*

- **Step 5**—Abstract other information required from the patient's record, including age, sex, discharge status, length of stay, and birth weight if the patient is a neonate.

Grouper Program

MS-DRG assignment is generally performed using a computer program called a "grouper." The **MS-DRG grouper program** is a computer software program designed to use information regarding the patient's condition, treatment, and other factors to follow the logic of the MDC decision-making tree to assign a MS-DRG to the hospital inpatient case, as outlined below:

- **Step 1**—The HIM coding professional enters information about the patient's age, sex, birth weight of

BOX 13-13 ■ KEY POINTS

MS-DRG Grouper

The MS-DRG grouper is a computer program designed to use information regarding the patient's condition, treatment, and other factors to follow the logic of the MDC decision-making tree to assign a MS-DRG to the hospital inpatient case.

a neonate, and discharge status and the number of hospital days. The program uses all information and follows the logic through the decision-making tree to assign a MS-DRG for the hospital inpatient case.

- **Step 2**—The HIM coding professional enters basic information and the principal diagnosis and all other diagnoses, including complications and co-morbidities. The program assigns the MDC based on the principal diagnosis.
- **Step 3**—The HIM coding professional enters the significant procedures (principal and other procedures) for the hospital inpatient case. The program determines whether the medical or surgical partition should be followed.

Figures 13-10 and 13-11 illustrate MS-DRG assignment using the Clinical Coding Expert, a computer program designed to provide correct and accurate reimbursement to each acute care facility in the United States. The figures illustrate the correct and incorrect MS-DRG assignments discussed earlier in this chapter, MS-DRG Patient Case 1 (see Figure 13-8). This program used a test national average calculation to calculate reimbursement for this example.

OUTPATIENT PROSPECTIVE PAYMENT SYSTEM (OPPS)

The implementation of the IPPS in 1983 proved to be successful in helping to control costs and in increasing provider incentives to manage care more efficiently. Since implementation of the IPPS, the focus has shifted to the development and implementation of a PPS for hospital outpatient services, as mandated in the BBA of 1997. The BBA of 1997 required CMS to replace the existing cost-based outpatient payment system with a PPS for hospital outpatient services. The Medicare OPPS was implemented in August of 2000. Legislation leading to the implementation of Medicare's PPS is outlined in Table 13-1.

The **Outpatient Prospective Payment System (OPPS)** was implemented in August 2000 by CMS to provide reimbursement for hospital outpatient services, including hospital-based ambulatory surgery. The system implemented under OPPS is known as Ambulatory Payment Classifications (APC). Payments under OPPS are predetermined fixed amounts, based on the service or procedure performed. This system encourages hospitals to control costs for the delivery of outpatient and ambulatory surgery care because payments are a set amount, regardless of the total charges accrued. As discussed earlier in this chapter, PPS Systems were implemented to control the rising cost of health care. Since implementation of the OPPS payment system for Medicare, other government and private payers have adopted similar systems. In order to understand services reimbursed under OPPS, it is necessary to differentiate between hospital-based outpatient services and non–hospital-based services.

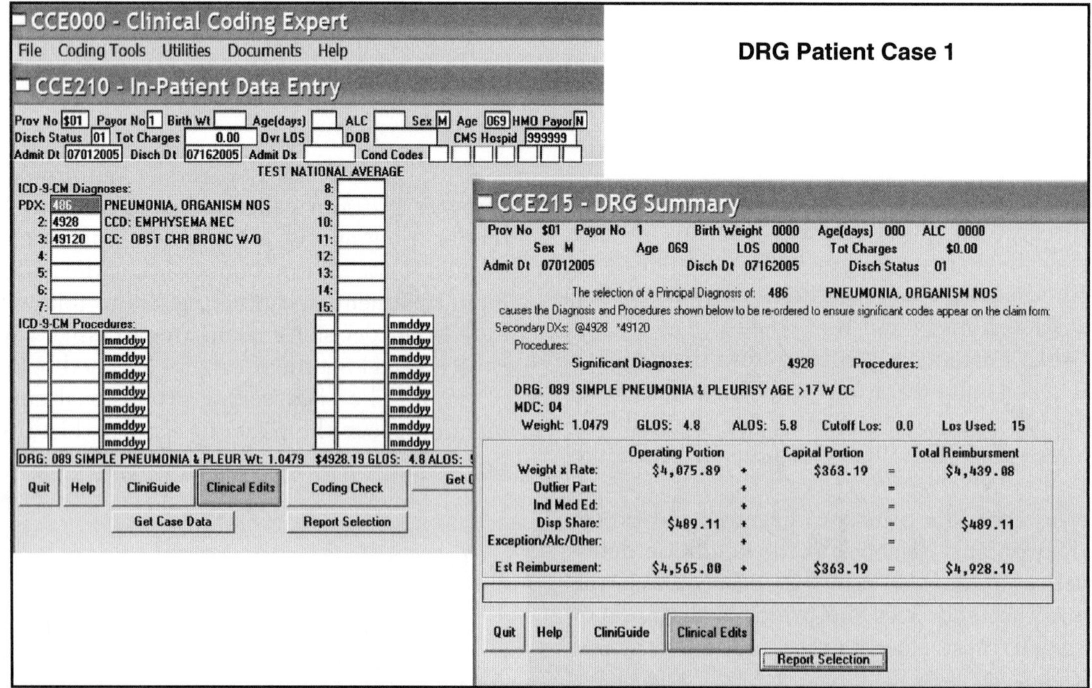

Figure 13-10 Correct DRG assignment. *(Screen shot from Clinical Coding Expert [CCE], used with permission from Innovative Health Solutions, LLC, www.ihsinfo.com/myihs.)*

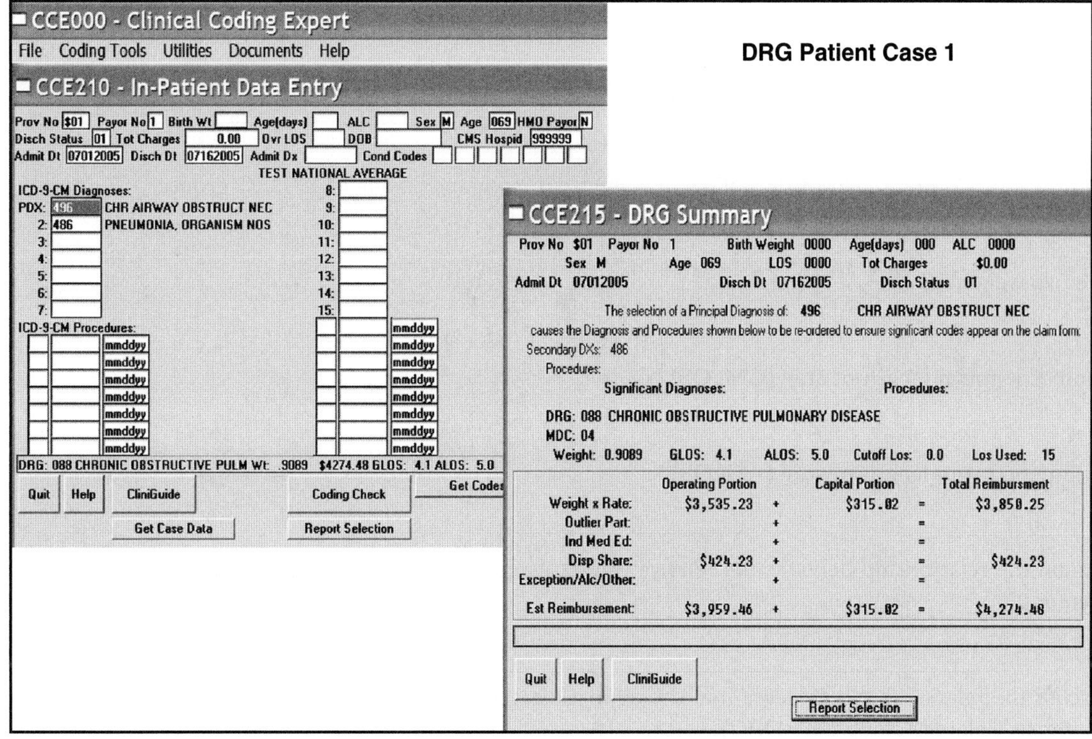

Figure 13-11 Incorrect DRG assignment. *(Screen shot from Clinical Coding Expert [CCE], used with permission from Innovative Health Solutions, LLC, www.ihsinfo.com/myihs.)*

BOX 13-14 ■ KEY POINTS

Outpatient Prospective Payment System (OPPS)

- The OPPS was implemented by CMS to provide reimbursement for hospital outpatient services, including ambulatory surgery performed in a hospital-based ambulatory surgery center (ASC).
- Payments under OPPS are predetermined fixed amounts, based on the service or procedure performed.

Hospital Outpatient Services

Outpatient services are those provided to patients who are not admitted to the hospital for an inpatient stay; the patient is released the same day. Outpatient services are provided by many different providers, such as physicians, chiropractors, social workers, and physical therapists. Services are provided in a variety of outpatient areas such as a clinic, imaging center, and ASC. Hospitals are also providers of many outpatient services. Hospital outpatient services are provided in many different areas such as a clinic, laboratory, imaging or ambulatory surgery center (ASC), Emergency Department, and many ancillary departments. Outpatient service providers and hospital-based outpatient service areas are illustrated in Figure 13-12. Many hospitals today have hospital-based outpatient service areas such as the following:

- Primary care physician office
- Urgent care or walk-in clinic
- Imaging center
- ASC
- Ancillary departments

Outpatient Service Providers

Physician
Chiropractor
Social worker
Physical therapist

Clinic (urgent care, walk in)
Laboratory
Imaging center
Ambulatory surgery center
Rehabilitation center

Hospital-Based Outpatient Service Areas

Physician office
Clinic (urgent care, primary care, walk in)
Laboratory
Imaging center
Ambulatory surgery center
Rehabilitation center
Emergency Department
Observation
(ancillary department such as Radiology, Pathology/Laboratory)

Figure 13-12 Outpatient service providers and hospital-based outpatient service areas.

TEST YOUR *Knowledge* BOX 13-3

MS-DRG: STRUCTURE, ASSIGNMENT, AND CODING

Provide an explanation of each of the following, which are assigned to each MS-DRG group:

1. Relative weight (RW)
2. Geometric mean length of stay (GMLOS)
3. Arithmetic mean length of stay (AMLOS)
4. Explain the relationship between the relative weight assigned to a MS-DRG and the MS-DRG payment.
5. Discuss the relationship between a major diagnostic category (MDC) and a Medicare Severity Diagnosis Related Group (MS-DRG).
6. Describe how MS-DRGs are further categorized within each MDC.
7. Explain the purpose of the decision-making tree within the MDC.
8. Describe when the surgical or the medical partitions within an MDC are followed.
9. List the variable information used to classify hospital inpatient cases into MS-DRG groups.
10. Discuss the effect that complications and co-morbidities have on MS-DRG assignment.
11. Discuss the three basic steps in assigning a MS-DRG.
12. How is the MDC determined?
13. State what form(s) and software may be used by a hospital for coding and MS-DRG assignment.
14. What coding systems are used to describe procedures and diagnoses for inpatient cases?
15. Provide a description of the grouper, and explain its relationship to MS-DRG assignment.

Historically all surgical procedures were performed in a hospital setting, typically on an inpatient basis. Medical advances improved the performance of surgical procedures in several ways:

- New techniques are less invasive
- Less-invasive procedures minimize the risk for infection and complications
- The recovery period is greatly reduced

Improvements in anesthesia and other pharmaceuticals minimize risk and reduce recovery time. These advances, combined with efforts to provide more efficient health care, led to the performance of same day surgeries, commonly referred to as ambulatory surgery. **Ambulatory surgery** is defined as surgery performed on a patient who is released the same day. Specialty facilities called Ambulatory Surgery Centers (ASC) were created to provide ambulatory surgery services.

Ambulatory Surgery Center (ASC)

An **ambulatory surgery center (ASC)** is a facility designed for the sole purpose of providing ambulatory surgery services. ASC can be hospital-based or independent facilities. It is imperative for hospital billing and coding personnel to understand the difference between a hospital-based ASC and an independent ASC, because different billing and coding rules apply and reimbursement is based on different payment systems.

Hospital-Based Ambulatory Surgery Centers

Hospital-based ASC are affiliated with or owned by a hospital. They may be freestanding or located within the hospital. ASCs are generally included in the hospital's cost reports, unless it has been legally structured as an independent ASC. Table 13-3 illustrates the differences between a hospital-based ASC and an independent ASC.

Medicare reimburses hospitals for all outpatient services under the OPPS APC, including ambulatory surgeries. Medicare and other payers require claims to be submitted via the UB-04 (CMS-1450) claim form. HCPCS and ICD-9-CM Volume I and II diagnosis codes are required for submission of outpatient claims.

Independent Ambulatory Surgery Centers

Independent ASCs are not hospital based or associated (legally or financially) with a hospital as outlined in Table 13-3. Because they are not hospital based, they are not included in a hospital's costs reports. Independent ASC are typically freestanding facilities that are privately owned. They are incorporated and structured within the legal definitions of an independent ASC. Independent ASC are required to obtain an employer identification number (also referred to as a tax identification number [TIN]) from the U.S. Internal Revenue Service (IRS).

Independent ASC are reimbursed by Medicare according to ASC payment groups. Although ASC payment groups are based on predetermined fixed payments for ambulatory surgeries, they are not incorporated under the OPPS. It is anticipated that reimbursement for freestanding ASC will be included under the OPPS in the near future. Many payers require

TABLE 13-3 Ambulatory Surgery Center (ASC)

Hospital-Based Ambulatory Surgery Center	Independent Ambulatory Surgery Center
Structure	
Hospital-affiliated or hospital-owned ambulatory surgery center (ASC) ASC can be located within the hospital, or it can be freestanding, but hospital based Legal arrangement determines whether the hospital qualifies for true freestanding ASC status—as an independent facility	Not integrated as part of the hospital Independent facility that offers ambulatory surgical services or day surgery Self-funded; not associated directly with a hospital Not included in hospital's cost reports
Billing and Coding	
Medicare and other payers require claims for ambulatory surgery to be submitted on the CMS-1450 (UB-04) claim form. HCPCS codes are required for reporting services, procedures and items. ICD-9-CM codes are required to report the patient's condition(s).	Some payers require claims to be submitted on the CMS-1450 (UB-04) claim form. Other payers may require claims to be submitted on the CMS-1500. HCPCS codes are generally required for reporting services, procedures and items. ICD-9-CM codes are required to report the patient's condition(s).
Reimbursement	
Billed and reimbursed as an outpatient hospital department Reimbursed under Hospital Outpatient Prospective Payment System (OPPS) under the Ambulatory Payment Classification (APC)	Independent freestanding ASC are reimbursed based on Medicare's "ASC List," which includes nine payment groups Reimbursed according to ASC payment groups

TEST YOUR *Knowledge* BOX 13-4

OUTPUTPATIENT PROSPECTIVE PAYMENT SYSTEMS (OPPS) AND HOSPITAL OUTPATIENT SERVICES

1. What legislation mandated the implementation of an Outpatient Prospective Payment System (OPPS)?
2. When was the OPPS implemented by CMS?
3. What services are reimbursed under OPPS?
4. How does the OPPS encourage providers to control cost of delivery of outpatient services?
5. Provide a brief description of outpatient services.
6. Define ambulatory surgery.
7. Describe a hospital-based ambulatory surgery center (ASC).
8. State the difference between hospital-based and independent ASCs.
9. Reimbursement for a hospital-based ASC is made under what payment system?
10. State the payment system used to reimburse independent ambulatory surgery centers (ASC).

independent ASCs to submit claims on a CMS-1500 form, using HCPCS codes to report services and procedures and ICD-9-CM Volumes I and II diagnosis codes to report patient conditions.

OUTPATIENT PROSPECTIVE PAYMENT SYSTEM (OPPS) AMBULATORY PAYMENT CLASSIFICATIONS (APC)

CMS published the final rule in the *Federal Register* regarding implementation of the OPPS on April 7, 2000, as illustrated in Figure 13-13. The payment system implemented by CMS under the OPPS in August 2000 is called Ambulatory Payment Classifications (APC). The **Ambulatory Payment Classification (APC)** is the OPPS implemented by CMS to provide reimbursement for hospital outpatient services. Under APC, the facility is paid a fixed fee based on the resources utilized to provide the service or procedure. Figure 13-14 outlines services covered under OPPS APC:

- Outpatient services (all services provided in hospital outpatient areas, including ambulatory surgeries)
- Certain Part B services furnished to hospital inpatients who have no Part A coverage
- Partial hospitalization services furnished by community mental health centers (CMHC)

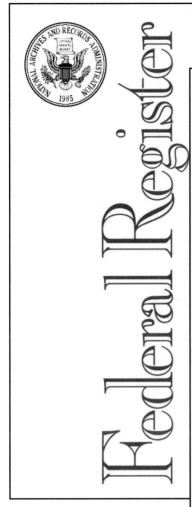

Friday,
April 7, 2000

18434 Federal Register / Vol. 65, No. 68 / Friday, April 7, 2000 / Rules and Regulations

DEPARTMENT OF HEALTH AND HUMAN SERVICES

Health Care Financing Administration

42 CFR Parts 409, 410, 411, 412, 413, 419, 424, 489, 498, and 1003

[HCFA–1005–FC]

RIN 0938–AI56

Office of Inspector General; Medicare Program; Prospective Payment System for Hospital Outpatient Services

AGENCY: Health Care Financing Administration (HCFA), HHS, and Office of Inspector General (OIG), HHS.

ACTION: Final rule with comment period.

SUMMARY: This final rule with comment period implements a prospective payment system for hospital outpatient services furnished to Medicare beneficiaries, as set forth in section 1833(t) of the Social Security Act. It also establishes requirements for provider departments and provider-based entities, and it implements section 9343(c) of the Omnibus Budget Reconciliation Act of 1986, which prohibits Medicare payment for nonphysician services furnished to a hospital outpatient by a provider or supplier other than a hospital, unless the services are furnished under an arrangement with the hospital. In addition, this rule establishes in regulations the extension of reductions in payment for costs of hospital outpatient services required by section 4522 of the Balanced Budget Act of 1997, as amended by section 201(k) of the Balanced Budget Refinement Act of 1999.

DATES: *Effective date:* July 1, 2000, except that the changes to § 412.24(d)(6), new § 413.65, and the changes to § 489.24(h), § 498.2, and § 498.3 are effective October 10, 2000.

Applicability date: For Medicare services furnished by all hospitals, including hospitals excluded from the inpatient prospective payment system, and by community mental health centers, the applicability date for implementation of the hospital outpatient prospective payment system is July 1, 2000.

Comment date: Comments on the provisions of this rule resulting from the Balanced Budget Refinement Act of 1999 will be considered if we receive them at the appropriate address, as provided below, no later than 5 p.m. on June 6, 2000. We will not consider comments concerning provisions that remain unchanged from the September 8, 1998 proposed rule or that were revised based on public comment.

See section VIII for a more detailed discussion of the provisions subject to comment.

ADDRESSES: Mail written comments (one original and three copies) to the following address ONLY: Health Care Financing Administration, Department of Health and Human Services, Attention: HCFA–1005–FC, P.O. Box 8013, Baltimore, MD 21244–8013.

If you prefer, you may deliver, by courier, your written comments (one original and three copies) to one of the following addresses:

Room 443–G, Hubert H. Humphrey Building, 200 Independence Avenue, SW., Washington, DC 20201, or

C5–14–03, Central Building, 7500 Security Boulevard, Baltimore, MD 21244–1850.

Comments mailed to those addresses may be delayed and could be considered late.

Because of staffing and resource limitations, we cannot accept comments by facsimile (FAX) transmission. In commenting, please refer to file code HCFA–1005–FC.

Comments received timely will be available for public inspection as they are received, generally beginning approximately 3 weeks after publication of a document, in Room 443–G of the Department's offices at 200 Independence Avenue, SW., Washington, DC, on Monday through Friday of each week from 8:30 a.m. to 5 p.m. (Phone (202) 690–7890).

For comments that relate to information collection requirements, mail a copy of comments to:

Health Care Financing Administration, Office of Information Services, Security and Standards Group, Division of HCFA Enterprise Standards, Room N2–14–26, 7500 Security Boulevard, Baltimore, MD 21244–1850, Attn: John Burke, HCFA–1005–FC; and

Lauren Oliven, HCFA Desk Officer, Office of Information and Regulatory Affairs, Room 3001, New Executive Office Building, Washington, DC 20503.

Copies: To order copies of the **Federal Register** containing this document, send your request to: New Orders, Superintendent of Documents, P.O. Box 371954, Pittsburgh, PA 15250–7954. Specify the date of the issue requested and enclose a check or money order payable to the Superintendent of Documents, or enclose your Visa or Master Card number and expiration date. Credit card orders can also be placed by calling the order desk at (202) 512–1800 or by faxing to (202) 512–2250. The cost for each copy is $8. As an alternative, you can view and photocopy the **Federal Register** document at most libraries designated as Federal Depository Libraries and at many other public and academic libraries throughout the country that receive the **Federal Register**.

FOR FURTHER INFORMATION CONTACT:

Janet Wellham, (410) 786–4510 or Chuck Braver, (410) 786–6719 (for general information)

Joel Schaer (OIG), (202) 619–0089 (for information concerning civil money penalties)

Kitty Ahern, (410) 786–4515 (for information related to the classification of services into ambulatory payment classification (APC) groups)

George Morey (410) 786–4653 (for information related to the determination of provider-based status)

Janet Samen (410) 786–9161 (for information on the application of APCs to community mental health centers)

SUPPLEMENTARY INFORMATION: To assist readers in referencing sections contained in this document, we are providing the following table of contents. Within each section, we summarize pertinent material from our proposed rule of September 8, 1998 (63 FR 47552) followed by public comments and our responses.

Table of Contents

Figure 13-13 *Federal Register,* Volume 65, No. 68, highlighting provisions of the final rule for implementation of the Hospital Outpatient Prospective Payment System (HOPPS). *(From the U.S. Federal Register, www.gpoaccess.gov/fr/index.html.)*

- Specified services and supplies provided by comprehensive outpatient rehabilitation facilities (CORF)
- Specified supplies furnished by home health agencies (HHA).

Reimbursement under the APC system is a fixed predetermined payment based on national median cost for procedures. The APC payment represents the total payment to the hospital, which includes the patient's coinsurance amount. Hospitals may receive payment for services rendered under multiple APC. Information regarding payment for multiple APC is discussed later in this chapter.

Ambulatory Payment Classification (APC) Development

The Health Care Financing Administration (HCFA), now known as CMS, was responsible for the development and implementation of the OPPS. APC is the

Ambulatory Payment Classifications (APC) Covered Services

Outpatient services (ambulatory surgeries and other services provided in hospital outpatient departments) such as:

- Medical clinic and emergency department visits
- Radiology procedures (some paid separately)
- Diagnostic services and tests
- Surgical pathology
- Observation services (for patients who meet specific criteria)
- Specific dental procedures
- Surgical and medical procedures
- Medical and surgical supplies and equipment (not integral to providing the service).

Certain Part B services furnished to hospital inpatients who have no Part A coverage.

Partial hospitalization services furnished by community mental health centers (CMHC).

Specified services and supplies provided by comprehensive outpatient rehabilitation facilities (CORF).

Specified supplies furnished by home health agencies (HHAs).

Figure 13-14 Hospital outpatient services covered under Ambulatory Payment Classifications (APC). *(Data from Ingenix:* APC expert, *Eden Prairie, Minn., 2005, Ingenix.)*

BOX 13-15 ■ key points

Ambulatory Surgery Center (ASC)

ASCs are facilities designed for the sole purpose of providing ambulatory surgery services.

- Hospital-based—owned by or affiliated with a hospital; may be freestanding or located within the hospital. Hospital-based ASCs are included in the hospital's cost reports and are reimbursed under the OPPS Ambulatory Payment Classification (APC).
- Independent—privately owned, freestanding facility that is structured in accordance with laws that define independent ASCs and is assigned its own Employer Identification Number. Reimbursement is determined under ASC payment groups.

OPPS system implemented by CMS. The system provides reimbursement based on the procedure performed, unlike the MS-DRG system, in which reimbursement is determined based on the patient's condition and treatment. Similar to the MS-DRG system, APC payment rates are determined based on the analysis of a large number of actual hospital outpatient claims. The development of the APC payment system began with a classification system called Ambulatory Patient Groups (APG). The APG classification system used actual hospital outpatient data for analysis and development of groups of procedures and services that were clinically similar and that required similar resources. Criteria set by CMS for grouping procedures and services into APC groups included:

BOX 13-16 ■ KEY POINTS

Ambulatory Payment Classification (APC)

The APC system is the Outpatient Prospective Payment System (OPPS) used by Medicare to provide reimbursement for hospital outpatient services. The APC system provides a predetermined fixed payment based on the service provided.

APC are assigned based in the service, procedure, or item provided.

APC Development

Development of APC began with Ambulatory Patient Groups (APG). The APG classification system used actual hospital outpatient data for analysis and development of groups of procedures and services that were clinically similar and that required similar resources. These groups are Ambulatory Payment Classifications.

APC Development Criteria

Criteria set by CMS for grouping procedures and services into APC involved:

- Clinical similarity
- Resource similarity
- Provider concentration
- Service frequency
- Upcoding and code fragmentation

Clinical Similarity: Procedures within each APC group should be similar clinically and relate to the same or a similar organ system. Procedures and services within the group require comparable treatment methods, and the level of complexity for treatment is similar.

Resource Similarity: Procedures or services included in an APC group require a comparable level of hospital resources to provide the service or perform the procedure.

Provider Concentration: Determination of payment levels for services provided by a limited number of hospitals. CMS created separate APC groups for services and procedures that are performed by a limited number of hospitals.

Service Frequency: Separate APC groups were not created for services and procedures that were not performed frequently. Codes representing services performed infrequently were assigned to the APC groups that were comparable based on resource use and clinical similarities.

Upcoding and Code Fragmentation: The APC groups are defined to limit opportunities to increase payments through minor upcoding. For example, if unique APC groups existed for excising a lesion of 1.0 cm on the arm (Current Procedural Terminology [CPT] code 11401) and a lesion of 1.1 cm (CPT code 11402), an incentive would exist to exaggerate the size of lesions to receive higher payment. APC groups were defined to capture resource consumption and clinical similarities. CMS groups similar procedures such as CPT 11401 and 11402 into the same APC group. CMS kept the APC groups as broad and inclusive as possible, without sacrificing resources or clinical similarity, to minimize the opportunity for upcoding. In general, nonspecific HCPCS codes (e.g., 20999, "unlisted procedure, musculoskeletal system, general") were assigned to the lowest-paying APC group with consistent clinical characteristics.

CMS classified outpatient procedures and services, represented by HCPCS codes, into more than 600 APC groups. Analysis of actual hospital outpatient data provided a basis for the conversion of billed charges to a median cost for each group. APC group payments were determined based on the following elements:

Relative weight (RW): An RW is assigned to each APC group by CMS that represents the relative value of resources used to provide the service or procedure.

Regional wage index: Regional differences are captured by incorporating the regional wage index into the formula used to calculate the national payment rate.

Conversion factor (CF): The CF is a national dollar amount, determined by CMS, used to convert the RW into an APC payment amount. The RW is multiplied by the CF to establish APC payment amounts.

Services and procedures included within the group: Annual review of services and procedures is performed to reflect new procedures, services, and items.

Once the classification system was used to group clinically similar services and procedures, each APC group was assigned an RW. The RW reflects the median

TEST YOUR *Knowledge* BOX 13-5

AMBULATORY PAYMENT CLASSIFICATIONS (APC) AND AMBULATORY PAYMENT CLASSIFICATION (APC) DEVELOPMENT

1. State the name of the Outpatient Prospective Payment System (OPPS) implemented by CMS.
2. When was the APC system implemented?
3. List the services that are covered under OPPS.
4. Describe reimbursement under APC.
5. Can a hospital receive payment for multiple APC?
6. What is the basis of payment under the APC system?
7. How does the basis of payment vary between the DRG and APC systems?
8. List four criteria required by Medicare in the development of the APC system.
9. How did CMS minimize the opportunity for upcoding and fragmentation in the development of the APC classification system?
10. Explain the purpose of the relative weight assigned to each APC group.

cost of providing the service, including operating and capital costs of services and procedures within the APC group. RWs for each APC group are used to calculate the actual national APC payment rate for the group. National payment rates established for each group are wage adjusted to reflect geographic differences. CMS performs annual reviews and updates of the system that are implemented on January 1 of following year. However, changes, deletions, and additions may be made on a quarterly basis.

BOX 13-17 ■ KEY POINTS

Elements of Ambulatory Payment Classification (APC)

APC group payments were determined based on the following elements:

- Relative weight (RW)
- Regional wage index
- Conversion factor (CF)
- Services and procedures included within the group

Ambulatory Payment Classification (APC) Payment Calculations

Payment rates under the APC system are referred to as APC payments. The payment rate under each APC is determined by multiplying the RW for the APC by a CF. The CF is determined annually by CMS in accordance with federal regulations, and taking into account budgetary constraints. The conversion factor is a dollar amount used to translate the RW assigned to the APC into a national payment rate for the APC group. Geographic differences are considered, using a hospital wage index published annually in the Federal Register. Figure 13-15 illustrates the basic formula used to calculate an APC group payment. The APC payment rate of $42.61 in APC 0012 represents the total payment amount the hospital will receive and includes the patient's co-payment amount. APC payment rates and conversion factors are updated annually for use effective January 1 of the following year.

APC #0012 — **Relative Weight 0.7477**, **Conversion factor $56.989**

RW × CF = APC Payment

Relative weight (×) conversion factor = APC Payment

0.7477 × $56.989 = $42.61

Medicare payment =	$31.43
National unadjusted copayment =	$11.18
Total payment =	$42.61

Figure 13-15 APC payment calculations. *(Data from Ingenix:* APC expert, *Eden Prairie, Minn., 2005, Ingenix.)*

Ambulatory Payment Classification (APC) Outliers

APC outliers are outpatient cases that involve patient conditions and circumstances that result in higher cost for the hospital to perform the procedure or service—a cost that is in excess of the APC payment rate. Under the APC system, hospitals may receive additional payment for outlier situations when the costs for the case exceed 2.6 times the APC payment amount. Payment to hospitals for outlier situations is the full APC payment rate plus an additional payment that equals 50% of the costs exceeding 2.6 times the APC payment rate.

BOX 13-18 ■ KEY POINTS

Ambulatory Payment Classification (APC) Outliers

Outliers involve patient conditions and circumstances that result in higher cost for the hospital to perform the procedure or service—a cost that is in excess of the APC payment rate.

A hospital may receive additional payment under the APC system for outlier situations when the costs for the case exceed 2.6 times the APC payment amount.

APC payment for outlier situations is the full APC payment rate plus an additional payment that equals 50% of the costs exceeding 2.6 times the APC payment

Ambulatory Payment Classification (APC) Transitional Pass-Through Payments

Transitional pass-through payments provide hospitals with additional payment under the OPPS APC payment system for certain drugs, devices, or biologicals that are considered "new technologies." HCPCS codes for these items are assigned to APC Group #0738. APC transitional pass-through payments provide reimbursement at the rate of 95% of the average wholesale price of the new drug or item.

Ambulatory Payment Classification (APC) Structure

The APC classification system contained over 800 APC payment groups in 2006. Each APC payment group is represented by a four-digit number such as 0012. HCPCS codes representing services, procedures, and items are categorized into the APC payment groups. APC groups can be classified based on the following categories of service: Surgical, Significant Procedure, Medical, Ancillary, Partial Hospitalization, and Transitional Pass-Through Services and Drugs.

BOX 13-19 ■ KEY POINTS

Ambulatory Payment Classification (APC) Structure

- Each APC payment group is represented by a four-digit number, such as 0012.
- HCPCS Level I and II procedure codes are categorized into the APC payment groups.
- APC group classifications are grouped based on categories of services.

Ambulatory Payment Classification (APC) Categories

All services, procedures, and items performed in a hospital outpatient setting are classified into one of the following APC categories, as outlined in Figure 13-16:

1. **Surgical APC.** A significant procedure is one that is: 1. surgical in nature, or 2. carries a procedural risk, or 3. carries an anesthetic risk, or 4. requires specialized training, as defined in The Uniform Hospital Discharge Data Set (UHDDS), Item 12. Surgical procedures are significant procedures. Surgical procedures performed in a hospital outpatient setting are reimbursed based on Surgical APCs. Surgical APCs are assigned based on the CPT code representing the most comprehensive procedure performed. For example: repair of a rotator cuff, 23410, is assigned to APC 0052, as illustrated in Figure 13-16.
2. **Significant Procedures.** Nonsurgical significant procedures that are performed on an outpatient basis are reimbursed based on significant procedure APCs. For example: "Intralesional chemotherapy administration" coded 96405 is assigned to APC 0116.
3. **Medical.** Outpatient medical visits to a hospital-based setting such as an Emergency Department or hospital-based clinic for care not involving a significant procedure are paid based on Medical APCs. The Medical APC is determined by site of service and the level of resources required for treatment of the patient's condition. For example, a medical visit for an eye examination, code 92004, is assigned to APC 0602.
4. **Ancillary.** Departments such as Radiology, Rehabilitation, and Laboratory are considered ancillary departments, and they perform various ancillary services such as an X-ray examination, physical therapy, or a complete blood count. Outpatient services

APC Categories

APC Assignment Based on HCPCS Code

HCPCS	SI	CI	Description	APC	Relative Weight	Payment Rate	National Unadjusted Copayment	Minimum Unadjusted Copayment
Surgical APC								
11402	T		Exc ben lesion + marg 1.1-2 cm	0019	4.1481	246.86	71.87	49.37
14040	T		Adjacent Tissue Transfer	0686	13.4973	803.24		160.65
14060	T		Skin tissue rearrangement	0027	18.1956	1,082.84	329.72	216.57
19120	T		Removal of breast lesion	0028	19.4351	1,156.60	303.74	231.32
23410	T		Repair rotator cuff, acute	0052	43.5754	2483.06		496.61
Significant Procedure APC–Non Invasive								
96410	S		Chemotherapy, infusion method	0017	2.9533	168.29	42.54	33.66
Medical APC								
92004	V		Eye exam, new patient	0602	1.3977	79.65		15.93
Ancillary APC								
71552	S		MRI chest w/o & w/dye	0337	8.5070	506.26	202.50	101.25
72010	X		X-ray exam of spine	0261	1.3351	76.08		15.22
72052	X		X-ray exam, neck spine	0261	1.2416	73.89		14.78
73721	S		MRI jnt of lwr extre w/o dye	0336	5.8678	349.20	139.68	69.84
Partial Hospitalization APC								
G0176	P		OPPS/PHP; activity therapy	0033	4.9370	281.33		56.27
Transitional Pass-Through APC								
J2783	G		Rasburicase	0738		106.04		21.21

Figure 13-16 Services are categorized into one of the APC groups illustrated based on the procedure code assigned. *(Data from Ingenix: APC expert, Eden Prairie, Minn., 2005, Ingenix, and Centers for Medicare & Medicaid Services, Hospital outpatient PPS, 2005.)*

provided by ancillary departments are reimbursed based on Ancillary APCs. An example of an ancillary service is an X-ray examination of the spine, code 72010, which is assigned to APC 0261.

5. **Partial Hospitalization.** Services provided in a CMHC that are considered partial hospitalization services are reimbursed based on Partial hospitalization APCs. For example: Partial Hospitalization activity therapy, code G1076, is assigned to APC 0033.
6. **Transitional Pass-Through Services and Drugs.** Services, drugs, and medical devices that are new and therefore not considered in APC payment groups are reimbursed separately based on Transitional Pass-Through APCs. An example is Rasburicase, which is a drug represented by code J2783, and it is assigned to APC 0738.

BOX 13-20 ■ key points

Ambulatory Payment Classification (APC) Categories

- Surgical
- Significant Procedures
- Medical
- Ancillary
- Partial Hospitalization
- Transitional Pass-Through Services and Drugs

APC groups include HCPCS codes that are assigned to the group and all relative information, as outlined in Table 13-4. For example, APC 0012 lists HCPCS codes and descriptions of procedures and services assigned to the group:

TABLE 13-4 Ambulatory Payment Classification (APC) 0012

CPT/HCPCS	SI	Description	APC	Relative Weight	Payment Rate	National Unadjusted Co-payment	Minimum Unadjusted Co-payment
11001	T	**Debride infected skin add-on**	**0012**	**0.7477**	**42.61**	**11.18**	**8.52**
11055	T	Trim skin lesion	0012	0.7477	42.61	11.18	8.52
11056	T	Trim skin lesions, 2 to 4	0012	0.7477	42.61	11.18	8.52
11300	T	Shave skin lesion	0012	0.7477	42.61	11.18	8.52
11301	T	**Shave skin lesion**	**0012**	**0.7477**	**42.61**	**11.18**	**8.52**
11732	T	Remove nail plate, add-on	0012	0.7477	42.61	11.18	8.52
11900	T	Injection into skin lesions	0012	0.7477	42.61	11.18	8.52
11901	T	Added skin lesions injection	0012	0.7477	42.61	11.18	8.52
15788	T	Chemical peel, face, epiderm	0012	0.7477	42.61	11.18	8.52
15793	T	Chemical peel, nonfacial	0012	0.7477	42.61	11.18	8.52
16000	T	Initial treatment of burn(s)	0012	0.7477	42.61	11.18	8.52
17340	T	**Cryotherapy of skin**	**0012**	**0.7477**	**42.61**	**11.18**	**8.52**
54056	T	Cryosurgery, penis lesion(s)	0012	0.7477	42.61	11.18	8.52
69220	T	Clean out mastoid cavity	0012	0.7477	42.61	11.18	8.52

Data from Ingenix: APC expert, *Eden Prairie, Minn., 2005, Ingenix, and Centers for Medicare & Medicaid Services, Hospital outpatient PPS, 2005.*

11001 Debride infected skin add-on
11301 Shave skin lesion
17340 Cryotherapy of skin

APC groups are assigned an RW, payment rate, and a national unadjusted co-payment and minimum unadjusted co-payment amount as outlined in APC 0012:

- RW is 0.7477.
- Payment rate is $42.61—The payment rate is the total amount the hospital will receive from Medicare and the patient.
- National unadjusted co-payment amount for APC 0012 is $11.18.
- Minimum unadjusted co-payment amount for APC 0012 is $8.52.

Hospitals are required to collect at least the minimum co-payment amount, which represents 20% of the APC payment $42.61.

The Medicare payment for APC 0012 made to the hospital is $31.43, which represents the payment rate of $42.61 less the national unadjusted co-payment amount of $11.18.

Ambulatory Payment Classification (APC) Packaged Services

Each APC payment group bundles or packages all services and items that are directly related and integral to the performance of the procedure or service. The resources (costs) for bundled items are included in the APC group payment rate. The following are examples of services and items packaged into APC groups. Packaged services are not separately payable.

- Use of the recovery room
- Use of an observation bed (other than in the specific situations)
- Drugs, biologicals, and other pharmaceuticals; medical and surgical supplies and equipment; surgical dressings, splints, casts, and other devices used for reduction of fractures or dislocations
- Supplies and equipment used for administering and monitoring anesthesia or sedation
- Intraocular lenses (IOLs) and several other designated implants

Ambulatory Payment Classification (APC) Payment Status Indicators (SI)

Each HCPCS code listed within an APC payment group is assigned a payment status indicator that explains how the service, procedure, or item is paid, potentially discounted, or not paid under the OPPS APC system. Table 13-5 lists payment status indicators, descriptions, and explanation of payment under OPPS. Several examples of status indicators are as follows:

Status indicator C: HCPCS codes with a status indicator C represent procedures that are not paid under OPPS, in accordance with Medicare Inpatient Only Procedure guidelines as discussed in the next section.

Status indicator E: HCPCS codes with status indicator E are non-covered procedures, services, or items that are not reported in a hospital outpatient setting, as outlined in Figure 13-17. Some of the services listed may be payable under other payment systems.

Status indicator G or H: HCPCS codes with status indicator G or H represent items that can result in an additional reimbursement under a transitional pass-through APC group.

Status indicator N: HCPCS codes with status indicator N represent procedures, services, or items that are incidental and packaged into the APC group payment and are not separately billable as discussed previously.

Status indicator T: HCPCS codes with a status indicator T represent procedures that are reimbursed in accordance with Multiple Procedure Reduction guidelines, discussed in the following section.

Ambulatory Payment Classifications (APC) Non-Covered Services

Some services are paid under other payment systems, such as fee schedules. These services are not paid as part of the APC amount and are considered excluded from the APC payment. These excluded services include:

- Physician services
- Certain nonphysician practitioner services
- Therapy services (physical, occupational, speech)
- Screening mammography
- Rehabilitation services
- Ambulance services
- Durable medical equipment supplied by the hospital for the patient's home use
- Clinical diagnostic laboratory services (paid under the laboratory fee schedule)
- Dialysis services furnished to end-stage renal disease (ESRD) patients (paid under an ESRD composite rate)
- Procedures and services that are considered unsafe when performed or provided in the outpatient setting (inpatient only)
- Services specific to other sites of service, such as inpatient and home health services
- Services provided to inpatients of a skilled nursing facility (SNF), subsequent to the assessment or creation of the comprehensive care plan but billable and covered under the SNF PPS
- Services otherwise not covered by Medicare, including those deemed unreasonable and/or unnecessary for diagnosing or treating an illness or disease (non-covered).

Figure 13-17 Highlights services that are not covered under APC. *(Data from Ingenix:* Ingenix coding lab: facilities and ancillary services, *Eden Prairie, Minn., 2004, Ingenix.)*

TABLE 13-5 Outpatient Prospective Payment System (OPPS) Payment Status Indicators

SI	Description	Payment
A	Durable Medical Equipment, Prosthetics, and Orthotics (excluding implants)	DMEPOS Fee Schedule
A	Physical, Occupational, and Speech Therapy	Physician Fee Schedule
A	Ambulance	Ambulance Fee Schedule
A	EPO for End-Stage Renal Disease (ESRD) Patients	National Rate
A	Clinical Diagnostic Laboratory Services	Laboratory Fee Schedule
A	Physician Services for ESRD Patients	Physician Fee Schedule
A	Screening Mammography	Physician Fee Schedule
B	Codes that should not be used on an OPPS hospital outpatient bill	Not Paid Under OPPS
C	Inpatient Procedures	Admit Patient; Bill as Inpatient
D	Deleted Code	Codes are Deleted Effective with the Beginning of the Calendar Year
E	Non-Covered Items and Services; codes not reportable in hospital outpatient settings	Not Paid Under OPPS or When Performed in a Hospital Outpatient Setting
F	Acquisition of Corneal Tissue; orphan drugs	Paid at Reasonable Cost
G	Drug/Biological Pass-Through	Additional Pass-Through Payment
H	Device Pass-Through	Additional Pass-Through Payment
K	Non Pass-Through Drug/Biological, Radiopharmaceutical Agents, Certain Brachytherapy Seeds	Paid under OPPS; separate APC
L	Influenza Vaccine; Pneumococcal Pneumonia Vaccine	Paid Reasonable Cost; not subject to deductible or coinsurance
N	Incidental Services, Packaged into APC Rate	Packaged
P	Partial Hospitalization	Paid Per Diem APC
S	Significant Procedure, Not Discounted When Multiple	Paid under OPPS
T	Significant Procedure, Multiple Procedure Reduction Applies	Paid under OPPS
V	Visit to Clinic or Emergency Department	Paid under OPPS
X	Ancillary Service	Paid under OPPS
Y	Nonimplantable Durable Medical Equipment (DME)	Not Paid under OPPS

(Data from Ingenix: Ingenix coding lab: facilities and ancillary services, *Eden Prairie, Minn., 2004, Ingenix, and Centers for Medicare & Medicaid Services, Hospital Outpatient PPS, 2005.)*

BOX 13-21 ■ KEY POINTS

Ambulatory Payment Classification Status Indicators

Each HCPCS code listed within an APC payment group is assigned a payment status indicator that explains how the services, procedure, or item is paid, or not paid, under the OPPS APC system. For example, a status indicator C indicates the procedure is an inpatient procedure.

Ambulatory Payment Classification (APC) Inpatient Only Procedures

Inpatient Only procedures are those identified by CMS with a status indicator C. CMS indicates that these procedures would not be safe, appropriate, or considered to fall within the boundaries of acceptable medical practice if they were performed on other than a hospital inpatient basis for the following reasons:

- Invasive nature of the procedure
- Need for postoperative care (at least 24 hours)

- Underlying physical condition of the patient requiring surgery.

CMS lists procedures, outlined in Figure 13-18, that are considered Inpatient Only procedures. Examples of Inpatient Only procedures are breast reconstruction, radical resection of a tumor, and cranial reconstruction. Inpatient Only procedures are not reimbursed under APCs.

BOX 13-22 ■ KEY POINTS

Inpatient Only Procedures

Inpatient Only procedures are those identified by CMS with a status indicator C and must be performed on an inpatient basis for the following reasons:

- Invasive nature of the procedure
- Need for postoperative care (at least 24 hours)
- Underlying physical condition of the patient requiring surgery

Inpatient only procedures are not reimbursed under APCs.

Ambulatory Payment Classification (APC) Multiple Procedure Reduction

HCPCS procedures with status indicator T are surgical procedures that are reimbursed at a reduction when performed with other surgical procedures during the same operative session. Reimbursement under the APC Multiple Procedure Reduction is determined as follows:

- Primary procedure is reimbursed at the full APC payment amount.
- Secondary procedures are reimbursed at 50% of the Medicare-allowed amount.
- Patient is responsible for the full co-payment for the primary procedure and 50% of the co-payment for secondary procedures.

Inpatient Only Procedures

Examples of procedures that are considered to be Inpatient Only include, but are not limited to, the following:

- Breast reconstruction using myocutaneous flaps
- Radical resections of tumors of the mandible
- Open treatment of certain craniofacial fractures
- Osteotomies of the femur and tibia
- Sinus endoscopy with repair of cerebrospinal fluid leaks
- Cranial reconstructions
- Surgical thoracoscopy
- Pacemaker procedures by thoracotomy
- Certain thromboendarterectomies
- Excisions of mediastinal cysts and tumors
- Excisions of stomach tumors
- Enterostomies
- Hepatotomies
- Ureterotomies and ureteral endoscopies through ureterotomies
- Transcranial approaches to the orbit
- Laminectomies
- Any other service deemed to be too invasive, too extensive, or too risky by virtue of proximity to major organs to be performed on an outpatient basis according to the Medicare Modernization Act–contained provisions for the critical access hospitals (CAH).

Figure 13-18 Listing of procedures designated by CMS as Inpatient Only procedures. *(Data from* U.S. Department of Health and Human Services, *Centers for Medicare & Medicaid Services.)*

Ambulatory Payment Classification (APC) Assignment

APCs are developed based on services and procedures performed and resources used to perform those services. Under the OPPS, APC payment groups are assigned based on the HCPCS codes submitted. It is important to remember that coding under the APC system represents the technical portion of services rendered. The professional component is not billed by the hospital unless the physician or other provider is employed by or under contract with the hospital.

Coding for Ambulatory Payment Classification (APC) Assignment

It is critical for hospital coding professionals to code accurately to ensure patient conditions and procedures and services recorded in the patient's record are described accurately. Accurate coding is also essential to ensure compliance with guidelines and to obtain optimum reimbursement. Inaccurate selection of procedures codes can lead to an APC assignment that is incorrect, resulting in lost revenue. Figure 13-19 illustrates correct and incorrect APC assignment for Patient Case 1. Patient Case 1 illustrates the effect of coding the wrong procedure on the APC assignment and the dramatic effect on reimbursement. The coder selected a code for excision of malignant tumor, 11641. This code does not describe the adjacent tissue transfer performed. Based on this coding, APC 0019 is assigned,

Ambulatory Payment Classification (APC) Patient Case 1

Ambulatory surgery performed to excise a 1.0-cm malignant lesion on the nose bridge. Adjacent tissue transfer performed, defect area 4 sq. cm.

Correct APC Assignment		Incorrect APC Assignment	
Procedure code assignment	14060	Procedure code assignment	11641
APC	**0027**	**APC**	**0019**
Rate	$823.84	Rate	**$283.15**

Figure 13-19 How inaccurate coding can lead to an incorrect APC assignment, which can lead to incorrect reimbursement. *(Modified from Fordney MT:* Insurance handbook for the medical office, *ed 9, St Louis, 2005, Elsevier.)*

TEST YOUR *Knowledge* BOX 13-6

AMBULATORY PAYMENT CLASSIFICATION (APC) PAYMENT CALCULATIONS AND STRUCTURE

1. Explain the relationship between the conversion factor and the APC relative weight.
2. Discuss how CMS accounts for geographic differences when calculating APC payment rates.
3. APC payment rates and conversion factors are updated annually for use effective _______________ of the following year.
4. Provide an explanation of APC outliers.
5. Outline the purpose of transitional pass-through payments.
6. What coding system is used to categorize items and procedures into APC payment groups?
7. List four categories of APC.
8. Explain how nonsurgical and significant procedures are reimbursed under APC.
9. Provide an explanation of ancillary service APC.
10. Define transitional pass-through APC.
11. Describe APC packaged services, and provide one example.
12. Explain the purpose and function of payment status indicators.
13. Describe the APC payment for procedures with a payment status indicator C.
14. Explain the relationship between Inpatient Only procedures and APC reimbursement.
15. Discuss how multiple procedures with a payment status indicator T are reimbursed under the APC system.

which represents a reimbursement rate of $283.15. In accordance with coding guidelines, when an excision is performed followed by an adjacent tissue transfer, the adjacent tissue transfer should be coded, which includes the tumor excision. The correct code, 14060 leads to an APC assignment of 0027, which represents a reimbursement rate of $823.84. Coding systems used for outpatient services are ICD-9-CM Volumes I and II diagnosis codes and HCPCS codes.

BOX 13-23 ■ KEY POINTS

Coding Systems for Required Outpatient Services

Diagnosis

ICD-9-CM Volumes I and II codes

Procedure

HCPCS Level I CPT codes
HCPCS Level II Medicare National codes

ICD-9-CM Volumes I and II Diagnosis Coding

Diagnosis coding is still a critical factor considered in determining reimbursement under the APC system. As discussed previously, diagnosis codes serve to explain why the services provided were "medically necessary." diagnosis coding is generally performed by HIM coders; however, departmental coders may also be involved in coding diagnoses. Hospital coders should follow the ICD-9-CM "Diagnostic Coding and Reporting Guidlines for Outpatient Services" to code hospital outpatient services. These guidelines are found in the ICD-9-CM coding manual. HIM coders are required to identify and code the following:

- Admitting diagnosis
- E code explaining external cause of the admitting diagnosis
- Principal diagnosis—the condition determined after study to be chiefly responsible for the hospital visit
- Secondary diagnoses—all other conditions that were treated or affect treatment.

ICD-9-CM Volume III Procedure Coding

Historically, ICD-9-CM Volume III procedure codes were reported on the CMS-1450 (UB-04) claim form for outpatient services where appropriate. ICD-9-CM Volume III procedure codes are no longer required on Medicare outpatient claims, effective October 1, 2004. Hospital coding professionals may still be required to use Volume III procedure codes for outpatient claims to meet other payer requirements or for hospital statistical purposes.

Health Care Common Procedure Coding System (HCPCS)

HCPCS Level I CPT, Level II Medicare National codes, and modifiers are required by CMS to report hospital outpatient services, procedures, and items. These codes are directly tied to the assignment of an APC payment group and therefore have a direct impact on reimbursement. Many charges for services are posted through the chargemaster. HIM coders are generally responsible for coding services that are not posted through the chargemaster.

HCPCS Level I CPT Procedure Coding

HCPCS Level I CPT codes are used to report services and procedures on outpatient claims. CPT coding guidelines published by the American Medical Association (AMA) for physician and outpatient services are used for hospital outpatient services; however, there are some guidelines that do not apply to hospital outpatient coding. Variations in coding guidelines for hospital outpatient services include: evaluation and management (E/M), observation, and surgical services and the use of modifiers. The following section reviews some of the most significant variations.

BOX 13-24 ■ KEY POINTS

CPT Coding Guideline Variations for Hospital Outpatient Services

- Evaluation and management (E/M) services
- E/M observation services
- Surgery services
- Multiple procedures
- Sequencing of procedures
- Modifiers

Evaluation and Management (E/M)

Evaluation and management (E/M) codes were designed to represent the amount of physician effort required to perform the service. Evaluation and Management documentation guidelines were developed by CMS for reporting of physician and outpatient E/M levels of service. These guidelines could not be adopted for hospital outpatient E/M services because they do not reflect facility resource utilization. It is anticipated that CMS will develop a system similar to the guidelines used for physician evaluation and management services.

In accordance with the guidelines for reporting under the APC payment system, hospitals are required to develop criteria (based on resource utilization) for selection of E/M levels of services. Under the OPPS APC system, medical visits in hospital clinics or the Emergency Department are represented with CPT E/M codes. The hospital's criteria for assigning the E/M codes must accurately reflect the hospital's resources used for each E/M procedure. It is essential for hospital coding professionals to gain an understanding of the hospital-specific criteria developed for E/M coding in order to accurately assign E/M service codes.

E/M codes are assigned to various levels of APC. Clinic and Emergency Department E/M services are categorized in levels. Each E/M code is assigned to APC 0600, 0601, 0602, 0610, 0611, or 0612, which are based on three levels: low, mid, and high. Each code within the APC group is assigned a payment status indicator V, which indicates payment is made under OPPS. Figure 13-20 illustrates the three levels of APC for E/M services. For example: APC 0600 represents a low level clinic visit. E/M codes assigned to APC 0600 include 99201, 99202, 99211, 99212, 99241, 99242, 99271, and 99272.

E/M Observation Services

Under the outpatient OPPS system, hospitals may bill observation services separately, and receive reimbursement, when a patient admitted for observation meets specified criteria and has a diagnosis of chest pain, asthma, or congestive heart failure. Observation services are reported with HCPCS Level I CPT codes. In reporting observation services, CMS requires HCPCS Level II code G0244, which is assigned to APC 0339. Hospital observation services cannot be billed separately if a procedure with a payment status indicator T is performed 24 hours before admission for observation or during the observation stay.

APC Categories for Evaluation and Management Services

CPT	Status Indicator	Description
APC 0600 Low Level Clinic Visit		
99201	V	Office/outpatient visit, new
99202	V	Office/outpatient visit, new
99211	V	Office/outpatient visit, est
99212	V	Office/outpatient visit, est
99241	V	Office consultation
99242	V	Office consultation
99271	V	Confirmatory consultation
99272	V	Confirmatory consultation
APC 0601 Mid Level Clinic Visit		
99203	V	Office/outpatient visit, new
99213	V	Office/outpatient visit, est
99243	V	Office consultation
99273	V	Confirmatory consultation
APC 0602 High Level Clinic Visit		
99204	V	Office/outpatient visit, new
99205	V	Office/outpatient visit, new
99214	V	Office/outpatient visit, est
99215	V	Office/outpatient visit, est
99244	V	Office consultation
99245	V	Office consultation
99274	V	Confirmatory consultation
99275	V	Confirmatory consultation
APC 0610 Low Level Emergency Department Visit		
99281	V	Emergency dept visit
99282	V	Emergency dept visit
APC 0611 Mid Level Emergency Department Visit		
99283	V	Emergency dept visit
APC 0612 High Level Emergency Department Visit		
99284	V	Emergency dept visit
99285	V	Emergency dept visit

Figure 13-20 Evaluation and management (E/M) APC illustrating low-, mid-, and high-level clinic and Emergency Department visits. *(Data from Ingenix:* APC expert, *Eden Prairie, Minn., 2005, Ingenix, and Centers for Medicare & Medicaid Services, Hospital outpatient PPS, 2005.)*

Surgery Services

Hospital outpatient procedures and surgeries are coded using CPT coding guidelines with three major exceptions: surgical package, multiple procedures, and sequencing.

1. Surgical package. The CPT surgical package includes preoperative and postoperative care for a global surgical period. Preoperative and postoperative care concepts do not apply to hospital outpatient procedures because the patient is released the same day, and the surgeon assumes postoperative care of the patient.
2. Multiple procedures are reimbursed based on multiple procedure reduction guidelines, and the procedures are assigned a payment status indicator of T. Modifier 51 is not used to report multiple procedures in a hospital outpatient setting.
3. Sequencing of procedures is not required on the claim when reporting multiple procedures, because procedures are reduced based on the APC payment and RW related to the APC.

HCPCS Level I CPT Modifiers

A **modifier** is a one- or two-digit code used to communicate to the payer circumstances regarding the procedure, service, or item that are not explained in the HCPCS code description. HCPCS Level I and Level II coding systems contain modifiers. CPT modifiers are two numeric digits. Not all CPT modifiers are designated for use in coding hospital outpatient services. Specific CPT modifiers have been designated as approved for hospital outpatient services and ASCs as indicated in the CPT manual. As outlined in Figure 13-21 the following circumstances require a modifier:

Evaluation and Management (E/M)

Two circumstances involving evaluation and management services require the use of a modifier.

1. When a procedure is performed on the same day as a "significant, separately identifiable" E/M service, a modifier 25 is required to tell the payer the E/M was a separate and distinct E/M service. An example of this would be if a patient arrives

HCPCS Level I CPT Modifiers

Evaluation and Management

25 Significant, Separately Identifiable Evaluation and Management Service by the Same Physician on the Same Day of Procedure 1 or Other Service

27 Multiple Outpatient Hospital E/M Encounters on the Same Date

Same Procedure Performed on Both Sides

50 Bilateral Procedure

Service Reduced, Staged or Related Procedure

52 Reduced Services

58 Staged or Related Procedure or Service by the Same Physician during the Postoperative Period

Multiple Distinct Procedures

59 Distinct Procedural Service

Procedure Discontinued or Repeated

73 Discontinued Outpatient Hospital/ASC Procedure Prior to Anesthesia Administration

74 Discontinued Outpatient Hospital/ASC Procedure After Anesthesia Administration

76 Repeat Procedure by Same Physician

77 Repeat Procedure by Another Physician

Return to the Operating Room

78 Return to the Operating Room for a Related Procedure During the Postoperative Period

79 Unrelated Procedure or Service by the Same Physician During the Postoperative Period

Laboratory

91 Repeat Clinical Diagnostic Laboratory Test

Figure 13-21 HCPCS Level I CPT modifiers approved for hospital outpatient use. *(Data from AMA:* Hospital outpatient services CPT 2005, *Chicago, 2005, American Medical Association.)*

in the emergency room with a head wound. The emergency room services are required to evaluate the patient and determine the need for surgery. The repair of the wound is then performed.

2. When a second or subsequent E/M service is performed, for example in two different outpatient settings, on the same day, a modifier 27 is required to tell the payer they are separate E/M services. An example of this would be if a patient was seen in the hospital-based clinic for a condition that was treated and patient was sent home. Later that evening the condition deteriorated and the patient arrived at the Emergency Department for treatment.

Same Procedure Performed on Both Sides of the Body

Many times the same procedure is performed on both sides of the body. When this situation arises, a modifier 50 must be used to tell the payer the procedure was bilateral. An example of this is when a patient requires a breast biopsy on each breast.

Service Reduced, Staged, or Related

When a service described by a CPT code was not entirely performed, a modifier 52 is used to tell the payer the services are reduced. An example of this would be a procedure that normally includes closure of the wound, and the decision is made not to close the wound.

Staged or related procedures require the use of a modifier 58 to tell the payer the procedure is staged or related. An example of this would be a patient presenting with severe, full-thickness burns and planned reconstruction is performed after the debridement procedure.

Multiple Distinct Procedures

Modifier 59 is used to tell the payer that the procedures are distinct and separate. Procedures performed during the same session on different body areas are examples of when the 59 modifier is required. For example: A patient involved in a motor vehicle accident required repair of lacerations in the emergency room and then was taken to the operating room for abdominal surgery.

Procedure Discontinued or Repeated

Situations arise in which a procedure must be discontinued for reasons involving the patient's health or because the procedure cannot be completed. Two modifiers for these circumstances are 73 and 74. Modifier 73 is used when the procedure is discontinued before the administration of anesthesia. For example, a procedure discontinued before anesthesia because the patient has a rapid heartbeat and difficulty breathing would require a 73 modifier. Modifier 74 is used when a procedure is discontinued after anesthesia is administered. For example, a procedure discontinued after anesthesia because the patient became unstable would require a 74 modifier.

Return to the Operating Room

When reporting situations in which a patient is returning to the operating room for a related or unrelated procedure, modifier 78 or 79 is used.

Laboratory

Modifier 91 is required when diagnostic clinical laboratory tests are repeated. This modifier is not to be used for laboratory tests with multiple repeat portions. For example, glucose fasting, CPT 82951, would not be reported with a modifier 91.

HCPCS Level II Medicare National Codes

HCPCS Level II Medicare National codes are used to report hospital outpatient services, procedures, and items when no CPT code can be found that adequately describes the service or when the payer requires Level

II codes as opposed to Level I codes. These codes are also directly tied to the APC payment group and payments assigned for the group. HCPCS Level II coding guidelines for outpatient services should be followed when coding hospital outpatient services. HCPCS Level II codes are also used to code pass-through services and items.

HCPCS Level II Modifiers

HCPCS Level II modifiers are used to communicate to the payer circumstances regarding the procedure or service that vary from the CPT or National code description, when a Level 1 modifier does not adequately describe the circumstances. Not all Level II modifiers are designed for use in coding hospital outpatient services. Figure 13-22 outlines HCPCS Level II modifiers that are approved for use in a hospital outpatient setting. It is important to remember that an HCPCS Level II modifier can be used with a Level I or II code. An HCPCS Level I modifier can only be used with a Level I code.

BOX 13-25 ■ KEY POINTS

Modifiers

- Modifiers are used to communicate to the payer circumstances regarding the procedure, service, or item that vary from the code HCPCS code description.
- Not all modifiers are designated for use in coding hospital outpatient services.
- Carefully review modifiers in each coding system to ensure the appropriate use of modifiers when coding hospital outpatient services

HCPCS Level II Modifiers

Site of Body Area

LT	Left side (used to identify procedures performed on the left side of the body)
RT	Right side (used to identify procedures performed on the right side of the body)
CA	Procedure payable only in the inpatient setting when performed emergently on an outpatient who expires prior to admission
GA	Waiver of liability statement on file
GG	Performance and payment of a screening mammogram and diagnostic mammogram on the same patient, same day
GH	Diagnostic mammogram converted from screening mammogram on same day
LC	Left circumflex, coronary artery (hospitals use with codes 92980-92984, 92995, 92996)
LD	Left anterior descending coronary artery (hospitals use with codes 92980-92984, 92995, 92996)
RC	Right coronary artery (hospitals use with codes 92980-92984, 92995, 92996)

Eye

El	Upper left, eyelid
E2	Lower left, eyelid
E3	Upper right, eyelid
E4	Lower right, eyelid

Hand		Foot	
FA	Left hand, thumb	TA	Left foot, great toe
F1	Left hand, second digit	T1	Left foot, second digit
F2	Left hand, third digit	T2	Left foot, third digit
F3	Left hand, fourth digit	T3	Left foot, fourth digit
F4	Left hand, fifth digit	T4	Left foot, fifth digit
F5	Right hand, thumb	T5	Right foot, great toe
F6	Right hand, second digit	T6	Right foot, second digit
F7	Right hand, third digit	T7	Right foot, third digit
F8	Right hand, fourth digit	T8	Right foot, fourth digit
F9	Right hand, fifth digit	T9	Right foot, fifth digit

Ambulance

QM	Ambulance service provided under arrangement by a provider of services
QN	Ambulance service furnished directly by a provider of services

Figure 13-22 HCPCS Level II modifiers approved for hospital outpatient use. *(Data from AMA:* Hospital outpatient services CPT 2005, *Chicago, 2005, American Medical Association.)*

Outpatient Prospective Payment System (OPPS) Grouper Program

OPPS APC assignment is often performed using a computer program called a grouper. The **OPPS grouper** is a computer software program designed to use information regarding the outpatient services to assign the appropriate APC payment group and calculate reimbursement, per line item.

- **Step 1**—The HIM coding professional enters information about the patient's age and sex and the hospital visit days. The program uses all information and follows the logic of the CMS OPPS reimbursement system to assign an APC payment group for the hospital service.
- **Step 2**—The HIM coding professional enters basic information and the principal diagnosis and all other diagnoses, including complications and co-morbidities. The program assigns APC payment groups based on the HCPCS code. While diagnosis codes are not required to calculate reimbursement, most systems require entry of a valid principal diagnosis.
- **Step 3**—The HIM coding professional enters all HCPCS codes for the hospital outpatient services. The program determines whether there is a valid APC, per line item, and prices it accordingly.

Figure 13-23 illustrates APC assignment using the Clinical Coding Expert, software designed to provide correct and accurate reimbursement to each acute care facility in the United States. The figures illustrate the correct and incorrect APC assignment discussed earlier in the chapter. This program used a test national average calculation for reimbursement for this example.

TEST YOUR *Knowledge* BOX 13-7

AMBULATORY PAYMENT CLASSIFICATION (APC) ASSIGNMENT AND CODING

1. Explain how APC payment groups are assigned and why it is critical for hospital coding professionals to code accurately.

2. Coding under APC represents what portion of services provided in the hospital (technical or professional)?

3. Discuss how incorrect procedure coding can affect APC assignment and reimbursement.

4. Explain the importance of ICD-9-CM diagnosis coding for reimbursement under the APC payment system.

5. List and describe the coding system required for reporting outpatient services, procedures, and items under the OPPS APC payment system.

6. Discuss how ICD-9-CM Volume III codes are used for hospital outpatient services.

7. Describe two levels of codes under HCPCS.

8. List three areas in CPT coding in which guidelines for coding outpatient services under the APC are different.

9. What criteria do hospitals use for the selection of E/M levels for hospital outpatient services.

10. Discuss how guidelines regarding the surgical package apply to hospital outpatient coding.

11. Explain reimbursement under APC for multiple procedures.

12. How does modifier use vary when coding hospital outpatient services?

13. List two E/M modifiers used in hospital outpatient coding.

14. Provide a description of modifier 59 usage in hospital outpatient coding.

15. Describe OPPS grouper.

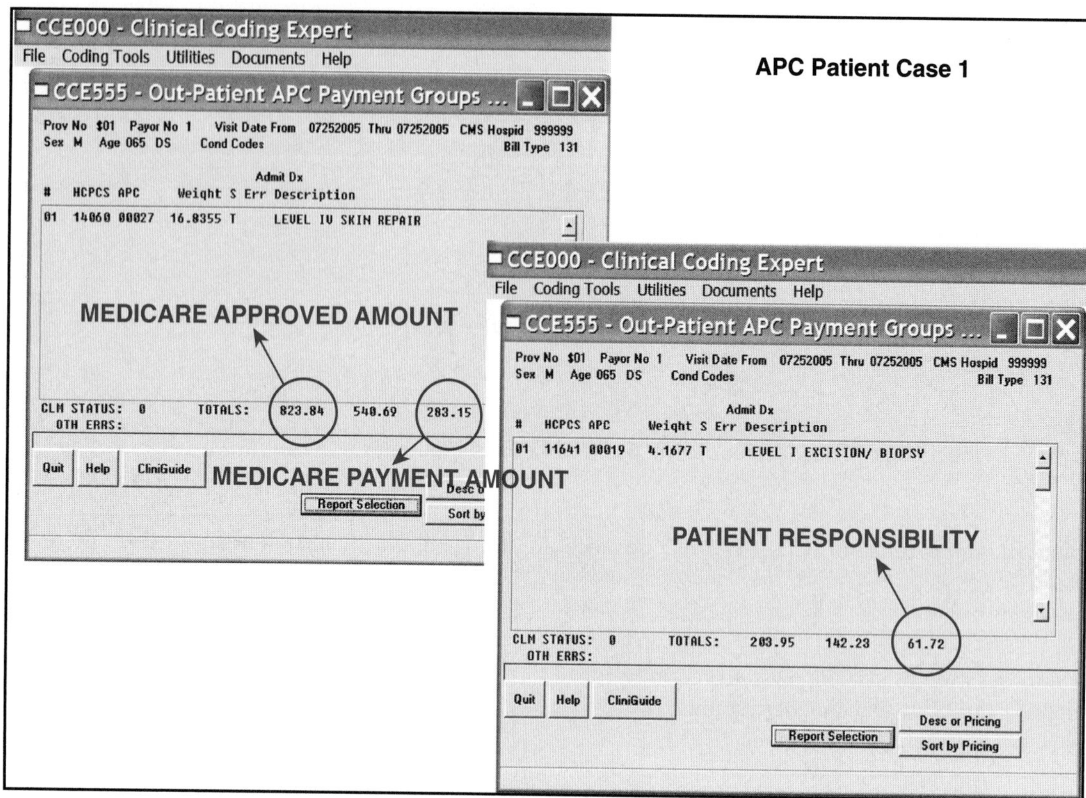

Figure 13-23 Correct and incorrect APC assignment. *(Screen shot from Clinical Coding Expert [CCE], used with permission from Innovative Health Solutions, LLC, www.ihsinfo.com/myihs.)*

CHAPTER SUMMARY

Changes in reimbursement systems have had a major impact on billing and coding for hospital services. Reimbursement systems have shifted from the traditional cost-based payment to a prospective payment system. Prospective Payment Systems (PPS) provide a predetermined fixed payment for services regardless of charges accrued by the hospital for those services. Each PPS brings with it different billing and coding requirements. The Medicare Severity Diagnosis Related Groups (MS-DRG) system is the IPPS implemented by CMS for reimbursement of hospital inpatient services. Payment under MS-DRG is based on coding that represents the patient's condition and procedures required to treat those conditions. The APC system is the Outpatient PPS (OPPS) implemented by CMS for reimbursement of hospital-based outpatient services. Payment under APC is based on coding that represents services performed and supporting diagnoses that explain medical necessity. Hospital billing and coding professionals today are required to understand the structure and basis of payment under these systems to ensure compliance with payer guidelines, and that appropriate payment is received. The significance of coding in today's health care industry is greater than ever. For hospitals the amount of payment received is directly related to coding. Inaccurate coding can represent revenue loss and noncompliance with payer guidelines.

CHAPTER REVIEW 13-1

True/False

1. PPSs were implemented to control the rising cost of health care. T F
2. PPSs provide predetermined fixed payments to hospitals regardless of the charges accrued. T F
3. Two PPS systems implemented by CMS are the MS-DRG and APC systems. T F
4. Coding has a direct impact on reimbursement. T F
5. The major difference between a hospital-based ambulatory surgery center and an Findependent ambulatory surgery center is that the independent ASC is not affiliated with or owned by a hospital. T F

Fill in the Blank

6. IPPS MS-DRG are based on the patient's ______________ and the ______________ required to treat the condition.
7. OPPS APC are based on the ______________ performed.
8. Additional payment may be received for inpatient cases that require more resources to treat a patient's condition. These situations are called ______________.
9. Hospitals may bill separately for observation services when a patient meets the following criteria: ______________.
10. The Uniform Hospital Discharge Data Set (UHDDS), Item 12, defines a ______________ procedure as one that is: 1. surgical in nature, or 2. carries a procedural risk, or 3. carries an anesthetic risk, or 4. requires specialized training.

Match the Following Definitions With the Terms at Right

11. ___ The coding system that drives MS-DRG assignment.
12. ___ A procedure that is considered surgical in nature, carries a high procedural or anesthetic risk, or requires specialized training.
13. ___ The coding system used to report services, items, and procedures for reimbursement under APC.
14. ___ Developed to categorize MS-DRG classifications according to body system.
15. ___ Assigned to APC to provide an explanation of how the service, procedure, or item will be paid.

A. HCPCS
B. Payment status indicator
C. Major diagnostic category (MDC)
D. Significant procedure
E. ICD-9-CM Volume I and II

CHAPTER REVIEW 13-2

Prospective Payment System (PPS) Payment Calculation

Part I

Use the MS-DRG calculator found at the following Web site: http://www.irp.com.

1. Identify the appropriate MS-DRG assignment and payment calculation for Case 10-3 in Chapter 10.

   MS-DRG # ______________

   Estimated MS-DRG payment rate ______________

   MDC______________

   MS-DRG weight ______________

   Average length of stay ______________

Part II

Using APC assignment data in Figure 13-16:

1. Identify the appropriate APC assignment for Case 10-1 and for the surgical procedure in Case 10-2 from Chapter 10. Record the following information:

   CASE 10-1

   APC group # ______________

   Payment rate ______________

   National or minimum adjusted co-pay ______________

   Status indicator ______________

   Explain what the status indicator means and how the procedure is paid.

   CASE 10-2

   APC group # ______________

   Payment rate ______________

   National or minimum adjusted co-pay ______________

   Status indicator ______________

   Explain what the status indicator means and how the procedure is paid.

2. Provide an example of incorrect APC assignment based on similar APC payment groups found in the APC data sheets.

GLOSSARY

Ambulatory Payment Classification (APC) The OPPS by CMS provide reimbursement for hospital outpatient services. Under APC, the facility is paid a fixed fee based on the resources utilized to provide the service or procedure.

Ambulatory Payment Classification (APC) outliers Outpatient cases that involve patient conditions and circumstances that result in higher cost for the hospital to perform the procedure or service, in excess of the APC payment rate.

Ambulatory surgery Surgery that is performed on a patient who is released the same day.

Ambulatory surgery center (ASC) A facility designed for the sole purpose of proving ambulatory surgery services.

Arithmetic mean length of stay (AMLOS) A value assigned to each MS-DRG to represent the average number of approved inpatient days for the MS-DRG.

Co-morbidity A preexisting condition that has an impact on the principal condition being treated.

Complications Conditions that arise during the admission that may require additional treatment and increased length of stay.

Conversion factor (CF) A national dollar amount, determined by CMS, used to convert the relative weight into an APC payment amount.

Geometric mean length of stay (GMLOS) A value assigned to each MS-DRG to represent an adjusted value of all cases, making allowances for Outliers, transfer cases, and negative Outlier cases that normally skew data. The GMLOS is used to calculate reimbursement for the MS-DRG.

Inpatient Prospective Payment System (IPPS) A prospective payment system established as mandated by the Tax Equity and Fiscal Responsibility Act (TEFRA) in 1983 to provide reimbursement for acute hospital inpatient services. The system implemented under IPPS is known as Diagnosis Related Groups (DRG).

Major Diagnostic Categories (MDC) The DRG System implemented in 1983 is now known as CMS-DRG. A grouping of hospital inpatient cases based on body system; used to further categorize MS-DRG.

Medicare Severity Diagnosis Related Groups (MS-DRG) The Inpatient Prospective Payment System (IPPS) implemented in 2009 to provide reimbursement for hospital inpatient services. MS-DRG is a payment classification system that defines patient categories based on diagnosis, procedure, and other clinical factors. Under MS-DRG, the facility is paid a fixed fee based on the patient's condition and relative treatments. MS-DRG replaced the CMS-DRG System from 1983.

Medicare Severity Diagnosis Related Groups (MS-DRG) grouper program A computer software program designed to use information regarding the patient's condition, treatment, and other factors to follow the logic of the MDC decision-making tree to assign a MS-DRG to the hospital inpatient case.

Medicare Severity Diagnosis Related Groups (MS-DRG) outliers Inpatient cases that involve circumstances that result in a patient case that requires a much longer length of stay or unusually high cost for treatment compared with most cases represented by the MS-DRG group.

Modifiers A one or two digit code used to communicate to the payer circumstances regarding the procedure, service, or item that are not explained in the HCPCS code description. HCPCS Level I and Level II coding systems contain modifiers. Not all CPT modifiers are designated for use in coding hospital outpatient services.

Outpatient Prospective Payment System (OPPS) Prospective Payment System implemented effective August 2000 by CMS that provides reimbursement for hospital outpatient services. The system implemented under OPPS is known as Ambulatory Payment Classifications (APC). OPPS payments are predetermined fixed amounts based on the service or procedure performed.

Outpatient Prospective Payment System (OPPS) grouper A computer software program designed to use information regarding the outpatient services to assign the appropriate APC payment group and calculate reimbursement, per line item.

Outpatient services Services provided to a patient who is not admitted to the hospital for an inpatient stay; the patient is released the same day.

Relative weight (RW) A value assigned to a MS-DRG or APC group or to a procedure code to reflect the relative resource consumption. The relative weight is utilized to calculate the total payment for the case. The higher the relative weight (RW) the higher the payment.

Transitional Pass-Through Payments Provide hospitals with additional payment for certain drugs, devices, or biologicals that are considered "new technologies." HCPCS codes for these items are assigned to APC group #0738.

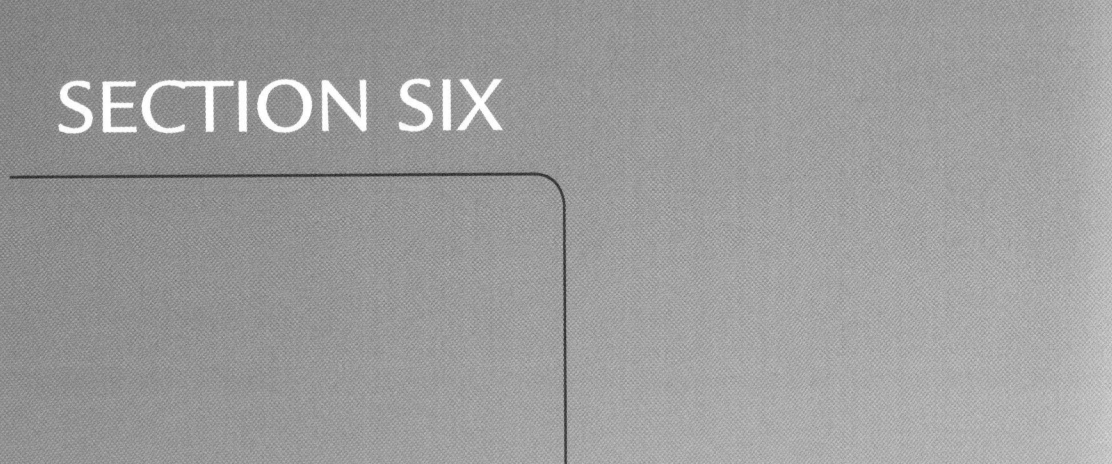

HIPAA and Compliance

Health Insurance Portability and Accountability Act (HIPAA)

Chapter 14

Health Insurance Portability and Accountability Act (HIPAA)

The objective of this chapter is to provide a basic understanding of the Health Insurance Portability and Accountability Act (HIPAA) of 1996. The implementation of HIPAA has and will continue to have a major impact on health care delivery and the processing of health care transactions. HIPAA includes provisions to improve the portability of health insurance, combat fraud and abuse, promote the use of medical savings accounts, and simplify the administration of health insurance. A detailed discussion of all HIPAA provisions is beyond the scope of this text. The chapter will provide a brief overview of the purpose and scope of HIPAA regulations. It is critical for hospital personnel to understand HIPAA regulations to ensure compliance. A discussion of HIPAA portability, administrative simplification, privacy, and security provisions will provide a basic understanding of the mandated standards and the consequence of non-compliance with those standards. The chapter will end with a discussion of the elements of a compliance plan.

Outline

Chapter Objectives

- Define terms, phrases, abbreviations, and acronyms related to HIPAA regulations and compliance.
- Discuss two major issues facing the health care industry leading to the implementation of HIPAA.
- Demonstrate an understanding of the purpose and content of HIPAA regulations.
- Explain the relationship between HIPAA privacy regulations and the patient's medical information.
- Demonstrate an understanding of the Administrative Simplification section of HIPAA and how it relates to claims processing.
- Describe provisions outlined under the Administrative Simplification section of HIPAA.
- Discuss provisions outlined under the Privacy section of HIPAA.
- Demonstrate an understanding of the HIPAA Privacy Rule and how it relates to patient medical information.
- Discuss provisions outlined under the HIPAA Security Rule.
- Discuss the importance of HIPAA Compliance.
- Provide an overview of the elements of a compliance plan.

Key Terms

Abuse
Authorization for Release of Medical Information
Business associate
Civil Monetary Penalties Law (CMP)
Clearinghouse
Compliance
Covered entity
De-identification
Disclosure of Protected Health Information (PHI)
Employer Identification Number (EIN)
Fraud
Health Insurance Portability and Accountability Act (HIPAA)
Health Insurance Portability and Accountability Act (HIPAA) Title I
Health Insurance Portability and Accountability Act (HIPAA) Title II
Individually Identifiable Health Information (IIHI)
Kassenbaum-Kennedy Legislation
National Provider Identifier (NPI)
Office of the Inspector General (OIG)
Office of Civil Rights
Protected Health Information (PHI)
Tax Identification Number (TIN)
Transaction
Use of PHI

Acronyms and Abbreviations

AHIMA—American Health Information Management Association
ANSI—American National Standards Institute
AS—Administrative Simplification
CMP—Civil Monetary Penalties Law
CMS—Centers for Medicare and Medicaid Services
CPT—Current Procedural Terminology
DHHS—Department of Health and Human Services
DOJ—Department of Justice
EDI—Electronic Data Interchange
EIN—Employer Identification Number
EPHI—Electronic Protected Health Information
HCPCS—Health Care Common Procedure Coding System
HIPAA—Health Insurance Portability and Accountability Act.
HIPAA (AS)—Health Insurance Portability and Accountability Act Title II: Administrative Simplification
ICD-9-CM—International Classification of Diseases, 9th Revision, Clinical Modification
IIHI—Individually Identifiable Health Information
MIP—Medical Integrity Program
NPI—National Provider Identifier
NPS—National Provider System
OCR—Office of Civil Rights
OIG—Office of the Inspector General
PHI—protected health information
TCS—Transaction Code Standards
TIN—Tax Identification Number

HIPAA OVERVIEW

During the 1990s major issues were facing the health care industry related to controlling the rising cost of health care. Legislators continued to develop and implement reimbursement methods designed to control the rising cost of health care. Health care leaders were called on to identify other issues that contributed to the rising cost of health care. Several contributing factors were identified. The limited access and portability of health insurance coverage was one factor identified. Many individuals did not have health insurance coverage or lost insurance coverage because of limited access or the inability to continue coverage after a job change. Another factor identified was fraud and abuse. The government estimates that billions of dollars are lost to fraud and abuse on an annual basis. The administrative cost of processing health care transactions was seen as yet another factor. It is estimated that billions of dollars annually are spent on the administration of health insurance. Legislation was developed and passed to address these factors that contributed to the rising cost of health care. The **Health Insurance Portability and Accountability Act (HIPAA),** also known as the **Kassenbaum-Kennedy Legislation,** was passed by Congress to improve access to health care; provide portability of health insurance coverage; combat waste, fraud, and abuse; and simplify the administration of health insurance.

BOX 14-1 ■ KEY POINTS

Health Insurance Portability and Accountability Act of 1996 (HIPAA), also Referred to as the Kassenbaum-Kennedy Legislation

Public Law 104-191 amends the Internal Revenue code of 1986. HIPAA was passed by Congress to improve access to health care, to provide portability of health insurance coverage, to combat waste, fraud, and abuse, and to simplify the administration of health insurance.

HIPAA LEGISLATION

HIPAA legislation is outlined under Public Law 104–191. HIPAA was passed by Congress in 1996 and was implemented in phases from 1996 to 2009. The purpose of the Act was to amend the Internal Revenue Code of 1986 to address many health care-related issues including the continuance of insurance coverage, fraud and abuse, and administrative simplification. HIPAA legislation is broken down into the following five sections, referred to as titles, as illustrated in Figure 14-1.

- Title I: Health Care Reform (Health Care Access, Portability, and Renewability)
- Title II: Preventing Health Care Fraud and Abuse, Administrative Simplification, and Medical Liability Reform
- Title III: Tax-Related Health Provisions
- Title IV: Application and Enforcement of Group Health Plan Requirements
- Title V: Revenue Offsets

This chapter will focus on HIPAA Titles I and II since they have the most significant impact today on health care providers and health insurers. The **Health Insurance Portability and Accountability Act (HIPAA) Title I** is referred to as Health Care Reform since its purpose is to ensure that individuals have access to health insurance coverage. Title I mandates improved access to health care and health coverage, and it imposes new regulations relating to the underwriting process performed by insurance companies to determine whether they will insure an individual. The **Health Insurance Portability and Accountability Act (HIPAA) Title II** is labeled Preventing Health Care Fraud and Abuse, Administrative Simplification, and Medical Liability Reform. Title II contains regulations aimed at protecting government programs from fraud and abuse. Another objective of Title II is to standardize and simplify the processing of health care transactions. Figures 14-2 and 14-3 highlight the primary objectives of HIPAA Title I and Title II provisions.

HIPAA Title I: Health Care Reform (Health Care Access, Portability, and Renewability)

The original focus of HIPAA was to ensure portability or continuation of health insurance coverage for workers who lost or changed jobs. Prior to the implementation of HIPAA insurance, companies could deny individuals coverage based on preexisting conditions or health status. Individuals who lost their jobs or changed employment often were unable to obtain health insurance coverage due to preexisting medical conditions. Individuals who presented with a catastrophic illness such as cancer or HIV infection could be denied coverage or insurance companies could elect to drop coverage because of the expense of treating such illnesses. HIPAA Title I is designed to reform health insurance to protect

Health Insurance Portability and Accountability Act (HIPAA) of 1996 Public Law 104-191

Title I Health Care Reform (Health Care Access, Portability, and Renewability)
Title II Preventing Health Care Fraud and Abuse Administrative Simplification Medical Liability Reform
Title III Tax-Related Health Provisions
Title IV Application and Enforcement of Group Health Plan Requirements
Title V Revenue Offsets

Figure 14-1 Titles of provisions implemented under the Health Insurance Portability and Accountability Act (HIPAA) of 1996, Public Law 104-191. *(Data from Health Insurance Portability and Accountability Act of 1996.)*

HIPAA Title I: Health Care Reform

Improve individual access to health care coverage
Access and continuity of insurance coverage
Preexisting condition clause
Prevent loss of coverage
Discrimination based on health status
Guarantee renewal of health insurance

Figure 14-2 Health Care Reform provisions. *(Data from Health Insurance Portability and Accountability Act of 1996.)*

HIPAA Title II: Fraud Prevention and Administrative Simplification

Combating waste, fraud, and abuse in health care
Increase funding to combat waste, fraud, and abuse
Amend penalties for fraudulent activities

Simplifying the administration of health insurance
HIPAA electronic transaction and code sets standards
HIPAA privacy requirements
HIPAA security requirements

Figure 14-3 Fraud Prevention and Administrative Simplification provisions. *(Data from Health Insurance Portability and Accountability Act of 1996.)*

BOX 14-2 ■ KEY POINTS

Health Insurance Portability and Accountability Act of 1996 (HIPAA) Title I: Health Care Reform

Title I of HIPAA includes provisions to achieve three major objectives that relate to portability and continuance of health insurance coverage as outlined below:

- Improve the continuation and portability of insurance coverage
- Prevent individuals from losing coverage or being denied coverage based on health status
- Guarantee individuals the ability to renew insurance coverage in multiemployer plans and multiple employer welfare arrangements.

health insurance coverage for millions of Americans when they change or lose their jobs; it guarantees health insurance access, portability, and renewal. Title I of HIPAA includes provisions to achieve three major objectives that relate to portability and continuance of health insurance coverage as outlined below:

- Improve the continuation and portability of insurance coverage by limiting the use of preexisting condition exclusions in health plans.
- Prevent individuals from losing coverage or being denied coverage based on health status by prohibiting insurance companies from discriminating against individuals based on health status.
- Guarantee individuals the ability to renew insurance coverage in multiemployer plans and multiple employer welfare arrangements.

HIPAA Title II: Preventing Health Care Fraud and Abuse and Administrative Simplification

Efforts to control the rising cost of health care led to the implementation of HIPAA legislation. Title II: Prevention of Health Care Fraud and Abuse and Administrative Simplification addresses two issues identified as contributing to the rising cost of health care: fraud and abuse and the cost of administering health insurance. One major objective of Title II is to save health care dollars through prevention of health care fraud and abuse. To accomplish this, Title II contains provisions to increase prevention and detection of fraud and abuse activities. Another objective is to standardize the health insurance administration process to reduce the cost of processing health care transactions. Health care leaders estimate that administrative costs could be reduced by billions of dollars annually by increasing the use of electronic data interchange (EDI) for health care transactions such as claim submission and payer remittance. Title II also contains provisions to standardize health care transactions for electronic processing.

BOX 14-3 ■ KEY POINTS

Health Insurance Portability and Accountability Act of 1996 (HIPAA) Title II: Fraud Prevention and Administrative Simplification—Two Major Objectives

Combating waste, fraud, and abuse in health care through the creation of several programs: The Health Care Fraud and Abuse Program, The Incentive Program for Fraud and Abuse, and the Medical Integrity Program

Simplifying the administration of health insurance provisions that mandate the adoption of national standards for electronic health transactions, including standard transactions and code sets and national identifiers for providers, health plans, and employers

Combating Waste, Fraud, and Abuse in Health Care

HIPAA Title II addresses the need to combat waste, fraud, and abuse in health care by increasing funding to support fraud detection activities, increasing civil monetary penalties for fraud and abuse, and through the creation of several programs: The Health Care Fraud and Abuse Program, The Incentive Program for Fraud and Abuse, and the Medical Integrity Program. Figure 14-4 illustrates the major initiatives outlined in Title II.

The Health Care Fraud and Abuse Program

The Health Care Fraud and Abuse Program was created under HIPAA to identify fraud and abuse in the Medicare and Medicaid programs and among private payers. HIPAA legislation established this program and allocated funds from the Medicare Part A Trust Fund to expand fraud and abuse control activities. HIPAA also expanded the definition of fraud to include language indicating that providers can be held liable if they knew or should have known that information on a claim was false. **Fraud** is defined as an intentional deception or misrepresentation that someone makes, knowing it is false, that could result in an unauthorized payment.

HIPAA Title II: Fraud and Abuse Initiatives

Increase activities to detect and prevent fraud and abuse activities within government programs through:

1. Increased funding to detect fraudulent activities.
2. Increased civil and monetary penalties for fraud violations.
3. Creation of programs to focus on fraud and abuse activities:
   The Health Care Fraud and Abuse Program
   The Incentive Program for Fraud and Abuse
   The Medical Integrity Program

Figure 14-4 Fraud and abuse initiatives. *(Data from Health Insurance Portability and Accountability Act of 1996.)*

BOX 14-4 ■ KEY POINTS

Health Care Fraud and Abuse Program

The Health Care Fraud and Abuse Program was created under HIPAA to identify fraud and abuse in the Medicare and Medicaid programs and among private payers. HIPAA legislation established this program and allocated funds from the Medicare Part A Trust Fund to expand fraud and abuse control activities.

HIPAA also expanded the definition of fraud to include language indicating that providers can be held liable if they knew or should have known that information on a claim was false.

The Centers for Medicare and Medicaid Services (CMS) outlines the following as the most common forms of fraud:

- Billing for services not furnished (phantom billing)
- Misrepresenting the diagnosis to justify payment
- Soliciting, offering, or receiving kickbacks
- Unbundling or "exploding" charges
- Falsifying certificates of medical necessity, plans of treatment, and medical records to justify payment

Figure 14-5 provides examples of the most common forms of fraud.

Abuse is defined as actions or practices of health care providers that are inconsistent with accepted sound business practice, which may result in improper payment. The Centers for Medicare and Medicaid Services (CMS) outlines the following as the most common forms of abuse:

- Claims for services not medically necessary
- Excessive charges for services or supplies
- Improper billing practices, including submission of claims to Medicare instead of third-party payers that are primary insurers for Medicare beneficiaries
- Unusually large payments in relation to services rendered by lawyers, consultants, agents, and others
- Increasing charges to Medicare beneficiaries but not to other patients.

Figure 14-6 provides examples of some of the most common forms of abuse.

The Incentive Program for Fraud and Abuse

The incentive program, also created under HIPAA, provides incentives to Medicare beneficiaries and others who report fraud and abuse in the Medicare program. Rewards are paid if the information leads directly to the recovery of Medicare funds.

The Medical Integrity Program (MIP)

The creation of a Medical Integrity Program (MIP) was authorized under HIPAA legislation. The primary objective of the program is to develop and implement systems to safeguard Medicare payments. One function is to identify and investigate suspicious claims throughout Medicare to ensure that Medicare does not pay claims other insurers should pay. MIP also ensures that Medicare pays only for covered services that are reasonable and medically necessary. HIPAA legislation also granted CMS authority to hire special fraud-fighting contractors to carry out audits, conduct medical reviews, and perform other essential program integrity activities that were previously performed by Medicare contractors who processed claims.

Fraud is defined as an intentional deception or misrepresentation that someone makes, knowing it is false, that could result in an unauthorized payment.

Examples of common forms of fraud:

☑ Submitting charges for hospital days after the patient is discharged.
This is known as "phantom billing."

☑ Adding a diagnosis not documented to obtain additional payment (such as diabetes or hypertensive heart disease).
This can be considered "upcoding."

☑ Paying providers for referrals to the hospital or practice.
This practice is against anti-kickback legislation.

☑ Using multiple codes to describe services that should be described with one code.
This is known as "unbundling."

☑ Documenting conditions not addressed during the visit to justify medical necessity, and thus to justify payment.
This can be considered "upcoding."

Figure 14-5 Examples of common forms of fraud. *(Data from Health Insurance Portability and Accountability Act of 1996.)*

Abuse is defined as actions or practices of health care providers that are inconsistent with accepted sound medical practice, which may result in improper payment

☑ Submission of a claims for a diagnostic procedures with diagnoses that do not meet medical necessity standards

☑ Submission of claims with charges that are excessive based on industry standards

☑ Submission of claims involving services related to a work-related injury to Medicare as the primary insurance

☑ Charging Medicare beneficiaries more than other patients are charged

Figure 14-6 Examples of common forms of abuse. *(Data from Health Insurance Portability and Accountability Act of 1996.)*

Simplifying the Administration of Health Insurance

The Title II: Administrative Simplification portion of the HIPAA regulations is designed to improve the efficiency and effectiveness of the nation's health care system by encouraging the widespread use of electronic data interchange (EDI). HIPAA Title II contains provisions that mandate the adoption of national standards

BOX 14-5 ■ KEY POINTS

The Medical Integrity Program (MIP)

The primary objective of the program is to develop and implement systems to safeguard Medicare payments by:

- Identifying and investigating suspicious claims throughout Medicare.
- Ensuring that Medicare does not pay claims other insurers should pay or pay for covered services that are not reasonable and medically necessary. Recruiting special fraud-fighting contractors to carry out audits, conduct medical reviews, and perform other essential program integrity activities.

BOX 14-6 ■ KEY POINTS

HIPAA Title II: Administrative Simplification (AS)

Administrative Simplification involves provisions to improve the efficiency and effectiveness of the nation's health care system by:

- Encouraging the widespread use of electronic data interchange.
- Mandating the adoption of national standards for electronic health transactions, including standard transactions and code sets and national identifiers for providers, health plans, and employers.
- Administrative Simplification also contains provisions to ensure the privacy and security of health care data.

for electronic health transactions, including standard transactions and code sets and national identifiers for providers, health plans, and employers. The increased use of electronic data exchange brought with it concerns regarding the security and privacy of health data. As illustrated in Figure 14-7, Title II also contains provisions to ensure the privacy and security of health care data. HIPAA administrative simplification, privacy, and security provisions will be discussed in detail later in this chapter.

HIPAA provisions were implemented in phases from 1996 to 2009 as follows:

- Title I: Health Care Reform was first to be implemented in 1996 and 1997.
- Title II: Fraud prevention provisions have been implemented.

Title II: Administrative Simplification provisions including privacy and security are scheduled through 2009, as illustrated in Table 14-1.

The implementation dates of HIPAA provisions are determined based on the publication date of the final rule. Before a rule (or law) becomes final, a preliminary draft is published in the *Federal Register* with a time frame for comments. After the comment period, the preliminary draft is revised to reflect the consensus of all comments received, and the final rule is published.

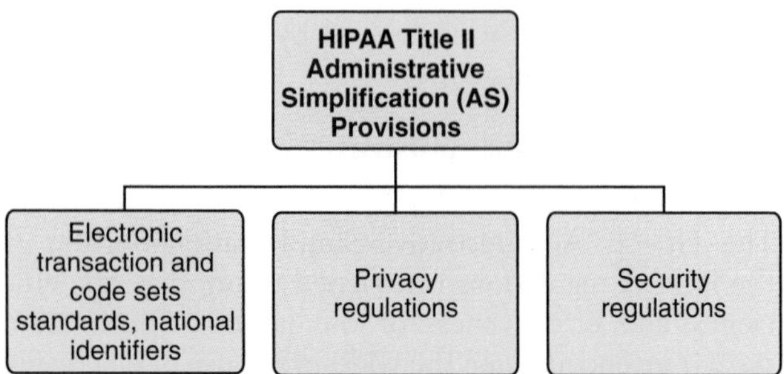

Figure 14-7 Provisions implemented under HIPAA Title II: Administrative Simplification (AS) provisions.

Generally, once the final rule is published there is a 2-year plus 60-day period before the rule becomes effective. All covered entities are required to comply with the HIPAA regulations on the effective date published in the *Federal Register*.

HIPAA REGULATIONS AND COMPLIANCE

The health care industry is governed and regulated in accordance with many state and federal regulations. Health care providers must implement systems to ensure compliance with all state and federal regulations. **Compliance** is the term used to describe the act of complying with state and federal regulations. A number of federal laws mandate compliance and have provisions for sanctions against individuals or organizations that do not comply, particularly in the areas of privacy and security of patient information, billing, and coding guidlines and claim submission requirements. For example, The **Civil Monetary Penalties Law (CMP)** of 1983 was passed for the purpose of prosecuting cases of Medicare and Medicaid fraud. This law contains provisions regarding the sanctions that can be imposed on individuals or organizations convicted of fraudulent activities as defined in the Federal False Claims Act. The sanctions that may be imposed under the Civil Monetary Penalties Law (CMP) are:

1. A penalty of up to $10,000 for each item or service wrongfully listed on a claim submitted to Medicare or Medicaid.
2. An assessment of up to triple the total amount improperly claimed.
3. Suspension from government programs for a period defined by the Department of Health and Human Services (DHHS).

HIPAA legislation mandates compliance with the standards and provisions involving administrative simplification, privacy and security.

TABLE 14-1 **Implementation of HIPAA Regulations**

Date	Implementation of HIPAA Regulations
August 21, 1996	HIPAA passed by Congress.
December 28, 2000	Final Rule published on privacy and confidentiality of all individually identifiable health information.
April 14, 2001	Final Rule on Privacy became effective.
August 17, 2001	Final Rule published on Transaction Standards and Code Sets.
October 15, 2002	Deadline to submit a compliance extension form for Electronic Health care Transactions and Code Sets.
October 16, 2002	Electronic Health care Transactions and Code Sets: all covered entities except those that filed for an extension and are not a small health plan.
April 14, 2003	Privacy: all covered entities except small health plans.
April 16, 2003	Electronic Health care Transactions and Code Sets: all covered entities must have started software and systems testing.
October 16, 2003	Electronic Health care Transactions and Code Sets: all covered entities that filed for an extension and small health plans.
October 16, 2003	Medicare will only accept paper claims under limited circumstances
April 14, 2004	Privacy–small health plans.
July 30, 2004	Employer Identifier Standard–all covered entities except small health plans.
April 20, 2005	Security Standards–all covered entities except small health plans.
August 1, 2005	Employer Identifier Standard–small health plans.
April 20, 2006	Security Standards–small health plans.
May 23, 2007	National Provider Identifier–all covered entities except small health plans
May 23, 2008	National Provider Identifier–small health plans

Data from Centers for Medicare and Medicaid Services, www.cms.hhs.gov/hipaa/hipaa2/general/deadlines.asp.

BOX 14-7 ■ KEY POINTS

Compliance

Compliance is the act of complying with state and federal regulations.

Federal and state laws mandate compliance with all provisions contained in the law such as:

- Health Insurance Portability and Accountability Act (HIPAA)—contains provisions related to preventing Health Care Fraud and Abuse, Administrative Simplification and Medical Liability Reform.
- The Federal False Claims Act—passed to prevent overuse of services and to uncover fraudulent activities in the Medicare and Medicaid programs.

A number of federal laws mandate compliance and have provisions for sanctions against individuals or organizations who are not in compliance such as the Civil Monetary Penalties Law (CMP)—passed for the purpose of prosecuting cases of Medicare and Medicaid fraud.

HIPAA Enforcement and Penalties

Compliance requirements are published in the Federal Register and include the date compliance must be met. Figure 14-8 illustrates enforcement agencies and penalties that can be imposed for non-compliance. Agencies responsible for enforcing standards and provisions include the Office of the Inspector General, the Centers for Medicare and Medicaid Services, and the Office of Civil Rights.

Office of the Inspector General (OIG)

The **Office of the Inspector General (OIG)** is an agency under the Department of Health and Human Services (DHHS) that is responsible for the detection and prevention of fraud and abuse. The OIG monitors compliance and enforces laws related to fraud and abuse. When a Medicare provider allegedly commits fraud, an investigation is conducted by the OIG. If evidence of

TEST YOUR *Knowledge* BOX 14-1

HIPAA OVERVIEW; HIPAA LEGISLATION

1. Provide another name for the Health Insurance Portability and Accountability legislation.
2. Explain why the Health Insurance Portability and Accountability Act of 1996 (HIPAA) was developed and implemented.
3. Describe the time frame for implementation of HIPAA legislation.
4. List the five titles of HIPAA that affect health care providers and health plans.
5. Discuss the original focus of HIPAA legislation.
6. List three objectives of HIPAA Title I.
7. State how HIPAA Title II is designed to combat fraud and abuse in health care.
8. Discuss the difference between fraud and abuse.
9. Provide a brief explanation of the purpose of Title II: Administrative Simplification.
10. Discuss the process followed for a rule to become final.

fraud or abuse is found by the OIG, the case is referred to the Department of Justice (DOJ) for prosecution. Criminal, civil, and/or administrative sanctions for fraud convictions may include (Figure 14-9):

- Civil penalties of up to $10,000 for each service or item falsely reported on the claim plus triple damages under the False Claims Act.
- Criminal fines and/or imprisonment of up to 10 years if there is a conviction of the crime of health care fraud as outlined in HIPAA or, for violations of federal anti-kickback statutes, imprisonment of up to 5 years and/or criminal fines of up to $25,000.
- Administrative sanctions such as exclusion from participation in Medicare and state programs may be imposed in addition to civil monetary penalties.

Centers for Medicare and Medicaid Services (CMS)

The Centers for Medicare and Medicaid Services (CMS) is an agency under the Department of Health and Human Services (DHHS) that oversees the Medicare and Medicaid programs. CMS enforces many laws related to the Medicare and Medicaid programs including the HIPAA standards transaction and code set provisions. Noncompliance with HIPAA standard transaction and code set provisions may result in monetary penalties. CMS may impose monetary penalties on the organization failing to comply, as follows:

- $100 per violation.
- $25,000 annual cap for a single standard.
- Exclusion from the program.

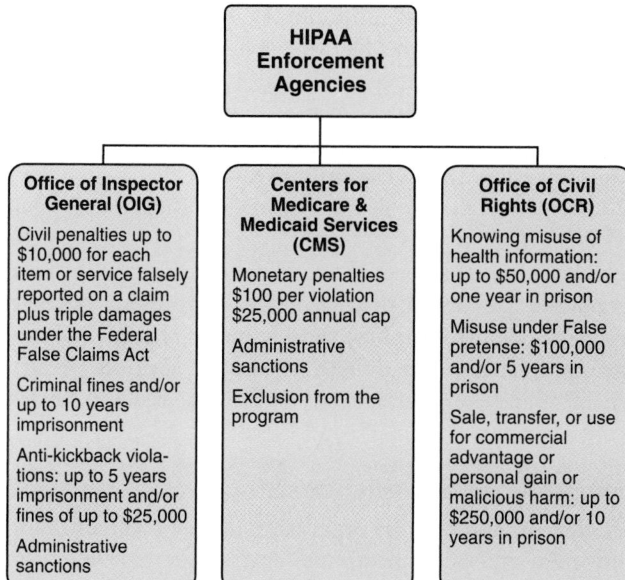

Figure 14-8 Civil Monetary Penalties (CMP) Law sanctions that may be imposed for HIPAA violations by various enforcement agencies such as the OIG, CMS, and OCR.

Office of Civil Rights (OCR)

The **Office of Civil Rights (OCR)** is an agency under the Department of Health and Human Services (DHHS) that is responsible for monitoring compliance and enforcement of HIPAA privacy standards. Complaints regarding privacy issues are submitted by individuals or other entities to the OCR in writing. The OCR conducts an investigation and determines required action. There are civil and criminal penalties for violating the rule. Civil penalties for HIPAA privacy violations can be up to $100 for each offense, with an annual cap of $25,000 for repeated violations of the same requirement. Penalties for violating the rule can be imposed only on covered entities, not on business associates. Criminal penalties are as follows:

- For knowing misuse of individually identifiable health information: up to $50,000 and/or 1 year in prison.
- For misuse under false pretenses: up to $100,000 and/or 5 years in prison.
- For offenses related to the sale, transfer, or use for commercial advantage or personal gain or malicious harm: up to $250,000 and/or ten years in prison.

BOX 14-8 ■ KEY POINTS

HIPAA Enforcement Agencies

Agencies responsible for enforcing HIPAA standards and provisions include the:

- Office of the Inspector General (OIG)
- Centers for Medicare and Medicaid Services (CMS)
- Office of Civil Rights (OCR).

Compliance requirements are published in the *Federal Register*, and they include the date compliance must be met.

State Laws and HIPAA

State laws may contain more stringent privacy protections that apply over and above the federal privacy standards. For example, states may have special privacy requirements for patients tested, diagnosed, or treated for alcohol and drug abuse, sexually transmitted diseases, or mental health disorders.

HIPAA regulations specify the organizations that are required to comply with all provisions; they are referred to as covered entities.

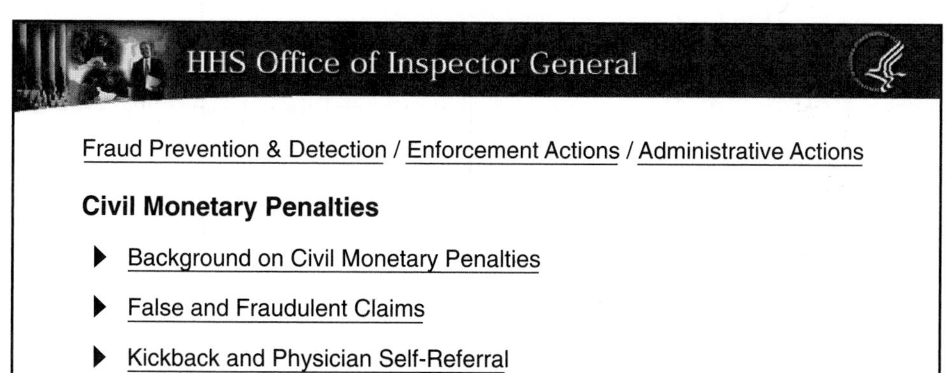

Figure 14-9 The Department of Health and Human Services, Office of the Inspector General Web site containing information on the Civil Monetary Penalties (CMP) Law. *(Data from* U.S. Department of Health and Human Services, *Office of Inspector General, www.oig.hhs.gov/fraud/enforcement/administrative/cmp/cmp.html#1, 2010.)*

BOX 14-9 ■ KEY POINTS

Covered Entities

A covered entity is an organization involved with health care delivery that provides health care services, submits claims for services, or provides health care coverage.

HIPAA identifies three types of covered entities that must follow the regulations:

- Health care providers
- Health plans
- All health care clearinghouses

Covered Entities

A **covered entity** is an organization involved with health care delivery that provides health care services, submits claims for services, or provides health care coverage. HIPAA identifies three types of covered entities that must follow the regulations: health care providers, health plans, and all health care clearinghouses, as outlined in Figure 14-10.

Health Care Providers

Health care providers are people or organizations that render health care services, bill for services rendered, and are paid for those services in the normal course of business. Examples of health care providers include hospitals, physicians, ambulatory surgery centers and other facilities, home health agencies, and ambulance services. In accordance with HIPAA regulations, CMS requires that Medicare claims be sent electronically from all providers with the exception of small practices that have less than 10 employees.

HIPAA Covered Entities

Health Care Providers

Individuals or organizations that render health care services including:

- Hospitals
- Physicians
- Ambulatory surgery centers and other facilities
- Home health agencies
- Ambulance services

Health Plans

Health plans that provide medical care or reimburse providers for health care services rendered including:

- Group health plans
- Health insurance carriers
- Health maintenance organizations
- Most federal health care agencies

Health Care Clearinghouses

Organizations that receive claim information from hospitals and other providers in various formats for conversion to a required format for submission to various payers. Clearinghouses as defined under HIPAA include:

- Billing service companies
- Repricing companies
- Value-added networks

Figure 14-10 Covered entities as outlined in HIPAA Title II: provisions. *(Data from Health Insurance Portability and Accountability Act of 1996.)*

Health Plans

Health plans that provide medical care or pay for care rendered by other providers are considered covered entities. Health plans outlined under HIPAA include group health plans, health insurance carriers, health maintenance organizations, and most federal health care agencies.

Health Care Clearinghouse

A **clearinghouse** is an organization that receives claim information from hospitals and other providers in various formats for conversion to a required format for submission to various payers. Health care clearinghouses as defined under HIPAA include billing service companies, repricing companies, and value added networks that process nonstandard data elements into standard data elements for the purpose of transmission of claims between health care providers and health plans.

BOX 14-10 ■ KEY POINTS

Clearinghouse

A **clearinghouse** is an organization that receives claim information from hospitals and other providers in various formats for conversion to a required format for submission to various payers.

Business Associates

HIPAA regulations also have an affect on many others in the health care field. For instance business associates are not covered entities and are not themselves required to comply with the law. However, they may need to make changes in order to do business with a covered entity. A **business associate** is an individual, organization, or entity that works with or for a covered entity but is not an employee of the covered entity. In accordance with HIPAA provisions, business associates is a category that includes billing companies, information technology contractors, consultants, collection agencies, law firms, and accountants. Covered entities are required to obtain a business associates agreement to ensure that the business associates perform their work within the parameters of HIPAA regulations. Figures 14-11, 14-12, and 14-13 illustrate a sample business associate agreement.

Business Associate Agreement

This Business Associate Contract ("Contract"), effective ____________, 200__ ("Effective Date"), is entered into by and between ______________________________ (the "Contractor"), with an address at ________________ ____ and ______________________________ (the "Hospital"), with an address at ________________________ (each a "Party" and collectively the "Parties").

WITNESSETH:

WHEREAS, the U.S. Department of Health and Human Services ("HHS") has issued final regulations, pursuant to the Health Insurance Portability and Accountability Act of 1996 ("HIPAA"), governing the privacy of individually identifiable health information obtained, created or maintained by certain entities, including healthcare providers (the "HIPAA Privacy Rule"); and

WHEREAS, the HIPAA Privacy Rule requires that the Hospital enter into this Agreement with Contractor in order to protect the privacy of individually identifiable health information maintained by the Hospital ("Protected Health Information", or "PHI", as defined in the HIPAA Privacy Rule); and

WHEREAS, Contractor and its employees, affiliates, agents or representatives may access paper and/or electronic records containing PHI in carrying out their obligations to the Hospital pursuant to either an existing or contemporaneously executed agreement for services ("Services Agreement"); and

WHEREAS, the Parties desire to enter into this Agreement to protect PHI, and to amend any agreements between them, whether oral or written, with the execution of this Agreement;

NOW, THEREFORE, for and in consideration of the premises and mutual covenants and agreements contained herein the parties agree as follows:

1. **Services Agreements**
   1.1. Existing Services Agreements. Hospital and Contractor are parties to the following Services Agreements executed prior to the Effective Date and currently in effect (if any):
   Agreement: Services: Date of Agreement:
   ____

   All existing Services Agreements between the Parties are incorporated into this Agreement. In the event of conflict between the terms of any Services Agreement and this Agreement, the terms and conditions of this Agreement shall govern.
   1.1. Contemporaneous Services Agreement. In the event that Hospital and Contractor are not parties to a Services Agreement existing prior to the Effective Date, but instead enter into a Services Agreement at the same time as executing this Agreement, such agreement shall be attached as **Exhibit A**, and incorporated here by reference. In the event of conflict between the terms of the Services Agreement and this Agreement, the terms and conditions of this Agreement shall govern.
   1.2. Use and Disclosure of PHI to Provide Services. The Contractor will not use or further disclose PHI (as such term is defined in the HIPAA Privacy Rule) other than as permitted or required by the terms of the Service Agreement or as required by law. Except as otherwise provided in this document, the Contractor may make any and all uses of PHI necessary to perform its obligations under the applicable Services Agreement. All other uses not authorized by this Agreement are prohibited.
2. **Additional Contractor Activities.** Except as otherwise provided in this Agreement, the Contractor may also:
   2.1. Use the PHI in its possession for its proper management and administration and/or to fulfill any present or future legal responsibilities of the Contractor, provided that such uses are permitted under state and federal confidentiality laws.
   2.2. Disclose the PHI in its possession for the purpose of its proper management and administration and/or to fulfill any present or future legal responsibilities of the Contractor. Contractor represents to Hospital that (i) any disclosure it makes will be permitted under applicable laws, and (ii) the Contractor will obtain reasonable written assurances from any person to whom the PHI will be disclosed that the PHI will be held confidentially and used or further disclosed only as required and permitted under the HIPAA Privacy Rule and other applicable laws, that any such person agrees to be governed by the same restrictions and conditions contained in this Agreement, and that such person will notify the Contractor of any instances of which it is aware in which the confidentiality of the PHI has been breached.
   2.3. Bring together the Hospital's PHI in Contractor's possession with the PHI of other covered entities that the Contractor has in its possession through its capacity as a contractor to such other covered entities, provided that the purpose of bringing the PHI information together is to provide the Hospital with data analyses relating to its Healthcare Operations, as such term is defined in the HIPAA Privacy Rule. The Contractor will not disclose the PHI obtained from Hospital to another covered entity without written authorization from Hospital.
   2.4. De-identify any and all PHI provided that the de-identification conforms to the requirements of applicable law as provided for in 42 C.F.R. § 164.514(b) and that Contractor maintains such documentation as required by applicable law, as provided for in 42 C.F.R. § 164.514(b). The Parties understand that properly de-identified information is not PHI under the terms of this Agreement.
3. 3.1 use or further disclose the minimum necessary PHI in performing the activities called for under the Services Agreement;
   3.2 use appropriate safeguards to prevent the use or disclosure of PHI other than as provided for in this Agreement;
   3.3 in conjunction with the requirements of **Section 2.2**, ensure that any subcontractors or agents to whom it provides PHI received from, or created or received by the Contractor on behalf of the Hospital, agree to the same restrictions and conditions that apply to the
   Contractor with respect to the PHI;

Figure 14-11 Page 1 of sample Business Associate Agreement used to ensure that business associates perform their work within the parameters of HIPAA Title II: regulations. Covered entities are required to obtain a business associate agreement. *(Courtesy American Medical Billers Association [AMBA].)*

HIPAA TITLE II: ADMINISTRATIVE SIMPLIFICATION (AS)

The Title II: Administrative Simplification (AS) portion of HIPAA mandates replacement of paper transactions submitted to government-sponsored programs with electronic transactions as a means of reducing the administrative cost of processing health care transactions. To accomplish the transition from paper to an electronic format for transactions, provisions require the adoption of national standards for electronic health transactions. The increase in use of electronic

BOX 14-11 ■ KEY POINTS

Business Associate

Individuals, organizations, and other entities that work with health care providers, health plans, and clearinghouses. In accordance with HIPAA, business associates include law firms, accountants, information technology (IT) contractors, billing companies, consultants, and collection agencies.

Business associates are not covered entities and are not themselves required to comply with the law. However, they may need to make changes in order to do business with a covered entity.

Business Associate Agreement

Page 2

1. **Contractor Covenants.** Contractor agrees to:
   - 3.4. within ten (10) days of a request by Hospital, report to Hospital all disclosures of PHI to a third party for a purpose other than Treatment, Healthcare Operations or Payment, as such terms are defined in the HIPAA Privacy Rule. The report to the Hospital shall identify: (i) the subject of the PHI (i.e., patient name or identifier), (ii) the PHI disclosed, and (iii) the purpose of the disclosure in accordance with the accounting requirements of 45 C.F.R. § 164.528;
   - 3.5. maintain the integrity of any PHI transmitted by or received from Hospital;
   - 3.6. comply with Hospital policies and procedures with respect to the privacy and security of PHI and other Hospital records, as well as policies and procedures with respect to access and use of Hospital's equipment and facilities;
   - 3.7. provide the rights of access, amendment, and accounting as set forth in **Sections 5, 6** and **7**.
4. **Hospital Covenants.** Hospital agrees to notify Contractor of material limitations to the consents or authorizations that have been obtained by Hospital from their patients and any other restrictions on the use or disclosure of PHI as agreed to by Hospital.
5. **Access to PHI.** Within five (5) days of a request by Hospital for access to PHI about a patient contained in a Designated Record Set, as such term is defined in the HIPAA Privacy Rule, the Contractor shall make available to Hospital, or the patient to whom such PHI relates or his or her authorized representative, such PHI for so long as such information is maintained in the Designated Record Set as defined in 45 C.F.R. § 164.524. In the event any patient requests access to PHI directly from the Contractor, the Contractor shall, within five (5) days, forward such request to Hospital. Any denials of access to the PHI requested shall be the responsibility of Hospital.
6. **Amendment of PHI.** Within ten (10) days of receipt of a request from Hospital for the amendment of patient's PHI or a record regarding a patient contained in a Designated Record Set the Contractor shall, as required by 45 C.F.R. § 164.526, incorporate any such amendments in the PHI; provided, however, that Hospital has made the determination that the amendment(s) is/are necessary because the PHI that is the subject of the amendment(s) has been, or foreseeable could be, relied upon by the Contractor or others to the loss of the patient who is the subject of the PHI to be amended. The obligation in this Section 6 shall apply only for so long as the PHI is maintained by Contractor in a Designated Record Set.
7. **Accounting for Disclosures of PHI.** Within thirty (30) days of notice by Hospital to the Contractor that it has received a request for an accounting of disclosures of PHI regarding an individual, the Contractor shall make available to Hospital such information as is in the Contractor's possession and is required for Hospital to make the accounting required by 45 C.F.R. § 164.528. In the event the request for an accounting is delivered directly to the Contractor, the Contractor shall, within five (5) days, forward the request to Hospital. It shall be Hospital's responsibility to prepare and deliver any such accounting requested.
8. **Access to Books and Records Regarding PHI.** The Contractor will make its internal Hospitals, books, and records relating to the use and disclosure of PHI received from, or created or received by the Contractor on behalf of, Hospital available to the Secretary of the U.S. Department of Health and Human Services for purposes of determining Hospital compliance with the HIPAA Privacy Rule.
9. **Disposition of PHI Upon Termination.** The Contractor will, at termination or expiration of the Services Agreement, if feasible, return or destroy all PHI received from, or created or received by the Contractor on behalf of, Hospital which the Contractor and/or its subcontractors or agents still maintain in any form, and will not retain any copies of such information. If such return or destruction is not feasible, the Contractor will notify Hospital of such event in writing, and will therefore extend the protections of this Agreement to the PHI and limit further uses and disclosures to those purposes that make the return or destruction of the PHI not feasible.
10. **Representations and Warranties**
    - 10.4. Mutual Representations and Warranties of the Parties. Each Party represents and warrants to the other Party:
    - (a) that it is duly organized, validly existing, and in good standing under the laws of the jurisdiction in which it is organized or licensed, it has the full power to enter into this Agreement and to perform its obligations described in this Agreement, and that the performance by it of its obligations under this Agreement have been duly authorized by all necessary corporate or other actions and that such performance will not violate any provision of any organizational charter or bylaws.
    - (b) that neither the execution of this Agreement, nor its performance, will directly or indirectly violate or interfere with the terms of another agreement to which it is a party, or give any governmental entity the right to suspend, terminate, or modify any of its governmental authorizations or assets required for its performance.
    - (c) that all of its employees, agents, representatives and members of its workforce, whose services may be used to fulfill obligations under this Agreement are or shall be appropriately informed of the terms of this Agreement and are under legal obligation to each Party, respectively, by contract or otherwise, sufficient to enable each Party to fully comply with all provisions of this Agreement.
    - (d) that it will reasonably cooperate with the other Party in the performance of the mutual obligations under this Agreement.
11. **Term.** Unless otherwise terminated as provided in Section 12, this Agreement shall become effective on the Effective Date and shall have a term that shall run concurrently with that of all relevant Services Agreement(s).

Figure 14-12 Page 2 of sample Business Associate Agreement used to ensure that business associates perform their work within the parameters of HIPAA Title II: regulations. Covered entities are required to obtain a business associate agreement. *(Courtesy American Medical Billers Association [AMBA].)*

transmission also required standards to ensure the privacy and security of health information. Figure 14-14 outlines a summary of the provisions contained in Title II. HIPAA Title II: Administrative Simplification (AS) standards are specified in three specific sections: HIPAA electronic transactions and code set standards (TCS), HIPAA Privacy Regulations, and HIPAA Security Regulations.

- HIPAA electronic transaction and code sets standards (TCS): these standards require all providers and payers who conduct business electronically to use the same health care transactions, code sets, and identifiers.
- HIPAA privacy regulations: the privacy requirements outline the necessary measures to ensure the privacy and confidentiality of patient health information.
- HIPAA security regulations: the security requirements outline the administrative, technical, and physical safeguards that are required to protect patients' health information.

HIPAA-AS Standard Transactions and Code Sets (TCS)

Standardizing the electronic transmission of administrative and financial information will reduce the number of forms and methods used in the claims processing cycle and reduce the nonproductive effort that goes into

Business Associate Agreement
Page 3

12. **Termination**
    12.1. Generally. This Agreement will automatically terminate without any further action of the Parties upon the termination or expiration of all relevant Services Agreement(s); provided, however, certain provisions and requirements of this Agreement shall survive such expiration or termination in accordance with **Section 13**.
    12.2. Termination by the Hospital. As provided for under 45 C.F.R. § 164.504(e)(2)(iii), the Hospital may immediately terminate this Agreement, all relevant Services Agreement(s) and any related agreements if the Hospital makes the determination that Contractor has breached a material term of this Agreement. Alternatively, and in the sole discretion of Hospital, Hospital may choose to provide Contractor with written notice of the existence of the breach and provide Contractor with thirty (30) calendar days to cure said breach upon mutually agreeable terms. In the event that mutually agreeable terms cannot be reached within this thirty (30) day period, Contractor shall cure said breach to the satisfaction of the Hospital within an additional fifteen (15) days. Failure by Contractor to cure said breach or violation in the manner set forth above shall be grounds for immediate termination of the Services Agreement by the Hospital. If termination is not feasible, Hospital has the right to report the problem to the Secretary of the U.S. Department of Health and Human Services.
    12.3. Termination by the Contractor. If Contractor determines that Hospital has breached a material term of this Agreement, then the Contractor shall provide Hospital with written notice of the existence of the breach and shall provide Hospital with thirty (30) calendar days to cure said breach upon mutually agreeable terms. In the event that mutually agreeable terms cannot be reached within this thirty (30) day period, Hospital shall cure said breach to the satisfaction of the Contractor within an additional fifteen (15) days. Failure by Hospital to cure said breach or violation in the manner set forth above shall be grounds for immediate termination of the Services Agreement by the Contractor.
13. **Effect of Termination.** Upon termination pursuant to Section 12, Contractor agrees to return or destroy all PHI pursuant to 45 C.F.R. § 164.504(e)(2)(I), if it is feasible to do so. Prior to doing so, the Contractor further agrees to recover any PHI in the possession of its subcontractors or agents. If it is not feasible for the Contractor to return or destroy all PHI, the Contractor will notify the Hospital in writing. Such notification shall include: (i) a statement that the Contractor has determined that it is infeasible to return or destroy the PHI in its possession, and (ii) the specific reasons for such determination. Contractor further agrees to extend any and all protections, limitations and restrictions contained in this Agreement to the Contractor's use and/or disclosure of any PHI retained after the termination of this Agreement, and to limit any further uses and/or disclosures to the purposes that make the return or destruction of the PHI not feasible. If it is not feasible for the Contractor to obtain from a subcontractor or agent any PHI in the possession of the subcontractor or agent, the Contractor must provide a written explanation to the Hospital and require the subcontractors and agents to agree to extend any and all protections, limitations and restrictions contained in this Agreement to the subcontractors' and/or agents' use and/or disclosure of any PHI retained after the termination of this Agreement, and to limit any further uses and/or disclosures to the purposes that make the return or destruction of the PHI not feasible.

INTENDING TO BE LEGALLY BOUND, the Parties hereto have duly executed this Agreement as of the Effective Date.

____
Hospital Name

____
Signature Date
Name/Title
Address
Phone Number

____
Contractor

____
Signature Date
Name/Title
Address
Phone Number

Figure 14-13 Page 3 of sample Business Associate Agreement used to ensure that business associates perform their work within the parameters of HIPAA Title II: regulations. Covered entities are required to obtain a business associate agreement. *(Courtesy American Medical Billers Association [AMBA].)*

processing paper or nonstandard electronic claims. Prior to the implementation of HIPAA, it is reported that more than 400 versions of a National Standard Format existed to submit a claim for payment. Transaction and code set standards (TCS) eliminate the variety of formats and create one single set of standards. The adoption of these standards enables providers to submit electronic claims in the same format, using standard codes, regardless of the payer. Every health plan must accept the standard format and standard codes and send electronic messages back to the provider, also in standard formats, advising the provider of claim status, payment, and other key information. The Department of Health and Human Services (DHHS) has estimated that by implementing transaction and code set standards (TCS), almost $30 billion dollars over 10 years would be saved. The benefits of transaction and code set standards and electronic claim submission are outlined in Table 14-2. Three areas of standardization are: standard transactions, standard code sets and unique identifiers.

BOX 14-12 ■ KEY POINTS

HIPAA Title II: Administrative Simplification (AS) Standards

HIPAA electronic transaction and code sets standards (TCS)
HIPAA Privacy regulations
HIPAA Security regulations

HIPAA Title II: Administrative Simplification (AS)

Standards for electronic health information transactions. The Secretary of HHS is required to adopt standards from among those already approved by private standards developing organizations for certain electronic health transactions, including claims, enrollment, eligibility, payment, and coordination of benefits.

Privacy. The Secretary is required to recommend privacy standards for health information to Congress 12 months after enactment. If Congress does not enact privacy legislation within 3 years of enactment, the Secretary shall promulgate privacy regulations for individually identifiable electronic health information.

Security. The standards adopted by the Secretary of HHS must also contain provisions to ensure the security of electronic health information systems.

Mandate on providers and health plans, and timetable. Providers and health plans are required to use the standards for the specified electronic transactions by the compliance deadline outlined in the regulations. Plans and providers may comply directly, or may use a health care clearinghouse. Certain health plans, in particular workers' compensation, are not covered.

Penalties. The bill imposes civil money penalties and prison for certain violations

Preemption of state law. The bill supersedes state laws, except where the Secretary determines that the state law is necessary to prevent fraud and abuse, to ensure appropriate state regulation of insurance or health plans, addresses controlled substances, or for other purposes. If the Secretary promulgates privacy regulations, those regulations do not preempt state laws that impose more stringent requirements. These provisions do not limit a state's ability to require health plan reporting or audits.

Figure 14-14 Summary of Administrative Simplification provisions. (*Data from Centers for Medicare & Medicaid Services: Summary of Administrative Simplification Provisions, www.cms.hhs.gov/hipaa/hipaa2/general/background/h3103sum.asp, 2005.*)

Administrative Information

Referral certification and authorizations for services

Enrollment and disenrollment of individuals into a health plan

Health plan eligibility

Financial Information

Health care claim submission for services

Process health plan premium payment

Check status of a claim submitted previously

Health care payment and remittance advice

Coordination of benefits

Figure 14-15 Examples of administrative and financial information as outlined under HIPAA Title II: provisions. *(Data from Health Insurance Portability and Accountability Act of 1996.)*

BOX 14-13 ■ KEY POINTS

HIPAA-AS Standard Transactions and Code Sets (TCS)

HIPAA provisions include three areas of standardization:

- Standard transactions
- Standard code sets
- Standard unique identifiers.

Standard Transactions

The HIPAA transactions standards apply to the financial and administrative information that is regularly exchanged between providers and health plans. Figure 14-15 illustrates examples of administrative and finan-

TABLE 14-2 HIPAA Title II: Standard Transaction Code Sets (TCS) and Electronic Claims Submission

Benefit	Explanation
Increased reliability and timely processing	Fast eligibility evaluation; reduced accounts receivable; industry averages for claim turnarounds are 9–15 days for electronic claim versus 30–45 days for paper claims
Quicker reimbursement from payer	Improves cash flow for the health care organization
Improved accuracy of data	Decreases processing time, increases data quality, and leads to better reporting
Easier and more efficient access to information	Improved patient support
Improved tracing of transactions	Facilitates tracking information regarding transactions to improve monitoring; for example, monitoring of outstanding claims can improve collections
Reduction of data entry and manual labor	Electronic transactions facilitate automated processes such as automatic payment posting
Reduction of office expenses	Reduces expenses for office supplies, postage, and telephone

Data from Burton BK: Quick guide to HIPAA, *ed 1, St Louis, 2004, Saunders.*

TEST YOUR *Knowledge* BOX 14-2

HIPAA REGULATIONS AND COMPLIANCE

1. Explain the relationship between HIPAA regulations and compliance.
2. List and discuss one law that mandates compliance and has provisions for sanctions for noncompliance.
3. Discuss penalties than can be imposed by the CMS on organizations that are in violation of HIPAA regulations.
4. What agency is responsible for detection of fraud and abuse in health care?
5. Discuss the involvement of the Centers for Medicare and Medicaid Services with enforcing HIPAA regulations.
6. What portion of HIPAA regulations is the Office of Civil Rights (OCR) responsible for enforcing?
7. What laws take precedence over federal privacy standards?
8. Provide an explanation of a covered entity.
9. List three examples of covered entities.
10. Discuss the relationship between business associates and covered entities.

cial information. The term transaction refers to the transmission of information between two parties to carry out financial and administrative activities related to health care. The following types of transmissions are considered transactions.

- Health care claims or equivalent encounter information
- Health care payment and remittance advice
- Coordination of benefits
- Health care claim status
- Enrollment and disenrollment in a health plan
- Eligibility for health plan
- Health plan premium payments
- Referral certification and authorization
- First report of injury
- Health claim attachments

The transactions outlined above have adopted formats as illustrated in Table 14-3.

The adopted standard formats were developed by the American National Standards Institute (ANSI). Each transaction is labeled with both the transaction number and the name. Standard formats are labeled with the numbers ANSI X12 and three more digits to define the transaction format further. For example, ANSI X12 837 is the standardized format required for submission of an electronic claim.

BOX 14-14 ■ KEY POINTS

Transactions

The term transaction refers to the transmission of information between two parties to carry out financial and administrative activities related to health care. Types of transactions are as follows:

- Health care claims and attachments, payments and remittance advice, and claim status inquiries
- Coordination of benefits
- Enrollment and disenrollment in a health plan and eligibility for a health plan
- Health plan premium payments
- Referral certification and authorization
- First report of injury

Standard Code Sets

HIPAA standard code sets are used in conjunction with the standard electronic transactions. Under HIPAA, a code set is any group of codes used for encoding data elements, such as terms, medical concepts, diagnoses, or procedures. Medical code sets used in the health care industry to process health care transactions include coding systems for medical data elements such as diseases; treatments and procedures; and supplies or other items provided, as illustrated in Table 14-4. Standard coding systems adopted under HIPAA for hospital services are outlined below.

- ICD-9-CM
- HCPCS Level I: CPT
- HCPCS Level II: Medicare National codes

TABLE 14-3 HIPAA Title II: Transactions and Standard Formats

Standardized Transaction	Format
Health care claim submission or equivalent encounter	ANSI X12 837
Health care payment and remittance advice	ANSI X12 835
Coordination of benefits (COB)	ANSI X12 837
Health care claim status inquiry and response	ANSI X12 276–277
Claim status request	ANSI X12 276
Unsolicited claim status notification	ANSI X12 277
Request for additional information	ANSI X12 277
Claim status response	ANSI X12 277
Health plan enrollment and disenrollment	ANSI X12 834
Eligibility for health plan inquiry and response	ANSI X12 270–271
Health plan premium payments	ANSI X12 820
Referral authorization inquiry and response	ANSI X12 278
Health claim attachments	No standard format developed to date

Data from Burton BK: Quick guide to HIPAA, *ed 1, St Louis, 2004, Saunders.*

TABLE 14-4 HIPAA Title II: Standard Code Sets Adopted

Standard Code Set	Medical Data Element
International Classification of Diseases, 9th Revision, Clinical Modification (ICD-9-CM) codes, Volumes I, II, and III	Volume I and II utilized to report the reason services were rendered, such as sign, symptom, condition, disease, illness, injury, or other reason for the visit. Volume III utilized to report significant procedures and services performed by a facility.
HCPCS Level I: CPT	To report physician and outpatient services, procedures, and items.
HCPCS Level II: Medicare National	To report services, procedures, and items when no CPT code provides an adequate description or when the payer indicates Level II codes should be used instead of Level I CPT codes.
National Drug Codes (NDC)	To report pharmaceuticals and biologics for retail pharmacy transactions.

Data from Burton BK: Quick guide to HIPAA, *ed 1, St Louis, 2004, Saunders.*

Supporting Code Sets

In addition to the major code sets outlined above, there are several supporting code sets that encompass both medical and nonmedical data, as illustrated in Table 14-5. You will not need to know all these specific codes, but it will be helpful to know they exist, especially if you are involved in the claims process in your facility. When constructing a claim, the supporting code sets are made up of required and situational data elements, similar to those on the paper claim form. These supporting code sets are embedded in data elements identified by the HIPAA standard electronic formats. "Required" refers to data elements that must be used to meet HIPAA transaction compliance standards. "Situational" means that the item depends on the data content or context. For example, a baby's birth weight is situational when you are submitting a claim for the delivery of the infant. Determining the required and situational data elements not currently collected for the claim form is complex, and you will become familiar with this process when you are performing claims processing duties. In addition to elements outlined in Table 14-5 required under HIPAA, the following supporting code sets have been developed:

- Taxonomy codes: provider specialty codes assigned to each health care provider.
- Patient account number: to be assigned to every claim.
- Relationship to patient: 25 different relationships including indicators such as grandson, adopted child, mother, and life partner.
- Facility code value: facility-related element that identifies the place of service, with at least 29 to choose from, including office, ambulance, air or water transport, and end-stage renal disease treatment facility.
- Patient signature source code: indicates how the patient or subscriber signatures were obtained for authorization and how signatures are retained by the provider. Codes include letters such as B for "signed signature authorization form or forms are on file" and P for "signature generated by provider" because the patient was not physically present for services such as pathology services.

TABLE 14-5 HIPAA Title II: Supporting Code Sets

Adjustment Reason Code	Entity Identifier Code	Product/Service Procedure Code
Agency Qualifier Code Amount	Exception Code	Prognosis Code
Qualifier Code	Facility Type Code	Provider Code
Ambulatory Patient Group Code	Functional Status Code	Provider Organization Code
Attachment Report Type Code	Hierarchical Child Code	Provider Specialty Certification Code
Attachment Transmission Code	Hierarchical Level Code	Provider Specialty Code
Claim Adjustment Group Code	Hierarchical Structure Code	Record Format Code
Claim Filing Indicator Code	Immunization Status Code	Reject Reason Code
Claim Frequency Code Claim	Immunization Type Code	Related-Causes Code
Payment Remark Code	Individual Relationship Code	Service Type Code
Claim Submission Reason Code	Information Release Code	Ship/Delivery or Calendar Pattern Code
Code List Qualifier Code	Insurance Type Code	Ship/Delivery Pattern Time Code
Condition Codes	Measurement Reference ID Code	Student Status Code
Contact Function	Code Medicare Assignment Code	Supporting Document Response Code
Contract Code	Nature of Condition Code	Surgical Procedure Code
Contract Type Code	Non-Visit Code Note	Transaction Set Identifier Code
Credit/Debit Flag Code	Reference Code	Transaction Set Purpose Code
Currency Code	Nutrient Administration Method Code	Unit or Basis Measurement Code
Disability Type Code	Nutrient Administration Technique Code	Version Identification Code X-Ray
Discipline Type Code	Place of Service Code	Availability Indicator Code
Employment Status Code Entity	Policy Compliance Code	

Data from Burton BK: Quick guide to HIPAA, *ed 1, St Louis, 2004, Saunders.*

BOX 14-15 ■ KEY POINTS

HIPAA-AS Supporting Code Sets

HIPAA provisions also require the following supporting code sets for use in claim form preparation:

- Taxonomy codes
- Patient account number
- Relationship to patient
- Facility code value
- Patient signature source code.

Standard Unique Identifiers

The Administrative Simplification provisions mandated the creation of HIPAA National Identifiers for employers, health care providers, health plans, and patients. Identifiers are numbers of predetermined length and structure, such as a person's Social Security number. They are important because the unique numbers can be used in electronic transactions as a standard system. There is discussion of establishing standard unique identifiers for health plans and patients; however, proposed rules have not been published to date. The following two standard unique identifiers have been developed.

Employer Identification Number (EIN)

HIPAA standards require the Employer Identification Number (EIN) for electronic transactions to identify the provider or employer. An **Employer Identification Number (EIN)** is a number assigned by the Internal Revenue Service to hospitals and other employers, and it is used for tax reporting purposes. The employer identification number is also known as the Tax Identification Number (TIN). Under HIPAA guidelines, the EIN number is used to identify employers on all electronic transactions, including those involving premium payments to health plans for employees, for the enrollment or disenrollment of employees in a health plan and to identify employers on claims.

BOX 14-16 ■ KEY POINTS

HIPAA-AS Standard Unique Identifiers

Employer Identification Number (EIN)

HIPAA guidelines mandate the use of the EIN to identify employers on all electronic transaction.

National Provider Identifier (NPI)

HIPAA mandates that the standard unique health identifier for health care providers when filing and processing health care claims and other transactions should be the NPI.

National Provider Identifier (NPI)

The **National Provider Identifier (NPI)** is the standard unique health identifier for health care providers to use in filing and processing health care claims and other transactions. NPIs are being issued through the National Provider System (NPS), which is being developed by CMS. The NPI will replace all identifiers that are currently being used. All health care providers are eligible for an NPI assignment. The NPI is ten positions in length, with nine numbers plus a check digit in the last position. The numbers will be assigned to individuals, such as doctors, nurses, and hygienists. NPI numbers will also be assigned to organizations, such as hospitals, pharmacies, and clinics. For example, if a physician is in a group practice, both the individual and the practice will have NPIs.

Enforcement and Penalties

CMS enforces the transaction and code set standards. Failure to comply with the transaction and code set rule may result in monetary penalties. CMS may impose a penalty of not more than $100 per violation on the entity failing to comply, with a cap of $25,000 for violations of a single standard in a calendar year.

HIPAA TITLE II: PRIVACY RULE

The HIPAA Privacy final rule was published by the Department of Health and Human Services (DHHS) in December of 2000 and it became effective on April 14, 2001. Compliance of HIPAA privacy standards was required two years after the effective date, April 14, 2003. The regulations are intended to protect the privacy and confidentiality of health information. Traditionally, there has been a focus on protecting the paper medical record and documentation that contained patient health information, such as progress notes and laboratory and radiology reports. HIPAA Privacy regulations expand these protections to apply to all forms of protected health information (PHI). The HIPAA Privacy Rule also expands patients' rights regarding access to and control of their health information. Under HIPAA, every person in the country has at least the same basic rights and protections, although some may have additional rights depending on state law. The HIPAA Privacy Rule contains provisions to adopt national standards to ensure the protection of health information and to give all patients the same basic rights regarding access to and control of their health information. Figure 14-16 provides a summary of HIPAA Privacy Rule mandates, which can be summarized as follows:

- To adopt privacy practices to ensure that patient rights are protected.
- To provide patients with a notice of privacy practices and obtain acknowledgement.

TEST YOUR *Knowledge* BOX 14-3

HIPAA TITLE II: ADMINISTRATIVE SIMPLIFICATION (AS)

1. Provide a brief explanation of the objectives of HIPAA Title II Administrative Simplification legislation.
2. List the three sections of HIPAA Title II Administrative Simplification.
3. Explain the purpose of HIPAA standard transactions and code sets.
4. Discuss the purpose of standard code sets required for health care transactions.
5. Discuss two significant benefits of standard transaction code sets and electronic claims submission for providers.
6. Outline two types of information to which HIPAA-(AS) transaction standards apply.
7. Explain the meaning of the term transaction.
8. List five examples of transactions.
9. Outline the coding systems that are listed as the standard coding systems adopted under HIPAA.
10. List and discuss two types of standard unique identifiers that have been developed under HIPAA.

Covered entities are required to:

- Adopt a set of privacy practices to ensure private rights are protected
- Provide notice of privacy practices
- Obtain required authorizations
- Obtain appropriate authorizations for use and disclosure of protected health information
- Allow patients access and changes to health information
- Provide accounting of nonroutine uses and disclosures

Figure 14-16 Provisions that must be followed by covered entities as outlined under the HIPAA Title II: Privacy Rule. *(Data from Health Insurance Portability and Accountability Act of 1996.)*

- To obtain appropriate authorizations for use and disclosure of protected health information (PHI).
- To allow patients access to their health information and the ability to request changes and to correct errors.
- To provide an account of nonroutine uses and disclosures to patients.

Protected Health Information (PHI)

HIPAA includes provisions to protect a patient's individually identifiable health information. **Individually identifiable health information (IIHI)** is any part of an individual's health information including demographic and medical information collected from the individual or received by a covered entity including information:

- Regarding the individual's past, present, or future physical or mental health or condition.
- Related to the provision of health care.
- Pertaining to past, present, or future payment for the provision of health care.

HIPAA Administrative Simplification provisions work to simplify and standardize health care transactions to increase the use of electronic data exchange. Protection of data that are transmitted electronically is a major focus of the HIPAA Privacy Rule, and these data are referred to as protected health information. **Protected health information (PHI)** refers to individually identifiable health information (IIHI) that is transmitted by electronic media, maintained in electronic form, or transmitted or maintained in any other form or medium.

De-Identified Information

The HIPAA Privacy Rule does not apply to information that has been de-identified. **De-identification** refers to the elimination of information that can be used to identify an individual. Identifiers of the individual, relatives, employers, and household members must be removed for the data to be de-identified. HIPAA recognizes the following data elements as information that can be used to identify an individual:

- Name, address, telephone number, fax number, and e-mail address(s).
- Social Security number, medical record number, account number, and health plan identification number.
- Certificate number, license number, and vehicle and device numbers.
- Web page URLs, Internet provider (IP) address(s), biometric identifiers, and facial photographs.
- Any other unique identifying number, characteristic, or code.

HIPAA Privacy Practices

HIPAA Privacy regulations require covered entities to adopt privacy practices that are appropriate for its health care services. Privacy practices should include guidelines regarding authorizations, privacy notification, patient access, an accounting of disclosures, employee training, and the appointment of a privacy officer, as outlined below:

- Authorizations: obtain authorization to disclose health information in nonroutine situations.
- Notification of privacy practices: informs patients of their rights to privacy and how the organization can use or disclose patient information. Patient acknowledgment of receipt of the notice of privacy practices is required.
- Access: allows patients access to their health information and the ability to request changes and to correct errors.
- Accounting: provides patients with an accounting of nonroutine uses and disclosures of their health information upon request.
- Employee training: educates employees on the organization's privacy practices.
- Privacy official: the organization must appoint a privacy official who is responsible for the adoption of privacy practices and the monitoring of compliance.

Notice of Privacy Practices

Under the HIPAA Privacy Rule, covered entities are required to inform patients of the organization's privacy

BOX 14-17 ■ KEY POINTS

De-identification

De-identification refers to the elimination of information that can be used to identify an individual. Identifiers of the individual, relatives, employers, and household members must be removed for the data to be de-identified. HIPAA recognizes specified data elements as information that can be used to identify an individual. Examples of identifying information include:

- Patient's name, address, telephone number, fax number, and e-mail address(s)
- Social Security number, medical record number, account number, health plan identification number
- Certificate number, license number, vehicle, device numbers

BOX 14-18 ■ KEY POINTS

HIPAA Privacy Notice

Covered entities are required to inform patients of the organization's privacy practices. The Notice of Privacy Practices informs patients of their rights and how health information may be used and disclosed. Under HIPAA, a Notice of Privacy Practices must explain the following:

- Use and disclosure of PHI by the organization
- Responsibility of provider to protect PHI
- Patient's rights regarding PHI
- The process for filing complaints with the office and the DHHS
- Contact individual for further information (usually the privacy officer)
- The date the Notice is effective.

practices. Compliance with this standard requires the covered entity to provide each patient with Notice of Privacy Practices. A signed acknowledgement of receipt of the notice must be obtained from the patient and kept on file. The Notice of Privacy Practices informs the patient of their rights and how health information may be used and disclosed, as shown in Figure 14-17. Under HIPAA a Notice of Privacy Practices must explain the following:

- How PHI may be used and disclosed by the organization.
- The health care provider's duties to protect PHI.

HIPAA REGULATIONS
NOTICE OF PRIVACY PRACTICES

THIS NOTICE DESCRIBES HOW INFORMATION ABOUT YOU MAY BE USED AND DISCLOSED AND HOW YOU CAN GET ACCESS TO THIS INFORMATION. PLEASE REVIEW IT CAREFULLY.

Please review and sign below to acknowledge receipt of this notice.

My signature below indicates that I have been provided with a copy of the notice of privacy practices.

Signature: ____________________

Date: ____________________

Signature of Patient or Legal Representative:

COMMUNITY GENERAL HOSPITAL

NOTICE OF PRIVACY PRACTICES

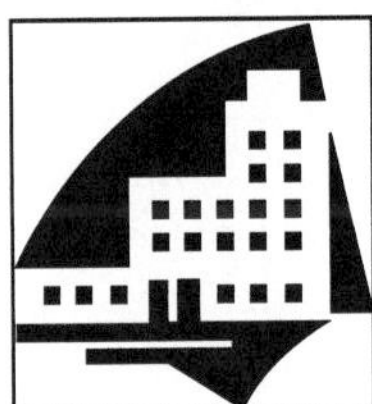

UNDERSTANDING YOUR HEALTH RECORD/ INFORMATION

Each time you visit a hospital, physician, or other healthcare provider, a record of your visit is made. Typically, this record contains your symptoms, examination and test results, diagnoses, treatment, and a plan for future care or treatment. This information, often referred to as your health or medical record, serves as a:

- means of communication among the many health professionals who contribute to your care
- legal document describing the care you received
- means by which you or a third-party payer can verify that services billed were actually provided
- a tool in educating health professionals
- a source of data for medical research
- a source of information for public health officials charged with improving the health of the nation
- a source of data for facility planning and marketing and a tool with which we can assess and continually work to improve the care we render and the outcomes we achieve. Understanding what is in your record and how your health information is used helps you to:
- ensure its accuracy
- better understand who, what, when, where and why others may access your health information make more informed decisions when authorizing disclosure to others.

YOUR HEALTH INFORMATION RIGHTS:
Although your health record is the physical property of the healthcare practitioner or facility that compiled it, the information belongs to you. You have the right to:

- request a restriction on certain uses and disclosures of your information as provided by 45 CFR 164.522
- obtain a paper copy of the notice of inform-ation practices upon request
- inspect and copy your health record as pro-vided for in 45 CFR 164.524
- amend your health record as provided in 45 CFR 164.528
- obtain an accounting of disclosures of your health information as provided in 45 CFR 164.528 request communications of your health information by alternative means or at alternative locations revoke your authorization to use or disclose health information except to the extent that action has already been taken.

OUR RESPONSIBILITIES
This organization is required to:

- maintain the privacy of your health information
- provide you with a notice as to our legal duties and privacy practices with respect to information we collect and maintain about you
- abide by the terms of this notice
- notify you if we are unable to agree to a requested restriction accommodate reasonable requests you may have to communicate health information by alternative means or at alternative locations.

We reserve the right to change our practices and to make the new provisions effective for all protected health information we maintain. Should our information practices change, we will mail a revised notice to the address you've supplied us.

We will not use or disclose your health infor-mation without your authorization, except as described in this notice.

FOR MORE INFORMATION OR TO REPORT A PROBLEM
If you have questions and would like additional information, you may contact the Director of Health Information Management at (747) 722-1800. If you believe your privacy rights have been violated, you can file a complaint with the Director of Health Information Management or with the Secretary of Health and Human Services. There will be no retali-ation for filing a complaint.

EXAMPLES OF DISCLOSURES FOR TREATMENT, PAYMENT AND HEALTH OPERATIONS
We will use your health information for treat-ment. For example: Information obtained by a nurse, physician or other member of your healthcare team will be recorded in your record and used to determine the course of treatment that should work best for you. Your physician will document in your record his expectations of the members of your health-care team. Members of your healthcare team will then record the actions they took and their observations. In that way the physician will know how you are responding to treatment. We will also provide your physician or a subsequent healthcare provider with copies of various reports that should assist him/her in treating you once you're discharged from this hospital.

Figure 14-17 Sample HIPAA Title II: Notice of Privacy Practices used to inform patients of the organization's privacy practices. *(Modified from American Health Information Management Association: Sample Notice of Health Information Practices, http://library.ahima.org.)*

- The patient's rights regarding PHI.
- How complaints may be filed with the office and the Department of Health and Human (DHHS) services if the patient believes his or her privacy rights have been violated.
- Who to contact for further information (usually the privacy officer).
- Effective date of the Notice.

In addition to providing a patient with the Notice of Privacy Practices, HIPAA requires the notice to be posted in a prominent area where patients can see it. If the organization has a Web site, HIPAA also requires that the notice be posted on the Web site. HIPAA regulations clearly indicate that covered entities are not allowed to request patients to waive their rights as a condition of receiving treatment.

Patient Privacy Rights

HIPAA Privacy regulations expand patients' rights to include access to health information and control over how PHI can be used or disclosed. Patient rights outlined under HIPAA include:

- Right to Notice of Privacy Practices.
- Right to request restrictions on certain uses and disclosures of PHI.
- Right to request confidential communications.
- Right to access (inspect and obtain a copy of) PHI.
- Right to request an amendment of PHI.
- Right to receive an account of disclosures of PHI.

Use and Disclosure of Protected Health Information (PHI)

The general rule is that a covered entity may not use or disclose protected health information without an individual's written authorization, except if permitted or required by the Privacy Rule. **Use of PHI** refers to sharing of protected health information (PHI) with health care professionals within the hospital as required to diagnose and treat the patient. **Disclosure of PHI** refers to releasing protected health information (PHI) to individuals or organizations outside the hospital. HIPAA regulations define exceptions to the privacy rule when no authorization is required to release or use protected health information.

Exceptions to the Privacy Rule

Covered entities such as a hospital may be required to use or disclose protected health information for several reasons, as illustrated in Figure 14-18. The Privacy Rule contains provisions for covered entities to use or disclose PHI for the purposes described below, and such entities are not required to obtain a written authorization for release of the information.

Treatment, Payment and Health Care Operations

Hospitals use and disclose PHI to individuals within the organization as required to diagnose and treat the patient. For example, health records are used by various ancillary departments within the organization to perform diagnostic and therapeutic services required to treat the patient. To obtain payment for services rendered, the hospital must send information regarding the diagnosis and treatment of patient conditions to health plans. This exception also applies to the release of information to the Workers' Compensation administration board for review and determination of a Workers' Compensation cases. During the course of providing health care services and billing for those services, there are various hospital operational and management functions that may require the use or disclosure of PHI.

Health Care Oversight and Regulation

Hospitals are regulated by several federal and state agencies. Oversight activities including audits, investigations, and site visits may require the use and disclosure of protected health information.

BOX 14-19 ■ KEY POINTS

HIPAA Use and Disclosure of Protected Health Information (PHI)

Use of PHI refers to sharing of PHI with health care professionals within the hospital as required to diagnose and treat the patient. **Disclosure of PHI** refers to releasing PHI to individuals or organizations outside of the hospital. The Privacy Rule contains provisions outlining:

- Exceptions to the Privacy Rule
- Authorization for release of health information
- Minimum necessary standard
- Designated Record Set
- Enforcement and penalties.

HIPAA Title II: Privacy Rule

Exceptions

(covered entities are not required to obtain authorization from the patient to use or disclose protected health information)

Treatment, Payment, and Health Care Operations

Health Care Oversight and Regulations

Public Health Safety and Protection

Administrative and Judicial Proceedings

Figure 14-18 Exceptions to the Privacy Rule as outlined under HIPAA Title II. Covered entities are not required to obtain authorization when information release is for the specified purposes. *(Data from Health Insurance Portability and Accountability Act of 1996.)*

Public Health Safety and Protection

Information regarding patient care is often used or disclosed to various federal and state agencies for the purposes of health safety and protection. For example, hospitals are required to report acts of violent crimes such as gunshot wounds to law enforcement agencies. Another example is reporting of information related to abuse or domestic violence. Use or disclosure of PHI is also required to monitor public health for the purpose of identifying epidemics or health hazards.

Administrative and Judicial Proceedings

A hospital may be required to release PHI as a part of an administrative or judicial proceeding, for example, when records are released in response to a subpoena.

Authorization for Release of Health Information

HIPAA regulations require covered entities to obtain written authorization to use or disclose PHI. An **authorization for release of medical information** is a written document signed by the patient that grants permission to the hospital to use or disclose PHI for specified purposes that are generally other than treatment, payment, or health care operations. Exceptions to this rule were outlined earlier in this section. Authorizations must contain the following information to meet HIPAA requirements:

- A description of the information to be used or disclosed.
- The name or other specific identification of the person (s) authorized to use or disclose the information.
- The name of the person(s) or group of people to whom the covered entity may make the use or disclosure.
- A description of each purpose of the requested use or disclosure.
- Expiration date.
- Signature of the individual (or authorized representative) and date.

Valid authorizations as defined under HIPAA must also include a statement regarding use of the information and revocation of the authorization, as outlined below (Figure 14-19):

- A statement of the individual's right to revoke the authorization in writing.
- A statement about whether the covered entity is able to base treatment, payment, enrollment, or eligibility for benefits on the authorization.
- A statement that information used or disclosed after the authorization may be disclosed again by the recipient and may no longer be protected by the rule.

BOX 14-20 ■ KEY POINTS

Authorization for Release of PHI

HIPAA regulations require covered entities to obtain a written authorization to disclose PHI.

The Authorization must contain specified information regarding the following:

- The person(s) authorized to use or disclose information
- The group of people to whom the covered entity may make the use or disclosure
- The information to be used or disclosed and the purpose

The authorization must include an expiration date and must be signed and dated by the patient to grant permission to the hospital to use or disclose.

Valid authorizations as defined under HIPAA must also include a statement regarding the following:

- Individual's right to revoke the authorization in writing.
- Whether the covered entity is able to base treatment, payment, enrollment, or eligibility for benefits on the authorization.
- Information used or disclosed after the authorization may be disclosed again by the recipient and may no longer be protected by the rule.

Minimum Necessary Standard

When using or disclosing PHI, a covered entity must try to limit the information shared to the minimum amount of PHI necessary to accomplish the intended purpose. The minimum necessary standard means taking reasonable safeguards to protect PHI from incidental disclosure. For example, a hospital billing professional may not disclose a patient's history of cancer on a Workers' Compensation claim for a sprained ankle. Only the information the recipient needs to know is appropriate.

Designated Record Set (DRS)

A covered entity must disclose an individuals' PHI to them (or their personal representative) when access is requested (or an accounting of disclosures of) PHI. According to the AHIMA Practice Brief: Defining the Designated Record Set, "patients' rights apply to a designated record set (DRS)." For a provider, the DRS includes medical and billing records the provider maintains. It does not include appointment and surgery schedules, requests for lab tests, or birth and death records. It also does not include mental health information, psychotherapy notes, and genetic information. For a health plan, the DRS includes enrollment, payment, claim decisions, and medical management systems of the plan.

Enforcement and Penalties

The HIPAA Privacy Rule requires compliance of all provisions by covered entities: health care providers,

Patient Authorization for Release of Protected Information

By signing this authorization, I authorize ______________________ to use and/or disclose
(Hospital Name)

certain protected health information (PHI) about me to or for the party or parties listed below.

This authorization permits ______________________ to use or disclose to
(Hospital Name)

______________________ the following individually identifiable health information (specifically
(Person or Entity to Receive the Information)

describe the information to be released, such as date(s) of service, level of detail to be released,

origin of information, etc.). ______________________

____

____

This authorization will expire on ______________________ .
(Expiration Date or Defined Event).

When my information is used or disclosed pursuant to this authorization, it may be subject to

redisclosure by the recipient and may no longer be protected by the federal HIPAA Privacy Rule.

I have the right to revoke this authorization in writing except to the extent that

______________________ has acted in reliance upon this authorization. My written revocation
(Hospital Name)

must be submitted to ______________________'s Privacy Officer at (*Street Address, City, State Zip*).

Signed by:

Signature of Patient or Legal Guardian ______ Relationship to Patient ______

Patient's Name ______ Date ______

Print Name of Patient or Legal Guardian ______

Figure 14-19 Sample patient authorization for release of protected health information as required under the HIPAA Privacy Rule. (Modified from American Health Information Management Association: *Patient Authorization for Hospital to Release Protected Health Information to Third Parties, http://library.ahima.org.)*

health plans, and health care clearinghouses. Failure to comply with HIPAA regulations may result in civil or criminal penalties. As discussed earlier in the chapter, the Office of Civil Rights (OCR) identifies and investigates potential HIPAA Privacy violations. Civil penalties for HIPAA Privacy violations, which can be imposed only on covered entities, not on business associates, can be up to $100 for each offense, with an annual cap of $25,000 for repeated violations of the same requirement. The first conviction for HIPAA violations occurred in August 2004, and the convicted individual could have received a sentence of 10 to 16 months in prison, home, or community confinement, as illustrated in Figure 14-20. The criminal and civil penalties that may result from an investigation are as follows:

- For knowing misuse of individually identifiable health information: up to $50,000 and/or 1 year in prison.
- For misuse under false pretenses: up to $100,000 and/or 5 years in prison.
- For offenses involving selling for profit or malicious harm: up to $250,000 and/or 10 years in prison.

BOX 14-21 ■ KEY POINTS

Designated Record Set (DRS)

According to the "AHIMA Practice Brief: Defining the Designated Record Set," includes medical and billing records the provider maintains.

Information not included in the DRS include:

- Appointment and surgery schedules
- Requests for lab tests
- Birth or death records
- Mental health information

AUGUST 19, 2004

UNITED STATES ATTORNEY'S OFFICE
Western District of Washington
PRESS ROOM

RICHARD W. GIBSON, age 42, of SeaTac, Washington pleaded guilty today in federal court in Seattle to wrongful disclosure of individually identifiable health information for economic gain. This is the first criminal conviction in the United States under the health information privacy provisions of the Health Insurance Portability and Accountability Act (HIPAA) which became effective in April, 2003. Those provisions made it illegal to wrongfully disclose personally identifiable health information.

As set forth in the Plea Agreement (also view information), GIBSON admitted that he obtained a cancer patient's name, date of birth and Social Security number while GIBSON was employed at the Seattle Cancer Care Alliance, and that he disclosed that information to get four credit cards in the patient's name. GIBSON also admitted that he used several of those cards to rack up more than $9,000 in debt in the patient's name. GIBSON admitted he used the cards to purchase various items, including video games, home improvement supplies, apparel, jewelry, porcelain figurines, groceries and gasoline for his personal use. GIBSON was fired shortly after the identity theft was discovered.

The Government and GIBSON agreed as part of the Plea Agreement, that GIBSON should be sentenced to a term of 10 to 16 months. Under these terms, the Court could order that the term be served either wholly in federal prison, or in a combination of federal prison and either home confinement or community confinement. GIBSON has also agreed to pay restitution to the credit card companies, and to the patient for expenses he incurred as a result of GIBSON's use of his identity.

At a hearing scheduled for November 5, 2004, U.S. District Court Judge Ricardo S. Martinez will determine whether to accept the Plea Agreement, and if accepted, will determine GIBSON's sentence within the 10-16 month range set forth in the Plea Agreement and the length of any supervised release following his prison term. If the Court rejects the Plea Agreement and the agreed upon sentence, GIBSON will have an opportunity to withdraw his guilty plea.

"Too many Americans have experienced identity theft and the nightmare of dealing with bills they never incurred. To be a vulnerable cancer patient, fighting for your life, and having to cope with identity theft is just unconscionable," stated United States Attorney John McKay. "This case should serve as a reminder that misuse of patient information may result in criminal prosecution."

The case was investigated by the Federal Bureau of Investigation (FBI) and is being prosecuted by Assistant United States Attorney Susan Loitz. For further information please contact Emily Langlie, Public Affairs Officer for the United States Attorney's Office at (206) 553-4110.

Figure 14-20 Press Notice from the United States Attorney General's office summarizing the specifics of the "First Ever Conviction for HIPAA Rules Violation." *(Modified from U.S. Attorney's Office Western District of Washington, Seattle Man Pleads Guilty in First Ever Conviction for HIPAA Rules Violation, www.usdoj.gov.)*

HIPAA TITLE II: SECURITY RULE

The final HIPAA Security Rule was published by the Department of Health and Human Services (DHHS) in the Federal Register on February 20, 2003. The Security regulations became effective on April 21, 2003, and compliance was required for most covered entities by April 20, 2005. The HIPAA Security Rule was implemented to protect electronic health information. As illustrated in Figure 14-21, the general provisions of the Security Rule require covered entities to:

- Ensure the confidentiality, integrity, and availability of all electronic protected health information (EPHI) the covered entity creates, receives, maintains, or transmits.
- Protect against any reasonably anticipated threats or hazards to the security or integrity of such information.
- Protect against any reasonably anticipated uses or disclosures of such information that are not permitted or required by the Privacy Rule.
- Ensure compliance by its workforce.
- Adopt standards and specifications required to implement provisions of the general rule.

HIPAA Security provision outline standards for administrative, technical, and physical safeguards required to ensure the security of electronic protected health information (EPHI).

Administrative Safeguards

Administrative safeguards concentrate on the security management policies and procedures required to prevent, detect, contain, and correct security violations. HIPAA security standards are designed to prevent unauthorized use or disclosure of EPHI through administrative actions and policies and procedures to manage

TEST YOUR *Knowledge* BOX 14-4

HIPAA TITLE II: PRIVACY RULE

1. State the date the HIPAA Privacy Rule became effective and the date required for compliance.
2. Discuss the purpose of the HIPAA Privacy Rule.
3. Explain how the HIPAA Privacy Rule expanded patients' rights.
4. Outline and discuss five HIPAA Privacy Rule mandates.
5. Discuss the difference between individually protected health information and protected health information.
6. The HIPAA Privacy Rule does not apply to information that has been de-identified. Explain what de-identified information is.
7. List and discuss privacy practice guidelines.
8. Explain the purpose of a Notice of Privacy Practices.
9. Discuss the Privacy Rule and how it relates to use and disclosure of health information.
10. Outline four exceptions to the Privacy Rule.
11. Provide an explanation of the purpose of an authorization for release of protected health information.
12. A valid authorization, as defined under HIPAA, must contain what information?
13. Explain what minimum necessary standard means.
14. State the purpose of the designated record set.
15. List the agency that identifies and investigates potential HIPAA privacy violations and discuss the penalties that can be imposed.

HIPAA Title II: Security Rule

General Rule Provisions

Section 164.306, the statement of the general rule, requires covered entities to:

- Ensure the confidentiality, integrity, and availability of all electronic protected health information (EPHI) the covered entity creates, receives, maintains, or transmits
- Protect against any reasonably anticipated threats or hazards to the security or integrity of such information
- Protect against any reasonably anticipated uses or disclosures of such information that are not permitted or required by the Privacy Rule
- Ensure compliance by its workforce

Covered entities are required to adopt standards and specifications required to implement provisions of the general rule.

Figure 14-21 Highlights of general provisions contained in the HIPAA Title II: Security Rule. *(Data from Health Insurance Portability and Accountability Act of 1996.)*

BOX 14-22 ■ KEY POINTS

HIPAA Title II: Security Rule

The HIPAA Security Rule became effective on April 21, 2003 and compliance was required for most covered entities by April 20, 2005. The rule was implemented to protect electronic health information.

HIPAA Security provisions outline standards for administrative, physician, and technical safeguards required to ensure the security of electronic protected health information (EPHI).

the selection, development, implementation, and maintenance of security measures to protect EPHI. HIPAA regulations outline the following required implementation specifications related to management controls to guard data integrity, confidentiality, and access: risk analysis and management, information system activity review, and procedures for security violations.

Risk Analysis and Management

Analyzing risk refers to the process that assesses the privacy and security risks of various safeguards and the implications of not having safeguards in place. This process has been newly introduced into health care compliance, and each organization must evaluate its vulnerabilities and the associated risks and decide how to reduce those risks. Reasonable safeguards must be implemented to protect against known risks.

Information System Activity Review

Review of system activities is critical to the prevention and detection of security violations. Internal audits and

BOX 14-23 ■ KEY POINTS

HIPAA Title II: Security Rule Administrative Safeguards

Administrative safeguards concentrate on the security management policies and procedures required to prevent, detect, contain, and correct security violations, as follows:

- Risk analysis and management
- Information system activity review
- Procedures for security violations.

information access controls are two ways an organization can review system activity:

Internal Audits

Audits conducted internally allow the organization to review who has had access to EPHI to ensure that there is no intentional or accidental inappropriate access, in both the practice management software system and the paper records or charges. Access controls are utilized to monitor system activity.

Information Access Controls

Access controls authorize each employee's physical access to EPHI. Implementation of password and access codes for separate employees allows management to restrict employees' access to records in accordance with their responsibility in the health care organization. For example, the medical records clerk who has an authorization to retrieve medical records will probably not have access to billing records located in the computer.

Termination procedures should be formally documented in the policies and procedures manual that outlines procedures for terminating the employee's access to EPHI. Other procedures would probably include changing office security pass codes, deleting user access to computer systems, deleting terminated employee's e-mail account, and collecting any access cards or keys from terminated employees.

Procedures for Security Violations

Policies and procedures are required to address security incidents, including required specifications, response, and reporting. This provision calls for covered entities to identify and respond to suspected security incidents that are known to the covered entity and to document security incidents and outcomes.

Technical Safeguards

Technical safeguards are technological controls in place to protect and control access to information on computers in the health care organization. Examples of technical safeguards are: access controls, audit controls, automatic log-offs and unique identifier ("user name").

BOX 14-24 ■ KEY POINTS

HIPAA Title II: Security Rule Technical Safeguards

Technical safeguards that concentrate on the protection and control of access to PHI on computers are as follows:

- Access to controls
- Audit of controls
- Automatic log-offs
- Unique identifier ("username")

Access Controls

Access controls consist of user-based access (the system is set up to place limitations on access to data tailored to each staff member) and role-based access (involves limitations created for each job category, e.g., scheduling, billing, or clinical).

Audit Controls

Audit controls are designed to keep track of log-ins to the computer system, administrative activity, and changes to data. This includes changing passwords, deleting user accounts, or creating new user accounts.

Automatic Log-Offs

Standards regarding automatic log-offs are required to prevent unauthorized users from accessing a computer when it is left unattended. The computer system or software program should automatically log off after a predetermined period of inactivity. Practice management software may have this useful feature; if not, the feature may be temporarily mimicked using a screensaver and a password.

Unique Identifier ("Username")

Each user should have a unique identifier or "username" and an unshared, undisclosed password to log into any computer with access to PHI. Identifying each unique user allows the functions of auditing and access controls to be implemented. Other authentication techniques involve more sophisticated devices, such as a magnetic card or fingerprints. Most organizations utilize passwords to control access. Passwords for all users should be changed on a regular basis and should never be common names or words. Passwords should never be shared with others. Many organizations consider sharing passwords grounds for termination.

BOX 14-25 ■ KEY POINTS

HIPAA Title II: Security Rule Physical Safeguards

Physical safeguards concentrate on prevention of unauthorized access to PHI. Physical safeguards include provisions related to protecting electronic information systems and related buildings and equipment from natural and environmental hazards and unauthorized intrusion:

- Media and equipment
- Physical access
- Secure workstations

Physical Safeguards

Physical safeguards also prevent unauthorized access to PHI. These physical measures and policies and procedures protect a covered entity's electronic information systems and related buildings and equipment from natural and environmental hazards and unauthorized intrusion. Appropriate and reasonable physical safeguards are described below.

Media and Equipment

Control measures should be documented in the organization's policies and procedures to protect EPHI recorded on various forms of media and equipment. Typical safeguard policies include how the organization handles the retention, removal, and disposal of paper records, as well as the recycling of computers and destruction of obsolete data disks or software programs containing PHI.

Physical Access

Controls should be implemented to limit unauthorized access to areas where equipment is stored as well as medical records. Locks on doors are the most common type of control.

Secure Workstations

Workstations should be secured to minimize the possibility of unauthorized viewing of PHI. As discussed earlier, log-off procedures are implemented to prevent unauthorized access at workstations. This includes making sure that password-protected screensavers are in use on computers when they are unattended and that desk drawers are locked.

HIPAA security regulations also mandate other standards to ensure compliance of all requirements, including the following:

- A security official must be assigned responsibility for the entity's security.
- All staff members must receive security awareness training.
- Organizations must control and monitor staff access to patients records.
- Organizations must limit physical access to facilities that contain EPHI.

- Organizations must determine where they have information security risks and vulnerabilities to illegal access.

Enforcement and Penalties

HIPAA security regulations are enforceable, and violation can result in civil and criminal actions and penalties.

HIPAA COMPLIANCE

HIPAA fraud prevention, standard transaction and code set, privacy, and security regulations apply to all covered entities. Noncompliance can lead to serious consequences for covered entities. Organizations are encouraged to develop and implement a compliance program to prevent, identify, and correct violations. To assist covered entities with the development and implementation of a compliance program, the Office of the Inspector General (OIG) has published sample compliance plans for various types of covered entities such as hospitals, billing companies, and small physician practices or hospitals. Sample compliance plans can be accessed on the OIG's Web site at www.oig.hhs.gov.

BOX 14-26 ■ KEY POINTS

Seven Components of an Effective Compliance Plan

Written standards, policies, and procedures
Compliance officer
Education and training
Effective lines of communications
Enforcement standards
Compliance evaluation
Problem resolution

OIG Model Compliance Plan

The presence of an OIG model compliance program can significantly diminish imposed penalties in the event of an OIG audit or other discovery of violations or noncompliance. Compliance programs can become a "meeting of the minds" for individuals within the organization and for business associates. An organization should consider a compliance program as a way to integrate regulatory requirements directly into policies and procedures.

The OIG's model compliance plan for hospitals contains seven basic components: written standards, policies, and procedures; compliance officer; education and training; effective lines of communication; enforcement standards; and compliance evaluation and problem resolution. The OIG's model compliance plan for hospitals can be viewed at www.oig.gov.

Written Standards, Policies, and Procedures

Written polices and procedures should be developed to incorporate regulatory requirements, and they should include standards of conduct, risk areas, claim development and submission process, medical necessity, anti-kickback and self-referral concerns, bad debts, and credit balances.

Compliance Officer

The designation of a compliance officer and compliance committee is required for the development, implementation, and monitoring of policies and procedures. The compliance officer can be someone within the organization or an individual outside the organization, depending on the size of the organization.

Education and Training

Effective training and education procedures must be developed and implemented. Training and education policies ensure that all hospital professionals understand all aspects of policies and procedures and regulatory issues. Education and training should be documented. Many employers utilize employee sign-in sheets or certificates of attendance.

Effective Lines of Communications

Effective lines of communications need to be developed to allow compliance issues to be identified and addressed within the organization. Policies related to communications should include provisions to allow access to the compliance officer and a formal process for submitting potential compliance issues. Many organizations have included hotlines to open lines of communications where employees can report potential compliance issues in confidence. All reports must be investigated and resolved.

Enforcement Standards

The disciplinary guidelines for enforcing standards should be communicated to all hospital personnel. The policies should also include provisions for new employees.

Compliance Evaluation

To ensure that the compliance program is effective, auditing and monitoring procedures should be conducted periodically.

Problem Resolution

Compliance procedures must include actions in response to detected compliance violations. Reports should be maintained.

TEST YOUR *Knowledge* BOX 14-5

HIPAA TITLE II: SECURITY RULE; HIPAA COMPLIANCE

1. Discuss the purpose of the HIPAA Title II Security Rule.
2. HIPAA security provisions contain standards for ______________, ______________, and ______________ safeguards.
3. Provide an explanation of administrative safeguards.
4. Technical safeguards address what security issues?
5. Outline three areas of physical safeguards that should be addressed for security purposes.
6. List three HIPAA provisions that apply to all covered entities.
7. Why are organizations encouraged to develop a compliance plan?
8. Explain why the Office of the Inspector General (OIG) developed sample compliance plans.
9. State how the presence of a compliance plan may be beneficial in the event of an audit.
10. List seven elements of an effective compliance plan.

CHAPTER SUMMARY

This chapter provides an overview of regulations under the Health Insurance Portability and Accountability Act (HIPAA) that were implemented in phases from 1996 to 2009. Title I: Health Care Reform of HIPAA focused on improving the continuation and portability of health insurance and ensuring that individuals would have the ability to renew insurance coverage in multiemployer plans. Although the original focus of HIPAA was to improve the portability and continuity of health care coverage, major changes were seen in the insurance billing and coding arena as a result of HIPAA. HIPAA Title II: Administrative Simplification (AS) was designed to standardize transactions to accomplish increased electronic transmission of transactions. The government estimates that billions of dollars can be saved annually by shifting from paper transactions to electronic transactions. HIPAA Title II also includes provisions regarding the privacy and security of health information. Title II requires covered entities to implement privacy and security policies and procedures that ensure a patient's rights to confidentiality are not breached. To ensure compliance, it is imperative for hospital personnel to understand the provisions of HIPAA as they relate to the day-to-day performance of their jobs.

CHAPTER REVIEW 14-1

True/False

1. HIPAA was implemented to improve the portability and continuity of health care coverage and to protect patient information. T F
2. Prior to HIPAA, individuals were denied coverage based on health status. T F
3. HIPAA Administrative Simplification focuses entirely on the standardization of health care transactions. T F
4. Noncompliance with HIPAA regulations does not result in civil and criminal penalties. T F
5. The Office of the Inspector General (OIG) developed model compliance plans to assist covered entities with the development of a compliance plan. T F

Fill in the Blank

6. List the name of the law that outlines penalties for fraudulent activities as defined in the Federal False Claims Act ____________________.
7. Covered entities, as defined under HIPAA, include the following three types of organizations: ____________________, ____________________, and ____________________.
8. Three agencies involved in enforcing HIPAA provisions are: ____________________, ____________________, and ____________________.
9. Standards developed under HIPAA Title II include: standard transactions, standard code sets, supporting code sets, and ____________________.
10. Compliance refers to ____________________.

Match the Following Definitions With the Terms at Right

11. ____ Provisions outlined in HIPAA legislation that require covered entities to adopt standard transaction and code sets.
12. ____ All patient individually identifiable information including information that is transmitted electronically.
13. ____ Provisions outlined in HIPAA legislation that require covered entities to adopt privacy standards to protect patient health information.
14. ____ A statement provided to patients that explains their privacy rights and how protected information may be used.
15. ____ Provisions outlined under HIPAA legislation that requires covered entities to adopt security standards to ensure the security of patient information transmitted electronically.

A. Protected health information (PHI)
B. Notice of Privacy Practices
C. HIPAA Title II: Administrative Simplification (AS)
D. HIPAA Title II: Privacy Rule
E. HIPAA Title II: Security Rule

Research Project

Perform research on the Internet or through contact with compliance professionals on HIPAA regulations and compliance. Provide an explanation of compliance requirements and prepare an outline of a hospital compliance plan. The outline should list each section in the plan with a brief description of the content of the section.

GLOSSARY

Abuse Actions or practices of health care providers that are inconsistent with accepted sound medical practice, which may result in improper payment.

Authorization for release of medical information A written document signed by the patient that grants permission to the hospital to use or disclose protected health information (PHI) for specified purposes that are generally other than treatment, payment, or health care operations.

Business associate An individual organization or entity that works with or for a covered entity but is not an employee of the covered entity. A billing company is an example of a business associate.

Civil Monetary Penalties Law of 1983 Legislation passed in 1983, for the purpose of prosecuting cases of Medicare and Medicaid fraud.

Clearinghouse An organization that receives claim information from hospitals and other providers in various formats for conversion to a required format for submission to various payers.

Compliance The act of complying with state and federal regulations.

Covered entity An organization involved with health care delivery that provides health care services, submits claims for services, or provides health care coverage.

De-identification Refers to the elimination of information that can be used to identify an individual.

Disclosure of protected health information (PHI) Refers to releasing protected health information to individuals or organizations outside the hospital.

Employer Identification Number (EIN) A number assigned by the Internal Revenue Service to hospitals and other employers and used for tax reporting purposes. The Employer Identification Number (EIN) is also referred to as the Tax Identification Number (TIN)

Fraud An intentional deception or misrepresentation that someone makes, knowing it is false, that could result in an unauthorized payment.

Health Insurance Portability and Accountability Act (HIPAA) Legislation passed by Congress and enacted in 1996 to improve access to health care; provide portability of health insurance coverage; combat waste, fraud, and abuse; and simplify the administration of health insurance. HIPAA legislation is also known as the Kassenbaum-Kennedy legislation.

Health Insurance Portability and Accountability Act (HIPAA) Title I Referred to as Health Care Reform since its purpose is to ensure that individuals have access to health insurance coverage.

Health Insurance Portability and Accountability Act (HIPAA) Title II HIPAA Title II contains regulations aimed at protecting government programs from fraud and abuse and to standardize and simplify the processing of health care transactions. HIPAA Title II is labeled Preventing Health Care Fraud and Abuse, Administrative Simplification, and Medical Liability Reform.

Individually identifiable health information (IIHI) Any part of an individual's health information including demographic and medical information collected from the individual or received by a covered entity including information.

Kassenbaum-Kennedy Legislation Also known as the Health Insurance Portability and Accountability Act (HIPAA), it was passed by Congress and enacted in 1996 to improve access to health care; to provide portability of health insurance coverage; to combat waste, fraud, and abuse; and to simplify the administration of health insurance.

National Provider Identifier (NPI) The standard unique health identifier for health care providers to use in filing and processing health care claims and other transactions.

Office of Civil Rights (OCR) An agency under the Department of Health and Human Services (DHHS) that is responsible for monitoring compliance and enforcement of HIPAA privacy standards.

Office of the Inspector General (OIG) An agency under the Department of Health and Human Services (DHHS) that is responsible for the detection and prevention of fraud and abuse.

Protected health information (PHI) Refers to individually identifiable health information (IIHI) that is transmitted by electronic media, maintained in electronic form, or transmitted or maintained in any other form or medium.

Transaction Refers to the transmission of information between two parties to carry out financial and administrative activities related to health care.

Use of PHI Refers to sharing of protected health information with health care professionals within the hospital as required to diagnose and treat the patient.

SECTION SEVEN

Appendixes

Appendix A: Cases

Appendix B: Claim Form Data

Appendix C: List of Web Resources

Appendix A

Cases

CASE 1: HOSPITAL OUTPATIENT LABORATORY

Summary

Patient Name: Myra Singerson **Date:** 03/19/20__

Established patient, 39 years of age, presents today for a follow-up visit for anemia. She indicates she is feeling extremely tired and run down. History and exam performed. I ordered an automated CBC and hepatic function tests to assess the patient's viral hepatitis B and progressive anemia. Patient to return in 5 days to discuss the results.

Johnathan Jamar, M.D.

Case 1: Hospital Outpatient Laboratory

Directions:

The patient face sheet/charge detail, laboratory requisition, and laboratory report are included in this case. Complete this case and prepare a CMS-1450 (UB-04) as follows:

Step 1: Assign revenue codes (see Appendix B) to each category of service listed on the patient face sheet/charge detail.

Submit your patient face sheet/charge detail to your instructor for review.

Step 2: The Coding Worksheet included in this case must be completed before data can be entered on the computer. Complete the Case 1 Coding Worksheet as follows:

a. Record the code(s) describing the admitting, principal, and other diagnoses.
b. Record HCPCS code(s) describing the laboratory procedures.
c. Record the code(s) for the items listed below the charge detail.

All other charges listed on the patient face sheet have been coded and posted by other departments.

d. Assign UB data codes (see Appendix B) to other information, as required, on the Coding Worksheet.

Submit your Coding Worksheet to your instructor for review.

Step 3: Complete a CMS-1450 (UB-04) claim form for this case. Claim forms can be completed manually or utilizing the software. Your instructor will advise if a manual claim is required. Otherwise begin completing the Student Software Case.

Student Software Case 1
Directions:

Use your completed Coding Worksheet and the software program located on Evolve to produce a completed CMS-1450 (UB-04). Follow these instructions to complete Student Software Case 1.

Step 1: The Coding Worksheet should be completed before entering data into the software. Use your completed Coding Worksheet and the patient face sheet/charge detail (after they are reviewed by your instructor) to enter information into the proper fields on the software. Follow the software screen by screen.

Step 2: Once you have completed each screen, preview your completed CMS-1450 (UB-04). Make required corrections before printing.

Step 3: Print your completed claim form and submit to your instructor for review, and keep a copy for your records.

Community General Hospital
Federal Tax ID# 62-1026428 NPI 1234567890
Case 1: Hospital Outpatient Laboratory—Myra Singerson

8192 South Street
Mars, Florida 37373
(747) 722-1800

PATIENT FACE SHEET AND CHARGE DETAIL

Admit/Discharge Date	Admit/Discharge Hour	Admission Source	Admission Type	Med Record / Soc Sec #	Patient Control #
Admit: 03/19/20__ Disch: 03/19/20__	Admit: 09:45 AM Disch: 10:45 AM	Physician Referral	Elective	MR# S654379821	15364572

Patient Name	DOB	Release Info	Assignment Ben	Discharge Status	Sex	Marital Status
Myra Singerson	02/26/1967	Y	Y	Discharge to Home	F	M

Patient Address	City, ST Zip	Phone
157 Main St.	Mars, Florida 37373	747 549-3176

INSURANCE INFORMATION

Primary Carrier	Insured's Name	Identification# 05148263 / Group Name and #	Provider #
Blue Cross/Blue Shield	Myra Singerson		00356572

Secondary Carrier	Insured's Name	Identification # / Group Name and #	Provider #

Pt Relationship	Employer Name	Employer Location	Treatment Authorization #
Self	Target	1716 Santana Street, Mars, Florida 37373	

Pt Relationship	Employer Name	Employer Location	Treatment Authorization #

PHYSICIANS/CLINICAL INFORMATION

Attending/Referring/Ordering Physician/ID#	Other Physician/ID #	Occurrence Date Date of Birth Insured	Condition/Value Info
Johnathan Jamar MD NPI: 1534612349	Johanna Sangchung MD NPI: 1527437692	02/26/1967	

CHARGE DETAIL

Revenue Code	Service Description	HCPCS/Rates	Service Units	Total Charges	Non -Covered Charges
	LAB/CHEMISTRY		1	114.00	
	LAB/HEMATOLOGY		1	48.00	
	TOTAL CHARGE		2	162.00	

OTHER CHARGES TO BE CODED, POSTED, AND ADDED TO CHARGE DETAIL ABOVE
NONE

Community General Hospital
Federal Tax ID# 62-1026428
NPI 1234567890

8192 South Street
Mars, Florida 37373
(747) 722-1800

LABORATORY REQUISITION

PATIENT NAME: Myra Singerson
DOB: 02/26/1967
INDICATIONS: Progressive Anemia, Viral Hepatitis B

ORDERING PHYSICIAN: Johnathan Jamar, M.D.
ACCOUNT # 24756
DATE: 03/19/20__

PHYSICIAN SIGNATURE: *Johnathan Jamar, M.D.*

CHEMISTRY
__ Acetone
__ Acid phos.
__ ACE level
__ ACTH
__ A/G ratio
✓ Albumin
__ Aldolase
✓ Alk Phos.
__ Amylase
✓ ALT (SGPT)
__ Amino acid screen
✓ Bilirubin, total
  ✓ Direct
  __ Indirect
__ BMP
__ BUN
__ Calcium
__ Cardiac Enzymes
  __ CK (CPK)
  __ LDH
  ✓ AST (SGOT)

__ Citrate
__ CKMB
__ CKMB Panel
__ Cholesterol
__ CMP
__ C-reactive Protein
__ Creatinine
__ Cortisol
__ Electrolytes
  __ Sodium
  __ Potassium
  __ Chloride
  __ Carbon Dioxide
__ Folic Acid
__ Folate
__ FSH
__ Glucose
__ Glucose, ____ Hr PP
__ Glucose Tolerance ___
__ Iron
__ Lactic Acid

__ LDH Isoenzymes
__ LH
__ Lipase
__ Magnesium
__ Osmolality
__ Phosphorus
✓ Protein Total
__ Protein Electrophoresis
__ TBG
__ Triglycerides
__ Troponin
__ TSH
__ T_3
__ T_4
__ Uric Acid
  __ VMA

HEMATOLOGY
__ Bleeding Time, Ivy
✓ CBC c Diff-Automated
__ CBC c Manual Diff
__ Factor VIII
__ Fibrinogen
__ HCT
__ HGB
  __ H&H
__ Eosinophil Ct Absolute
__ Eosinophil Smear
__ ESR
__ LE Cell Prep
__ Platelet Ct
__ PT
__ PTT (APTT)
__ RBC
__ RBC Indices
__ Reticulocyte Ct
__ Sickle Cell Prep
__ WBC

Community General Hospital
Federal Tax ID# 62-1026428
NPI 1234567890

8192 South Street
Mars, Florida 37373
(747) 722-1800

PATIENT NAME: Myra Singerson
DOB: 02/26/1967
INDICATIONS: Progressive Anemia, Viral Hepatitis B
EXAM DATE: 03/19/ 20__

ORDERING PHYSICIAN: Johnathan Jamar, M.D .
ATTENDING PHYSICIAN: Johanna Sangchung, M.D.
ACCOUNT #: S654379821
TIME: 9:45 AM

LABORATORY RESULTS

Test Name	In Range	Out of Range	Reference Range
CBC AUTOMATED (INCLUDES AUTOMATED DIFFERENTIAL/PLATELET)			
WBC-WHITE BLOOD CELL COUNT			3.8
RBC-RED BLOOD CELL COUNT			3.80
HEMOGLOBIN			11.7
HEMATOCRIT			35.0
MCV		101.3 (H)	
MCH		34.9 (H)	
MCHC	34.4		32.0
RDW	13.7		11.0
PLATELET COUNT	325		140
ABSOLUTE NEUTROPHILS	4240		1500
ABSOLUTE LYMPHOCYTES	2679		850
ABSOLUTE MONOCYTES	333		200
ABSOLUTE EOSINOPHILS	133		15
ABSOLUTE BASOPHILS	15		0–20 CELLS/MCL
NEUTROPHILS	57.3		%
LYMPHOCYTES	36.2		%
MONOCYTES	4.5		%
EOSINOPHILS	1.8		%
BASOPHILS	0.2		%

Test Name	In Range	Out of Range	Units	Reference Range
HEPATIC FUNCTION				
PROTEIN, TOTAL	7.2		G/DL	6.0-8.3
ALBUMIN	4.3		G/DL	3.5-4.9
BILIRUBIN, TOTAL	0.5		MG/DL	0.2-1.3
BILIRUBIN, DIRECT	0.1		MG/DL	0.0-0.3
ALKALINE PHOSPHATASE	49		U/L	20-125
TRANSFERASE, ALANINE AMINO (AST)	15		U/L	2-35
TRANSFERASE, ASPARTATE AMINO (ALT)	11		U/L	2-40

HEALTH INFORMATION MANAGEMENT CODING WORKSHEET

STUDENT NAME:		**DATE:**
PATIENT NAME:		**CASE #1:**
DEMOGRAPHICS		
Medical Record Number:	**Bill Type#:**	
Patient Name: Last, First, Middle Init:	Admit Hour Code:	Discharge Hour Code:
	Admit Type Code:	Discharge Status Code:
	Admit Source Code:	Patient Relationship Code:
Condition Code(s)	Occurrence Span Code and Date:	Value Code and Amount:

ADMISSION INFORMATION

Type of admission:	**ER**	**Facility**	**Physician Referral**	**Other**	**Unknown**

Admitting Diagnosis		**HIM Code(s)**
Principal Diagnosis (Including complications and co-morbidities if applicable)		**HIM Code**
Other Secondary Diagnosis (Including complications and co-morbidities if applicable)		**HIM Code(s)**
Procedure(s)	**Date:**	**HIM Code(s)**
Medications, supplies, equipment or other item(s)	**Date:**	**HIM Code(s)**

DISCHARGE INFORMATION

Home	Facility	AMA	Deceased	Other

DRG ASSIGNMENT		**APC ASSIGNMENT**		
MDC:	Surgical/Medical:			

CONTRIBUTING FACTORS

Age	Sex	Discharge Status	Complications/Comorbidities	Birthweight

Questions/Need Clarification:

CASE 2: HOSPITAL OUTPATIENT RADIOLOGY

Summary

Patient Name: James V. Thomas **Date:** 10/15/20__

Established patient, 69 years of age, presents today complaining of shortness of breath and dizziness. He states he has experienced loss of consciousness. History and exam reveals the patient's heart rate is slow and his abdomen is extremely tender. I ordered a chest X-ray and a CT of the abdomen. Patient to return in 5 days to discuss the results.

David Sanchez, M.D.

Case 2: Hospital Outpatient Radiology

Directions:

The patient face sheet/charge detail, radiology requisition, and radiology reports are included in this Case 2. Complete this case and prepare a CMS-1450 (UB-04) as follows:

Step 1: Assign revenue codes (see Appendix B) to each category of service listed on the patient face sheet/charge detail.

Submit your patient face sheet/charge detail to your instructor for review.

Step 2: The Coding Worksheet included with this case must be completed before data can be entered on the computer. Complete the Case 2 Coding Worksheet as follows.

a. Record the code(s) describing the admitting, principal, and other diagnoses.
b. Record HCPCS code(s) describing the radiology procedures.
c. Record the code(s) for the items listed below the charge detail.

All other charges listed on the patient face sheet have been coded and posted by other department.

d. Assign UB data codes (see Appendix B) to other information, as required, on the Coding Worksheet.

Submit your Coding Worksheet to your instructor for review.

Step 3: Complete a CMS-1450 (UB-04) claim form for this case. Claim forms can be completed manually or utilizing the software. Your instructor will advise if a manual claim is required. Otherwise begin completing the Student Software Case.

Student Software Case 2
Directions:

Use your completed Coding Worksheet and the software program located on Evolve to produce a completed CMS-1450 (UB-04). Follow these instructions to complete Student Software Case 2.

Step 1: The Coding Worksheet should be completed before entering data into the software. Use your completed Coding Worksheet and the patient face sheet/charge detail (after they are reviewed by your instructor) to enter information into the proper fields on the software. Follow the software screen by screen.

Step 2: Once you have completed each screen, preview your completed CMS-1450 (UB-04). Make required corrections before printing.

Step 3: Print your completed claim form and submit to your instructor for review, and keep a copy for your records.

Community General Hospital
Federal Tax ID# 62-1026428 NPI 1234567890
Case 2: Hospital Outpatient Radiology—James V. Thomas

8192 South Street
Mars, Florida 37373
(747) 722-1800

PATIENT FACE SHEET AND CHARGE DETAIL

Admit/Discharge Date	Admit/Discharge Hour	Admission Source	Admission Type	Med Record / Soc Sec #	Patient Control #
Admit: 01/15/20__ Disch: 01/15/20__	Admit: 10:15 AM Disch: 12:45 PM	Clinic Referral		MR# T625485935	12474383

Patient Name	DOB	Release Info	Assignment Ben	Discharge Status	Sex	Marital Status
James V. Thomas	01/05/1937	Y	Y	Discharge to Home	M	

Patient Address	City, ST Zip	Phone
522 North Street	Ocala, Florida 32561	752 555 4761

INSURANCE INFORMATION

Primary Carrier	Insured's Name	Identification# 124569781B Group Name and #	Provider #
Medicare	James V. Thomas		00356563

Secondary Carrier	Insured's Name	Identification # Group Name and #	Provider #

Pt Relationship	Employer Name	Employer Location	Treatment Authorization #
Self	Retired	Mars, FL 37373	AZ5673452

Pt Relationship	Employer Name	Employer Location	Treatment Authorization #

PHYSICIANS/CLINICAL INFORMATION

Attending/Referring/Ordering Physician/ID#	Other Physician/ID #	Occurrence Date	Condition/Value Info
David Sanchez MD NPI: 1525737911	Milton Hayber, MD NPI: 1496324123		Beneficiary would not provide information regarding other insurance

CHARGE DETAIL

Revenue Code	Service Description	HCPCS/Rates	Service Units	Total Charges	Non-Covered Charges
	DRUGS/INCIDENT RAD		1	24.50	
	CHEST X-RAY		1	87.00	
	CT SCAN		1	918.00	
	TOTAL CHARGE		3	1029.50	

OTHER CHARGES TO BE CODED, POSTED, AND ADDED TO CHARGE DETAIL ABOVE
Diagnostic imaging contrast material, radiopharmaceutical (DRUGS/INCIDENT RAD) 1 @ 24.50

Community General Hospital
Federal Tax ID# 62-1026428
NPI 1234567890

8192 South Street
Mars, Florida 37373
(747) 722-1800

RADIOLOGY REQUISITION

PATIENT NAME: James V. Thomas	**ORDERING PHYSICIAN:** David Sanchez, M.D.
DOB: 01/05/1937	**ACCOUNT #** JT432
PHYSICIAN SIGNATURE: *David Sanchez, M.D.*	**DATE:** 01/12/20__
INDICATIONS: Abdominal tenderness, shortness of breath and dizziness	

PLEASE FAX SCRIPT PRIOR TO PATIENTS SCEHDUELD APPOINTMENT

PLEASE CHECK

GENERAL X-RAY
- ☐ 74415 IVP D
- ☐ 74000 KUB
- ☐ 74020 Abdominal Series (2V)
- ☐ 74022 Acute Abdominal Series (3V)
- ☐ 73610 Ankle L/R
- ☐ 72050 C-Spine (min 4V)
- ☐ 72040 C-Spine (max 3V)
- ☑ _____ Chest (2V)
- ☐ 73080 Elbow L/R
- ☐ 73550 Femur L/R
- ☐ 73630 Foot L/R
- ☐ 73090 Forearm L/R
- ☐ 73130 Hand L/R
- ☐ 73500 Hip L/R
- ☐ 73060 Humerus L/R
- ☐ 73564 Knee L/R
- ☐ 72110 L Spine (min. 4V)
- ☐ 72170 Pelvis
- ☐ 71100 Ribs - Unilat L/R
- ☐ 71110 Ribs-Bilat
- ☐ Other________________

MRI
- ☐ 74181 Abd wo/contrast
- ☐ 74182 Abd w/contrast
- ☐ 74183 Abd w/wo contrast
- ☐ 70551 Brain wo/contrast
- ☐ 70552 Brain w/contrast
- ☐ 70553 Brain w/wo contrast
- ☐ 72141 C-Spine w/o contrast
- ☐ 72156 C-Spine w/wo contrast
- ☐ 71550 Chest wo/contrast
- ☐ 71551 Chest w/contrast
- ☐ 71552 Chest w/wo contrast
- ☐ 73721 Lower Extremity (jt.) R/L
- ☐ 73718 Lower Extremity (no jt.) R/L
- ☐ 72148 L-Spine wo/contrast
- ☐ 72158 L-Spine w/wo contrast

MRA ☐ **MRV** ☐
- ☐ 74185 Abd w/wo contrast
- ☐ 71555 Chest w/wo contrast (Exc Myocardium)
- ☐ 70544 Head wo/contrast
- ☐ 70546 Head w/wo contrast
- ☐ 70545 Head w/contrast
- ☐ 73725 Lower Ext. w/wo contrast
- ☐ 70547 Neck wo/contrast
- ☐ 70548 Neck w/contrast
- ☐ 70549 Neck w/wo contrast
- ☐ 73225 Upr. Ext. w/wo contrast
- ☐ Other__________________

CT SCAN
- ☐ _____ Abd wo/contrast
- ☑ _____ Abd w/wo contrast
- ☐ 70450 Brain wo/contrast
- ☐ 70470 Brain w/wo contrast
- ☐ 72125 C-Spine wo/contrast
- ☐ 71250 Chest wo/contrast
- ☐ 71260 Chest w/contrast
- ☐ 71270 Chest w/wo contrast
- ☐ 70482 IAC's, Orbits, Pituitary w/wo cont.
- ☐ 72131 L-Spine wo/contrast
- ☐ 70486 Maxiofacial (Sinus) wo/contrast
- ☐ 72192 Pelvis wo/contrast
- ☐ 72193 Pelvis w/contrast
- ☐ 72194 Pelvis w/wo contrast
- ☐ 70491 Soft Tissue Neck w/contrast
- ☐ 72128 T-Spine wo/contrast
- ☐ 74150/72192 Urogram

ULTRASOUND
- ☐ 76700 Abd Total
- ☐ 76705 Abd, Single Organ/Quadrant
- ☐ 93925 Arterial Lower Ext.-Bilat.
- ☐ 93926 Arterial Lower Ext.-Unilat. L/R
- ☐ 93930 Arterial Upper Ext. - Bilat.
- ☐ 93931 Arterial Upper Ext. - Unilat. L/R
- ☐ 76645 Breast L/R
- ☐ 93880 Carotid
- ☐ 76880 Extremity, Non Vascular L/R
- ☐ 76801 OB - 1st Trimester
- ☐ Other___________________

MAMMOGRAPHY
- ☐ 76092 Screening mammography
- ☐ 76091 Diagnostic mammography - Bilat
- ☐ 76090 Diagnostic mammography - Unil L/R

DEXA SCAN
- ☐ 76075 Bone Density, DEXA

ECHOCARDIOGRAM
- ☐ 93307/93320/93325 Echo, Dop. Echo w/pulsect wave and color flow

PET SCAN

Specify Area___________________

STRESS TEST
- ☐ 78465 Dual Isotope Nuclear Stress Test
  ___ Adenosine/Dubutamine

☐ CORRELATION OR ☑ COMPARISON
Please compare with exam done on
__________ _____ _____

Community General Hospital
Federal Tax ID# 62-1026428
NPI 1234567890

8192 South Street
Mars, Florida 37373
(747) 722-1800

RADIOLOGY REPORT

PATIENT NAME: James V. Thomas
DOB: 01/05/1937
INDICATIONS: Abdominal tenderness
EXAM: CT Abdomen W/WO Contrast

ORDERING M.D.: David Sanchez, M.D.
RADIOLOGY #: 432765
EXAM DATE: 01/15/20__

TECHNICAL INFORMATION: The patient received oral contrast, and CT imaging through the upper abdomen was followed by IV contrast, and further imaging throughout the abdomen was performed utilizing helical acquisition.

FINDINGS: A small amount of ascites surrounds the liver. The liver and spleen are otherwise unremarkable. The pancreas and abdominal aorta appear within normal limits. Both kidneys are unremarkable.

IMPRESSION: 1. SMALL AMOUNT OF ASCITES SURROUNDING THE LIVER. NO OTHER FINDINGS ARE NOTED.

Milton Hayber, M.D.

Community General Hospital
Federal Tax ID# 62-1026428
NPI 1234567890

8192 South Street
Mars, Florida 37373
(747) 722-1800

RADIOLOGY REPORT

PATIENT NAME: James V. Thomas
DOB: 01/05/1937
INDICATIONS: Shortness of breath and dizziness
EXAM: Chest X-ray PA and Lateral

ORDERING M.D.: David Sanchez, M.D.
RADIOLOGY #: 432779
EXAM DATE: 01/15/20__

Two views of the chest demonstrate the lungs to be clear. The cardiac and mediastinal silhouettes are of normal size and contour. The central pulmonary vasculature appears normal. I see no osseous abnormalities.

IMPRESSION: 1. NEGATIVE CHEST EXAMINATION.

Milton Hayber, M.D.

HEALTH INFORMATION MANAGEMENT
CODING WORKSHEET

STUDENT NAME:			**DATE:**
PATIENT NAME:			**CASE #2:**
DEMOGRAPHICS			
Medical Record Number:		**Bill Type#:**	
Patient Name: Last, First, Middle Init:	Admit Hour Code:		Discharge Hour Code:
	Admit Type Code:		Discharge Status Code:
	Admit Source Code:		Patient Relationship Code:
Condition Code(s)	Occurrence Span Code and Date:	Value Code and Amount:	

ADMISSION INFORMATION					
Type of admission:	**ER**	**Facility**	**Physician Referral**	**Other**	**Unknown**

Admitting Diagnosis		**HIM Code(s)**
Principal Diagnosis (Including complications and co-morbidities if applicable)		**HIM Code**
Other Secondary Diagnosis (Including complications and co-morbidities if applicable)		**HIM Code(s)**
Procedure(s)	**Date:**	**HIM Code(s)**
Medications, supplies, equipment or other item(s)	**Date:**	**HIM Code(s)**

DISCHARGE INFORMATION				
Home	Facility	AMA	Deceased	Other

DRG ASSIGNMENT		**APC ASSIGNMENT**		
MDC:	Surgical/Medical:			

CONTRIBUTING FACTORS				
Age	Sex	Discharge Status	Complications/Comorbidities	Birthweight

Questions/Need Clarification:

CASE 3: EMERGENCY DEPARTMENT VISIT

Summary

Patient Name: Tyron J. Sampson **Date:** 09/12/20__

This 53-year-old male, from out of town was driving his truck this morning and, while sitting at a light, had total loss of vision in his left eye. This continued for about 4 to 5 minutes, and then he had 50% loss of vision in his right eye which again lasted 4 to 5 minutes. He came right to the Emergency Department.

Dr. Noah Drake

Case 3: Emergency Department Visit

Directions:

The patient face sheet/charge detail, history and physical exam, EKG, Radiology, and Laboratory reports are included in this Case. Complete this case and prepare a CMS-1450 (UB-04) as follows:

Step 1: Assign revenue codes (see Appendix B) to each category of service listed on the patient face sheet/charge detail.

Submit your patient face sheet/charge detail to your instructor for review.

Step 2: The Coding Worksheet included with this case must be completed before data can be entered on the computer. Complete the Case 3 Coding Worksheet as follows:

a. Record the codes describing the admitting, principal, and other diagnoses.
b. Record the codes describing the emergency department visit, laboratory, radiology, and EKG services.
c. Record the codes for the items listed below the charge detail.

All other charges listed on the patient face sheet have been coded and posted by other departments.

d. Assign UB data code (see Appendix B) to other information on the Coding Worksheet.

Submit your Coding Worksheet to your instructor for review.

Step 3: Complete a CMS-1450 (UB-04) claim form for this case. Claim forms can be completed manually or utilizing the software. Your instructor will advise if a manual claim is required. Otherwise begin completing the Student Software Case.

Student Software Case 3
Directions:

Use your completed Coding Worksheet and the software program located on Evolve to produce a completed CMS-1450 (UB-04). Follow these instructions to complete Student Software Case 3.

Step 1: The Coding Worksheet should be completed before entering data into the software. Use your completed Coding Worksheet and the patient face sheet/charge detail (after they are reviewed by your instructor) to enter information into the proper fields on the software. Follow the software screen by screen.

Step 2: Once you have completed each screen, preview your completed CMS-1450 (UB-04). Make required corrections before printing.

Step 3: Print your completed claim form and submit to your instructor for review, and keep a copy for your records.

Community General Hospital

Federal Tax ID# 62-1026428 NPI 1234567890

Case 3: Emergency Department Visit—Tyron J. Sampson

8192 South Street
Mars, Florida 37373
(747) 722-1800

PATIENT FACE SHEET AND CHARGE DETAIL

Admit/Discharge Date	Admit/Discharge Hour	Admission Source	Admission Type	Med Record / Soc Sec #	Patient Control #
Admit: 09/12/20__ Disch: 09/12/20__	Admit: 10:27 AM Disch: 2:10 PM		Urgent	MR# S846195253	49237521

Patient Name	DOB	Release Info	Assignment Ben	Discharge Status	Sex	Marital Status
Tyron J. Sampson	10/17/1953	Y	Y	Discharge to Home	M	M

Patient Address	City, ST Zip	Phone
424 State Highway 12	West Springs, Florida 32433	(407) 323-7979

INSURANCE INFORMATION

Primary Carrier	Insured's Name	Identification# 202672985	Provider #
Health Network of Orlando	Tyron J. Sampson	Group Name and # HN 76532	N24922
Secondary Carrier	Insured's Name	Identification #	Provider #
		Group Name and #	

Pt Relationship	Employer Name	Employer Location	Treatment Authorization #
Self	Unemployed		HN 792113
Pt Relationship	Employer Name	Employer Location	Treatment Authorization #

PHYSICIANS/CLINICAL INFORMATION

Attending/Referring/Ordering Physician/ID#	Other Physician/ID #	Occurrence Date	Condition/Value Info
Noah Drake, M.D. NPI: 1439231679		Onset of Symptoms/ illness 09/12/20__	*Patient & spouse- unemployed *Deductible = $250.00

CHARGE DETAIL

Revenue Code	Service Description	HCPCS/Rates	Service Units	Total Charges	Non -Covered Charges
	PHARMACY		3	1233.75	
	LAB/CHEMISTRY		1	150.00	
	LAB/UROLOGY		1	89.75	
	DX X-RAY/CHEST		1	132.25	
	EMERG ROOM		1	504.50	
	EKG/ECG		1	81.00	
	TOTAL CHARGE		8	2191.25	

OTHER CHARGES TO BE CODED, POSTED, AND ADDED TO CHARGE DETAIL ABOVE
NONE

HISTORY, PHYSICAL FINDINGS, AND TREATMENT

CHIEF COMPLAINT:

This 53-year-old, single male from out of town was driving his truck this morning and, while sitting at a light, had total loss of vision in his left eye. This continued for about 4 to 5 minutes, and then he had 50% loss of vision in his right eye which again lasted 4 to 5 minutes. He came right to the Emergency Department.

ALLERGIES:

The patient lists aspirin as an allergy

VITALS

Temp:	Pulse:	Resp:	BP:	Pulse OX
99.2	88	18	140/93 rechecked 112/68	95

CURRENT MEDICATIONS:

1. Celebrex 200 mg daily
2. Triamterene/hydrochlorothiazide 50/25 mg/daily
3. Norvasc 10 milligrams daily
4. Additional hydrochlorothiazide 12.5 mg/daily
5. Hyzaar was started on the day of his visual obscuration

Patient in by (name of person or ambulance)
Patient drove himself to ED

Patient Signature – Release record/Assignment of benefits:
Tyron J. Sampson 09/12/20__

PHYSICIAN ORDERS:
✓ O2 ✓ EKG 12 lead ✓ Comp Metabolic Panel ✓ C.C. URINE
✓ RADIOLOGY *Chest X-ray, single portable* ✓ PULSE OX

PAST MEDICAL HISTORY:

Status post coronary artery bypass graft. Last admitted in April of this year for Rotablator atherectomy and stenting of the saphenous vein graft to the circumflex. He is supposed to be on an aspirin a day. He has not taken that for the last 2½ months because it makes him bleed. He has had no other neurologic symptoms during the day. There was no headache or other acute problems.

PHYSICAL EXAM:

Emergency Department Level 4 evaluation and management performed. The patient's blood pressure is so high he is about to have a stroke. Alert male. No substernal chest pain or pressure. He does have back and chest wall pains which are chronic. He worked as a plumber, digging ditches, etc., and is a very hard-working gentleman. He is currently unemployed and was in town on job interviews. Head and neck exam is unremarkable. Ocular exam is normal. Visual acuity is normal. Visual fields by confrontation. Retinas are pink. There are mild to moderate AV crossing changes. No hemorrhages or exudates are appreciated. Mental status is normal. Cranial nerves II-XII intact. Motor and sensory exams are normal and symmetrical. Cerebellar exam is normal. No drift or pathologic reflexes. Gait normal. Deep tendon reflexes normal. Chest is clear. Cardiovascular exam: SI and S2 normal. No S3 or S4. Normal murmur. No pleural or pericardial friction rubs. No peripheral edema, cyanosis, or clubbing. Abdominal exam is benign. He is well hydrated. No rashes are present. The remainder of the neurologic exam is entirely normal.

EKG demonstrates normal sinus rhythm with occasional premature ventricular complexes, left atrial enlargement, T-wave abnormality. Comprehensive metabolic panel and CC urine normal. Chest X-ray reveals stable appearance of the chest post coronary bypass with no acute process and no change since the previous study in February

TREATMENT:

Administered 10 milligrams of Norvasc and started on Hyzaar, Triamterene, and hydrochlorothiazide. Plavix 75 mg po. Discussed patient status with patient's cardiologist in his home town. Cardiologist recommends an ultrasound and MRI of the brain and MRA of the neck. The patient wants to pursue further treatment with home-town cardiologist. Patient was stabilized and with clearance from the patient's cardiologist the patient is discharged to home.

Assessment:

1. Sudden Loss of Vision
2. High Blood Pressure
3. Coronary Artery Disease
4. Status Post Coronary Artery Bypass (Native Artery)

Community General Hospital
Federal Tax ID# 62-1026428
NPI 1234567890

8192 South Street
Mars, Florida 37373
(747) 722-1800

PATIENT NAME: Tyron J. Sampson
DATE: 09/12/20__
12 SEPT 20__ ER HR 11:02 PM VPB 8 SINUS RHYTHM MULTIFORM 2020

ATTENDING M.D.: Noah Drake, M.D.
EXAM: EKG, 12 Lead

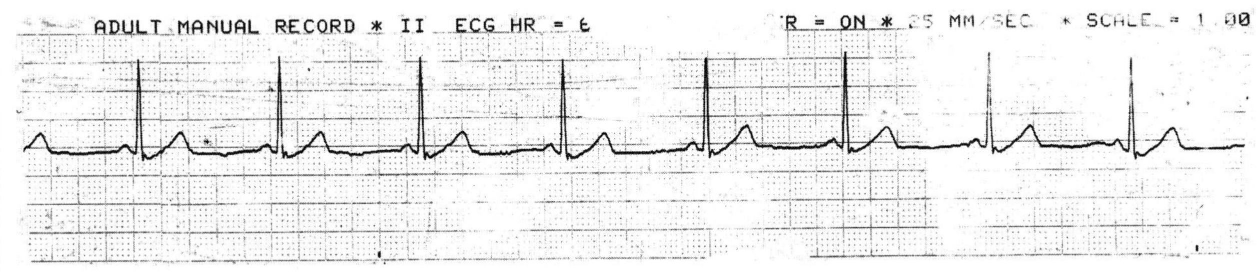

(From Brooks MA, Gillingham EA: Health unit coordinating, *ed 5, St Louis, 2004, Saunders.)*

12 SEPT 20__ ER HR 11:02 PM VPB 8 SINUS RHYTHM MULTIFORM 2020

Community General Hospital
Federal Tax ID# 62-1026428
NPI: 1234567890

8192 South Street
Mars, Florida 37373
(747) 722-1800

RADIOLOGY REPORT

PATIENT NAME: Tyron J. Sampson
DOB: 10/17/1953
INDICATIONS: Loss of Vision
EXAM DATE: 09/12/20__

ATTENDING M.D.: Noah Drake, M.D.
ORDERING M.D.: Andrew James Jr., M.D.
ACCOUNT #: S846195253

PORTABLE CHEST:

Stable appearance of the chest post coronary bypass with no acute process and no change since the previous study of February.

REPORT SIGNATURE ON FILE 09/12/20__

REPORTED AND SIGNED BY: Andrew James, Jr., M.D.

Community General Hospital
Federal Tax ID# 62-1026428
NPI 1234567890

8192 South Street
Mars, Florida 37373
(747) 722-1800

LABORATORY RESULTS				
CHEMISTRY	**Results**		**Units**	**Reference Range**
GLUCOSE	160	H	mg/dL	65–110
ALBUMIN	4.3		g/dL	2.6–5.2
SODIUM	138		mmol/L	137–145
POTASSIUM	4.7		mmol/L	3.6–5.0
BILIRUBIN TOTAL	0.2		mg/dL	0.1–1.1
PROTEIN, TOTAL	7.2		g/dL	6.0–8.3
CHLORIDE	103		mmol/L	98–107
CARBON DIOXIDE	25		mmol/L	22–31
ALK PHOS TOTAL	89		IU/L	30–115
BUN	17		mg/dL	7–21
CREATININE	1.0		mg/dL	0.7–1.5
ALT (SGPT)/AST (SGOT	22		IU/L	7–40
CALCIUM, TOTAL	9.5		mg/dL	8.5–10.6

URINALYSIS			
COLOR	:YELLOW		YELLOW
CLARITY	:CLEAR		CLEAR
SPECIFIC GRAVITY	:>=1.030 :5.0		1.005 1.030
PH	:100 mg/dL		4.5 8.0
PROTEIN	:NEGATIVE		>30
GLUCOSE	:NEGATIVE		NEG
KETONES	:NEGATIVE		NEG
BILIRUBIN	:NEGATIVE		NEG
BLOOD,UR	:NEGATIVE		NEG
UROBILINOGEN	:0.2 E.U./dL		0.2 1.0
NITRITES	:NEGATIVE		NEG
LEUKOCYTE ESTERASE	:NEGATIVE		NEG
MICROSCOPIC			
WBC			
EPITHELIAL CELLS	:0 - 1		
GRANULAR CASTS/LPF	:OCC	/HPF	0-5
	:3-6 FINELY GRANULAR, OCC		
MUCUS	COARSELY GRANULAR		

HEALTH INFORMATION MANAGEMENT CODING WORKSHEET

STUDENT NAME:			**DATE:**
PATIENT NAME:			**CASE #3:**
DEMOGRAPHICS			
Medical Record Number:	**Bill Type#:**		
Patient Name: Last, First, Middle Init:	Admit Hour Code:		Discharge Hour Code:
	Admit Type Code:		Discharge Status Code:
	Admit Source Code:		Patient Relationship Code:
Condition Code(s)	Occurrence Span Code and Date:	Value Code and Amount:	
ADMISSION INFORMATION			
Type of admission: **ER**	**Facility**	**Physician Referral**	**Other** **Unknown**

Admitting Diagnosis		**HIM Code(s)**
Principal Diagnosis (Including complications and co-morbidities if applicable)		**HIM Code**
Other Secondary Diagnosis (Including complications and co-morbidities if applicable)		**HIM Code(s)**
Procedure(s)	**Date:**	**HIM Code(s)**
Medications, supplies, equipment or other item(s)	**Date:**	**HIM Code(s)**

DISCHARGE INFORMATION				
Home	Facility	AMA	Deceased	Other

DRG ASSIGNMENT		**APC ASSIGNMENT**		
MDC:	Surgical/Medical:			

CONTRIBUTING FACTORS				
Age	Sex	Discharge Status	Complications/Comorbidities	Birthweight

Questions/Need Clarification:

CASE 4: HOSPITAL EMERGENCY DEPARTMENT

Summary

Patient Name: Lucy L. Richards | **Date:** 08/08/20__

An 83-year-old, single female was brought in by firemen from the scene of an accident in which a tree hit her in the head. There was a significant amount of bleeding. She lost consciousness for about 5 minutes, before paramedics arrived. Per paramedics she was hemodynamically stable on transport with altered mental status. Her neck was immobilized by firemen, no collar was in place. She arrived in the emergency room with trauma team present. On arrival she complained of shortness of breath. O2 administered.

Marie Martino, M.D.

Case 4: Emergency Department Visit

Directions:

The patient face sheet/charge detail, history and physical exam, radiology, and laboratory reports are included in this Case. Complete this case and prepare a CMS-1450 (UB-04) as follows:

Step 1: Assign revenue codes (see Appendix B) to each category of service listed on the patient face sheet/charge detail.

Submit your patient face sheet/charge detail to your instructor for review.

Step 2: The Coding Worksheet included with this case must be completed before data can be entered on the computer. Complete the Case 4 Coding Worksheet as follows:

a. Record the codes describing the admitting, principal, and other diagnoses.
b. Record the codes describing the emergency department visit, laboratory, and radiology services.
c. Record the codes for the items listed below the charge detail.

All other charges listed on the patient face sheet have been posted and coded by other departments.

d. Assign UB data code (Appendix B) to other information on the Coding Worksheet.

Submit your Coding Worksheet to your instructor for review.

Step 3: Complete a CMS-1450 (UB-04) claim form for this case. Claim forms can be completed manually or utilizing the software. Your instructor will advise if a manual claim is required. Otherwise begin completing the Student Software Case.

Student Software Case 4
Directions:

Use your completed Coding Worksheet and the software program located on Evolve to produce a completed CMS-1450 (UB-04). Follow these instructions to complete Student Software Case 4.

Step 1: The Coding Worksheet should be completed before entering data into the software. Use your completed Coding Worksheet and the patient face sheet/charge detail (after they are reviewed by your instructor) to enter information into the proper ›elds on the software. Follow the software screen by screen.

Step 2: Once you have completed each screen, preview your completed CMS-1450 (UB-04). Make required corrections before printing.

Step 3: Print your completed claim form and submit to your instructor for review, and keep a copy for your records.

Community General Hospital
Federal Tax ID# 62-1026428 NPI 1234567890
Case 4: Emergency Department—Lucy L. Richards

8192 South Street
Mars, Florida 37373
(747) 722-1800

PATIENT FACE SHEET AND CHARGE DETAIL

Admit/Discharge Date	Admit/Discharge Hour	Admission Source	Admission Type	Med Record / Soc Sec #	Patient Control #
Admit: 08/08/20__ Disch: 08/08/20__	Admit: 3:30 PM Disch: 7:15 PM	Info Not Avail	Emergency	MR# R217594264	51742167

Patient Name	DOB	Release Info	Assignment Ben	Discharge Status	Sex	Marital Status
Lucy L. Richards	02/07/1923	Y	Y	Discharge to Home	F	S

Patient Address	City, ST Zip	Phone
241 Mocking Lane	Ocala, Florida 34721	741 428-5179

INSURANCE INFORMATION

Carrier	Insured's Name	Identification# / Group Name and #	Provider #
Primary Carrier Medicare	Insured's Name Lucy L. Richards	Identification# 513714275B Group Name and #	00375471
Secondary Carrier	Insured's Name	Identification # Group Name and #	Provider #

Pt Relationship	Employer Name	Employer Location	Treatment Authorization #
Self	Retired		
Pt Relationship	Employer Name	Employer Location	Treatment Authorization #

PHYSICIANS/CLINICAL INFORMATION

Attending/Referring/Ordering Physician/ID#	Other Physician/ID #	Occurrence Date Accident-No Medical Liability Coverage:	Condition/Value Info
Marie A Martino, M.D NPI: 1653476902	Melvin Wong, M.D. NPI: 1653260001	08/08/20__	*Co-insurance Payer A $100.00

CHARGE DETAIL

Revenue Code	Service Description	HCPCS/Rates	Service Units	Total Charges	Non-Covered Charges
	MED-SUR SUPPLIES		35	565.95	
	PROSTH/ORTH DEV		1	85.00	
	LAB/HEMATOLOGY		1	140.00	
	X-RAY CHEST		1	192.25	
	CT SCAN/HEAD		1	648.00	
	EMERG ROOM		1	224.00	
	EMERG ROOM		1	250.00	
	TOTAL CHARGE		41	2105.20	

OTHER CHARGES TO BE CODED, POSTED, AND ADDED TO CHARGE DETAIL ABOVE
Cervical Collar, Philly

HISTORY, PHYSICAL FINDINGS, AND TREATMENT

CHIEF COMPLAINT:

An 83-year-old, single female was brought in by firemen from the scene of an accident in which a tree hit her in the head. There was a significant amount of bleeding. She lost consciousness for about 5 minutes, before paramedics arrived. Per paramedics she was hemodynamically stable on transport with altered mental status. Her neck was immobilized by firemen, no collar was in place. She arrived in the emergency room with trauma team present. On arrival she complained of shortness of breath. O2 administered.

Marie Martino, M.D.

ALLERGIES:	*VITALS*
No allergies	**Temp:** 99.2 · **Pulse:** 100 · **Resp:** 18, rechecked · **BP:** 150/100, 112/68 · **Pulse OX** 100% after nasal cannula oxygen was administered
LAST TETANUS:	Patient in by (name of person or ambulance) *Brought in by firemen from scene of an accident*
CURRENT MEDICATIONS *No medications*	Patient Signature – Release record/Assignment of benefits: Lucy L. Richards *08/08/20__*
PHYSICIAN ORDERS:	✓ RADIOLOGY *Chest X-ray 2 views* ✓ IMAGING *CT head without contrast* ✓ LABS

PAST MEDICAL HISTORY:

The patient denied any significant medical illnesses.

PHYSICAL EXAM:

Emergency Department Level 2 was performed. The patient answered questions appropriately with slight disorientation for a Glasgow of 14. Primary survey revealed airway to be open, lung sounds bilaterally. Patient's breathing normal after oxygen administered. There is obviously a laceration across the scalp which was bleeding significantly but controlled by direct pressure. Remainder of primary survey showed no other evidence of exsanguinations or no instability and neurologic exam showed a Glasgow of 14; this is nonfocal.

There were no known drug allergies. She stated the last time she had eaten was approximately 12 hours ago. Although patient was disoriented this information appeared reliable. Lab and chest x-ray negative.

Secondary survey, continued with pupils equal and reactive to 4 to 2, brisk. No jaw lesions. Pupils move bilaterally. TMs were bilaterally clear. The neck was immobilized. The patient denied neck pain. No crepitus in the chest wall. Heart regular rate and rhythm. No pelvic instability. Rectal exam – Tone normal. Bilateral extremities without fracture deformity. Pulses equal and full centrally.

CT scan of the head showed no evidence of cephalhematoma of the right scalp and face region. No obvious facial fracture. No obvious skull fracture. No intracranial bleed noted. Basal cisterns well preserved. Ventricles slightly decreased in size suggestive of generalized swelling.

TREATMENT:

Repair of superficial laceration across the scalp extending from 3 cm proximal to the hairline across the parietal aspects of the scalp to the occiput; total length approximately 30 cm. Under local anesthesia, the laceration was repaired with 2-0 vicryl interrupted stitches. The wound was dressed with antibiotic ointment and dressing was applied. A Philadelphia collar was placed keeping her head and C-spine precautions.

ASSESSMENT:

1. Head Trauma, Open
2. Scalp Laceration
3. Shortness of Breath

Community General Hospital
Federal Tax ID# 62-1026428
NPI 1234567890

8192 South Street
Mars, Florida 37373
(747) 722-1800

LABORATORY RESULTS

PATIENT NAME: Lucy L. Richards

CHEMISTRY

TEST NAME	RESULTS		UNITS	REFERENCE RANGE
GLUCOSE	160	H	mg/dL	65–110
SODIUM	138		mmol/L	137–145
POTASSIUM	4.7		mmol/L	3.6–5.0
CHLORIDE	103		mmol/L	98–107
CARBON DIOXIDE	25		mmol/L	22–31
ANION GAP	9			6–22
BUN	17		mg/dL	7–21
CREATININE	1.0		mg/dL	0.7–1.5
BUN/CREAT RATIO	16.3			8.0–20.0
CALCIUM	102		U/L	30–110

Community General Hospital
Federal Tax ID# 62-1026428
NPI 1234567890

8192 South Street
Mars, Florida 37373
(747) 722-1800

RADIOLOGY REPORT

PATIENT NAME: Lucy L Richards
DOB: 02/07/1923
EXAM DATE: 08/08/20__

ORDERING M.D.: Marie A Martino, M.D.
ACCOUNT #: R217594264
RADIOLOGY #: 458267

INDICATIONS: Shortness of breath
CHEST, PA AND LATERAL

Two views of the chest demonstrate the lungs to be clear. The cardiac and mediastinal silhouettes are of normal size and contour. The central pulmonary vasculature appears normal. I see no abnormalities.

IMPRESSION: NEGATIVE CHEST EXAMINATION.

Melvin Wong, M.D.

Community General Hospital
Federal Tax ID# 62-1026428
NPI 1234567890

8192 South Street
Mars, Florida 37373
(747) 722-1800

RADIOLOGY REPORTS

PATIENT NAME: Lucy L Richards
DOB: 02/07/1923
EXAM DATE: 08/08/20__

ORDERING M.D.: Marie A Martino, M.D.
ACCOUNT #: R217594264
RADIOLOGY #: 458239

INDICATIONS: Patient struck in the head by a tree, loss of consciousness
CT HEAD/BRAIN WITHOUT CONTRAST

TECHNIQUE: Transaxial sections from skull base to vertex without the use of IV contrast material.

FINDINGS: There is a large amount of atrophy in the left parietal area. Focal area of low density is seen in the left periventricular zone. There is also a focal old lacunar infarct in the right thalamus. Some encephalomalacia is also seen in the right parietooccipital region. Encephalomalacia is also seen in the right parietooccipital region consistent with an old area of infarct. Basal ganglia calcifications are noted bilaterally, which are of no clinical significance. There is a large amount of soft tissue swelling in the right frontoorbital region. Bone windows to that area do not show any fracture. Basal ganglia calcifications are seen.

Brainstem and cerebellum are intact. There is some mucosal thickening in the left maxillary antrum consistent with chronic sinusitis.
IMPRESSION:
1. Marked soft tissue swelling in the right frontoorbital region without underlying bleed
2. No acute intracranial pathology
3. Encephalomalacia in both parietooccipital regions consistent with old areas of infarction
4. Old lacunar infarct in several other areas
5. Moderate diffuse atrophy

Melvin Wong, M.D.

HEALTH INFORMATION MANAGEMENT CODING WORKSHEET

STUDENT NAME:			**DATE:**
PATIENT NAME:			**CASE #4:**
DEMOGRAPHICS			
Medical Record Number:	**Bill Type#:**		
Patient Name: Last, First, Middle Init:	Admit Hour Code:		Discharge Hour Code:
	Admit Type Code:		Discharge Status Code:
	Admit Source Code:		Patient Relationship Code:
Condition Code(s)	Occurrence Span Code and Date:	Value Code and Amount:	
ADMISSION INFORMATION			

Type of admission:	**ER**	**Facility**	**Physician Referral**	**Other**	**Unknown**

Admitting Diagnosis		**HIM Code(s)**
Principal Diagnosis (Including complications and co-morbidities if applicable)		**HIM Code**
Other Secondary Diagnosis (Including complications and co-morbidities if applicable)		**HIM Code(s)**
Procedure(s)	**Date:**	**HIM Code(s)**
Medications, supplies, equipment or other item(s)	**Date:**	**HIM Code(s)**

DISCHARGE INFORMATION				
Home	Facility	AMA	Deceased	Other

DRG ASSIGNMENT		**APC ASSIGNMENT**		
MDC:	Surgical/Medical:			

CONTRIBUTING FACTORS				
Age	Sex	Discharge Status	Complications/Comorbidities	Birthweight

Questions/Need Clarification:

CASE 5: HOSPITAL AMBULATORY SURGERY

Summary

Patient Name: Kamika J. Lotaman **Date:** 08/22/20__

This is a 41-year-old with two children who has a history of two previous cesarean sections and a long and very significant past medical history of leiomyoma. She has been suffering from abdominal pain, discomfort, and excessive menstruations that are disabling since January. She has been treated with conservative medical management but is still complaining of severe right lower quadrant pain and discomfort and frequent and excessive menstruation. She states on a scale of 1 to 10 that it is approximately an 8 in discomfort. The patient is scheduled at Community General Hospital for Ambulatory Surgery on August 22nd for a hysterectomy.

Michael Jefferson, M.D.

Case 5: Hospital Ambulatory Surgery

Directions:

The patient face sheet/charge detail, progress note, and operative report are included in this Case. Complete this case and prepare a CMS-1450 (UB-04) as follows:
Step 1: Assign revenue codes (see Appendix B) to each category of service listed on the patient face sheet/charge detail.

Submit your patient face sheet/charge detail to your instructor for review.

Step 2: The Coding Worksheet included in this case must be completed before data can be entered on the computer
Complete the Case 5 Coding Worksheet as follows:

a. Record the codes describing the admitting, principal, and other diagnoses
b. Record the codes describing the Ambulatory Surgery services.
c. Record the codes for the items listed below the charge detail.

All other charges listed on the patient face sheet have been coded and posted by other departments.

d. Assign UB data code (see Appendix B) to other information on the Coding Worksheet.

Submit your Coding Worksheet to your instructor for review.

Step 3: Complete a CMS-1450 (UB-04) claim form for this case. Claim forms can be completed manually or utilizing the software. Your instructor will advise if a manual claim is required. Otherwise begin completing the Student Software Case.

Student Software Case 5
Directions:

Use your completed Coding Worksheet and the software program located on Evolve to produce a completed CMS-1450 (UB-04). Follow these instructions to complete Student Software Case 5:

Step 1: The Coding Worksheet should be completed before entering data into the software. Use your completed Coding Worksheet and the patient face sheet/charge detail (after they are reviewed by your instructor) to enter information into the proper fields on the software. Follow the software screen by screen.

Step 2: Once you have completed each screen, preview your completed CMS-1450 (UB-04). Make required corrections before printing.

Step 3: Print your completed claim form and submit to your instructor for review, and keep a copy for your records.

Community General Hospital
Federal Tax ID# 62-1026428
Case 5: Hospital Ambulatory Surgery—Kamika L. Lotaman

8192 South Street
Mars, Florida 37373
(747) 722-1800

PATIENT FACE SHEET AND CHARGE DETAIL

Admit/Discharge Date	Admit/Discharge Hour	Admission Source	Admission Type	Med Record / Soc Sec #	Patient Control #
Admit: 08/22/20__ Disch: 08/22/20__	Admit: 7:00 AM Disch: 3:30 PM	Physician Referral	Elective	MR# L002829614	60997906

Patient Name	DOB	Release Info	Assignment Ben	Discharge Status	Sex	Marital Status
Kamika J. Lotaman	10/25/1965	Y	Y	Discharge to Home	F	S

Patient Address	City, ST Zip	Phone
721 Second Street	Mars, Florida 37373	747 721 5142

INSURANCE INFORMATION

Primary Carrier	Insured's Name	Identification# DA46854X / Group Name and #	Provider #
Medicaid	Kamika J. Lotaman		00356563

Secondary Carrier	Insured's Name	Identification # / Group Name and #	Provider #

Pt Relationship	Employer Name	Employer Location	Treatment Authorization #
Self			

Pt Relationship	Employer Name	Employer Location	Treatment Authorization #

PHYSICIANS/CLINICAL INFORMATION

Attending/Referring/Ordering Physician/ID#	Other Physician/ID #	Occurrence Date	Condition/Value Info
Michael Jefferson, M.D. NPI: 1943742907	Anthony Tom, M.D. NPI: 1847394279	Last menstrual period 08/15/20__	

CHARGE DETAIL

Revenue Code	Service Description	HCPCS/Rates	Service Units	Total Charges	Non-Covered Charges
	DRUGS/NONPSCRPT		7	190.36	
	IV SOLUTIONS		5	353.57	
	MED-SUR SUPPLIES		36	6301.67	
	STERILE SUPPLY		1	177.56	
	OR SERVICES		6	3410.08	
	ANESTHESIA		6	1097.89	
	RECOVERY ROOM		4	1213.49	
	TOTAL CHARGES		65	12744.62	

OTHER CHARGES TO BE CODED, POSTED, AND ADDED TO CHARGE DETAIL ABOVE

Surgical Trays 1 $177.56
Pelvic Laparoscopy Tray

PHYSICIAN PROGRESS NOTES

Patient Name: Kamika J. Lotaman **Date:** 08/19/20__

This is a 41-year-old with two children who has a history of two previous cesarean sections and a long and very significant past medical history of leiomyoma. She has been suffering from abdominal pain, discomfort, and excessive menstruations that have been disabling since January. She has been treated with conservative medical management using GnRH agonist. In addition she has had a myomectomy in the past. She presented to my office today with worsening complaints of severe right lower quadrant pain and discomfort and frequent and excessive menstruation that affects her ability to work and her relationship with her spouse. She states on a scale of 1 to 10 that it is approximately an 8 in discomfort. No other significant medical problems were noted.

The patient is scheduled at Community General Hospital for ambulatory surgery on 8/22/20__ for a hysterectomy.

Michael Jefferson, M.D.

Community General Hospital
Federal Tax ID# 62-1026428

8192 South Street
Mars, Florida 37373
(747) 722-1800

OPERATIVE REPORT

PATIENT NAME:	Kamika J. Lotaman
MEDICAL RECORD:	# L002829614
DATE OF PROCEDURE:	August 22, 20__
SURGEON:	Michael Jefferson, M.D.
ASSISTANT:	Anthony Tom, M.D.
PREOPERATIVE DIAGNOSIS:	Abdominal Pain, Excessive and frequent menstruation, Leiomyomata Uteri
POSTOPERATIVE DIAGNOSIS:	Leiomyomata Uteri
PROCEDURE:	Hysterectomy

OPERATIVE PROCEDURE:
The patient was placed on the operating room table and placed under general anesthetic without complications. The abdomen and perineum were prepped and draped in sterile fashion. Bladder was emptied. An infraumbilical incision was made vertically and extended down to the fascia. The fascia was incised and the peritoneal cavity was entered. Stay sutures were placed on the angles of the stitch, and a blunt port was then put into place and tied down. A trocar was inserted through the laparoscope and the abdomen was insufflated. The patient was placed in Trendelenburg position. Prior to this, vaginal instruments were placed for uterine manipulation.

The uterus was used in order to adequately visualize the pelvis using the vaginal instruments. Both right and left lower quadrant port sites were placed atraumatically. Next, a Babcock was used to grasp the infundibulopelvic ligament on the right with the Endo GIA and was fired across the infundibulopelvic ligament with great care to identify the ureter out of the operative field. Second and third bites were taken on this side which incorporated the round ligament down to the uterine vessels. The same procedure was done on the opposite side.

The bladder flap and peritoneum was developed using graspers and hot scissors. At this point, the procedure was taken vaginally and the legs were rotated superiorly, and a weighted speculum was placed in the posterior vault of the vagina. The vaginal instruments that were placed for uterine mobility were removed and Lahey clamps were then used on the uterine cervix. The vaginal mucosa was then circumferentially injected with 0.5% Xylocaine with 1:200,000 epinephrine and then the vaginal mucosa was mobilized.

The posterior cul-de-sac was entered atraumatically. Heaney clamps were used on uterosacral ligaments bilaterally. These were clamped, cut, tied, and held. Second bites were then taken on each side and these were clamped, cut, and tied. The weighted speculum was replaced with a duckbill weighted speculum and the anterior cul-de-sac was entered. Third bites were then taken on each side which incorporated uterine vessels. At this point, the uterus was flipped. The remaining pedicle was grasped, clamped, and cut and the uterus and tubes and ovaries were removed. The weight of the uterus is less then 250 gm.

The peritoneum was closed using a pursestring-type suture using chromic suture and the uterosacral ligaments were plicated in the midline using #0 Vicryl suture. The incisions were closed using interrupted figure-of-eight 2-0 Vicryl suture. At this point, the gloves were changed and the patient was repositioned and we went back above to look at the port sites and reviewed the pelvic anatomy. It was completely hemostatic. Nezhat suction irrigator was used to irrigate the pelvis. At this point, each port site was removed and inspected and not bleeding. The umbilical port site was closed first by closing the fascia with #0 Vicryl suture and then stapling with two skin staples. The port sites on each side were then stapled and the wounds were dressed. A Foley catheter was placed, and the patient was awakened and taken to the recovery room in stable condition.

#78573409 T: 08/22/20__
DICTATION # M2664JJK

Michael Jefferson, M.D.

HEALTH INFORMATION MANAGEMENT CODING WORKSHEET

STUDENT NAME:		**DATE:**	
PATIENT NAME:		**CASE #5:**	
DEMOGRAPHICS			
Medical Record Number:	**Bill Type#:**		
Patient Name: Last, First, Middle Init:	Admit Hour Code:	Discharge Hour Code:	
	Admit Type Code:	Discharge Status Code:	
	Admit Source Code:	Patient Relationship Code:	
Condition Code(s)	Occurrence Span Code and Date:	Value Code and Amount:	

ADMISSION INFORMATION					
Type of admission:	**ER**	**Facility**	**Physician Referral**	**Other**	**Unknown**

Admitting Diagnosis		**HIM Code(s)**
Principal Diagnosis (Including complications and co-morbidities if applicable)		**HIM Code**
Other Secondary Diagnosis (Including complications and co-morbidities if applicable)		**HIM Code(s)**
Procedure(s)	**Date:**	**HIM Code(s)**
Medications, supplies, equipment or other item(s)	**Date:**	**HIM Code(s)**

DISCHARGE INFORMATION				
Home	Facility	AMA	Deceased	Other

DRG ASSIGNMENT		**APC ASSIGNMENT**		
MDC:	Surgical/Medical:			

CONTRIBUTING FACTORS				
Age	Sex	Discharge Status	Complications/Comorbidities	Birthweight

Questions/Need Clarification:

CASE 6: AMBULATORY SURGERY VISIT

Summary

Patient Name: Sofia M. Steinberg **Date:** 04/03/20__

This is a 43-year-old female scheduled for a colonoscopy as she has been experiencing nausea, severe stomach pains. and diarrhea. She indicates these episodes generally occur within 20 minutes of when she eats. The episodes of pain and diarrhea continued after she resumed a regular diet and last week she noticed blood in her stool.

Jeffery Barnes, M.D.

Case 6: Ambulatory Surgery Visit

Directions:
The patient face sheet/charge detail; patient history, physical exam, and operative report are included in the Case 6 file in Appendix A. Complete this case and prepare a CMS-1450 (UB-04) as follows.
Step 1: Assign revenue codes (see Appendix B) to each category of service listed on the patient face sheet/charge detail.

Submit your patient face sheet/charge detail to your instructor for review.

Step 2: The Coding Worksheet included with this case must be completed before data can be entered on the computer. Complete the Case 6 Coding Worksheet as follows:

a. Record the codes describing the admitting, principal, and other diagnoses.
b. Record the HCPCS Level I CPT code(s) describing the ambulatory surgery services (including pathology) in addition to the ICD-9-CM Volume III procedure code(s) as required by this payer.
c. Record the code(s) for the items listed below the charge detail.

All other charges listed on the patient face sheet have been coded and posted by other departments.

d. Assign UB data code (see Appendix B) to other information on the Coding Worksheet.

Submit your Coding Worksheet to your instructor for review.

Step 3: Complete a CMS-1450 (UB-04) claim form for this case. Claim forms can be completed manually or utilizing the software. Your instructor will advise if a manual claim is required. Otherwise begin completing the Student Software Case.

Student Software Case 6
Directions:

Use your completed Coding Worksheet and the software program located on Evolve to produce a completed CMS-1450 (UB-04). Follow these instructions to complete Student Software Case 6.

Step 1: The Coding Worksheet should be completed before entering data into the software. Use your completed Coding Worksheet and the patient face sheet/charge detail (after they are reviewed by your instructor) to enter information into the proper fields on the software. Follow the software screen by screen.

Step 2: Once you have completed each screen, preview your completed CMS-1450 (UB-04). Make required corrections before printing.

Step 3: Print your completed claim form and submit to your instructor for review, and keep a copy for your records.

Community General Hospital

Federal Tax ID# 62-1026428 NPI 1234567890
Case 6: Hospital Ambulatory Surgery—Sofia M. Steinberg

8192 South Street
Mars, Florida 37373
(747) 722-1800

PATIENT FACE SHEET AND CHARGE DETAIL

Admit/Discharge Date	Admit/Discharge Hour	Admission Source	Admission Type	Med Record / Soc Sec #	Patient Control #
Admit: 04/03/20__ Disch: 04/03/20__	Admit: 8:00 AM Disch: 12:00 PM	Physician Referral	Elective	MR# S155321876	51734271

Patient Name	DOB	Release of Info	Assignment Ben	Discharge Status	Sex	Marital Status
Sofia M. Steinberg	06/14/1962	Y	N	Discharge to Home	F	S

Patient Address	City, ST Zip	Phone
512 Johns Highway	Orlando, Florida 32853	404 724 5146

INSURANCE INFORMATION

Primary Carrier	Insured's Name	Identification# SS172321 / Group Name and #	Provider #
Aetna	Sofia M. Steinberg		0046781
Secondary Carrier	Insured's Name	Identification # / Group Name and #	Provider #

Pt Relationship	Employer Name	Employer Location	Treatment Authorization #
Self	Universal Studios	International Dr Orlando FL 32854	X7953278
Pt Relationship	Employer Name	Employer Location	Treatment Authorization #

PHYSICIANS/CLINICAL INFORMATION

Attending/Referring/Ordering Physician/ID#	Other Physician/ID #	Occurrence Date	Condition/Value Info
Jeffrey Barnes, M.D. NPI: 1584732144	Joseph Johns, M.D. NPI: 1539441100		*Estimated Patient Responsibility A $500.00

CHARGE DETAIL

Revenue Code	Service Description	HCPCS/Rates	Service Units	Total Charges	Non-Covered Charges
	DRUGS		10	150.00	
	IV SOLUTIONS		2	2.30	
	MED-SUR SUPPLIES		6	629.30	
	STERILE SUPPLY		20	534.20	
	PATHOL/BIOPSY		3	375.00	
	OR SERVICES		1	1094.00	
	ANESTHESIA		2	222.00	
	RECOVERY ROOM		2	222.00	
	TOTAL CHARGE		46	3248.80	

OTHER CHARGES TO BE CODED, POSTED, AND ADDED TO CHARGE DETAIL ABOVE
NONE

PROGRESS NOTE

Patient Name: Sofia M. Steinberg **Date:** 03/29/20__

This is a 43-year-old female patient who was seen in the office 2 weeks ago with chief complaints of nausea, severe stomach pains, and diarrhea. She noted the episodes generally occur within 20 minutes of when she eats. I prescribed Prevacid 3 mg and placed on a bland diet for 2 weeks. The patient returned to the office today indicating she is still experiencing nausea, severe stomach pains, and diarrhea, and she has noticed blood in her stool. States the onset of symptoms occurs within 10 to 15 minutes after a meal. Discussed other treatments involving medications and or diet and a colonoscopy. The patient decided to proceed with the colonoscopy and she is scheduled for the procedure on April 3rd at Community General Hospital.

Jeffery Barnes, M.D.

Community General Hospital
Federal Tax ID# 62-1026428
NPI 1234567890

8192 South Street
Mars, Florida 37373
(747) 722-1800

OPERATIVE REPORT

PATIENT NAME: Sofia M. Steinberg
MEDICAL RECORD: S155321876
DATE OF PROCEDURE: 04/03/20__
SURGEON: Jeffrey Barnes, M.D.
ASSISTANT: Joseph Johns, M.D.
PREOPERATIVE DIAGNOSIS: Stomach pain, diarrhea, nausea, blood in stool
POSTOPERATIVE DIAGNOSIS:
1. Two polyps in the splenic flexure, status post biopsy.
2. One polyp in the sigmoid colon, status post biopsy.
3. Small non-bleeding internal hemorrhoids

PROCEDURE: COLONOSCOPY

DESCRIPTION OF PROCEDURE:
After an informed consent the patient was prepped and draped in the usual sterile fashion. The colonoscope was introduced under direct visualization up to the cecum. The prep was fair.

FINDINGS: Cecum, ascending colon, and transverse colon appeared normal. In the splenic flexure area, there were two polyps; both of these polyps were about 2 cm each in size. They were removed with hot biopsy forceps. In the sigmoid colon, there was another polyp, which was about 1 cm in size. That was also biopsied with the cold biopsy forceps. No diverticulosis was noted. Small non-bleeding internal hemorrhoids were present. The patient tolerated the procedure well.

#27921365 T: 04/04/20__
DICTATION # Z6123GMT

Jeffrey Barnes, M.D.

Community General Hospital
Federal Tax ID# 62-1026428
NPI 1234567890

8192 South Street
Mars, Florida 37373
(747) 722-1800

PATHOLOGY REPORT

PATIENT NAME:	Sofia M. Steinberg	MEDICAL RECORD:	S155321876
PATHOLOGIST:	Martin Marcus, M.D.		

SPECIMEN SUBMITTED: Polyps

GROSS DESCRITPION: Specimen consists of three colon polyps ranging in size from 1 cm to 2 cm.

MICROSCOPIC DESCRIPTION: Sections reveal two polyps from the splenic flexure measuring 2 cm and 1 from sigmoid colon measuring 1 cm. Examination of the polyps show surface epithelium and underlying glands lined by a serrated feathery surface epithelium.

DIAGNOSIS: Benign polyps.

HEALTH INFORMATION MANAGEMENT CODING WORKSHEET

STUDENT NAME:		**DATE:**
PATIENT NAME:		**CASE #6:**
DEMOGRAPHICS		
Medical Record Number:	**Bill Type#:**	
Patient Name: Last, First, Middle Init:	Admit Hour Code:	Discharge Hour Code:
	Admit Type Code:	Discharge Status Code:
	Admit Source Code:	Patient Relationship Code:
Condition Code(s)	Occurrence Span Code and Date:	Value Code and Amount:

ADMISSION INFORMATION		
Type of admission: ER Facility Physician Referral Other Unknown		
Admitting Diagnosis		**HIM Code(s)**
Principal Diagnosis (Including complications and co-morbidities if applicable)		**HIM Code**
Other Secondary Diagnosis (Including complications and co-morbidities if applicable)		**HIM Code(s)**
Principal Procedure (Significant procedure performed for definitive treatment or that most closely relates to the principal diagnosis)	**Date:**	**HIM Code(s)**
Other Procedure(s)	**Date:**	**HIM Code(s)**
Medications, supplies, equipment or other item(s)	**Date:**	**HIM Code(s)**

DISCHARGE INFORMATION				
Home	Facility	AMA	Deceased	Other

DRG ASSIGNMENT		**APC ASSIGNMENT**		
MDC:	Surgical/Medical:			

CONTRIBUTING FACTORS				
Age	Sex	Discharge Status	Complications/Comorbidities	Birthweight

Questions/Need Clarification:

CASE 7: HOSPITAL OUTPATIENT CARDIAC CATHETERIZATION

Summary

Patient Name: Donald M. Matthews **Date:** 04/28/20__

57-year-old male patient with progressive unstable angina and malignant hypertension undergoes a left heart catheterization. Patient had an MI 3 months ago. Cardiac catheterization is performed with coronary angiography.

James Moya, M.D.

Case 7: Hospital Outpatient Cardiac Catheterization

Directions:

The patient face sheet/charge detail; patient history, physical exam, and operative report are included in the Case 7 file in Appendix A. Complete this case and prepare a CMS-1450 (UB-04) as follows.
Step 1: Assign revenue codes (see Appendix B) to each category of service listed on the patient face sheet/charge detail.

Submit your patient face sheet/charge detail to your instructor for review.

Step 2: The Coding Worksheet included in this case must be completed before data can be entered on the computer. Complete the Case 7 Coding Worksheet as follows.

a. Record the codes describing the admitting, principal, and other diagnoses.
b. Record the codes describing the outpatient services.
c. Record the codes for the items listed below the charge detail.

All other charges listed on the patient face sheet have been posted and coded by other departments.

d. Assign UB data code (see Appendix B) to other information on the Coding Worksheet.

Submit your Coding Worksheet to your instructor for review.

Step 3: Complete a CMS-1450 (UB-04) claim form for this case. Claim forms can be completed manually or utilizing the software. Your instructor will advise if a manual claim is required. Otherwise begin completing the Student Software Case.

Student Software Case 7

Directions:

Use your completed Coding Worksheet and the software program located on Evolve to produce a completed CMS-1450 (UB-04). Follow these instructions to complete Student Software Case 7.

Step 1: The co Coding Worksheet should be completed before entering data into the software. Use your completed Coding Worksheet and the patient face sheet/charge detail (after they are reviewed by your instructor) to enter information into the proper fields on the software. Follow the software screen by screen.

Step 2: Once you have completed each screen, preview your completed CMS-1450 (UB-04). Make required corrections before printing.

Step 3: Print your completed claim form and submit to your instructor for review, and keep a copy for your records.

Community General Hospital
Federal Tax ID# 62-1026428 NPI 1234567890
Case 7: Hospital Outpatient Cardiac Catheterization—Donald M. Matthews

8192 South Street
Mars, Florida 37373
(747) 722-1800

PATIENT FACE SHEET
AND CHARGE DETAIL

Admit/Discharge Date	Admit/Discharge Hour	Admission Source	Admission Type	Med Record / Soc Sec #	Patient Control #
Admit: 04/28/20__ Disch: 04/28/20__	Admit: 12:00 PM Disch: 3:15 PM	Physician Referral	Elective	MR# M567932176	7621583

Patient Name	DOB	Release of Info	Assignment Ben	Discharge Status	Sex	Marital Status
Donald M. Matthews	07/15/1949	Y	Y	Discharge to Home	M	M

Patient Address	City, ST Zip	Phone
214 5th Street North	Orlando, Florida 32853	404 724 5217

INSURANCE INFORMATION

Primary Carrier	Insured's Name	Identification# 276547131B	Provider #
Medicare		Group Name and #	562417
Secondary Carrier	**Insured's Name**	**Identification # 23541764**	**Provider #**
Travelers	Donald M. Matthews	Group Name and #	00617159

Pt Relationship	Employer Name	Employer Location	Treatment Authorization #
Self	Dean Witter	2561 Main Street Orlando FL 39524	
Pt Relationship	Employer Name	Employer Location	Treatment Authorization #

PHYSICIANS/CLINICAL INFORMATION

Attending/Referring/Ordering Physician/ID#	Other Physician/ID #	Occurrence Date	Condition/Value Info
James Moya, M.D. NPI: 1556982121			*Patient &/or Spouse Employed; No Other Coverage Exists *Deductible Payer A $250.00

CHARGE DETAIL

Revenue Code	Service Description	HCPCS/Rates	Service Units	Total Charges	Non-Covered Charges
	PHARMACY		4	1145.80	
	DRUGS/OTHER		3	77.50	
	MED-SUR SUPPLIES		5	740.82	
	CARDIAC CATH LAB		1	2736.50	
	CARDIAC CATH LAB		1	390.00	
	CARDIAC CATH LAB		1	554.00	
	TOTAL CHARGE		15	5644.62	

OTHER CHARGES TO BE CODED, POSTED, AND ADDED TO CHARGE DETAIL ABOVE
NONE

PROGRESS NOTES	
Patient Name: Donald M. Matthews	**Date:** 04/28/20__

57-year-old male patient with unstable angina. Patient is being treated for malignant hypertension. Patient had an MI 3 months ago. A heart catheterization was recommended at that time, but the patient did not want to undergo the procedure then. About 2 weeks ago the patient began experiencing marked progression of his angina in frequency and severity. Patient has been experiencing a sudden onset of chest pain. The pain is substernal, to the left chest, up to the left shoulder and behind the left scapula, down his left arm. The pain is more severe with deep breath. The patient presents today for a scheduled left heart catheterization.

James Moya, M.D.

Community General Hospital
Federal Tax ID# 62-1026428
NPI 1234567890

8192 South Street
Mars, Florida 37373
(747) 722-1800

CARDIAC CATHETERIZATION

PATIENT NAME:	Donald M. Matthews	MEDICAL RECORD#:	M567932176
DATE OF PROCEDURE:	04/28/20__	PHYSICIAN:	James Moya, M.D.
INDICATIONS FOR PROCEDURE:	Unstable Angina		
PRE-PROCEDURE DIAGNOSIS:	Unstable Angina, Malignant Hypertension, Myocardial Infarction		
POST PROCEDURE DIAGNOSIS:	Coronary Artherosclerosis		

PROCEDURE: LEFT HEART CATHETERIZATION INCLUDING SELECTIVE CORONARY ANGIOGRAPHY.

CATH TECHNIQUE: After written consent was obtained, the patient was given Benadryl 50 mg p.o. The patient was prepped and draped in the usual fashion. Using 1% Lidocaine, local anesthesia was applied to the right groin. The right femoral artery was entered using 18-gauge Cook needle and the guide wire was passed through the needle without any resistance; 6-French sheath system was placed. Selective coronary angiography was performed using 6-French right Judkins catheter for the right coronary artery and 6-French left Judkins catheter for the left coronary artery. The catheter was withdrawn using a wire and the patient was taken to the holding area where the sheaths were removed and direct pressure was applied to the right groin until hemostasis was obtained.

During the right and left coronary angiography, a guide wire was used to exchange the catheters. The pedal pulses were obtained and they were unchanged from the precatheterization status. The patient tolerated the procedure well and left the cath lab in good condition.

RESULTS:
1. Right coronary artery is a nondominant vessel and has 70% mid-segment lesion.
2. Left main is a normal-caliber vessel proximally, posteriorly and for about 30% to 40% distal lesion and then it divided into left anterior descending and left circumflex.
3. Left circumflex is a dominant vessel and gave rise to multiple obtuse marginal branches, and then gave rise to posterior descending artery. There is an 80% lesion in the distal part of the left circumflex before it gives rise to the posterior descending artery and the rest of the left circumflex has nonobstructive disease.
4. Left anterior descending artery is a small vessel and has a 60% mid-segment lesion with good distal flow and gave rise to multiple diagonal branches that have some luminal irregularities.

IMPRESSION:
1. Coronary artery disease, three vessel, with 30% left main disease.

RECOMMENDATIONS: The patient needs to have IV Persantine scan. If there is ischemia in the distribution of the left anterior descending then he needs to have coronary artery bypass surgery. However, if there is no ischemia, medical treatment could be tried at the present time. Angioplasty of the left circumflex could not be done because of the distal left main disease.

#9265394 T: 05/01/20__
DICTATION # P5133MMN

James Moya, M.D.

HEALTH INFORMATION MANAGEMENT CODING WORKSHEET

STUDENT NAME:		**DATE:**
PATIENT NAME:		**CASE #7:**
DEMOGRAPHICS		
Medical Record Number:	**Bill Type#:**	
Patient Name: Last, First, Middle Init:	Admit Hour Code:	Discharge Hour Code:
	Admit Type Code:	Discharge Status Code:
	Admit Source Code:	Patient Relationship Code:
Condition Code(s)	Occurrence Span Code and Date:	Value Code and Amount:

ADMISSION INFORMATION

Type of Admission: **ER** **Facility** **Physician Referral** **Other** **Unknown**

Admitting Diagnosis		**HIM Code(s)**
Principal Diagnosis (Including complications and co-morbidities if applicable)		**HIM Code**
Other Secondary Diagnosis (Including complications and co-morbidities if applicable)		**HIM Code(s)**
Procedure(s)	**Date:**	**HIM Code(s)**
Medications, supplies, equipment or other item(s)	**Date:**	**HIM Code(s)**

DISCHARGE INFORMATION

Home Facility AMA Deceased Other

DRG ASSIGNMENT		**APC ASSIGNMENT**		
MDC:	Surgical/Medical:			

CONTRIBUTING FACTORS

Age	Sex	Discharge Status	Complications/Comorbidities	Birthweight

Questions/Need Clarification:

CASE 8: HOSPITAL INPATIENT STAY

Summary

Patient Name: Tyron J. Sampson **Date:** 09/16/20__

This 53-year-old right-handed gentleman from out of town is being admitted through the emergency room with a severe chest pain, headache, confusion and loss of vision. The patient indicated he was in the emergency room 4 days ago for an episode of near blindness. It was recommended at that time that he have an ultrasound, MRI of the brain, and MRA of the neck. He noted that he was going to pursue care when he returned home. Ultrasound revealed carotid stenosis demonstrating a question of right carotid hemodynamically significant stenosis. Angiography revealed severe right internal carotid stenosis.

Franklin D. Harder, M.D.

Case 8: Hospital Inpatient Stay

Directions:

The patient face sheet/charge detail, admission history and physical, progress notes, vascular lab report, operative report, and discharge summary are included in this case. Complete this case and prepare a CMS-1450 (UB-04) as follows:

Step 1: Assign revenue codes (see Appendix B) to each category of service listed on the patient face sheet/charge detail.

Submit your patient face sheet/charge detail to your instructor for review.

Step 2: The Coding Worksheet included with this case must be completed before data can be entered on the computer. Complete the Case 8 Coding Worksheet as follows.

a. Record the codes describing the admitting, principal, and other diagnoses
b. Record the ICD-9-CM Volume III procedure code(s) describing the vascular lab service and surgery service
c. Record the code(s) for the items listed below the charge detail

All other charges listed on the patient face sheet have been coded and posted by other departments.

d. Assign UB data codes (see Appendix B) to other information on the coding worksheet

Note: when describing the type of bill the payer must be advised to Void/Cancel the prior claim submitted.

Submit your Coding Worksheet to your instructor for review.

Step 3: Complete a CMS-1450 (UB-04) claim form for this case. Claim forms can be completed manually or utilizing the software. Your instructor will advise if a manual claim is required. Otherwise begin completing the Student Software Case.

Student Software Case 8
Directions:

Use your completed Coding Worksheet and the software program located on Evolve to produce a completed CMS-1450 (UB-04). Follow these instructions to complete Student Software Case 8.

Step 1: The Coding Worksheet should be completed before entering data into the software. Use your completed Coding Worksheet and the patient face sheet/charge detail (after they are reviewed by your instructor) to enter information into the proper fields on the software. Follow the software screen by screen.

Step 2: Once you have completed each screen, preview your completed CMS-1450 (UB-04). Make required corrections before printing.

Step 3: Print your completed claim form and submit to your instructor for review, and keep a copy for your records.

Community General Hospital

Federal Tax ID# 62-1026428 NPI 1234567890

Case 8: Hospital Inpatient—Tyron J. Sampson

8192 South Street
Mars, Florida 37373
(747) 722-1800

PATIENT FACE SHEET AND CHARGE DETAIL

Admit/Discharge Date	Admit/Discharge Hour	Admission Source	Admission Type	Med Record / Soc Sec #	Patient Control #
Admit: 09/16/20__ Disch: 09/20/20__	Admit: 2:47 PM Disch: 12:17 PM	Emergency Room	Urgent	MR# S846195251	61008667

Patient Name	DOB	Release Info	Assignment Ben	Discharge Status	Sex	Marital Status
Tyron J. Sampson	10/17/1953	Y	Y	Discharge to home under the care of Home health service	M	M

Patient Address	City, ST Zip	Phone
424 State Highway 12	West Springs, Florida 32433	(407) 323-7979

INSURANCE INFORMATION

Primary Carrier	Insured's Name	Identification# / Group Name and #	Provider #
Health Network of Orlando	Tyron J. Sampson	Identification# 00005148263 Group Name and # WS FLA HN 76532	D54121
Secondary Carrier	Insured's Name	Identification # Group Name and #	Provider #

Pt Relationship	Employer Name	Employer Location	Treatment Authorization #
Self	Unemployed		HN 290473
Pt Relationship	Employer Name	Employer Location	Treatment Authorization #

PHYSICIANS/CLINICAL INFORMATION

Attending/Referring/Ordering Physician/ID#	Other Physician/ID #	Occurrence Date	Condition/Value Info
Franklin D. Harder, M.D. NPI: 1364309721	Ameila Torinson, D.O. NPI: 1006854321	Onset of Symptoms/illness 09/15/20__	*Patient & spouse-unemployed *Deductible = $250.00 *Common SemiPvt $679.75

CHARGE DETAIL

Revenue Code	Service Description	HCPCS/Rates	Service Units	Total Charges	Non-Covered Charges
	ROOM-BOARD/SEM	679.75	5	2719	
	PHARMACY		73	4515	
	IV SOLUTIONS		3	277.5	
	MED-SURG SUPPLIES		93	6260.5	
	LABORATORY		28	2206.5	
	DX X-RAY		4	6301.25	
	DX X-RAY/ARTER		1	1673	
	OR SERVICES		3	6848.75	
	ANESTHESIA		10	1919.5	
	EMERG ROOM		1	504.5	
	RECOVERY ROOM		1	633.25	
	EKG/ECG		1	81	
	PERI VASCUL LAB		3	1450	
	TOTAL CHARGE		225	$35389.75	

OTHER CHARGES TO BE CODED, POSTED, AND ADDED TO CHARGE DETAIL ABOVE
9/17 Single A Line with Heparin (implantable access catheter) Qty 1 price ea $156.25

ADMISSION HISTORY AND PHYSICAL

Patient Name: Tyron J. Sampson **Date:** 09/16/20__

HISTORY OF PRESENT ILLNESS:

This 53-year-old right-handed gentleman from out of town is being admitted through the emergency room with a severe chest pain, headache, confusion, and loss of vision. The patient indicated he was in the emergency room 4 days ago for an episode of near blindness. It was recommended at that time that he have an ultrasound, MRI of the brain, and MRA of the neck. He noted he was going to pursue care when he returned home. He has had three or four episodes in the last 3 months of brief lightheadedness not associated with his numbness or with this visual disturbance. The patient's blood pressure is so high he is about to have a stroke. He is alert and does have back and chest wall pains. The chest pain has subsided since he was admitted.

ALLERGIES:

He lists aspirin because of rectal bleeding episode

VITALS

Temp:	Pulse:	Resp:	BP:	O2 sats:
99	86	14	116/80	

CURRENT MEDICATIONS:
1. Celebrex 200 mg daily.
2. Triamterene/hydrochlorothiazide 50/25 mg/daily
3. Norvasc 10 milligrams daily
4. Additional hydrochlorothiazide 12.5 mg/daily
5. Hyzaar was started on the day of his visual obscuration.

Patient in by (name of person or ambulance)
Patient drove himself to ED

Patient Signature – Release record/Assignment of benefits:
Tyron J. Sampson *09/12/20__*

PHYSICIAN ORDERS:
✓ Basic Metabolic Panel
✓ Lipid Panel ✓ Protime, PTT
✓ Urtinalysis ✓ EKG

PAST MEDICAL HISTORY:

Patient has severe hypertension and is post coronary artery bypass graft of a native vessel. Approximately 3 months ago he stopped taking aspirin because of rectal bleeding. He did have a proctoscopic examination which revealed hemorrhoids. He follows his cardiologist regarding his cardiac disease and has had an irregular heartbeat but never atrial fibrillation.

He indicates that approximately 3 months ago he was pulling strongly on a pipe wrench at work and ever since has had discomfort in the shoulder girdle area, intermittent numbness bilaterally in the hands, a more constant numbness in the ulnar aspect of the right hand, and a wasting of the right arm. Some numbness in the left side of the chest, which he related to previous coronary artery surgery, seems to be expanded in size. He had appointment with his family physician, under Workers' Compensation regarding these particular issues. The pain he has been experiencing has been much alleviated by Celebrex. Intermittent numbness occurred more commonly initially in the right hand but is now more common in the left hand and follows patterns typical for carpal tunnel syndrome with increase while driving and brief episodes of worsening while sleeping.

EXAMINATION:

GENERAL EXAMINATION
No distress. Muscular, well-dressed. Head and neck exam is unremarkable. Ocular exam is normal. Visual acuity is normal. Visual fields by confrontation. Retinas are pink. There are mild to moderate AV crossing changes. No hemorrhages or exudates are appreciated. Mental status is normal. Cranial nerves II-XII intact. Motor and sensory exams are normal and symmetrical. Cerebellar exam is normal. No drift or pathologic reflexes. Gait normal. Deep tendon reflexes normal. Chest is clear. Cardiovascular exam: SI and S2 normal. No S3 or S4. Normal murmur. No pleural or pericardial friction rubs. No peripheral edema, cyanosis, or clubbing. Abdominal exam is benign. He is well hydrated. No rashes are present.

NEUROLOGICAL EXAMINATION
Mental status is normal. Cranial nerves demonstrate first-degree nystagmus. The fundus is normal. Fields are full. Face is symmetrical. Motor examination is normal and strong throughout including the APBs. Reflexes are 1 to absent throughout. The plantars are flexor. Sensory examination: Decreased pinprick in the left median nerve distribution.

EKG demonstrates normal sinus rhythm with occasional premature ventricular complexes, left atrial enlargement, T-wave abnormality. Labs: CBC, basic metabolic, lipid panel, and urinalysis normal. Chest X-ray reveals stable appearance of the chest post coronary bypass with no acute process and no change since the previous study in February.

ASSESSMENT/PLAN OF CARE:

Probable carotid stenosis. Carotid ultrasound scheduled for the AM.

PHYSICIAN PROGRESS NOTES

Patient Name: Tyron J. Sampson

9/17/20__ Carotid and cerebral artery ultrasound reveals hemodynamically significant stenotic lesion right internal carotid artery. Cardiologist recommended an MRI of the brain and MRA of the head and neck. The MRI/MRA revealed proximal right internal carotid severe stenosis. Probable additional severe stenosis paraclinoid and supraclinoid segment of right internal carotid and possibly some degree of stenosis posterior genu cavernous right internal carotid. Carotid angiography scheduled for the AM.

09/18/20__ Angiogram reveals proximal right internal carotid severe stenosis, 90%. Discussed surgical options with the patient. Patient consent to endarterectomy in the am.

Community General Hospital
Federal Tax ID# 62-1026428
NPI 1234567890

8192 South Street
Mars, Florida 37373
(747) 722-1800

VASCULAR LAB REPORT

PATIENT NAME: Tyron J. Sampson
DOB: 10/17/1953
EXAM DATE: 09/18/20__
ATTENDING: Franklin D. Harder, M.D.
ACCOUNT #: S846195251

CLINICAL INDICATIONS: Visual Obscuration, Carotid stenosis
PROCEDURE: RIGHT COMMON CAROTID ANGIOGRAM

The procedure and/or need for sedation was discussed with the patient, or other responsible party who understands the procedure and/or need for sedation including the reason for having it, the benefits, risks, side effects, and alternatives. The patient or other responsible party agrees to proceed and signed written informed consent was obtained.

Following right femoral artery access, catheter is advanced through the aorta; a second order right common carotid was selectively catheterized with cervical and cranial filming. There were no complications.

Right common carotid artery is of normal caliber with shallow plaque posteriorly at its bifurcation. Proximal right internal carotid has extremely severe stenosis, approximately 90%. The right internal carotid fills slowly but quite well distal to the stenosis. The external carotid system filling in advance of internal carotid. Right cavernous internal carotid has shallow plaque inferiorly with only 15% to 20% stenosis. The right ophthalmic artery fills well and is unremarkable. Right middle cerebral also fills well, although slowly and is only mildly reduced in its caliber.

IMPRESSION: Proximal right internal carotid severe (90%) stenosis with small ulceration distal to the stenosis

Dr. Terence Thomas

Community General Hospital
Federal Tax ID# 62-1026428
NPI 1234567890

8192 South Street
Mars, Florida 37373
(747) 722-1800

OPERATIVE REPORT

PATIENT NAME:	Tyron J. Sampson
MEDICAL RECORD:	# S846195251
DATE OF PROCEDURE:	09/19/20__
SURGEON:	Franklin D. Harder, M.D.
ASSISTANT:	Amelia Torinson, M.D.
PREOPERATIVE DIAGNOSIS:	Stenosis
POSTOPERATIVE DIAGNOSIS:	Severe systemic right internal carotid stenosis
PROCEDURE:	Carotid endarterectomy

INDICATIONS FOR OPERATION
This is a 53-year-old white male who is status post coronary artery bypass grafting, who presented with loss of vision in both eyes. He was noted to be hypertensive and subsequently bruits were noted as well. This led to carotid ultrasound that showed tight stenosis of the right internal carotid. A carotid arteriogram was obtained which showed a very tight stenosis. Because of his symptomatic status and degree of stenosis, it was felt that he would benefit from carotid endarterectomy. The risks, benefits, indications, and alternatives were explained to the patient and his family and they desired to proceed with surgical intervention.

DESCRIPTION OF OPERATION
The patient was taken to the main operating room and placed in the supine position under general endotracheal anesthesia with the appropriate monitoring devices. He was prepped and draped. An incision was made just to the right of his sternocleidomastoid and dissection carried down through the fatty tissues with the Bovie electrocautery. The facial vein was identified, ligated and divided. We identified the common carotid, internal carotid, and external carotid. 7500 units of Heparin was administered. Clamps were sequentially applied to the internal carotid, common carotid, and external carotid. An arteriotomy was made and extended using Potts scissors. A Javid shunt was flushed, placed, and secured with shunt clamps.

Endarterectomy was started with the freer elevator and the proximal edge divided with Potts scissors. We continued and extracted the plaque and a thrombus from the internal carotid. We proceeded distally and noted good feathering at the distal margin. One 7-0 prolene suture was used to tack the plaque. A Dacron Finess patch was then tailored and we used 6-0 prolene to secure the patch in place. The shunt was removed. The artery deaired and closure completed. The clamps were removed and we checked for hemostasis. Bleeding points were secured with 6-0 prolene. A Blake drain was placed about the stab incision and carried through the skin.

The deep tissues were closed with a running 3-0 Vicryl. The platysma was closed with a running 3-0 Vicryl and the skin was closed with 4-0 Vicryl subcuticular. The patient tolerated the procedure well and was taken to the postanesthesia care unit in good condition.

#326646543 T 09/21/20__
DICTATION # M97623DPL

Franklin Harder, M.D.

DISCHARGE SUMMARY

Patient Name: Tyron J. Sampson **Date:** 9/20/20__

This 53-year-old right-handed gentleman from out of town was admitted through the emergency room with a severe chest pain, headache, confusion, and loss of vision. The patient indicated he was in the emergency room 2 weeks ago for an episode of near blindness. It was recommended at that time that he have an ultrasound, MRI of the brain, and MRA of the neck. He decided to wait and pursue care when he returned home.

Carotid ultrasound performed indicated stenosis of the right carotid. Findings are not typical, therefore, the radiologist suggested an MRI/MRA and angiography which revealed proximal right internal carotid severe (90%) stenosis with small ulceration distal to the stenosis. Right cavernous carotid segment with shallow plaque and only mild stenosis.

Carotid endarterectomy was performed, patient tolerated the procedure well, no complications.

Postop: Patient vitals good, in stable condition. Discharge home under the care of a home health organization. Follow-up 1 week.

Franklin D. Harder, M.D.

HEALTH INFORMATION MANAGEMENT CODING WORKSHEET

STUDENT NAME:		**DATE:**
PATIENT NAME:		**CASE #8:**
DEMOGRAPHICS		
Medical Record Number:	**Bill Type#:**	
Patient Name: Last, First, Middle Init:	Admit Hour Code:	Discharge Hour Code:
	Admit Type Code:	Discharge Status Code:
	Admit Source Code:	Patient Relationship Code:
Condition Code(s)	Occurrence Span Code and Date:	Value Code and Amount:

ADMISSION INFORMATION

Type of Admission: **ER** **Facility** **Physician Referral** **Other** **Unknown**

Admitting Diagnosis		**HIM Code(s)**
Principal Diagnosis (Including complications and co-morbidities if applicable)		**HIM Code**
Other Secondary Diagnosis (Including complications and co-morbidities if applicable)		**HIM Code(s)**
Principal Procedure (Significant procedure performed for definitive treatment or that most closely relates to the principal diagnosis)	**Date:**	**HIM Code(s)**
Other Significant Procedure(s)	**Date:**	**HIM Code(s)**
Medications, supplies, equipment or other item(s)	**Date:**	**HIM Code(s)**

DISCHARGE INFORMATION

Home Facility AMA Deceased Other

DRG ASSIGNMENT		**APC ASSIGNMENT**		
MDC:	Surgical/Medical:			

CONTRIBUTING FACTORS

Age	Sex	Discharge Status	Complications/Comorbidities	Birthweight

Questions/Need Clarification:

CASE 9: HOSPITAL INPATIENT STAY

Summary

Patient Name: Donald Hostenburg **Date:** 12/23/20__

Mr. Hostenburg is a 40-year-old male with severe and persistent pain involving his neck and left upper extremity unresponsive to conservative treatment. MRI Scan showed disc herniation C5-6. Patient admitted for complete cervical diskectomy.

Stephanie Merle, M.D.

Case 9: Hospital Inpatient Stay

Directions

The patient face sheet/charge detail, admission history and physical, operative report, progress notes, and discharge summary are included in this case. Complete this case and prepare a CMS-1450 (UB-04) as follows:

Step 1: Assign revenue codes (see Appendix B) to each category of service listed on the patient face sheet/charge detail.

Submit your patient face sheet/charge detail to your instructor for review.

Step 2: The Coding Worksheet included with this case must be completed before data can be entered on the computer. Complete the Case 9 Coding Worksheet as follows.

a. Record the codes describing the admitting, principal, and other diagnoses.
b. Record the ICD-9-CM Volume III procedure code(s) describing the principal and other significant procedures.
c. Record the code (s) for the items listed below the charge detail.

All other charges listed on the patient face sheet have been coded and posted by other departments.

d. Assign UB data codes (Appendix B) to other information on the Coding Worksheet.

Submit your Coding Worksheet to your instructor for review.

Step 3: Complete a CMS-1450 (UB-04) claim form for this case. Claim forms can be completed manually or utilizing the software. Your instructor will advise if a manual claim is required. Otherwise begin completing the Student Software Case.

Student Software Case 9
Directions:

Use your completed Coding Worksheet and the software program located on Evolve to produce a completed CMS-1450 (UB-04). Follow these instructions to complete Student Software Case 9:

Step 1: The Coding Worksheet should be completed before entering data into the software. Use your completed Coding Worksheet and the patient face sheet/charge detail (after they are reviewed by your instructor) to enter information into the proper fields on the software. Follow the software screen by screen.

Step 2: Once you have completed each screen, preview your completed CMS-1450 (UB-04). Make required corrections before printing.

Step 3: Print your completed claim form and submit to your instructor for review, and keep a copy for your records.

Community General Hospital

Federal Tax ID# 62-1026428 NPI 1234567890

Case 9: Hospital Inpatient Stay—Donald Hostenberg

8192 South Street
Mars, Florida 37373
(747) 722-1800

PATIENT FACE SHEET
AND CHARGE DETAIL

Admit/Discharge Date	Admit/Discharge Hour	Admission Source	Admission Type	Med Record / Soc Sec #	Patient Control #
Admit: 12/23/20__ Disch: 12/25/20__	Admit: 10:52 AM Disch: 11:15 AM	HMO Referral	Urgent	MR# H089016814	30126792

Patient Name	DOB	Release Info	Assignment Ben	Discharge Status	Sex	Marital Status
Donald Hostenburg	01/15/1966	Y	Y	Discharge to home	M	M

Patient Address	City, ST Zip	Phone
1717 Circle Street	Oldsmar, Florida 34677	(813) 962-4443

INSURANCE INFORMATION

Carrier	Insured's Name	Identification# / Group Name and #	Provider #
Primary Carrier State Worker's Comp Ins	Insured's Name Donald Hostenburg	Identification# 127395326 Group Name and # W72943	Provider # 55432722
Secondary Carrier Aetna	Insured's Name Alice Hostenburg	Identification # 462603089 Group Name and # C0695	Provider # 9247243J

Pt Relationship	Employer Name	Employer Location	Treatment Authorization #
Self	Walmarts, Inc	141 17th Street, Oldsmar, Florida 34677	1589820494 Covered days=2
Pt Relationship Spouse	Employer Name City of Oldsmar	Employer Location 1716 South Street, Oldsmar, Florida 34677	Treatment Authorization #

PHYSICIANS/CLINICAL INFORMATION

Attending/Referring/Ordering Physician/ID#	Other Physician/ID #	Occurrence Date	Condition/Value Info
Stephanie Merle, M.D. NPI: 1104724241	Thomas Stromb, M.D. NPI: 1976524129	Accident Employment Related 02/14/20__	1) Employment related 2) Private Room@725.00 No semiprivate rooms available

CHARGE DETAIL

Revenue Code	Service Description	HCPCS/Rates	Service Units	Total Charges	Non-Covered Charges
	ROOM-BOARD/PVT	725.00	2	1450	
	PHARMACY		37	2392	
	IV SOLUTIONS		8	490	
	MED–SUR SUPPLIES		19	5299	
	SUPPLY/IMPLANT		1	808	
	LABORATORY		3	312	
	DX X-RAY		1	1034	
	OR SERVICES		6	7305	
	ANESTHESIA		5	1980	
	RESPIRATORY SVC		1	140	
	RECOVERY ROOM		2	894	
	EKG/ECG		1	137	
	TOTAL CHARGE		86	22,241.00	

OTHER CHARGES TO BE CODED, POSTED, AND ADDED TO CHARGE DETAIL ABOVE

*Four post collar, occipital, mandibular

ADMISSION HISTORY AND PHYSICAL

HISTORY OF PRESENT ILLNESS:
Mr. Hostenburg is admitted today for a cervical diskectomy. He was seen in the office last week for a follow-up on the neck injury he sustained when he fell off a ladder at work in February of this year. After 2 months of physical therapy he was doing relatively well until recently, when he began having pain involving his neck; about 1 month ago, he began having pain radiating to his left upper extremity. His complaints included persistent and severe pain involving his neck and left upper extremity, some numbness involving his left hand, no difficulty with ambulation, no difficulty with bowel or bladder control. MRI scan showed a displaced intervertebral disc C5-6. He is scheduled for surgery in the morning since conventional treatments are not resolving the pain.

ALLERGIES:	**VITALS**				
NONE	**Temp:** 98.9	**Pulse:** 73	**Resp:** 18	**BP:** 132/90	**O2 sats:** Normal

LAST TETANUS: *Not known*	Patient in by (name of person or ambulance) Accompanied by his wife
CURRENT MEDICATIONS: *Reglan 10 mg* *Zantac 150 mg*	Patient Signature – Release record/Assignment of benefits: *Donald Hostenburg* 12/23/20__

Physician Orders:

PREOP ORDERS: ✓ CBC ✓ Chest Xray ✓ EKG Labs: ✓ CBC ✓ Basic Metabolic Panel
ADMIT ORDER: ✓ Private Room Med/Surg Unit ✓ Diet NPO MN ✓ IV D5 .45 NS (1000ml)

PAST MEDICAL HISTORY:

He has had the usual childhood diseases without complications. Operations- Back surgery In 1981, 1985, and 1986. Currently taking Reglan and Zantac for gastroesophageal reflux disease.

PHYSICAL EXAM:

REVIEW OF SYSTEMS: Generally he has been in good health.

PHYSICAL EXAMINATION: This is a well-developed, well-nourished male, with pain involving his neck and left upper extremity. He does appear to be in discomfort.

HEENT: His head is normocephalic.

NECK: Examination of his neck reveals no evidence of paracervical muscle spasm, he has some moderate limitation of neck flexion and extension, secondary to pain, which he localizes in the base of his neck and left shoulder. Spurlings test is positive on the left, negative on the right. Carotid pulsations are symmetrical, there are no carotid bruits.

CHEST: Clear to auscultation.

HEART: Examination reveals a regular rhythm, there are no murmurs heard.

ABDOMEN: Soft, there are no masses felt.

EXTREMITIES: He has good peripheral pulses.

BACK: Examination of his back reveals no evidence of paravertebral muscle spasm, he has some moderate limitation of back flexion and extension, secondary to pain, which he localizes in his lower back, it is non-radicular.

NEUROLOGICAL EXAMINATION: He is alert and oriented, speech and comprehension are normal. Cranial nerve exam is within normal limits. Motor exam–he has some mild weakness of his left biceps. Reflexes are equal and symmetrical, except for diminished left biceps reflex. Sensory exam shows decreased appreciation of sensation to pin prick involving the dorsum of his left hand.

MRI scan of the cervical spine revealed evidence of a herniated disc of C5-C6.

ASSESSMENT:

1. Neck Pain, Radiating to left upper extremity   2. Herniated Cervical Disc of C5-C6

PLAN:

Patient admitted for complete diskectomy C5-C6. Continue administration of current medications Reglan and Zantac as indicated on the orders.

Community General Hospital
Federal Tax ID# 62-1026428
NPI 1234567890

8192 South Street
Mars, Florida 37373
(747) 722-1800

OPERATIVE REPORT

PATIENT NAME:	Donald Hostenburg
MEDICAL RECORD #:	H089016814
DATE OF PROCEDURE:	12/24/20__
SURGEON:	Stephanie Merle, M.D.
ASSISTANT:	Thomas Stromb, M.D.
PREOPERATIVE DIAGNOSIS:	Neck pain radiating to the left upper extremity, persistent and severe. Unresponsive to conservative treatment. Cervical disc herniation at C5-6.
POSTOPERATIVE DIAGNOSIS:	Cervical disc herniation at C5-6.
PROCEDURE:	Complete diskectomy C5-6 with removal of spondylitic bar C5-6 Disc fusion C5-6

PROCEDURE: The patient was brought to the operating where anesthesia was administered. He was then placed in halter traction utilizing 5 pounds traction. Head and neck remained in neutral position. The upper chest and neck were prepped and draped in the routine manner. An incision was made approximately 4 cm in length centered over the C5-6, bleeding controlled utilizing the cautery. The platysma was then split in the direction of its fibers, the anterior border of the sternocleidomastoid was identified. Utilizing blunt dissection, two bundles were developed, the lateral bundle consisting of the sternocleidomastoid muscle, carotid artery and jugular vein. The medial bulb consisting of the esophagus and trachea.

The anterior border of the vertebral body was identified. The C5-6 disc space was identified with the aid of C-arm fluoroscopy. The colli longus muscle was mobilized and retracted the colli longus muscle. The operating microscope was brought in. A diskectomy was performed at C5-6 without difficulty. Extruded disc fragment on the left was removed without difficulty. The cartilaginous ligament was decorticated. A spondylitic bar was removed with a Hall microdrill. Bone plug was cut, shaped, and formed for the fit of the fibular strut graft and placed under fluoroscopy control. An Orion plate was then placed at C5-6 under fluoroscopy control.

The wound was irrigated with saline and Bacitracin solution. Hemostasis was checked with the use of a cautery. Platysma was then closed using interrupted #3-0 Dexon. SubQ was then closed with interrupted #3-0 Dexon. The skin was closed using running subcuticular stitch of #4-0 Dexon. There were no operative complications. Needle and sponge counts were correct. The patient was taken to recovery.

#74253257 T: 12/26/20__
DICTATION # K4625TMG

Stephanie Merle, M.D.

PROGRESS NOTES

Patient Name: Donald Hostenburg

12/23/20__ Admit to surgical unit for cervical diskectomy with fusion. Administered preop meds and Reglan and Zantac.

12/24/20__ Patient tolerated procedure well. No complications. Postoperatively patient resting well, pain level is moderate. Cervical collar applied.

12/25/20__ Patient resting at present. No distress noted. IV and PCA infusing well. Anterior neck dressing is clean and in tact. A four-post C-collar in place. Denies numbness or tingling of extremities, grips strong. Reviewed discharge instructions. Patient discharged to home.

DISCHARGE SUMMARY

Patient Name: Donald Hostenburg

This is a 40-year-old male with severe and persistent pain involving his neck and left upper extremity unresponsive to conservative treatment. MRI scan showed disc herniation C5-6. Admitted on 12/23/20__ for surgery.

He was taken to the OR on 12-24 where the following surgical procedures were performed:
1. Complete diskectomy C5-6.
2. Removal of spondylitic bars C5-6.
3. Cut, shave, and form plug from fibular strut graft.
4. Anterior cervical fusion C5-6 using fibular strut graft and Orion plate under fluoroscopy control.

Following surgery he has done well with significant improvement in his preoperative symptomatology. He has been fitted with a 4-post collar and has been ambulatory. There was minimal neck pain and no arm pain, no numbness, paresthesias, or difficulty with bladder or bowel control. The incision looks good, there is no evidence of infection, he is afebrile.

He is discharged today on 12/25/20__ with discharge instructions regarding care of the incision and on a program of gradually increasing activity. I have given a prescription today for Lortab 10/40 1 q6h prn. Flexeril 10 mg 1 PO tid. He is to call the office to make an appointment to see me in 1 week. If he has any problems prior to that time or any questions he is to call us immediately.

FINAL DIAGNOSIS:
1. Herniated disc C5-6.

Stephanie Merle, M.D.

HEALTH INFORMATION MANAGEMENT CODING WORKSHEET

STUDENT NAME:		**DATE:**
PATIENT NAME:		**CASE #9:**
DEMOGRAPHICS		
Medical Record Number:	**Bill Type#:**	
Patient Name: Last, First, Middle Init:	Admit Hour Code:	Discharge Hour Code:
	Admit Type Code:	Discharge Status Code:
	Admit Source Code:	Patient Relationship Code:
Condition Code(s)	Occurrence Span Code and Date:	Value Code and Amount:

ADMISSION INFORMATION

Type of admission: **ER** **Facility** **Physician Referral** **Other** **Unknown**

Admitting Diagnosis		**HIM Code(s)**
Principal Diagnosis (Including complications and co-morbidities if applicable)		**HIM Code**
Other Secondary Diagnosis (Including complications and co-morbidities if applicable)		**HIM Code(s)**
Principal Procedure (Significant procedure performed for definitive treatment or that most closely relates to the principal diagnosis)	**Date:**	**HIM Code(s)**
Other Significant Procedure(s)	**Date**	**HIM Code(s)**
Medications, supplies, equipment or other item(s)	**Date:**	**HIM Code(s)**

DISCHARGE INFORMATION

Home Facility AMA Deceased Other

DRG ASSIGNMENT		**APC ASSIGNMENT**		
MDC:	Surgical/Medical:			

CONTRIBUTING FACTORS

Age	Sex	Discharge Status	Complications/Comorbidities	Birthweight

Questions/Need Clarification:

CASE 10: HOSPITAL INPATIENT STAY

Summary

Patient Name: Charles M. Santos **Date:** 06/09/20__

Mr. Santos is a 73-year-old male who has history of chronic biliary lithiasis and is noted to have some obstruction of the left intrahepatic biliary system. A percutaneous cholangiogram performed in May demonstrated stenosis of the left hepatic duct in the intrahepatic portion. The patient was diagnosed with cholangiocarcinoma in March of last year. The patient is admitted for a left hepatic lobectomy and common bile duct excision. A cholangiogram was performed on 6/18/20__. The patient was discharged on 6/20/20__.

James J. Wortheyton, M.D.

Case 10: Hospital Inpatient Stay

Directions

The patient face sheet/charge detail; admission history and physical; operative report, radiology report, and discharge summary are included in this Case. Complete this case and prepare a CMS-1450 (UB-04) as follows.

Step 1: Assign revenue codes (see Appendix B) to each category of service listed on the patient face sheet/charge detail.

Submit your patient face sheet/charge detail to your instructor for review.

Step 2: The Coding Worksheet included with this case must be completed before data can be entered on the computer. Complete the Case 10 Coding Worksheet as follows:

a. Record the code(s) describing the admitting, principal, and other diagnoses.
b. Record the ICD-9-CM Volume III procedure code(s) describing the radiology and surgical services.
c. Record the code(s) for the items listed below the charge detail.

All other charges listed on the patient face sheet have been coded and posted by other departments.

d. Assign UB data code options (see Appendix B) to other information on the Coding Worksheet.

Submit your Coding Worksheet to your instructor for review.

Step 3: Complete a CMS-1450 (UB-04) claim form for this case. Claim forms can be completed manually or utilizing the software. Your instructor will advise if a manual claim is required. Otherwise begin completing the Student Software Case.

Student Software Case 10
Directions:

Use your completed Coding Worksheet and the software program located on Evolve to produce a completed CMS-1450 (UB-04). Follow these instructions to complete Student Software Case 10:

Step 1: The Coding Worksheet should be completed before entering data into the software. Use your completed Coding Worksheet and the patient face sheet/charge detail (after they are reviewed by your instructor) to enter information into the proper fields on the software. Follow the software screen by screen.

Step 2: Once you have completed each screen, preview your completed CMS-1450 (UB-04). Make required corrections before printing.

Step 3: Print your completed claim form and submit to your instructor for review, and keep a copy for your records.

Community General Hospital

Federal Tax ID# 62-1026428 NPI 1234567890

Case 10: Hospital Inpatient Laboratory—Charles M. Santos

8192 South Street
Mars, Florida 37373
(747) 722-1800

PATIENT FACE SHEET AND CHARGE DETAIL

Admit/Discharge Date	Admit/Discharge Hour	Admission Source	Admission Type	Med Record / Soc Sec #	Patient Control #
Admit: 06/09/20__ Disch: 06/20/20__	Admit: 11:15 AM Disch: 12:23 PM	Physician Referral	Elective	MR# S006912347	42683144

Patient Name	DOB	Release Info	Assignment Ben	Discharge Status	Sex	Marital Status
Charles M. Santos	12/08/1933	Y	Y	Left Against Medical Advise (AMA)	M	M

Patient Address	City, ST Zip	Phone
72 Apricot Lane	Orlando, Florida 32853	404 724 2391

INSURANCE INFORMATION

Carrier	Insured's Name	Identification# / Group Name and #	Provider #
Primary Carrier Medicare	Insured's Name Charles M. Santos	Identification# 706432721A Group Name and #	Provider # 5720591
Secondary Carrier FLA First (Medigap)	Insured's Name Charles M. Santos	Identification # 5442374132 Group Name and # 3427605	Provider #

Pt Relationship	Employer Name	Employer Location	Treatment Authorization #
Self	Retired		AZ43259667 Covered days = 11
Pt Relationship	Employer Name	Employer Location	Treatment Authorization #

PHYSICIANS/CLINICAL INFORMATION

Attending/Referring/Ordering Physician/ID#	Other Physician/ID #	Occurrence Date	Condition/Value Info
James J. Wortheyton, M.D. NPI: 1697255462	William Tatterburg, M.D. NPI: 1892434321		Semi-Private Room@510.00

CHARGE DETAIL

Revenue Code	Service Description	HCPCS/Rates	Service Units	Total Charges	Non -Covered Charges
	MED-SUR-GY-2BED	510.00	11	5610	
	PHARMACY		216	6632.78	
	MED-SUR SUPPLIES		238	5331.6	
	LABORATORY		107	2522.67	
	PATHOL/BIOPSY		11	789.01	
	DX X-RAY		9	523	
	OR SERVICES		504	8540	
	ANESTHESIA		40	2277	
	RESPIRATORY SVC		72	1187	
	PHYSICAL THERP		8	516	
	PULMONARY FUNC		5	90	
	RECOVERY ROOM		7	2653	
	EKG/ECG		3	141	
	TOTAL CHARGE		1231	$36813.06	

OTHER CHARGES TO BE CODED, POSTED, AND ADDED TO CHARGE DETAIL ABOVE
NONE

ADMISSION HISTORY AND PHYSICAL

Patient Name: Charles M. Santos

HISTORY OF PRESENT ILLNESS:
A 73-year-old white male with cholangiocarcinoma, intermediate cardiovascular risk, and moderate risk of pulmonary complications postoperatively admitted for a left hepatic lobectomy.

The patient's biliary symptoms date back 5 years, at which time he had choledocholithiasis and subsequently had an open cholecystectomy. He was asymptomatic until about 2 years ago when he had jaundice and abdominal pain. Endoscopic retrograde cholangiopancreatography with placement of a stent along with a biliary drain was performed at that time. However, he still experienced periodic jaundice requiring restenting times three, the most recent in December of last year.

He has had increasing epigastric pain, most prevalent after eating and at night. Prior to this admission, cardiology and pulmonology consults were obtained for perioperative risk classification. CT of the abdomen revealed no dominant masses and a left hepatic duct that was obstructed with left lobar atrophy. The right lobe was within normal limits. There were no enlarged lymph nodes. An angiogram was performed which revealed no vascular encasement and the portal vessels were patent. The left hepatic artery was noted to fill by the gastroduodenal artery.

Pulmonary consultation indicates the patient at a moderate risk of pulmonary complications due to his chronic obstructive pulmonary disease. They recommended optimizing his pulmonary medications prior to surgery. Cardiology consultation concluded that the patient had an intermediate risk of perioperative complications secondary to the patient's atrial fibrillation and coronary artery disease of a native artery, which required percutaneous transluminal coronary angioplasty in October 2005. They recommended postoperative electrocardiogram assessment, low dose Lopressor, and fasting lipid profile to evaluate his further cardiac risks.

ALLERGIES:	**Vitals**				
No allergies	**Temp:** 97.9	**Pulse:** 100–110	**Resp:** 12–13	**BP:** 100/60	**O2 sats:** Normal

Patient in by (name of person or ambulance)	Patient Signature – Release record/Assignment of benefits:
Wife brought paitent in	Charles M. Santos 06/09/20__

CURRENT MEDICATIONS:

K-Dur 20 mEq p.o. q.d. Dyazide 40 mg p.o. q.d.	Furosemide 40 mg p.o. q.d. Lisinopril 20 mg p.o. q.d.	Aerobid MDI 2 puffs b.i.d. Combivent MDI 2 puffs bi.d.

PHYSICIAN ORDERS:
✓ LABS ✓ Electrocardiogram ✓ NPO midnight ✓ IV Fluids midnight ✓ Pulmonary meds to be administered ✓ D/C'd coumadin 1 week

PAST MEDICAL HISTORY:

Atrial fibrillation, which he has had for years, treated with Coumadin and Cardizem. Note he has been off Coumadin for the past week. Coronary artery disease status post percutaneous transluminal coronary angioplasty in October 2005. Chronic obstructive pulmonary disease for 28 years, associated with his long standing tobacco abuse and malignant hypertension.

The patient underwent subtotal gastrectomy for peptic ulcer disease in 1958. He had an open cholecystectomy performed last year. He has had biliary stents placed and biliary drains placed, as well. The last biliary drain was changed out in May of this year. A percutaneous cholangiogram performed in May demonstrated stenosis of the left hepatic duct in the intrahepatic portion.

(*Continued*)

ADMISSION HISTORY AND PHYSICAL—*cont'd*
PHYSICAL EXAM:
REVIEW OF SYSTEMS: He has had some weight loss, shortness of breath which is increased in the morning. No chest pain and no recent nausea and vomiting. The patient denies jaundice, stool is without bile, dark urine, hematuria, dysuria, melena, or bright red blood per rectum. GENERAL: The patient is awake, alert and appropriate, oriented times three, in no acute distress. HEENT: Normocephalic, atraumatic, pupils are equal, round, and reactive to light, sclerae nonicteric, extraocular movements intact. Oropharynx clear. No icterus sublingually. Moist mucous membranes. NECK: Supple, no lymphadenopathy, no carotid bruits. PULMONARY: Clear to auscultation bilaterally. No wheezes, however, a prolonged expiratory phase. HEART: Irregular heart beat, rate is controlled. ABDOMEN: Right subcostal scar, nondistended, minimally tender in the epigastrium, no tenderness in the right upper quadrant, he has good bowel sounds. His abdomen is soft. EXTREMITIES: No clubbing, cyanosis and edema. 2 + peripheral pulses. Extremities are warm and dry. NEUROLOGICAL: Grossly intact, non-focal. LABORATORY DATA: Labs are pending. Electrocardiogram is pending. The preoperative evaluation is complete.
ASSESSMENT/PLAN: Admission to general surgery service for preoperative preparation for a left hepatic lobectomy. He will be n.p.o. with intravenous fluids after midnight. He will be given his pulmonary medications to optimize his pulmonary status preoperatively. His Coumadin was held 1 week prior to this admission.

Community General Hospital
Federal Tax ID# 62-1026428
NPI 1234567890

8192 South Street
Mars, Florida 37373
(747) 722-1800

OPERATIVE REPORT

PATIENT NAME:	Charles M. Santos	MEDICAL RECORD#:	S006912347
DATE OF PROCEDURE:	06/10/20__	SURGEON:	James Wortheyton, M.D.
ASSISTANT:	William Tatterburg, M.D.	ANESTHESIA:	General Endotracheal
PREOPERATIVE DIAGNOSIS:	Obstruction of the left intrahepatic biliary system		
POSTOPERATIVE DIAGNOSIS:	Cholangiocarcinoma		
PROCEDURE:	Left Hepatic lobectomy		

INDICATIONS FOR SURGERY: Mr. Santos is a 73-year-old male with a history of chronic biliary lithiasis who was noted to have some obstruction of the left intrahepatic biliary system. A percutaneous cholangiogram demonstrated stenosis of the left hepatic duct in the intrahepatic portion. The presumptive diagnosis of cholangiocarcinoma was made.

TECHNICAL PROCEDURES USED: Patient was placed on the OR table in supine position. Pressure points were padded. ASA monitoring devices were in place, sequential compression devices were placed on both lower extremities. Inhalational IV anesthesia was delivered and the patient intubated under controlled conditions.

The abdomen was sterilely prepped and draped in the usual fashion for a procedure of this sort. Bilateral subcostal incision was made through the skin using the cold knife and carried through subcutaneous tissue using Bovie cautery device. The incision was made through his previous subcostal incisions for previous cholecystectomy and antrectomy. Incision was carried through the anterior abdominal wall in layers. The peritoneal cavity was entered in the area that had not had previous operation. There were adhesions of the omentum to the underside of the anterior abdominal wall where the previous incision had been closed. These were taken down using Bovie cautery device. Adhesions of the omentum and transverse mesocolon to the edge of the liver and stomach were taken down using Bovie cautery and sharp dissection.

We then ran the small bowel from the ligament of Treitz up to the ileocecal valve and the colon from the ileocecal valve to the rectum. There were no identifiable masses. There was no lymphadenopathy. Next, adhesions were taken down from the porta hepatis. We identified the hepatic artery and pleural vein. Control was made of both of these with vessel loops. Next, the left hepatic triannular ligament was taken down using Bovie cautery. The left hepatic lobe was then fully mobilized. We then continued the dissection along the cardiac portion of the diaphragm, taking down the broad ligament at that point. The left, right, and middle hepatic veins were identified. Control was gained with the left and middle hepatic vein using vessel loops. Once vascular control was achieved, we identified the biliary ducts; the bile duct was quite large and ectatic. I then gained control of the left hepatic duct. The left hepatic duct was then divided. The proximal end was suture ligated and the segment of the distal end was sent for frozen section. This was read to be free of any malignancy. The distal end was oversewn using running #4-0 Prolene suture.

We then divided the left hepatic artery and left portal vein and suture ligated the ends. Next we turned attention to outflow. The left and middle hepatic veins were clamped with C-clamps and divided with a significantly long stump. The hepatic ends of the veins were suture ligated; the distal ends of the veins were oversewn with a running #4-0 Prolene suture. C-clamps were removed. We then rotated the left hepatic lobe to the right side of the body. Small venous attachments to the cava were taken down, divided between clamps, and suture ligated. Once the left hepatic lobe was freed from the cava we began combination of Bovie cautery and finger fracture to divide the right lobe from the left lobe. Larger vessels and bile ducts were controlled and suture ligated before being divided. This was continued throughout the liver.

Once the liver had been divided the specimen was passed off the field. Bleeding from the raw surface of the liver was then controlled using the Argon beam coagulator. Bleeding from the liver edge, and leaks from any major vessels or any bile ducts were controlled by suture ligating with #3-0 silk stick tie. Surgicel was placed on the raw surface of the liver and effectively welded to the raw surface of the liver using the argon beam coagulator. A 10-mm JP drain was then placed along the raw surface of the liver and brought out through a separate stab incision. A second 10-JP was placed underneath the porta hepatis and brought out through a separate stab incision in the right flank.

The abdominal cavity was copiously irrigated and the effluent was suctioned dry. The fascial layer was closed en masse with a running #1 loop PDS. Skin was closed with staples. Sterile dressings were place on the wound. The drains were held in place with #2-0 silk drain stitches. Sterile dressings were applied to the wound. There were no complications. Counts correct times-two. Patient was then taken to the 5E ICU in good and stable condition, but intubated. Plan will be to extubate him in the morning.

SPECIMENS REMOVED: 1. Left hepatic lobe. 2. Distal hepatic duct margin.

James J. Wortheyton, M.D.

DICTATION # K4625TMG
BY: cam-112392 06/16/20__ 1:43 PM

Community General Hospital
Federal Tax ID# 62-1026428
NPI 1234567890

8192 South Street
Mars, Florida 37373
(747) 722-1800

RADIOLOGY REPORT

PATIENT NAME:	Charles M. Santos	MEDICAL RECORD#:	S006912347
DOB:	12/08/1933	EXAM DATE:	06/18/20__
ATTENDING M.D.:	James Wortheyton, M.D.	RADIOLOGY #:	76932457
ORDERING M.D.:	James Wortheyton, M.D.		
INDICATIONS:	Left intrahepatic hepatic duct cholangiocarcinoma		

EXAM: T-TUBE CHOLANGIOGRAM

PROCEDURE: A cholangiogram was performed through the patient's existing transhepatic biliary drain using Hypaque contrast. Fluoroscopic spot and overhead films were obtained. Comparison is made to a previous study.

FINDINGS: Scout image of the right upper quadrant demonstrates mottled air overlies the right upper quadrant. A biliary drain, Davol drain, and surgical clips are identified. The visualized intrahepatic bile ducts have normal caliber and arborization. The loop end of the biliary drain lies within the extrahepatic biliary duct, this is a change from the previous study where the loop appears to lie within small bowel. The intrahepatic biliary duct is somewhat dilated and irregular where the Davol drain lies. The 20-minute postdrainage film demonstrates normal bile duct emptying. A small amount of contrast refluxes into the stomach.

IMPRESSION:
1. Transhepatic biliary drain with Cope loop present within the extrahepatic bile duct; this is a change from the previous study in May, at which time the loop was present within small bowel.
2. Moderate extrahepatic biliary duct dilatation and irregularity, unchanged.
3. No evidence of extravasation or obstruction. T-TUBE CHOLANGIOGRAM

James J. Wortheyton, M.D.

DISCHARGE SUMMARY

Patient Name: Charles M. Santos **Date:** 6/20/20__

REASON FOR ADMISSION: Mr. Santos is a 73-year-old male who was diagnosed with cholangiocarcinoma in March of last year. He was noted to have some obstruction of the left intrahepatic biliary system. A cholangiogram performed in May demonstrated stenosis of the left hepatic duct in the intrahepatic portion. He is now admitted for left hepatic lobectomy and common bile duct excision. He was cleared by both pulmonary and cardiology services prior to his operation. He had a moderate risk of pulmonary complications secondary to intermediate cardiovascular risk perioperatively due to his COPD and CAD.

HOSPITAL COURSE: The patient was admitted to the general surgery service. The patient was taken to the operating room on 6/10/200_ where a left hepatic lobectomy with common bile duct excision was performed. His estimated blood loss was 1.5 liters. His replacement was 7 liters of crystalloid, 1 liter of Hespan, and three units of packed cells. Postoperatively, the patient was in stable condition. Surgical pathology revealed: 1. Liver, Left Lobe, Biopsy: Adenocarcinoma, consistent with Cholangiocarcinoma 2. Hepatic duct, excision: Negative for carcinoma

Labs on postoperative day number two within normal limits. The patient was hemodynamically stable. His lungs had occasional expiratory wheezes, otherwise he had good air movement. He was cardiovascularly stable. He was tolerating sips of clears on postoperative day number 3 and in stable condition. Postoperative days 4 through 10 he was given physical therapy to help mobilize and ambulate. He was given respiratory therapy to maximize his pulmonary status. His diet was advanced to a regular diet by postoperative day number 5. The patient had a T-tube cholangiogram 2 days ago which revealed good filling of the biliary tree and small bowel without any leak. His final Jackson-Pratt drain was then pulled. The patient continued to do well. His wound was intact and clean with no infection. He had good bowel sounds and was tolerating a regular diet, passing gas, and having bowel movements. Prior to discharge his lab results were better but not within normal limits. Patient was advised to remain in the hospital for one more day but declined.

DISCHARGE INSTRUCTIONS: Patient was discharged against medical advise. Schedule follow-up in 5 days. His diet was regular, activity was ad lib with no heavy lifting or straining. He was to flush his biliary drain catheter with 5 cc of sterile normal saline three times a day. He is to pack the wounds with wet to dry normal saline and gauze b.i.d. He is to take Augmentin times 5 more days. He has prescriptions for Percocet for pain and Prevacid. He was placed on a prednisone taper. He is to resume his Coumadin this week.

James J. Wortheyton, M.D.

HEALTH INFORMATION MANAGEMENT CODING WORKSHEET

STUDENT NAME:			**DATE:**
PATIENT NAME:			**CASE #10:**
DEMOGRAPHICS			
Medical Record Number:		**Bill Type#:**	
Patient Name: Last, First, Middle Init:	Admit Hour Code:		Discharge Hour Code:
	Admit Type Code:		Discharge Status Code:
	Admit Source Code:		Patient Relationship Code:
Condition Code(s)	Occurrence Span Code and Date:		Value Code and Amount:
Relationship to Insured Code:			
ADMISSION INFORMATION			
Type of admission: **ER** **Facility** **Physician Referral** **Other** **Unknown**			

Admitting Diagnosis		**HIM Code(s)**
Principal Diagnosis (Including complications and co-morbidities if applicable)		**HIM Code**
Other Secondary Diagnosis (Including complications and co-morbidities if applicable)		**HIM Code(s)**
Principal Procedure (Significant procedure performed for definitive treatment or that most closely relates to the principal diagnosis)	**Date**	**HIM Code**
Procedure(s)	**Date:**	**HIM Code(s)**
Medications, supplies, equipment or other item(s)	**Date:**	**HIM Code(s)**

DISCHARGE INFORMATION				
Home	Facility	AMA	Deceased	Other

DRG ASSIGNMENT		**APC ASSIGNMENT**		
MDC:	Surgical/Medical:			

CONTRIBUTING FACTORS				
Age	Sex	Discharge Status	Complications/Comorbidities	Birthweight

Questions/Need Clarification:

Appendix B

Claim Form Data

CONTENTS

SECTION I: CMS-1450 (UB-04) COMPLETION INSTRUCTIONS FOR PAPER CLAIMS

Form Locator (FL) #/Line #	DESCRIPTION (Numbers/Letters in each FL description designate the line/field where information is recorded)
1 (1–4)	**Billing Provider Name, Address, Phone.** Line 1) PROVIDER NAME; 2) STREET ADDRESS; 3) CITY, STATE, ZIP CODE; 4) AREA CODE AND TELEPHONE NUMBER; AREA CODE AND FAX NUMBER; AND COUNTRY CODE: *(US for United States)*
2 (1–4)	**Provider's Pay to Name and Address** if different from provider in FL 1.*Three lines:* 1) PAY TO NAME; 2) STREET ADDRESS; 3) CITY, STATE, ZIP (if different from FL 1); 4) Reserved.
3 (A-B)	**Patient Control Number (PCN)/Medical/Health Record Number (MRN/HRN).** 3A) PCN that is assigned by facility to identify the patient account for the claim. 3B) MRN/HCN that is assigned to the patient's medical or health record by the facility.
4	**Type of Bill.** Four-digit code with leading number "0" and three additional digits to identify the type of facility, type of care, and frequency of the bill.
5	**Federal Tax ID Number (TIN) or Employer ID Number (EIN).** A number assigned by the federal government to the provider for tax reporting purposes. Displayed as XX-XXXXXXX.
6	**Statement Covers Period.** Date services began and ended. Displayed as MMDDYY.
7	**Reserved for assignment by the National Uniform Billing Committee (NUBC).**
8 (A-B)	**Patient Name/Identifier.** 8A) PATIENT IDENTIFIER (if different from the insured ID in FL 60). 8B) PATIENT NAME (last, first, middle initial).
9 (A-E)	**Patient Address.** 9A) PATIENT STREET ADDRESS; 9B) CITY; 9C) STATE; 9D) ZIP; 9E) COUNTRY CODE (US for United States). Enter patient's full mailing address (should be permanent address), including street number or PO box.
10	**Patient Birth Date.** Displayed as MMDDCCYY. If unknown, enter all zeros.
11	**Patient Sex.** A single character that represents PATIENT'S sex as recorded at the time of admission, outpatient service, or start of care. M-Male, F-Female, U-Unknown.
12	**Admission/Start of Care Date.** Enter the date of the hospital visit or inpatient admission. Displayed as MMDDYY.
13	**Admission Hour.** Enter two-digit hour code that represents the hour of admission for inpatient care.
14	**Priority/Type of Admission Visit.** Enter a one-digit code indicating the priority of the admission/visit. 1-Emergency, 2-Urgent, 3-Elective, 4-Newborn, 5-Trauma, 6–8 Reserved, 9-Information not available.
15	**Point of Origin for Admission or Visit.** Enter a one-digit alphanumeric code to explain the source or referral for the admission/visit. Below are some common sources of referral (not inclusive). 1-Non-Health Care facility, 2-Clinic, 3-Reserved, 4-Transfer from a hospital (different facility), 5-Transfer from a skilled nursing facility (SNF), 6-Transfer from other health care facility, 7-Emergency Department/Room (ED/ER), 8-Court/law enforcement, 9-Information not available.
16	**Discharge Hour.** Enter a two-digit code indicating the hour the patient is discharged from inpatient care.
17	**Patient Discharge Status.** Enter a two-digit code that explains the patient status at the time of discharge/ end of service period reported in FL 6. 01-Discharge home, 02-Discharged/transferred to short-term general hospital, 03-Discharged/transferred to skilled nursing facility (SNF), 04-Discharged/transferred to an intermediate care facility (ICF).
18–28	**Condition Code(s).** Enter two-digit alphanumeric condition code(s) to describe conditions or events relating to the claim when they may have an affect on processing. *Refer to Section II: Data Code Options in Appendix B.*
29	**Accident State.** Enter a two-digit state abbreviation explaining where the accident occurred, when applicable.
30	**Reserved for assignment by the NUBC**

Form Locator (FL) #/Line #	DESCRIPTION (Numbers/Letters in each FL description designate the line/field where information is recorded)
31–34 (A-B)	**Occurrence Codes and Dates**. Enter two-digit code(s) and date(s) to explain an event that happened associated with the claim that may affect payer processing. The date is displayed as MMDDYY. *Refer to Section II: Data Code Options in Appendix B.*
35–36 (A-B)	**Occurrence Span Codes and Dates**. Enter two-digit code(s) and date(s) to identify an event that relates to payment of the claim. The date is displayed as MMDDYY. *Refer to Section II: Data Code Options in Appendix B.*
37	**Reserved for assignment by the NUBC.**
38 (1–5)	**Responsible Party**. NAME AND ADDRESS OF PARTY RESPONSIBLE FOR THE BILL. Line 1) First, middle, last name. 2) Street address. 3) City, state, zip.
39–41 (A-B)	**Value Codes and Amounts**. Enter a two-digit code to describe data necessary for claim processing as required by the payer. 01-Most common semiprivate room rate, 02-Hospital has no semiprivate rooms, 05-Professional component. *Refer to Section II: Data Code Options in Appendix B.*
42 (1–23)	**Revenue Code**. Enter four-digit code "0250" used to identify categories of items and services. The leading digit is "0". Revenue code 0001–Total Charge is entered on line 23. *Refer to Section III Revenue Code Listing in Appendix B.*
43 (1–23)	**Revenue Code Description**. Enter the standard abbreviated description for each revenue code. Line 23–enter the page numbers for the claim. *Refer to Section III: Revenue Code Listing in Appendix B for revenue code standard abbreviated descriptions.*
44 (1–22)	**Health Care Common Procedure Coding System (HCPCS)/Accommodation Rates/Health Insurance Prospective Payment System (HIPPS) Rate Codes**. 1) Enter the HCPCS Level I or Level II code, modifier, and rate; accommodation rate for inpatient claims; and the HIPPS rate code. Dollar amount is displayed as 750.50.
45 (1–23)	**Service Date**. Enter the date service is provided for outpatient claims only. The date is displayed as MMDDYY. Line 23–enter the date the claim was created. The date is displayed as MMDDYY.
46 (1–22)	**Units of Service**. Enter the total number of units for the revenue code category, such as the number of days of accommodations, pints of blood, x-ray procedures, or laboratory procedures.
47 (1–23)	**Total Charges**. Enter the total charges (covered and noncovered services) for the revenue code category. Line 23–enter the total charges for the claim.
48 (1–23)	**Noncovered Charges**. Enter the total of noncovered charges for the revenue code category. Line 23–enter the total of noncovered charges for the claim.
49	**Reserved for assignment by the NUBC.**
50–65	**Enter information in 50–65 (A-C) pertaining to related health plan (Payer).** Line A–Primary payer, Line B–Secondary Payer, Line C–Tertiary (third) payer.
50 (A-C)	**Payer Name**. Enter name of the health plan. Line A–Primary payer, Line B–Secondary Payer, Line C–Tertiary payer.
51 (A-C)	**Health Plan Identification Number (HIN)**. Enter the health plan ID number.
52 (A-C)	**Release of Information Certification Indicator**. Enter a single letter that indicates whether there is a signed release of information statement on file. I-Informed consent not obtained. Y-signed statement on file.
53 (A-C)	**Assignment of Benefits Certification Indicator.** Enter the letter that indicates that the provider has a signed assignment of benefits form on file. N-No, W-Not applicable (when patient refuses to assign benefits), and Y-Yes.
54 (A-C)	**Prior Payments From Payer**. Enter the amount collected (to date) from the health plan for this claim.
55 (A-C)	**Estimated Amount Due From Payer**. Enter the estimated amount due from the health plan (estimated responsibility less any prior payments).

Form Locator (FL) #/Line #	DESCRIPTION (Numbers/Letters in each FL description designate the line/field where information is recorded)
56 (A-C)	**National Provider Identifier (NPI)**. Enter the NPI for the provider submitting the claim.
57 (A-C)	**Other (Billing) Provider Identifier.** Enter the NPI for the other provider.
58 (A-C)	**Insured's Name**. Enter the name of the individual who carries the insurance. Record last and first names. Use a space to separate last and first names. The name recorded should match the name on the insurance card, such as Evelyn Brown or Thomas James III. Displayed as Brown Evelyn; James III Thomas.
59 (A-C)	**Patient's Relationship to Insured**. Enter two-digit code that indicates the relationship. 01-Spouse *(Patient is the spouse of insured)*, 18-Self *(Patient is the insured)*, 19-Child; 20-Employee; 21-Unknown.
60 (A-C)	**Insured's Unique Identifier**. Enter the unique number assigned to the insured by the payer.
61 (A-C)	**Insured's Group Name.** Enter the group or plan name found on the insurance card.
62 (A-C)	**Insured's Group Number.** Enter the group number found on the insurance card.
63 (A-C)	**Treatment Authorization Code**. Enter the number provided when preauthorization is obtained from the payer.
64 (A-C)	**Document Control Number (DCN).** Enter the internal control number assigned to the claim by the payer.
65 (A-C)	**Employer Name of the Insured.** Enter the insured's employer name when coverage is provided by the employer.
66	**Diagnosis and Procedure Code Qualifier (*International Classification of Diseases* [ICD], Version Indicator)**. Enter the digit that represents the version of ICD. 9-Ninth Revision, 0-Tenth Revision.
67	**Principal Diagnosis Code and Present on Admission (POA) Indicator**. Enter the ICD code that describes the principal diagnosis (the condition determined after study to be chiefly responsible for the admission). Do not enter a period between the third and fourth digits. **POA indicator.** Enter a single letter that indicates the condition was present at the time of admission, including those clearly present but not diagnosed until after admission. Y-The condition was present at the time of admission, N-Not present at time of admission, U-Documentation insufficient to determine presence; no information in the record, W-Clinically undetermined. *Example:* 530 81 Y
67 (A-Q)	**Other Diagnosis Codes.** Enter the ICD code(s) for conditions that coexist at the time of admission or developed subsequently that were treated or had an effect on treatment or length of stay. Do not enter a period between the third and fourth digits. **POA indicator**. Enter a single letter that indicates the condition was present at the time of admission.
68	**Reserved for assignment by the NUBC.**
69	**Admitting Diagnosis Code.** Enter the ICD code(s) that describes the patient's diagnosis at the time of inpatient admission.
70 (A-C)	**Patient Reason for Visit**. Enter the ICD code(s) that describe the patient's condition at the time of outpatient registration.
71	**Prospective Payment System (PPS) Code.** Enter the PPS MS-DRG code assigned to the inpatient admission.
72 (A-C)	**External Cause of Injury (ECI) Code.** Enter the ICD code(s) that describes the external cause of injury.
73	**Reserved for assignment by the NUBC.**

Form Locator (FL) #/Line #	DESCRIPTION (Numbers/Letters in each FL description designate the line/field where information is recorded)
74	**Principal Procedure Code and Date.** Enter the ICD VOL III procedure code for the significant procedure performed for definitive treatment of the principal diagnosis or the procedure that closely relates to the principal diagnosis and the date the procedure was performed. **EXAMPLE:** 00 66 The date is displayed as MMDDYY.
74 (A-E)	**Other Procedure Codes and Dates.** Enter the ICD Volume III procedure code(s) for all significant procedures *(other than the principal procedure)* performed during the stay and the date they were performed, displayed as MMDDYY.
75	**Reserved for assignment by the NUBC.**
76 (1–2)	**Attending Provider Name and Identifiers.** Line 1) Enter the national provider identifier (NPI) of the attending physician. Line 2) Enter the attending physician name (last, first, middle). Some payers may still require the secondary identifier. Secondary identifier qualifiers: OB-State license number, 1G-Unique provider identification number (UPIN), G2-Provider commercial number.
77 (1–2)	**Operating Physician Name and Identifiers.** Line 1) Enter the national provider identifier (NPI) of the operating physician. Line 2) Enter the operating physician name (last, first, middle). Some payers may still require the secondary identifier. Secondary identifier qualifiers: OB-State license number, 1G-Unique provider identification number (UPIN), G2-Provider commercial number.
78–79 (1–2)	**Other Provider Names and Identifiers.** Line 1) Enter the national provider identifier (NPI) and provider type qualifier. Provider type qualifier: DN-Referring provider, ZZ-Other operating physician, 82-Rendering provider. Line 2) Enter name of other physician (last, first, middle initial). Some payers may still require the secondary identifier. Secondary identifier qualifiers: OB-State license number; 1G-Unique provider identification number (UPIN), G2-Provider commercial number.

SECTION II: CMS-1450 (UB-04) DATA CODE OPTIONS

FL 4: Types of Bill Codes

Listed below are some of the most common types of bill codes. This is not an all-inclusive list.

Bill Type and Description		IP/OP
0000–010x	Reserved for Assignment by NUBC	—
011x	Hospital Inpatient (Including Medicare Part A)	IP
012x	Hospital Inpatient (Medicare Part B only)	OP
013x	Hospital Outpatient	OP
014x	Hospital—Laboratory Services Provided to Non-patients	OP
018x	Hospital—Swing Beds	IP
021x	Skilled Nursing—Inpatient (Medicare Part A)	IP
022x	Skilled Nursing—Inpatient (Medicare Part B)	OP
023x	Skilled Nursing—Outpatient	OP
028x	Skilled Nursing—Swing Beds	IP
032x	Home Health—Inpatient (Part B only)	OP
033x	Home Health—Outpatient (Plan of treatment under Part A, DME Part A)	OP
034x	Home Health—Other (for medical and surgical services not under a plan of treatment)	OP
041x	Religious Non-medical Health Care Institutions—Hospital Inpatient	IP
043x	Religious Non-medical Health Care Institutions—Outpatient Services	OP
065x	Intermediate Care—Level I	IP
066x	Intermediate Care—Level II	IP
071x	Clinic—Rural Health	OP
072x	Clinic—Hospital Based or Independent Renal Dialysis Center	OP
073x	Clinic—Freestanding	OP
074x	Clinic—Outpatient Rehabilitation Facility (ORF)	OP
075x	Clinic—Comprehensive Outpatient Rehabilitation Facility (CORF)	OP
076x	Clinic—Community Mental Health Center	OP
077x	Clinic—Federally Qualified Health Center (FQHC)	OP
079x	Clinic—Other	OP
081x	Special Facility—Hospice (non-hospital based)	OP
082x	Special Facility—Hospice (hospital based)	OP
083x	Special Facility—Ambulatory Surgery Center	OP
084x	Special Facility—Freestanding Birthing Center	IP
085x	Special Facility—Critical Access Hospital	OP
086x	Special Facility—Residential Facility	IP
089x	Special Facility—Other	IP *or* OP

Reserved for Assignment by NUBC (015x-017x, 019x-020x, 024x-027x, 029x-031x, 035x-040x, 042x, 044x-064x).

FL 4: Types of Bill Frequency Codes (attach this digit to the type of bill code in place of the "X").

Listed below are some of the most common bill frequency codes. This is not an all-inclusive list.

Fourth-Digit Options

0-Non-payment/zero claim
1-Admit through discharge claim
2-Interim: First claim
3-Interim: Continuing claim
4-Interim: Last claim
5-Late charge only
6-Replacement of prior claim
7-Void/cancel of a prior claim
8-Final claim for home health PPS episode

FL 11: Patient Sex

Code	Description
M	Male
F	Female
U	Unknown

FL 13 and 16 Hour Codes

CODE	AM (MIDNIGHT)	CODE	PM (NOON)
00	12:00–12:59	12	12:00–12:59
01	01:00–01:59	13	01:00–01:59
02	02:00–02:59	14	02:00–02:59
03	03:00–03:59	15	03:00–03:59
04	04:00–04:59	16	04:00–04:59
05	05:00–05:59	17	05:00–05:59
06	06:00–06:59	18	06:00–06:59
07	07:00–07:59	19	07:00–07:59
08	08:00–08:59	20	08:00–08:59
09	09:00–09:59	21	09:00–09:59
10	10:00–10:59	22	10:00–10:59
11	11:00–11:59	23	11:00–11:59

FL 14: Priority (Type) of Visit

1-Emergency
2-Urgent
3-Elective
4-Newborn
5-Trauma center
6–8-Reserved for assignment by the NUBC
9-Information not available

FL 15: Source of Admission Codes

1-Non–health care facility point of origin
2-Clinic
3-Reserved for assignment by the NUBC
4-Transfer from hospital (different facility)

5-Transfer from skilled nursing facility (SNF) or intermediate care facility (ICF)
6-Transfer from another health care facility
7-Emergency room
8-Court/law enforcement
9-Information not available
A-Reserved for assignment by the NUBC
B-Transfer from another home health agency (HHA)
C-Readmission to same home health agency (HHA)
D-Transfer from one distinct unit of the hospital to another distinct unit of the same hospital, resulting in a separate claim to the payer
E-Transfer from ambulatory surgery center
F-Transfer from Hospice and is under a hospice plan of care or enrolled in a hospice program
G–Z-Reserved for assignment by the NUBC

Code Structure for Newborn

1–4-Reserved for assignment by the NUBC
5-Born inside this hospital
6-Born outside this hospital
7–9-Reserved for assignment by the NUBC

FL 17: Patient Discharge Status Codes

Code	Description	Code	Description
01	Discharged to home or self-care (routine discharge)	42	Expired; place unknown
02	Discharged/transferred to another short-term general hospital for inpatient care	43	Discharged/transferred to a federal health care facility
03	Discharged/transferred to a skilled nursing facility (SNF) with Medicare certification of anticipation of skilled care	44–49	Reserved for assignment by the NUBC
04	Discharged/transferred to an intermediate care facility (ICF)	50	Discharged to hospice-home
05	Discharged/transferred to designated cancer center or children's hospital	51	Discharged to hospice; medical facility (certified) providing hospice level of care
06	Discharged/transferred to home under care of organized home health service organization in anticipation of covered skilled care	52–60	Reserved for assignment by the NUBC
07	Left against medical advice (AMA) or discontinued care	61	Discharged/transferred to a hospital-based Medicare-approved swing bed
08	Reserved for assignment by the NUBC	62	Discharged/transferred to an inpatient rehabilitation facility (IRF) including Rehabilitation Distinct Part Unit of a Hospital
09	Admitted as an inpatient to this hospital	63	Discharged/transferred to a Medicare-certified long-term care hospital (LTCH)
10-19	Reserved for assignment by the NUBC	64	Discharged/transferred to a nursing facility certified under Medicaid but not certified under Medicare
20	Expired	65	Discharged/transferred to a psychiatric hospital or Psychiatric Distinct Part Unit of a Hospital
21–29	Reserved for assignment by the NUBC	66	Discharged/transferred to a critical access hospital (CAH)
30	Still patient	67–69	Reserved for assignment by the NUBC
31–39	Reserved for assignment by the NUBC	70	Discharged/transferred to another type of health care institution not defined elsewhere in this code list
40	Expired at home (Medicare and TRICARE hospice claims only)	71–99	Reserved for assignment by the NUBC
41	Expired in a medical facility, such as a hospital, SNF, ICF, or freestanding hospice (Medicare and TRICARE hospice claims only)		

FL 18 to 28: Condition Codes

Code **Description**
01-Military service related
02-Condition is employment related
03-Patient covered by insurance not reflected here
04-Information-only bill
05-Lien has been filed
06-End-stage renal disease (ESRD) patient in the first 30 months of coverage by employer group health plan
07-Treatment of non-terminal condition for hospice patient
08-Beneficiary would not provide information concerning other insurance coverage
09-Neither patient nor spouse is employed
10-Patient and/or spouse is employed but no employer group health plan (EGHP) exists

FL 31 to 34 (A-B): Occurrence Codes and Dates

This is not an all-inclusive list.

Code	Description
01	Accident/medical coverage
02	No-fault insurance, including auto accident/other
03	Accident/tort liability
04	Accident/employment related
05	Accident/no medical liability coverage
06	Crime victim
07–08	Reserved for assignment by the NUBC
09	Start of infertility treatment cycle
10	Last menstrual period
11	Onset of symptoms/illness
A0	Reserved for assignment by the NUBC
A1	Birth date-Insured A policy
A2	Effective date-Insured A policy
A3	Benefits exhausted–Payer A
A4	Split bill date
A5–AZ	Reserved for assignment by the NUBC

FL 35 to 36 (A-B) Occurrence Span Codes and Dates

Code	Description	Code	Description
70	Qualifying stay dates for SNF use only	80	Prior same-SNF stay dates for payment ban purposes
71	Prior stay dates	81–99	Reserved for assignment by the NUBC
72	First/last visit dates	MO	QIO/UR-approved stay dates
73	Benefit eligibility period	M1	Provider liability-no utilization
74	Non-covered level of care/leave of absence dates	M2	Inpatient respite care dates
75	SNF level of care dates	M3	Intermediate care facility (ICF) level of care
76	Patient liability	M4	Residential level of care
77	Provider liability period	M5–MQ	Reserved for assignment by the NUBC
78	SNF prior stay dates	MR–ZZ	Reserved for assignment by the NUBC
79	Payer code		

FL 39 to 41 (A-D) Value Codes and Amount

This is not an all-inclusive list.

Code	Description
01	Most common semiprivate room rate
02	Hospital has no semiprivate rooms
05	Professional component
A1	Deductible payer A
A2	Co-insurance payer A
A3	Estimated patient responsibility payer A
A4	Covered self-administrable drugs: emergency
A5	Covered self-administrable drugs: not self-administrable in form and situation furnished by patient

FL 59 Patient's Relationship Codes

Code	Description
01	Spouse
18	Self
19	Child
20	Employee
21	Unknown
39	Organ Donor
40	Cadaver Donor
53	Life Partner
G8	Other relationship

SECTION III: CMS-1450 (UB-04) REVENUE CODE LISTING

Note: The following revenue code list is not all inclusive. This listing includes all data required to complete the cases in Appendix A.

A complete copy of the UB-04 revenue code listing can be obtained from the National Uniform Billing Committee (NUBC) or on the CMS Web site at www.cms.hhs.gov.

FL 42 Revenue Codes

Accommodation Revenue Codes (010X–021X)

010X **All-Inclusive Rate**

Subcategory	*Standard Abbreviation*
0-All-Inclusive Room and Board Plus Ancillary	ALL INCLUDE R&B/ANC
1-All-Inclusive Room and Board	ALL INCLUDE R&B

011X **Room and Board—Private (Medical or General)**

Subcategory	*Standard Abbreviation*
0-General Classification	ROOM-BOARD/PVT
1-Medical/Surgical/Gyn	MED-SUR-GY/PVT
2-OB	OB/PVT
3-Pediatric	PEDS/PVT
4-Psychiatric	PSYCH/PVT
5-Hospice	HOSPICE/PVT
6-Detoxification	DETOX/PVT
7-Oncology	ONCOLOGY/PVT
8-Rehabilitation	REHAB/PVT
9-Other	OTHER/PVT

012X **Room and Board—Semi-Private Two-Bed (Medical or General)**

Subcategory	*Standard Abbreviation*
0-General Classification	ROOM-BOARD/SEMI
1-Medical/Surgical/Gyn	MED-SUR-GY/2BED
2-OB	OB/2BED
3-Pediatric	PEDS/2BED
4-Psychiatric	PSYCH/2BED
5-Hospice	HOSPICE/2BED
6-Detoxification	DETOX/2BED
7-Oncology	ONCOLOGY/2BED
8-Rehabilitation	REHAB/2BED
9-Other	OTHER/2BED

013X **Semi-Private—Three and Four Beds**
014X **Private (Deluxe)**
015X **Room and Board—Ward (Medical or General)**
016X **Other Room and Board**
017X **Nursery**

018X **Leave of Absence**
Note: **Charges are billable for codes 2–5.**

Subcategory	*Standard Abbreviation*
0-General Classification	LEAVE OF ABSENCE or LOA
1-Reserved	
2-Patient Convenience	LOA/PT CONV
3-Therapeutic Leave	LOA/THERAPEUTIC
4-ICF Mentally Retarded—any reason	LOA/ICF/MR
5-Nursing Home (for Hospitalization)	LOA/NURS HOME
9-Other Leave of Absence	LOA/OTHER

019X **Subacute Care**

Code	Description	Standard Abbreviation
020X	**Intensive Care**	
	Subcategory	*Standard Abbreviation*
	0-General Classification	INTENSIVE CARE or ICU
	1-Surgical	ICU/SURGICAL
	2-Medical	ICU/MEDICAL
	3-Pediatric	ICU/PEDS
	4-Psychiatric	ICU/PSYCH
	6-Intermediate ICU	ICU/INTERMEDIATE
	7-Burn Care	ICU/BURN
	8-Trauma	ICU/TRAUMA
	9-Other Intensive Care	ICU/OTHER
021X	**Coronary Care**	
	Subcategory	*Standard Abbreviation*
	0-General Classification	CORONARY CARE or CCU
	1-Myocardial Infarction	CCU/MYO INFARC
	2-Pulmonary Care	CCU/PULMONARY
	3-Heart Transplant	CCU/TRANSPLANT
	4-Intermediate CCU	CCU/INTERMEDIATE
	9-Other Coronary Care	CCU/OTHER

Ancillary Revenue Codes (022X–099X)

Code	Description	Standard Abbreviation
022X	**Special Charges**	
023X	**Incremental Nursing Charge Rate**	
024X	**All-Inclusive Ancillary**	
	Subcategory	*Standard Abbreviation*
	0-General Classification	ALL INCLUDE ANCIL
	9-Other Inclusive Ancillary	ALL INCLUDE ANCIL/OTHER
025X	**Pharmacy**	
	Subcategory	*Standard Abbreviation*
	0-General Classification	PHARMACY
	1-Generic Drugs	DRUGS/GENERIC
	2-Nongeneric Drugs	DRUGS/NONGENERIC
	3-Take-Home Drugs	DRUGS/TAKEHOME
	4-Drugs Incident to Other	DRUGS/INCIDENT ODX
	5-Drugs Incident to Radiology	DRUGS/INCIDENT RAD
	6-Experimental Drugs	DRUGS/EXPERIMT
	7-Nonprescription	DRUGS/NONPSCRPT
	8-IV Solutions	IV SOLUTIONS
	9-Other Pharmacy	DRUGS/OTHER
026X	**Intravenous (IV) Therapy**	
	Subcategory	*Standard Abbreviation*
	0-General Classification	IV THERAPY
	1-Infusion Pump	IV THER/INFSN PUMP
	2-IV Therapy/Pharmacy Services	IV THER/PHARM/SVC
	3-IV Therapy/Drug/Supply/Delivery	IV THER/DRUG/SUPPLY DELV
	4-IV Therapy/Supplies	IV THER/SUPPLIES
	9-Other IV Therapy	IV THERAPY/OTHER
027X	**Medical/Surgical Supplies and Devices (See also 062X, an extension of 27X)**	
	Subcategory	*Standard Abbreviation*
	0-General Classification	MED-SUR SUPPLIES
	1-Nonsterile Supply	NONSTER SUPPLY
	2-Sterile Supply	STERILE SUPPLY
	3-Take-Home Supplies	TAKEHOME SUPPLY
	4-Prosthetic/Orthotic Devices	PROSTH/ORTH DEV
	5-Pacemaker	PACEMAKER
	6-Intraocular Lens	INTRAOC LENS

	7-Oxygen-Take-Home	O2/TAKEHOME
	8-Other Implants	SUPPLY/IMPLANTS
	9-Other Supplies/Devices	SUPPLY/OTHER

028X	**Oncology**	
	Subcategory	*Standard Abbreviation*
	0-General Classification	ONCOLOGY
	9-Other Oncology	ONCOLOGY/OTHER

029X	**Durable Medical Equipment (DME) (Other Than Renal)**	
	Subcategory	*Standard Abbreviation*
	0-General Classification	MED EQUIP/DURAB
	1-Rental	MED EQUIP/RENT
	2-Purchase of new DME	MED EQUIP/NEW
	3-Purchase of used DME	MED EQUIP/USED
	4-Supplies/Drugs for DME Effectiveness (HHAs Only)	MED EQUIP/SUPPLIES/DRUGS
	9-Other Equipment	MED EQUIP/OTHER

030X	**Laboratory**	
	Subcategory	*Standard Abbreviation*
	0-General Classification	LAB
	1-Chemistry	LAB/CHEMISTRY
	2-Immunology	LAB/IMMUNOLOGY
	3-Renal Patient (Home)	LAB/RENAL HOME
	4-Nonroutine Dialysis	LAB/NR DIALYSIS
	5-Hematology	LAB/HEMATOLOGY
	6-Bacteriology and Microbiology	LAB/BACT-MICRO
	7-Urology	LAB/UROLOGY
	9-Other Laboratory	LAB/OTHER

031X	**Laboratory Pathological**	
	Subcategory	*Standard Abbreviation*
	0-General Classification	PATHOLOGY LAB or PATH LAB
	1-Cytology	PATHOL/CYTOLOGY
	2-Histology	PATHOL/HISTOLOGY
	4-Biopsy	PATHOL/BIOPSY
	9-Other Laboratory—Pathological	PATHOL/OTHER

032X	**Radiology—Diagnostic**	
	Subcategory	*Standard Abbreviation*
	0-General Classification	DX X-RAY
	1-Angiocardiography	DX X-RAY/ANGIO
	2-Arthrography	DX X-RAY/ARTH
	3-Arteriography	DX X-RAY/ARTER
	4-Chest X-Ray	DX X-RAY/CHEST
	9-Other Radiology—Diagnostic	DX X-RAY/OTHER

033X	**Radiology—Therapeutic**	
	Subcategory	*Standard Abbreviation*
	0-General Classification	RX X-RAY
	1-Chemotherapy—Injected	CHEMOTHER/INJ
	2-Chemotherapy—Oral	CHEMOTHER/ORAL
	3-Radiation Therapy	RADIATION RX
	5-Chemotherapy—IV	CHEMOTHERP-IV
	9-Other Radiology—Therapeutic	RX X-RAY/OTHER

034X	**Nuclear Medicine**	
	Subcategory	*Standard Abbreviation*
	0-General Classification	NUCLEAR MEDICINE or NUC MED
	1-Diagnostic	NUC MED/DX
	2-Therapeutic	NUC MED/RX
	9-Other Nuclear Medicine	NUC MED/OTHER

Code	Subcategory	Standard Abbreviation
035X	**CT Scan**	
	Subcategory	*Standard Abbreviation*
	0-General Classification	CT SCAN
	1-Head Scan	CT SCAN/HEAD
	2-Body Scan	CT SCAN/BODY
	9-Other CT Scan	CT SCAN/OTHER
036X	**Operating Room Services**	
	Subcategory	*Standard Abbreviation*
	0-General Classification	OR SERVICES
	1-Minor Surgery	OR/MINOR
	2-Organ Transplant—other than kidney	OR/ORGAN TRANS
	7-Kidney Transplant	OR/KIDNEY TRANS
	9-Other Operating Room Services	OR/OTHER
037X	**Anesthesia**	
	Subcategory	*Standard Abbreviation*
	0-General Classification	ANESTHESIA
	1-Anesthesia Incident to Radiology	ANESTHE/INCIDENT RAD
	2-Anesthesia Incident to Other Diagnostic Services	ANESTHE/INCIDENT ODX
	4-Acupuncture	ANESTHE/ACUPUNC
	9-Other Anesthesia	ANESTHE/OTHER
038X	**Blood**	
	Subcategory	*Standard Abbreviation*
	0-General Classification	BLOOD
	1-Packed Red Cells	BLOOD/PKE RED
	2-Whole Blood	BLOOD/WHOLE
	3-Plasma	BLOOD/PLASMA
	4-Platelets	BLOOD/PLATELETS
	5-Leukocytes	BLOOD/LEUKOCYTES
	6-Other Components	BLOOD/COMPONENTS
	7-Other Derivatives (Cryoprecipitate)	BLOOD/DERIVATIVES
	9-Other Blood	BLOOD/OTHER
039X	**Blood Storage and Processing**	
	Subcategory	*Standard Abbreviation*
	0-General Classification	BLOOD/STOR-PROC
	1-Blood Administration	BLOOD/ADMIN
	9-Other Blood Storage and Processing	BLOOD/OTHER STOR
040X	**Other Imaging Services**	
	Subcategory	*Standard Abbreviation*
	0-General Classification	IMAGE SERVICE
	1-Diagnostic Mammography	MAMMOGRAPHY
	2-Ultrasound	ULTRASOUND
	3-Screening Mammography	SCR MAMMOGRAPHY/GEN MAMMO
	4-Positron Emission Tomography	PET SCAN
	9-Other Imaging Services	OTHER IMAG SVS
041X	**Respiratory Services**	
	Subcategory	*Standard Abbreviation*
	0-General Classification	RESPIRATORY SVC
	2-Inhalation Services	INHALATION SVC
	3-Hyperbaric Oxygen Therapy	HYPERBARIC O2
	9-Other Respiratory Services	OTHER RESPIR SVS

042X **Physical Therapy**

Subcategory	*Standard Abbreviation*
0-General Classification	PHYSICAL THERP
1-Visit Charge	PHYS THERP/VISIT
2-Hourly Charge	PHYS THERP/HOUR
3-Group Rate	PHYS THERP/GROUP
4-Evaluation or Reevaluation	PHYS THERP/EVAL
9-Other Physical Therapy	OTHER PHYS THERP

043X **Occupational Therapy**

Subcategory	*Standard Abbreviation*
0-General Classification	OCCUPATION THERP
1-Visit Charge	OCCUP THERP/VISIT
2-Hourly Charge	OCCUP THERP/HOUR
3-Group Rate	OCCUP THERP/GROUP
4-Evaluation or Re-evaluation	OCCUP THERP/EVAL
9-Other Occupational Therapy	OTHER OCCUP THERP

044X **Speech-Language Pathology**

Subcategory	*Standard Abbreviation*
0-General Classification	SPEECH PATHOL
1-Visit Charge	SPEECH PATH/VISIT
2-Hourly Charge	SPEECH PATH/HOUR
3-Group Rate	SPEECH PATH/GROUP
4-Evaluation or Re-evaluation	SPEECH PATH/EVAL
9-Other Speech-Language Pathology	SPEECH PATH/OTHER

045X **Emergency Room**

Subcategory	*Standard Abbreviation*
0-General Classification	EMERG ROOM
1-EMTALA Emergency Medical Screening Service	ER/EMTALA
2-ER Beyond EMTALA Screening	ER/BEYOND EMTALA
6-Urgent Care	URGENT CARE
9-Other Emergency Room	OTHER EMERG ROOM

046X **Pulmonary Function**

Subcategory	*Standard Abbreviation*
0-General Classification	PULMONARY FUNC
9-Other Pulmonary Function	OTHER PULMON FUNC

047X **Audiology**

Subcategory	*Standard Abbreviation*
0-General Classification	AUDIOLOGY
1-Diagnostic	AUDIOLOGY/DX
2-Treatment	AUDIOLOGY/RX
9-Other Audiology	AUDIOL/OTHER

048X **Cardiology**

Subcategory	*Standard Abbreviation*
0-General Classification	CARDIOLOGY
1-Cardiac Catheterization Lab	CARDIAC CATH LAB
2-Stress Test	STRESS TEST
3-Echocardiology	ECHOCARDIOLOGY
9-Other Cardiology	OTHER CARDIOLGY

049X **Ambulatory Surgical Care**

Subcategory	*Standard Abbreviation*
0-General Classification	AMBUL SURG
9-Other Ambulatory Surgical Care	OTHER AMBUL SURG

Note: Observation or hold beds are not reported under this code. They are reported under revenue code 0762, "Observation Room."

50X **Outpatient Services**
Subcategory — *Standard Abbreviation*
0-General Classification — OUTPATIENT SVS
9-Other Outpatient Services — OUTPATIENT/OTHER

051X **Clinic**
052X **Free-standing Clinic**
053X **Osteopathic Services**
054X **Ambulance**
055X **Skilled Nursing**
056X **Medical Social Services**
057X **Home Health Aide (Home Health)**
058X **Other Visits (Home Health)**
059X **Units of Service (Home Health) (Medicare—Required Code)**
060X **Oxygen (Home Health)**
061X **Magnetic Resonance Technology (MRT)/Angiography (MRA)**
062X **Medical/Surgical Supplies—Extension of 027X**
063X **Drugs Requiring Specific Identification—Extension of 025X**
064X **Home IV Therapy Services**
065X **Hospice Services**

066X **Respite Care (HHA Only)**
Subcategory — *Standard Abbreviation*
0-General Classification — RESPITE CARE
1-Hourly Charge/Skilled Nursing — RESPITE/SKILLED NURSE
2-Hourly Charge/Home Health Aide/Homemaker — RESPITE/HMEAID/HMEMKE
9-Other Respite Care — RESPITE/OTHER

067X **Outpatient Special Residence Charges**
Subcategory — *Standard Abbreviation*
0-General Classification — OP SPEC RES
1-Hospital Based — OP SPEC RES/HOSP BASED
2-Contracted — OP SPEC RES/CONTRACTED
9-Other Special Residence Charges — OP SPEC RES/OTHER

068X **Not Assigned**
069X **Not Assigned**
070X **Cast Room**

071X **Recovery Room**
Subcategory — *Standard Abbreviation*
0-General Classification — RECOVERY ROOM
9-Other Recovery Room — OTHER RECOV RM

072X **Labor/Delivery Room**

073X **EKG/ECG (Electrocardiogram)**
Subcategory — *Standard Abbreviation*
0-General Classification — EKG/ECG
1-Holter Monitor — HOLTER MONT
2-Telemetry — TELEMETRY
9-Other EKG/ECG — OTHER EKG-ECG

074X **EEG (Electroencephalogram)**
Subcategory — *Standard Abbreviation*
0-General Classification — EEG
9-Other EEG — OTHER EEG

075X **Gastrointestinal Services**
Subcategory — *Standard Abbreviation*
0-General Classification — GASTR-INTS SVS
9-Other Gastrointestinal — OTHER GASTRO-INTS

076X	**Treatment or Observation Room**
077X	**Preventive Care Services**
078X	**Telemedicine**
079X	**Lithotripsy**
080X	**Inpatient Renal Dialysis**
081X	**Organ Acquisition**
082X	**Hemodialysis—Outpatient or Home**
083X	**Peritoneal Dialysis—Outpatient or Home**
084X	**Continuous Ambulatory Peritoneal Dialysis (CAPD)—Outpatient or Home**
085X	**Continuous Cycling Peritoneal Dialysis (CCPD)—Outpatient or Home**
086X	**Reserved for Dialysis (National Assignment)**
087X	**Reserved for Dialysis (National Assignment)**
088X	**Miscellaneous Dialysis**
089X	**Reserved for Assignment by the NUBC**
090X	**Psychiatric/Psychological Treatments**
091X	**Psychiatric/Psychological Services**

092X Other Diagnostic Services

Subcategory	*Standard Abbreviation*
0-General Classification	OTHER DX SVS
1-Peripheral Vascular Lab	PERI VASCUL LAB
2-Electromyelogram	EMG
3-Pap Smear	PAPSMEAR
4-Allergy Test	ALLERGY TEST
5-Pregnancy Test	PREG TEST
9-Other Diagnostic Service	ADDITIONAL DX SVS

093X Not Assigned

094X Other Therapeutic Services

Subcategory	*Standard Abbreviation*
0-General Classification	OTHER RX SVCS
1-Recreational Therapy	RECREATION RX
2-Education/Training	EDUC/TRAINING
3-Cardiac Rehabilitation	CARDIAC REHAB
4-Drug Rehabilitation	DRUG REHAB
5-Alcohol Rehabilitation	ALCOHOL REHAB
6-Complex Medical Equipment—Routine	CMPLX MED EQUIP/ROUT
7-Complex Medical Equipment—Ancillary	CMPLX MED EQUIP
9-Other Therapeutic Services	ADDITIONAL RX SVS

095X	**Not Assigned**
096X	**Professional Fees**
097X	**Professional Fees (Extension of Code 096X)**
098X	**Professional Fees (Extension of Codes 096X and 097X)**

099X Patient Convenience Items

Subcategory	*Standard Abbreviation*
0-General Classification	PT CONVENIENCE
1-Cafeteria/Guest Tray	CAFETERIA
2-Private Linen Service	LINEN
3-Telephone/Telegraph	TELEPHONE
4-TV/Radio	TV/RADIO
5-Nonpatient Room Rentals	NONPT ROOM RENT
6-Late Discharge Charge	LATE DISCHARGE
7-Admission Kits	ADMIT KITS
8-Beauty Shop/Barber	BARBER/BEAUTY
9-Other Patient Convenience Items	PT CONV/OTHER

0001 Total Charge

Appendix C

List of Web Resources

CHAPTER 1

www.phatnav.com
www.christianhistory.com

CHAPTER 2

www.os.dhhs.gov/ocr/hburton.html
www.defenselink.mil
www.oig.hhs.gov
www.access.gpo.gov
www.fdhc.state.fl.us
www.jcaho.org
www.aapc.com
www.ahima.org
www.aaham.org

CHAPTER 3

www.passavanthospital.com
www.northside.com
www.poconocarecenter.com
www.cv.vccs.edu
www.stfrancismaryville.com

CHAPTER 4

www.cms.gov

CHAPTER 5

www.nubc.org

CHAPTER 6

www.cms.gov
www.fair-debt-collection.com
www.flsenate.gov

CHAPTER 7

www.cdc.gov
www.cms.hhs.gov
www.radcodeinc.com
www.census.gov

CHAPTER 10

www.cms.hhs.gov
www.claimsnet.com

CHAPTER 11

www.managingmanagedcare.com
www.hotinsurancehints.com

CHAPTER 12

www.insurancefinder.com
www.umd.nycpic.com
www.aap.org
www.tricare.osd.mil
www.usmil.com
www.medicare.gov
www.dtic.mil
www.ncsl.org
www.therubins.com

CHAPTER 13

www.irp.com
www.umanitoba.ca
www.stryker.com

CHAPTER 14

www.cpr.net
www.oig.hhs.gov
www.hipaadvisory.com
www.usdoj.gov
www.library.ahima.org

Index

Page numbers followed by *b* indicate boxes; those followed by *f* indicate figures; and those followed by *t* indicate tables.

D

E

F

I

J

Q

R